Oxford

Ophthalmology

About the Oxford American Handbooks in Medicine

The Oxford American Handbooks are pocket clinical books, providing practical guidance in quick reference, note form. Titles cover major medical specialties or cross-specialty topics and are aimed at students, residents, internists, family physicians, and practicing physicians within specific disciplines.

Their reputation is built on including the best clinical information, complemented by hints, tips, and advice from the authors. Each one is carefully reviewed by senior subject experts, residents, and students to ensure that content reflects the reality of day-to-day medical practice.

Key series features

- Written in short chunks, each topic is covered in a two-page spread to enable readers to find information quickly. They are also perfect for test preparation and gaining a quick overview of a subject without scanning through unnecessary pages.
- Content is evidence based and complemented by the expertise and judgment of experienced authors.
- The Handbooks provide a humanistic approach to medicine—it's more than just treatment by numbers.
- A "friend in your pocket," the Handbooks offer honest, reliable guidance about the difficulties of practicing medicine and provide coverage of both the practice and art of medicine.
- For quick reference, useful "everyday" information is included on the inside covers.

Published and Forthcoming Oxford American Handbooks

Oxford American Handbook of Clinical Medicine
Oxford American Handbook of Anesthesiology
Oxford American Handbook of Cardiology
Oxford American Handbook of Clinical Dentistry
Oxford American Handbook of Clinical Diagnosis
Oxford American Handbook of Clinical Pharmacy
Oxford American Handbook of Critical Care
Oxford American Handbook of Emergency Medicine
Oxford American Handbook of Geriatric Medicine
Oxford American Handbook of Nephrology and Hypertension
Oxford American Handbook of Neurology
Oxford American Handbook of Obstetrics and Gynecology
Oxford American Handbook of Oncology
Oxford American Handbook of Ophthalmology
Oxford American Handbook of Otolaryngology
Oxford American Handbook of Pediatrics
Oxford American Handbook of Physical Medicine and Rehabilitation
Oxford American Handbook of Psychiatry
Oxford American Handbook of Pulmonary Medicine
Oxford American Handbook of Rheumatology
Oxford American Handbook of Sports Medicine
Oxford American Handbook of Surgery
Oxford American Handbook of Urology

Oxford American Handbook of Ophthalmology

Edited by

James C. Tsai, MD, MBA

Robert R. Young Professor and Chairman
Department of Ophthalmology and Visual Science
Yale University School of Medicine
Chief of Ophthalmology,
Yale-New Haven Hospital
New Haven, Connecticut

Alastair K.O. Denniston, MA, MRCP, MRCOphth

Clinical Lecturer in Ophthalmology
University of Birmingham, UK

Philip I. Murray, PhD, FRCP, FRCS, FRCOphth

Professor of Ophthalmology
University of Birmingham, UK

John J. Huang, MD

Associate Professor of Ophthalmology and Visual Science
Director of Clinical Trials and Translational Research,
Yale Eye Center
Director of Uveitis and Ocular Immunology
Yale University School of Medicine
New Haven, Connecticut

Tamir S. Aldad, BA

Predoctoral Research Fellow
Yale University School of Medicine
New Haven, Connecticut

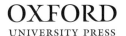

OXFORD
UNIVERSITY PRESS

OXFORD
UNIVERSITY PRESS

Oxford University Press, Inc. publishes works that further
Oxford University's objective of excellence
in research, scholarship and education.

Oxford New York

Auckland Cape Town Dar es Salaam Hong Kong Karachi
Kuala Lumpur Madrid Melbourne Mexico City Nairobi
New Delhi Shanghai Taipei Toronto

With offices in

Argentina Austria Brazil Chile Czech Republic France Greece
Guatemala Hungary Italy Japan Poland Portugal
Singapore South Korea Switzerland Thailand Turkey Ukraine Vietnam

Published by Oxford University Press Inc.
198 Madison Avenue, New York, New York 10016

www.oup.com

Oxford is a registered trademark of Oxford University Press

First published 2011

Library of Congress Cataloging in Publication Data

Oxford American handbook of ophthalmology/edited by James C. Tsai ... [et al.].
p. ; cm.
Other title: Handbook of ophthalmology
Includes index.
ISBN 978-0-19-539344-6
1. Ophthalmology—Handbooks, manuals, etc.   I. Tsai, James C.   II. Title:
Handbook of ophthalmology.
[DNLM: 1. Eye Diseases—Handbooks. WW 39]
RE48.9.O94 2011
617.7—dc22
2010028006

9 8 7 6 5 4 3 2 1

Printed in China
on acid-free paper

Preface and Acknowledgments

In this American edition of the popular *Oxford Handbook of Ophthalmology*, the editors have attempted to retain the essence of the original handbook while incorporating recent advances, current practice patterns, and state-of-the-art concepts in the wide-ranging field of ophthalmic disease. In doing so, we hope that this Handbook provides the eye care provider with timely information that is readily accessible and easy to incorporate into the everyday management of patients. As a rapid reference guide for practicing clinicians, trainees, students, and other ancillary health care professionals, the *Oxford American Handbook of Ophthalmology* greatly benefits from the expertise of accomplished clinicians in the various subspecialties in ophthalmology.

The editors of the *Oxford American Handbook of Ophthalmology* would like to express our deepest gratitude to the contributing chapter authors, all of whom are exceptional faculty members practicing in the Department of Ophthalmology and Visual Science at the Yale University School of Medicine. We also acknowledge and appreciate the advice and technical support of Andrea Seils and Staci Hou at Oxford University Press in New York, as well as Angela Luck for her anatomical illustrations. We are indebted to our mentors, colleagues, students, and patients for helping to shape and enhance our clinical and scholarly endeavors. We wish to thank Alastair Denniston and Philip Murray, the authors of the original UK edition of the *Oxford Handbook of Ophthalmology*, and acknowledge the extraordinary work they did. Finally, we wish to thank our families and friends for their incredible support and encouragement throughout the entire editorial process.

Contents

Contributors

C. Robert Bernardino, MD, FACS
Associate Professor of Ophthalmology and Visual Science
Residency Program Director
Yale-New Haven Hospital
Director, Ophthalmic Plastic and Orbital Surgery Section
Yale University School of Medicine
New Haven, Connecticut

Jimmy K. Lee, MD
Assistant Professor of Ophthalmology and Visual Science
Director, Cornea and Refractive Surgery Sections
Yale University School of Medicine
New Haven, Connecticut

Miguel A. Materin, MD
Assistant Professor of Ophthalmology and Visual Science
Director, Ophthalmic Oncology
Smilow Cancer Hospital at Yale-New Haven
Yale University School of Medicine
New Haven, Connecticut

Hylton R. Mayer, MD
Assistant Professor of Ophthalmology and Visual Science
Glaucoma Fellowship Director, Yale Eye Center
Director, Cataract Section
Yale University School of Medicine
New Haven, Connecticut

Daniel J. Salchow, MD
Assistant Professor of Ophthalmology and Visual Science
Director, Pediatric Ophthalmology and Strabismus Section
Yale University School of Medicine
New Haven, Connecticut

Symbols and abbreviations

↑, ↓	increased, decreased
→	leading to
Δ	prism diopter
5-FU	5-fluorouracil
AACG	acute angle-closure glaucoma
AAU	acute anterior uveitis
AC	anterior chamber
AC:A	accommodative convergence to accommodation ratio
ACE	angiotensin-converting enzyme
ACh	acetylcholine
ACIOL	anterior chamber intraocular lens
ACTH	adrenocorticotrophic hormone
AD	autosomal dominant
ADH	antidiuretic hormone
AF	atrial fibrillation
AIDS	acquired immune deficiency syndrome
AION	anterior ischemic optic neuropathy
ALT	argon laser trabeculoplasty
AMD	age-related macular degeneration
ANA	antinuclear antibody
ANCA	antineutrophil cytoplasmic antibody
APMPPE	acute posterior multifocal placoid pigment epitheliopathy
APTT	activated partial thromboplastin time
AR	autosomal recessive
ARC	abnormal retinal correspondence
ARDS	acute respiratory distress syndrome
ARN	acute retinal necrosis
ART	antiretroviral therapy
AS	anterior segment; ankylosing spondylitis
ASD	atrial septal defect
ASFA	anterior segment fluorescein angiography
AVM	arteriovenous malformation
AZOOR	acute zonal occult outer retinopathy
BAL	bronchoalveolar lavage
BCC	basal cell carcinoma
BCL	bandage contact lens
BCVA	best-corrected visual acuity
BDR	background diabetic retinopathy
BDUMP	bilateral diffuse uveal melanocytic proliferation

bid	twice daily
BM	basement membrane
BMI	body mass index
BP	blood pressure
BRAO	branch retinal artery occlusion
BRVO	branch retinal vein occlusion
BSS	balanced salt solution
BSV	binocular single vision
BUT	break-up time (of tear film)
BVD	back vertex distance
C3F8	perfluoropropane
CBC	complete blood count
CCF	carotid–cavernous (sinus) fistula
CCT	central corneal thickness
CCTV	closed-circuit television
C/D	cup–disc ratio
CEA	carotid endarterectomy
CF	counting fingers
CFEOM	chronic fibrosis of extraocular muscles
CHED	congenital hereditary endothelial dystrophy
CHRPE	congenital hypertrophy of retinal pigment epithelium
CHSD	congenital hereditary stromal dystrophy
CIN	conjunctival intraepithelial neoplasia
CL	contact lens
CME	cystoid macular edema
CMV	cytomegalovirus
CN II	optic nerve
CN III	oculomotor nerve
CN IV	trochlear nerve
CN V	trigeminal nerve
CN VI	abducens nerve
CN VII	facial nerve
CNS	central nervous system
CNV	choroidal neovascular membrane
COPD	chronic obstructive pulmonary disease
COWS	cold–opposite warm–same
CPEO	chronic progressive external ophthalmoplegia
CPSD	corrected pattern standard deviation
CRAO	central retinal artery occlusion
CRP	C-reactive protein
CRVO	central retinal vein occlusion
CSF	cerebrospinal fluid
CSLO	confocal scanning laser ophthalmoscopy

CSME	clinically significant macular edema
CSNB	congenital stationary night blindness
CSR	central serous (chorio)retinopathy
CT	computer tomography
CVA	cerebrovascular accident
CVS	cardiovascular system
CWS	cotton-wool spot
CXR	chest X-ray
D	diopter; diffusion
dB	decibel
DBP	diastolic blood pressure
DC	diopter cylinder
DCCT	Diabetes Control and Complication Trial
DCG	dacryocystogram
DCR	dacryocystorhinostomy
DD	disc diameter
DIC	disseminated intravascular coaguloathy
DICC	drug-induced cicatrizing conjunctivitis
DKA	diabetic ketoacidosis
DLEK	deep lamellar endothelial keratoplasty
DLK	deep lamellar kerotoplasty
DMV	Department of Motor Vehicles
DNA	deoxyribonucleic acid
DOT	directly observed therapy
ds	double-stranded (of nucleic acids)
DS	diopter sphere
DSEK	Descemet's stripping endothelial keratoplasty
DUSN	diffuse unilateral subacute neuroretinitis
DVD	dissociated vertical deviation
DVT	deep venous thrombosis
EBV	Epstein–Barr virus
ECC	enhanced corneal compensator
ECCE	extracapsular cataract extraction
ECG	electrocardiogram
EEG	electroencephalogram
ELISA	enzyme-linked immunosorbent assay
EMG	electromyogram
ENT	ear, nose, and throat specialist (otolaryngologist)
EOG	electro-oculogram
EOM	extraocular muscle
ERD	exudative retinal detachment
ERG	electroretinogram
ESR	erythrocyte sedimentation rate

EUA	examination under anesthesia
E-W	Edinger–Westphal (nucleus)
FA	fluorescein angiography
Fab	fragment antigen-binding
FAP	familial adenomatous polyposis
FAZ	foveal avascular zone
FB	foreign body
FBC	full blood count
FDA	Food and Drug Administration
FDP	frequency doubling perimetry
FED	Fuchs' endothelial dystrophy
FEF	frontal eye fields
FH	family history
FHI	Fuchs' heterochromic iridocyclitis
FLAIR	fluid-attenuated inversion recover
FML	fluorometholone
FNA	fine needle aspiration
FSH	follicle-stimulating hormone
GA	general anesthesia
GCA	giant cell arteritis
GCS	Glasgow Coma Scale
GDD	glaucoma drainage device
GEN	gaze-evoked nystagmus
GH	growth hormone
GI	gastrointestinal system
GU	genitourinary system
GVHD	graft-versus-host disease
HA	hyaluronic acid
HDL	high-density lipoprotein
HHV8	human herpes virus 8
HIV	human immunodeficiency virus
HLA	human leukocyte antigen
HM	hand movements
HPI	history of presenting illness
HPV	human papilloma virus
HRCT	high-resolution computed tomography
HRT	Heidelberg retinal tomography
HSV	herpes simplex virus
HTLV-1	human T-cell lymphotropic virus type 1
HVF	Humphrey visual field
HZO	herpes zoster ophthalmicus
IA	irrigation and aspiration
IBD	inflammatory bowel disease

ICA	internal carotid artery
ICCE	intracapsular cataract extraction
ICE	iridocorneal endothelial syndrome
ICGA	indocyanine green angiography
ICP	intracranial pressure
IFIS	intraoperative floppy iris syndrome
ILM	internal limiting membrane
IM	intramuscular
INO	internuclear ophthalmoplegia
IO	inferior oblique
IOFB	intraocular foreign body
IOL	intraocular lens
IOP	intraocular pressure
IPCV	idiopathic polypoidal choroidal vasculopathy
IR	inferior rectus
IRMA	intraretinal microvascular abnormalities
ISCEV	International Society for Clinical Electrophysiology of Vision
IV	intravenous
IVC	inferior vena cava
JIA	juvenile idiopathic arthritis
KCS	keratoconjunctivitis sicca
KP	keratic precipitate
LASEK	laser subepithelial keratomilieusis
LASIK	laser stromal in situ keratomilieusis
LCH	Langerhans cell histiocytosis
LFT	liver function tests
LGN	lateral geniculate nucleus
LH	luteinizing hormone
LHON	Leber's hereditary optic neuropathy
LOCS III	Lens Opacities Classification System III
LogMAR	logarithm of the minimum angle of resolution
LP	light perception; lumbar puncture
LPI	laser peripheral iridotomy
LPS	levator palpebrae superioris
LR	lateral rectus
LVA	low vision aid
MCP	multifocal choroiditis with panuveitis
MC&S	microscopy, culture, and sensitivities
MD	mean deviation
MEWDS	multiple evanescent white dot syndrome
M:F	male-to-female ratio
MG	myasthenia gravis
MI	myocardial infarction

min	minute
MLF	medial longitudinal fasciculus
MLN	manifest latent nystagmus
MLT	micropulse laser trabeculoplasty
MMC	mitomycin C
MR	medial rectus
MRA	magnetic resonance angiography
MRI	magnetic resonance imaging
MRV	magnetic resonance venography
MS	multiple sclerosis
Nd-YAG	neodymium-yttrium-aluminium-garnet laser
NF-1, -2	neurofibromatosis types 1 and 2
NFL	nerve fiber layer
NHL	non-Hodgkin's lymphoma
NLP	no light perception
NorA	noradrenaline
NPDR	nonproliferative diabetic retinopathy
NPO	nothing by mouth
NRR	neuroretinal rim
NSAID	nonsteroidal anti-inflammatory drug
NSF	nephrogenic systemic fibrosis
NTG	normal-tension glaucoma
NVD	neovascularization of the optic disc
NVE	neovascularization elsewhere
NVG	neovascular glaucoma
NVI	neovascularization of the iris
OA	osteoarthritis
OCP	ocular cicatricial pemphigoid
OCT	optical coherence tomography
OD	oculus dexter (right eye)
OHT	ocular hypertension
OKN	optokinetic nystagmus
OMMP	ocular mucous membrane pemphigoid
ONH	optic nerve head
OS	oculus sinister (left eye)
OVD	ophthalmic viscosurgical device
PACG	primary angle-closure glaucoma
PAM	pigmented acquired melanosis
PAN	polyarteritis nodosa; periodic alternating nystagmus
PAS	peripheral anterior synechiae; periodic acid–Schiff
PE	physical exam
PCO	posterior capsular opacification
PCIOL	posterior chamber intraocular lens

PCP	primary care physician
PCR	polymerase chain reaction
PCV	polypoidal choroidal vasculopathy
PDR	proliferative diabetic retinopathy
PDS	pigmentary dispersion syndrome
PDT	photodynamic therapy
PE	pulmonary embolism
PERG	pattern electroretinogram
PET	positron emission tomography
PF	preservative free
PFV	persistent fetal vasculature
PHMB	polyhexamethylene biguanide
PI	peripheral iridotomy
PIC	punctate inner choroidopathy
PK	penetrating keratoplasty
PMH	past medical history
PMMA	polymethyl methacrylate
PNS	peripheral nervous system
PO	per os (by mouth)
POAG	primary open-angle glaucoma
POH	past ophthalmic history
POHS	presumed ocular histoplasmosis syndrome
PORN	progressive outer retinal necrosis
POT	parieto-occipito-temporal (junction)
PPD	purified protein derivative
PPDR	preproliferative diabetic retinopathy
PPMD	posterior polymorphous corneal dystrophy
PPRF	paramedian pontine reticular formation
PRK	photorefractive keratectomy
PRP	panretinal photocoagulation
PS	posterior synechiae
PSD	pattern standard deviation
PSS	Posner–Schlossman syndrome
PTT	prothrombin time
PUK	peripheral ulcerative keratitis
PVD	posterior vitreous detachment
PVR	proliferative vitreoretinopathy
PXF	pseudoexfoliation syndrome
q	every (e.g., q1h = every 1 hour)
RA	rheumatoid arthritis
RAPD	relative afferent pupillary defect
RAST	radioallergosorbent test
Rb	retinoblastoma

RD	retinal detachment
RE	right eye
RES	recurrent erosion syndrome
RF	rheumatoid factor
RGP	rigid gas permeable (of contact lenses)
RK	refractive keratectomy
RNA	ribonucleic acid
RNFL	retinal nerve fiber layer
ROP	retinopathy of prematurity
ROS	review of systems
RP	retinitis pigmentosa
RPE	retinal pigment epithelium
RPR	rapid plasma reagin
RRD	rhegmatogenous retinal detachment
RS	respiratory system
rtPA	recombinant tissue plasminogen activator
SBP	systolic blood pressure
SBS	shaken baby syndrome
SC	subcutaneous
SCC	squamous cell carcinoma
sec	second(s)
SF	short-term fluctuation
SF6	sulfur hexafluoride
SH	social history
Si	silicone (of oil)
SINS	surgery-induced necrotizing scleritis
SITA	Swedish interactive threshold algorithm
SLE	systemic lupus erythematosus
SLK	superior limbic keratoconjunctivitis
SLP	scanning laser polarimetry
SLT	selective laser trabeculoplasty
SO	superior oblique
SR	superior rectus
SRF	subretinal fluid
SUN	Standardization of Uveitis Nomenclature (group)
SVC	superior vena cava
SVP	spontaneous venous pulsation
SWAP	short-wavelength automated perimetry
TB	tuberculosis
TED	thyroid eye disease
TEN	toxic epidermal necrolysis
TFT	thyroid function tests
TG	triglyceride

TI	transillumination defects
TINU	tubulointerstitial nephritis with uveitis
TLT	titanium:sapphire laser trabeculoplasty
TM	trabecular meshwork
TNF	tumor necrosis factor
tPA	tissue plasminogen activator
TPHA	treponema pallidum hemagglutination assay
TRD	tractional retinal detachment
TSH	thyroid-stimulating hormone
TTT	transpupillary thermotherapy
UA	urinalysis
UC	ulcerative colitis
U+E	urea and electrolytes
UGH	uveitis–glaucoma–hyphema syndrome
URTI	upper respiratory tract infection
US	ultrasound
UV	ultraviolet
$V_{1,2,3}$	ophthalmic, maxillary, and mandibular divisions of CN V
VA	visual acuity
VCC	variable corneal compensator
VDRL	venereal disease research laboratory test
VEGF	vascular endothelial growth factor
VEP	visual-evoked potential
VF	visual field
VHL	von Hippel–Lindau syndrome
VKC	vernal keratoconjunctivitis
VKH	Vogt–Koyanagi–Harada syndrome
VOR	vestibulo-ocular reflex
VSD	ventricular septal defect
VZV	varicella zoster virus
WHO	World Health Organization
X	X-linked
XD	X-linked dominant
yr	year

Orthoptic abbreviations

ACS	alternating convergent strabismus
ADS	alternating divergent strabismus
AHP	abnormal head posture
ARC	abnormal retinal correspondence
BD	base down (of prism)
BI	base in (of prism)
BO	base out (of prism)
BU	base up (of prism)
BSV	binocular single vision
CC	Cardiff cards
CI	convergence insufficiency
Conv XS	convergence excess
CSM	central, steady, and maintained (quality of fixation)
CT	cover test
DVD	dissociated vertical deviation
DVM	delayed visual maturation
Ecc fix	eccentric fixation
E	esophoria
ET	esotropia
E(T)	intermittent esotropia
FCPL	forced choice preferential looking
FL/FLE	fixing with left eye
FR/FRE	fixing with right eye
H	hyperphoria
HT	hypertropia
Ho	hypophoria
HoT	hypotropia
KP	Kay's pictures
LCS	left convergent strabismus
LDS	left divergent strabismus
MLN	manifest latent nystagmus
MR	Maddox rod
MW	Maddox wing
NPA	near point of accommodation
NPC	near point of convergence
NRC	normal retinal correspondence
o/a	overaction
Obj	objection

Occ	occlusion
OKN	optokinetic nystagmus
PCT	prism cover test
PFR	prism fusion range
PRT	prism reflection test
RCS	right convergent strabismus
RDS	right divergent strabismus
Rec	recovery
SG	Sheridan Gardiner test
Sn	Snellen chart
SP	simultaneous perception
Supp	suppression
u/a	underaction
VOR	vestibulo-ocular reflex
X	exophoria
XT	exotropia
X(T)	intermittent exotropia

More complex variations for intermittent strabismus include:

R(E)T	intermittent right esotropia predominantly controlled
RE(T)	intermittent right esotropia predominantly manifest

Adjust according to whether:
R (right), L (left), or A (alternating)
ET (esotropia), XT (exotropia), HT (hypertropia), or HoT (hypotropia).

These abbreviations are in common usage and are approved by the American Academy of Ophthalmology

Chapter 1

Clinical skills

Obtaining an ophthalmic history

One of the first and most vital skills acquired by those involved in eye care is the accurate and efficient taking of an ophthalmic history. In ophthalmology clinical examination is very rewarding, probably more so than in any other specialty. However, this is additional to, rather than instead of, the history.

Apart from the information gained, a rapport is established which should help the patients to tolerate the relatively invasive ophthalmic examination. The patients are also more likely to accept any subsequent explanation of diagnosis and ongoing management if they know they have been listened to.

Presenting illness (PI)

Why are they here?

The patient's initial illness (i.e., complaint) often helps to direct additional questioning and examination. Routine eye care referral has a valuable role in screening for asymptomatic disease (notably glaucoma) but may generate unnecessary referrals for benign variants (e.g., anomalous discs, early lens opacities).

History of presenting illness (HPI)

The analysis of most ophthalmic problems center around general questions regarding the onset, precipitants, associated features (e.g., pain, redness, discharge, photophobia, etc.), duration, relieving factors, recovery, and specific questions of the presenting illness (i.e., complaints) (Box 1.1). Even after clinical examination, further information may be needed to include or rule out diagnoses.

Although some of these processes can be formalized as algorithms, their limitations should be recognized; they cannot compare to the multivariate processing, recognition of exceptions, and calculation of diagnostic probabilities subconsciously practiced by an experienced clinician.

Past ophthalmic history (POH)

The background for each presentation is important. Inquire about previous surgery/trauma, previous/concurrent eye disease, and refractive error. The differential diagnosis of an acute red eye will be affected by knowing that the patient had complicated cataract surgery 2 days previously or has a 10-year history of recurrent acute anterior uveitis, or even that the patient wears contact lenses.

Past medical history (PMH)

Similarly, consider the entire patient. Ask generally about any medical problems. In addition, inquire specifically about relevant conditions that they may have forgotten to mention. The patients presenting with recurrently itchy eyes may not mention that they have eczema or asthma. Similarly, if they have presented with a vascular event, ask specifically about diabetes, hypertension, and hypercholesterolemia.

Box 1.1 Obtaining the history of the presenting illness (HPI)—an example

Patient presenting with loss of vision

Did the event occur suddenly or gradually?

Sudden loss of vision is commonly associated with a vascular occlusion (e.g., AION, CRAO, CRVO) or bleeding (e.g., vitreous hemorrhage, "wet" macular degeneration). Gradual loss of vision is commonly associated with degenerations or depositions (e.g., cataract, macular dystrophies or "dry" macular degeneration, corneal dystrophies).

Is the vision loss associated with pain?

Painful blurring of vision is most commonly associated with anterior ocular processes (e.g., keratitis, anterior uveitis), although orbital disease, optic neuritis, and giant cell arteritis may also cause painful loss of vision.

Is the problem transient or persistent?

Transient loss of vision is commonly due to temporary/subcritical vascular insufficiency (e.g., giant cell arteritis, amaurosis fugax, vertebrobasilar artery insufficiency), whereas persistent loss of vision suggests structural or irreversible damage (e.g., vitreous hemorrhage, macular degeneration).

Does the problem affect one or both eyes?

Unilateral disease may suggest a local (or ipsilateral) cause. Bilateral disease may suggest a more widespread or systemic process.

Is the vision blurred, dimmed or distorted?

Blurring or dimming of vision may be due to pathology anywhere in the visual pathway from cornea to cortex; common problems include refractive error, cataract, and macular disease. Distortion is commonly associated with macular pathology, but again may arise from high refractive error (high ametropia/astigmatism) or other ocular disease.

Where is the problem with their vision?

A superior or inferior hemispheric field loss suggests a corresponding inferior or superior vascular event involving the retina (e.g., retinal vein occlusion) or optic disc (e.g., segmental AION). Peripheral field loss may indicate retinal detachment (usually rapidly evolving from far periphery), optic nerve disease, chiasmal compression (typically bitemporal loss), or cortical pathology (homonymous hemianopic defects). Central blurring of vision suggests diseases of the macula (positive scotoma: a "seen" spot) or optic nerve (negative scotoma: an unseen defect).

When is there a problem?

For example, glare from headlights or bright sunlight is commonly due to posterior subcapsular lens opacities.

Family history (FH)

This is relevant both to diseases with a significant genetic component (e.g., retinitis pigmentosa, some corneal dystrophies) and to infectious conditions (e.g., conjunctivitis, TB, etc.).

Social history (SH)

Ask about smoking and alcohol intake if relevant to the ophthalmic disease (e.g., vascular event or unexplained optic neuropathy, respectively). Consider the social context of the patients. Will they be able to manage hourly drops? Can they even take the top off the bottle?

Drugs and allergies

Ask about concurrent medication and any allergies to previous medications (e.g., drops), since these may limit your therapeutic options. In addition to actual allergies, consider contraindications (e.g., asthma or chronic obstructive pulmonary disease [COPD] and β-blockers).

Assessment of vision: acuity (1)

Measuring visual acuity (VA)

Box 1.2 An approach to measuring visual acuity

Select (and document) appropriate test:	Consider age, language, literacy, general faculties of patient
Check distance acuity (for each eye):	Unaided with distance prescription with pinhole (if <20/30)
Check near acuity (for each eye) (where appropriate):	Unaided with near prescription

Selecting the appropriate clinical test

Table 1.1 Tests of visual acuity

Patient	Distance	Near
Adult: literate	Snellen LogMAR	Test type N chart
Adult: illiterate	Illiterate E Landholt ring Sheridan-Gardiner (single optotype)	Reduced Sheridan-Gardiner
Children: age ≥3 years	Sheridan-Gardiner (single optotype) Sonsken-Silver (multiple optotype)	
Children: age ≥2 years	Kay picture test (single optotype) Multiple picture test	Reduced Kay picture test
Babies/infants	Clinical tests: fix and follow, objection to occlusion, picking up fine objects Preferential looking tests: Keeler, Teller, Cardiff cards Electrodiagnostic tests: Visual-evoked potential (VEP) response to alternating checkerboard of varying frequency	

Distance acuity

Snellen charts (Fig. 1.1)

The optotypes subtend 5 min of arc if read at the distance ascribed to that line, with each component of the letter subtending just 1 min of arc. This is the denominator. The actual distance at which it is used (usually 20 feet) is the numerator. Thus, if only the top line (400 optotype letter) can be read at 20 feet, the Snellen acuity is 20/400. Normal visual acuity is 1 min of arc or 20/20, although Vernier acuity may be up to 5 sec of arc. A change of 2 lines should be regarded as significant.

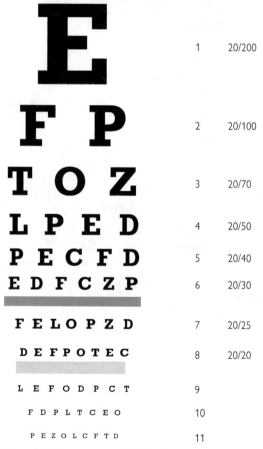

Figure 1.1 Schematic example of Snellen chart.

Assessment of vision: acuity (2)

Distance acuity (cont.)

LogMAR charts

This records the logarithm of the minimum angle of resolution (LogMAR). Based on the Bailey–Lovie logMAR chart, the actual chart in common usage is the Ferris modification known as the ETDRS chart (Fig. 1.2). LogMAR testing has marked advantages over Snellen, notably that 1) all letters are equally legible; 2) it controls the crowding phenomenon with 5 letters on each line and appropriate separation; and 3) there is a logical geometric progression of resolution. Starting with the LogMAR 1.0 line (Snellen 20/200), each letter is read. It is usually read at 20 feet. Each correct line (worth 0.1 units) or each correct letter (worth 0.02 units) is subtracted from 1.0 to give the final score.

Table 1.2 Distance acuity scoring systems

Snellen (US in feet)	LogMAR	Decimal	Snellen (UK in m)
20/200	1.0	0.1	6/60
20/80	0.6	0.25	6/24
20/40	0.3	0.5	6/12
20/20	0	1.0	6/6
20/10	−0.3	2.0	6/3

Crowding is a phenomenon by which neighboring targets interfere as proximity increases. Amblyopic patients are particularly susceptible and may score better with single optotype tests (e.g., Sheridan-Gardiner), than on a multiple test (e.g., Snellen). This has led to the use of multiple optotype forms of letter matching or picture tests.

Although other tests may approximate to a Snellen acuity reading, they are not exactly equivalent. It is therefore important to document which test has been used.

Pinhole acuity

A pinhole (stenopeic aperture, 1.2 mm diameter) can neutralize up to 3D of refractive error.

Near (reading) acuity

Various charts are available. Most have paragraphs of text that are read by the patient at his/her usual reading distance (usually around 30 cm). The notation used is N, this corresponding to the point size of the text being read. The range of the booklets is from N5 to N48.

Testing low visual acuity

If the vision is less then 20/200, walk the patient closer to the chart (or bring the chart to the patient). If it is less than 20/800, try counting fingers (scores CF), then hand movements (HM). If it is less than this, light perception (LP) is tested with a bright light. If light perception is present, try all four quadrants and ask the patient to point from which side the light is perceived (light projection).

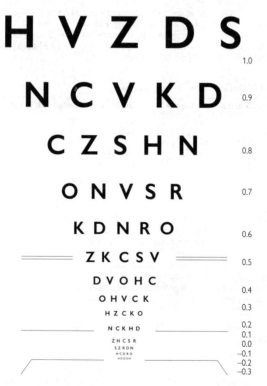

Figure 1.2 Schematic example of LogMAR chart.

Assessment of vision: clinical tests in children and tests of binocular status

Behavioral tests for babies/infants

Fix and follow

From 3 months of age, a baby should be able to fix and follow a target. Note whether fixation is central, steady, and maintained when the target is moved. Use of different-size targets can give an estimation of acuity.

Further information can be gained by observation of behavior. Do they respond to fine stimuli ("hundreds and thousands test")? Do they object to occlusion of one eye more than the other?

Preferential looking tests

These tests depend on the normal preference to look at the more visually interesting target, i.e., patterned rather than blank.

Keeler and Teller acuity cards comprise a series of cards, each of which has a black and white grating on a gray background of matching luminance (Fig. 1.3). The spatial frequency of the grating (i.e., the thinness of the lines) approximates to different acuity levels. The cards are presented so that the observer has to decide which direction the child has looked before knowing whether this corresponds to the position of the grating (i.e., it is a "forced choice").

Cardiff acuity cards have "vanishing optotypes." These are a series of pictures with increasingly fine outlines that are correspondingly difficult to see. These can be used as either a preferential looking test or a picture test (if verbal).

Recognition tests for older children

Picture tests

These include Cardiff acuity cards, Kay picture cards (single picture optotypes; optotypes vary in size), and multiple picture cards (similar but multiple optotypes on each card). The patient then selects the matching optotype on a handheld card or identifies the object verbally.

Sheridan-Gardiner test

This test has five booklets with single-letter optotypes that are presented at a distance of 20 feet (or, if necessary, 10 feet). The patient then selects the matching optotype on a handheld card. This is useful for children or others unable to use a Snellen or LogMAR chart.

Sonsken–Silver test

This is similar to the Sheridan-Gardiner test but has multiple-letter optotypes. Multiple optotype tests are generally only suitable for older children and are used more in this group than the equivalent test with single optotypes.

Tests of binocular status (see Table 1.3)

Binocular vision may be graded from simultaneous perception to fusion and finally to steropsis (a "3D" perception). These can be demonstrated on a synoptophore ranging from the simultaneous perception of two images (e.g., bird + cage → bird in a cage), to the fusion of two images (e.g., rabbit with tail + rabbit with flowers → rabbit with tail and flowers), and finally to the perception of depth in a fused image (e.g., two disparate images of a bucket → 3D bucket). Normal disparity perceived is 60 sec of arc but may be up to 15 sec.

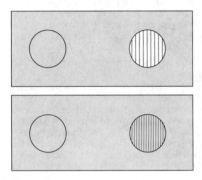

Figure 1.3 Schematic example of Keeler acuity cards.

Table 1.3 Tests of binocular status

Test	Icon	Mechanism	Monocular clues	Disparity
Titmus		Polaroid glasses	Yes	40–3000 sec of arc
TNO		Red-green glasses	No	15–480 sec of arc
Lang		Intrinsic cylinder lenses	Yes if not held perpendicular	550–1200 sec of arc
Frisby		Intrinsic plate thickness	Yes if not held perpendicular	15–600 sec of arc
Synoptophore		Separate eyepieces	No	90–720 sec of arc

Assessment of vision: contrast and color

Contrast sensitivity

While visual-acuity charts (e.g., Snellen) test high contrast (black letters on white background), most daily visual tasks require resolution of low to medium contrast. Contrast sensitivity may be reduced in the presence of normal Snellen acuity. It may be measured by a number of charts, all of which score the minimum contrast detectable for a specified target size.

The Vistech chart has rows of broken circles that decrease in contrast across the row and diminish in size from row to row. Identification of target orientation is plotted on a template to give a graph of contrast vs. spatial frequency. Charts are available for use at 1.5 feet and 10 feet.

Alternative charts maintaining a constant target size include the Pelli–Robson chart (triplets of capital letters, read until 2 or 3 mistakes in 1 triplet; Fig. 1.4) or Cambridge chart (square wave gratings, usually read at 20 feet, forced choice as to which of two luminance matched pages the grating is on).

Color vision

Red desaturation

The perception of redness (e.g., of a red pin) in both eyes is compared, occluding one at a time. This can be done for central vision (reduced in an optic neuropathy) or peripheral field (bitemporally reduced in a chiasmal lesion). An approximate score can be assigned by the patient to the washed-out image in relation to the normal image, e.g., 50%.

Ishihara pseudo-isochromatic plates

These are used at 2 feet under good illumination in patients with VA ≥20/60. The first test plate (seen even by achromats with sufficient acuity) is followed by a series of plates testing red–green confusion. Some of the plates differentiate whether the defect is of the protan (red) or deutan (green) system. It does not test the tritan (blue) system. Patients with congenital red–green color blindness (protanopia, deuteranopia) tend to make predictable mistakes, whereas in acquired disease (optic neuropathy), the mistakes do not follow a specific pattern.

Hardy–Rand–Rittler plates

These are less commonly used, but they have the advantage of testing tritan as well as protan and deutan discrimination.

Farnsworth-D15 test

This is a test of confusion, giving limited information on the protan, deutan, and tritan systems. It may be used as a screening test of color vision (e.g., for military personnel).

Farnsworth–Munsell 100-Hue test

This is a time-consuming test of color discrimination in which the patient attempts to order 85 colored caps by hue. When this is plotted onto a dedicated chart, it provides detailed information on protan, deutan, and tritan systems. This test is often used as the final arbitrator for color vision–requiring professions.

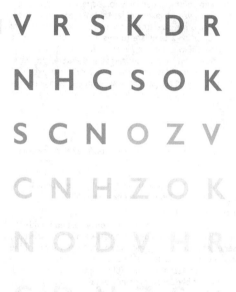

Figure 1.4 Schematic example of Pelli–Robson chart.

Biomicroscopy: slit-lamp overview

The slit lamp (biomicroscope) provides excellent visualization of both the anterior segment and, with the help of additional lenses, the posterior segment of the eye. Advantages of the slit-lamp view are that it is magnified (6–40×) and stereoscopic. Although basic slit-lamp skills are quickly gained, mastering its finer points enables one to use it to its full potential. Careful preparation of the slit lamp and patient is essential to optimize both quality of view and patient and clinician comfort.

Optical and mechanical features

The slit lamp consists of a binocular compound microscope and an adjustable illumination system. Since it has a fixed focal plane, objects are brought into focus by moving the slit lamp forward or backward. Movement of the slit lamp laterally (adjusted with the joystick) and vertically (a dial often attached to the joystick) permits visualization of each eye without having to adjust patient position.

Magnification

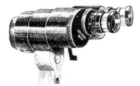

Figure 1.5 Eyepieces.

Most conventional slit lamps have two objective settings (1× and 1.6×) and two eyepiece options (10× and 16×). The total magnification thus ranges from 10× to 25×.

Others have a series of Galilean telescopes that can be dialed into position to give magnifications ranging from 6.3× to 40×. A zoom system is used less commonly.

Illumination: filters

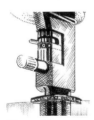

Figure 1.6 Illumination filters.

The illumination can be adjusted by use of a series of filters. Options include unfiltered, heat-absorbing filter, 10% gray filter, red-free filter, and cobalt blue filter (commonly from left to right).

In practice, the heat-absorbing filter is generally used for high illumination and the gray filter for lower illumination. The red-free and cobalt blue filters are used in specific situations. The red-free filter increases visualization of the vitreous and retinal nerve fiber layer and vasculature. The cobalt blue filter is mainly used to visualize fluorescein but also assists detection of iron lines.

The beam height and width are adjusted by apertures; the beam height is recorded (in mm) and may be useful in measurement (e.g., disc size, corneal ulcer, etc.).

Illumination: orientation and angulation

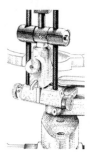

The orientation of the beam may be adjusted from vertical to horizontal (or any other angle) by swinging the superior aspect of the illumination arm to the left or right (useful for gonioscopy or in measuring lesions). Angulation of the beam is achieved by swinging the whole illumination arm to the side (horizontal) or tilting the illumination arm upward (vertical).

The alternative techniques of direct illumination, retroillumination, scleral scatter, and specular reflection (p. 18) require different angulations of the illumination arm, and some require the illumination arm to be unlocked, to displace the beam from the center of the field of view. Tilting the beam vertically may reduce troublesome reflections when using handheld lenses.

Figure 1.7 Illumination arm.

Illumination: mirrors

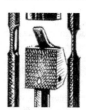

In certain situations, such as when using small angulations (3–10°), the standard long mirror may partially obscure the view. If this is troublesome, it can be replaced by the short mirror.

Figure 1.8 Mirror.

Fixation lamp

Many slit lamps have a fixation target, either a standard fixation lamp or an annular target with a focusing range of −15 to +10. This is adjusted to the patients' refractive error, enabling them to see the target clearly.

Stereovariator

Some slit lamps have a stereovariator that changes the angle of convergence from 13° to 4.5°. The conventional 13° provides better stereopsis, but the 4.5° provides a larger binocular field of view and thus improved acuity (binocular acuity > monocular acuity). This means that the 4.5° setting may be advantageous for detailed examination of certain ocular surfaces (e.g., corneal endothelium).

Biomicroscopy: use of the slit lamp

Box 1.3 Outline of slit-lamp examination

Set-up

- Adjust patient chair, slit lamp (Fig. 1.9), and your chair so that you and the patient can be comfortable during the examination.
- Adjust the chin rest until the patient's eyes are at the level of the marker (on the side of the head rest).
- Adjust the eyepieces:
  1) Dial in your refraction: use the nearer scale for the 10× eyepieces and the further scale for the 16× eyepieces;
  2) Fine-tune eyepieces: focus each eye in turn on a focusing rod placed in the central column (requires removal of the tonometer plate); this may be more "minus" than expected because of induced accommodation.
- Adjust the interpupillary distance.

Examination

- Start examination with lowest magnification (1× setting and 10× eyepieces) and low illumination. Rather than inadvertently dazzling your patient, first test brightness (e.g., on your hand).
- Start examination with direct illumination (usually fairly thin beam, angled 30–60°).
- Examine in a methodical manner from outside in, i.e., orbit/ocular adnexa, lids, anterior segment, posterior segment.
- Throughout the examination:
  1) Adjust illumination: adjust filter, orientation, and angulation and illumination technique (direct illumination, retroillumination, scleral scatter, specular reflection) to optimize visualization.
  2) Adjust magnification: to optimize visualization (e.g., of cells in the anterior chamber).
- At the end of the examination, do not leave your patient stranded on the slit lamp. Switch the slit lamp off (for the sake of the patient and the bulb) and encourage the patient to sit back.

Additional techniques

- *Tonometry:* Goldmann tonometer with fluorescein and blue light.
- *Gonioscopy and indirect funduscopy:* performed with appropriate handheld lenses.

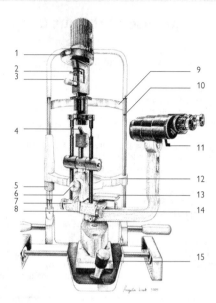

1	Indicator for beam height	9	Head band
2	Lever for selecting filters	10	Height marker (patient eye level)
3	Control for beam height	11	Lever for selecting magnification
4	Mirror	12	Chin rest
5	Control for chin rest height	13	Tonometer plate
6	Centering screw	14	Control for beam width
7	5° stops	15	Joystick
8	Latch for vertically tilting beam		

Figure 1.9 Slit lamp with key features identified.

Anterior segment examination (1)

Table 1.4 An approach to examining the anterior segment

Observe	Body habitus, face, orbits
Examine **lashes**.	Loss, color, position, crusting
Examine **lid margins**.	Position, contour, skin folds, defects, inflammation, lumps/bumps
Examine **palpebral conjunctiva**. • *Explain, then gently evert the lids.*	Papillae, follicles, exudate, membrane, pseudomembrane
Examine fornices	Loss of fornices, symblepharon, ankyloblepharon
Examine bulbar **conjunctiva/episclera**.	Hyperemia, hemorrhage, lumps/bumps, degenerations, foreign bodies/deposits
Examine **sclera**.	Hyperemia, thinning, perforation
Examine **cornea**. • *Use diffuse/direct illumination/ scleral scatter/specular reflection, as required.*	Diameter, thickness, shape; precorneal tear film, epithelium, Bowman's layer, stroma, Descemet's membrane, endothelium
Examine **anterior chamber**.	Grade flare/cells/depth; fibrin, pigment, depth
Examine iris. • *Use direct/retroillumination.*	Color, structure, movement, transillumination defects
Examine lens. • *Use direct/retroillumination.*	Opacity (pattern and maturity), size, shape, position, stability, capsule (anterior and posterior)
Examine **anterior vitreous**.	Cells, flare, lens-vitreous interface, degenerations
Stain cornea. • *Use fluorescein ± Rose Bengal.*	Tear film breakup time, Seidel's test
Check corneal sensation. • *Use topical anesthetic.*	
Perform applanation **tonometry**.	
Consider: gonioscopy, pachymetry, Schirmer's test	

Additional techniques for anterior segment examination

Illumination techniques

Although *direct illumination* is most commonly used, additional pathology may be revealed by using the following techniques:

- *Scleral scatter:* Unlock the light source so that the slit beam can be displaced laterally to fall on the limbus while the microscope remains focused on the central cornea. Total internal reflection results in a generalized glow around the limbus and the highlighting of subtle opacities within the cornea, e.g., early edema, deposits, etc.
- *Retroillumination:* Direct the light source at a relatively posterior reflecting surface (e.g., iris or retina) and focus on the structure of interest (e.g., cornea, or iris and lens). View undilated for iris transillumination defects; view dilated for lens opacities.
- *Specular reflection:* Focus on the area of interest and change the angle of illumination to highlight discontinuities in an otherwise smooth reflecting surface, e.g., examining the endothelium for guttata.

Tear film breakup time (BUT)

Place a drop of fluorescein into the lower fornix. Ask patient to blink once and then not to blink (or hold lids open if necessary). Observe with blue light the time taken until the tear film breaks up. A result <10 sec is abnormal.

Seidel's test

Place a drop of 2% fluorescein over the area of concern and observe with the cobalt blue light. The test is positive if there is a luminous green flow of aqueous. This results from local dilution of the stain by aqueous leaking from a surgical wound, penetrating injury or filtering bleb.

Schirmer's test

Whatman test paper is folded 5 mm from the end and inserted in the temporal fornix of both lower lids. After 5 min, the strips are removed and the length wetted is measured. This result is an indication of basic and reflex tearing. It is normal if >10 mm, borderline at 5–10 mm, and abnormal if <5 mm. Repeating the test after the addition of a topical anesthetic gives an indication of basic secretion alone.

Applanation tonometry

Place a combination of local anesthetic and fluorescein into the lower fornix. Rotate the tonometer dial and record the pressure at which the inner aspect of the two luminous green circles just touch. Usually, the white line on the prism is aligned with the horizontal merdian; however, in high astigmatism, the red line should be aligned with the minor axis. This is also affected by corneal thickness (p. 68).

Tonometer checks and calibration

Goldmann tonometers may be checked by using the metal bar and control weight supplied. With the weight exactly midway along the bar (central stop), the tonometer should read 0 mmHg. The next two stops correspond to 20 and 60 mmHg, respectively. Significant deviation from this indicates a need for formal recalibration by the manufacturer.

Anterior segment examination (2)

Anterior chamber (AC) depth measurement

Peripheral AC depth can be estimated using the Van Herick method: set the slit beam at 60° and directed just anterior to the limbus. If the AC depth is less than one-quarter of the corneal thickness, the angle is narrow and should be assessed on gonioscopy. A more central AC depth can be measured with a pachymeter.

Alternatively, use a horizontal beam set at 60 to the viewing arm, and measure the length of beam at which the image on the cornea just abuts the image on the iris. Multiply this by 1.4 to get the depth in mm.

AC reaction

In the presence of AC inflammation, grade both the flare (visible as haze illuminated by the slit-lamp beam; Table 1.5) and cells (seen as particles slowly moving through the beam; Table 1.6). This is important both in detecting intraocular inflammation and in monitoring response to treatment.

Table 1.5 Grading of AC flare

Grade	Description
0	None
1+	Faint
2+	Moderate (iris + lens clear)
3+	Marked (iris + lens hazy)
4+	Intense (fibrin or plastic aqueous)

Reprinted with permission from Jabs DA, et al. SUN Working Group (2005). *Am J Ophthalmol* 140:509–516.

Table 1.6 Grading of AC cells (counted with 1 × 1 mm slit)

Activity	Cells
0	<1
0.5+	1–5
1+	6–15
2+	16–25
3+	26–50
4+	>50

Reprinted with permission from Jabs DA, et al. SUN Working Group (2005). *Am J Ophthalmol* 140:509–516.

Gonioscopy

Use an indirect (Goldmann, Zeiss) or direct (Koeppe) goniolens to assess the iridocorneal angle, including the iris insertion, the iris curvature, and the angle approach. If the angle is closed, indent (with a Zeiss lens) to see if it can be opened ("appositional closure") or zippered shut ("synechial closure"). Describe according to the Shaffer (Table 1.7) or Spaeth (Table 1.8) grading system, recording which classification is being used (e.g., "4 = wide open" if using Shaffer) (see Fig. 1.10).

Shaffer classification

Table 1.7 Shaffer classification

Shaffer grade	Grade 4	Grade 3	Grade 2	Grade 1	Grade 0
Angular approach	40°	30°	20°	10°	0°
Most posterior structure clearly visualized	Ciliary body	Scleral spur	Trabeculum	Schwalbe's line	Cornea
Risk of closure	Closure not possible	Closure not possible	Closure possible	Closure probable	Closed
Summary	Wide open	Moderately open	Moderately narrow	Very narrow	Closed

Spaeth classification

Categorize according to iris insertion, angular approach, and iris curvature (e.g., D40R)

Table 1.8 Spaeth classification

Iris insertion	A	B	C	D	E
	Above Schwalbe's line	Below Schwalbe's line	Below scleral spur	Deep	Extremely deep
Angular approach	Estimate in degrees (°)				
Iris curvature	R		S		Q
	Regular convex		Steep convex		Queer (i.e., concave)

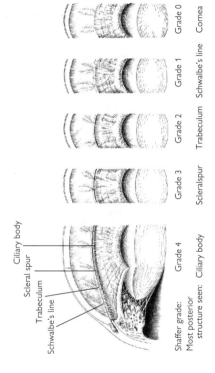

Figure 1.10 Anterior chamber angle with gonioscopic views. See Shaffer classification table for details.

Posterior segment examination (1)

Table 1.9 An approach to examining the posterior segment

Predilation perform RAPD, consider:	Amsler testing
Observe	Body habitus, face, orbits
Examine **iris**	Adequate dilation, aniridia, albinism
Examine **lens**	Clarity, position, aphakia/pseudophakia
Examine **vitreous** • *Use conventional/red-free illumination*	Cells, flare, pigment, hemorrhage, opacities, PVD, optical clarity
Examine **optic disc**	Size, vertical cup:disc ratio, color, flat/elevated/tilted, neuroretinal rim (inc. contour, notches, hemorrhages), pits/colobomata
Examine **optic disc margin**	Edema, capillaries, drusen
Examine **optic disc vessels**	Baring, bayonetting, anomalous vasculature, presence of spontaneous venous pulsation
Examine **peripapillary area** • *Use conventional/red-free illumination*	Hemorrhages, atrophy, pigmentation, retinal nerve fiber layer defects
Examine **macula**	Position, flat/elevated, fluid/hemorrhage/exudate, drusen/atrophy/gliosis, angioid streaks/lacquer cracks, retinal striae/choroidal folds, cherry-red spot
Examine **retinal vessels**	Attenuation/dilation, tortuosity, sheathing, emboli, IRMA/ neovascularization/telangiectasia/shunt vessels
Examine **peripheral fundus**	Degenerations/breaks/retinal detachments/dialysis/retinoschisis/ fluid/hemorrhage/exudate; pigmentary retinopathy, chorioretinal scars, tumors, laser/cryotherapy/buckles

At the slit lamp, consider choice of lens, Watzke–Allen test.
With the indirect ophthalmoscope, consider choice of lens, scleral indentation.
IRMA, intraretinal microaneurysms; PVD, posterior vitreous detachment; RAPD, relative afferent papillary defect.

Instruments used in posterior segment examination

Slit lamp
Most ophthalmologists examining the posterior segment use the slit lamp with a handheld lens (e.g., 90D).

Optical features
The choice of lens balances the advantages of greater magnification (e.g., 66D lens) against wider field of view (e.g., 90D lens). Some (e.g., super-field/super66) attempt to combine both these qualities.

Contact lenses provide the highest clarity and may be useful in assessing detail (e.g., area centralis for macular pathology) or where the view is poor (e.g., media opacities). The retinal view using these lenses is inverted. Three-mirror contact lenses (e.g., Goldmann) facilitate examination of the periphery; the views are mirror image rather than fully inverted.

Method

Ideally, the patient's eyes are dilated; the fundal view obtained without dilation is usually limited in both extent and stereopsis. Adjust the slit lamp so that it is coaxial and focused on the center of the cornea. Interpose the lens 1 cm in front of the eye and draw the slit lamp back until a clear fundal view is obtained.

To view the peripheral retina, ask the patient to look in the direction of the area you wish to examine (i.e., down to view inferior retina). Troublesome reflections can be reduced by moving the illumination beam slightly off axis.

Indirect ophthalmoscope and scleral indentor

The indirect ophthalmoscope (assisted by scleral indentation) is the instrument of choice for examination of the peripheral fundus.

Optical features

The choice of lens depends on the need for greater magnification (e.g., 3-fold with 20D lens but smaller field of view) vs. wider field of view (e.g., larger field of view with 28D lens but only 2-fold magnification). The retinal view is inverted.

Method

Ensure the patient is well dilated, positioned flat, and looking straight up at the ceiling. Have lens, indenter, and retinal chart/paper (for recording findings) available. Align eyepieces and illumination by viewing your outstretched thumb. Ensure that the headband is sufficiently tight that the ophthalmoscope will remain secure as you move around. Illumination brightness is adjusted according to quality of view and patient comfort.

View from above, with the ophthalmoscope directed downward toward the pupil and with the lens held directly in the line of illumination. Resting this hand lightly against the patient's face helps steady the lens at an appropriate focal distance for a clear fundal view. To view the peripheral retina, change the angulation by asking the patient to look in the direction of the area to be examined (i.e., down to view inferior retina) while angling your head and lens in the opposite direction.

Scleral indentation

To view, for example, the inferior ora, ask the patient to look straight up and place the indenter on the outside of the lower lid, resting tangentially against the area to be indented. Then ask the patient to look straight down, moving the indenter with the globe. Observe the area of interest while gently exerting pressure over it. Continue for 360°. Warn the patient that the procedure may be uncomfortable.

Posterior segment examination (2)

Instruments used in posterior segment examination (cont.)

Direct ophthalmoscope

For those who see patients in a non-ophthalmic setting, this may be the only option available for fundal examination. Ophthalmologists may also choose to use it where access to a slit lamp or indirect ophthalmoscopy is not possible (e.g., on intensive care unit patients).

- *Optical features:* There is high magnification (15×) but only a small field of view. The retinal view is not inverted.
- *Method:* Optimize your view with adequate dilation, dimmed room, and a fully charged ophthalmoscope. The field of view should be maximized by coming very near to the eye. Optimal view of the optic disc is achieved by approaching from 15° to 20° temporally while on the same horizontal level as the patient.

Additional examination techniques for posterior segment examination

Amsler grid

This is viewed at 1 foot. Ask the patient to fixate one eye at a time on the central dot and comment on whether any of the small squares are missing or distorted. There are seven charts, of which chart 1 is suitable for most patients (Table 1.10). It consists of a 20 × 20 grid of 5 mm squares each representing 1° of central field (if viewed at 1 foot).

Watzke–Allen test

While using the slit lamp and handheld lens to view the macula, project a thin strip of light across the fovea. Ask the patient whether the line he/she sees is broken, narrowed, or complete. A clear gap (Watzke–Allen positive) suggests a full-thickness macular defect or hole.

Goldmann 3-mirror lens

This contact lens is used with the slit lamp to examine the central and peripheral fundus. This is a mirror image rather than a rotated image of the peripheral fundus (cf. standard indirect ophthalmoscopy). It comprises four parts: central (view central 30°), equatorial mirror (largest; views 30° to equator), peripheral mirror (intermediate; views equator to ora), and gonioscopic mirror (smallest; views ora serrata, pars plana and angle).

Retinal charts

One standardized representation of vitreoretinal pathology uses the code presented in Table 1.11.

Table 1.10 Amsler charts

Chart	Design	Color	Use
1	Standard grid	White on black	Most patients
2	Standard grid with diagonals	White on black	Helps fixation
3	Standard grid	Red on black	Tests color scotoma, e.g., optic neuropathy, chloroquine toxicity
4	Random dots	White on black	Tests scotoma only (no lines to become distorted)
5	Horizontal lines	White on black	Tests in one meridian (standard horizontal lines)
6	Horizontal lines	Black on white	Tests in one meridian (standard/fine horizontal lines)
7	Standard/fine central grid	White on black	High sensitivity for central lesions

Table 1.11 Retinal chart key

Structure	Color
Detached retina	Blue
Flat retina	Red
Retinal veins	Blue
Retinal breaks	Red within a blue outline
Retinal thinning	Red hatching within a blue outline
Lattice degeneration	Blue hatching within a blue outline
Pigment	Black
Exudate	Yellow
Vitreous opacities	Green

Table 1.12 Optical properties of commonly used lenses

Lens	Field of view	Magnification of image	Magnification of laser spot
With indirect ophthalmoscope			
20D	46°/60°	3.1	0.3
28D	53°/69°	2.3	0.4
Non-contact lens with slit lamp			
60D	81°	1.2	0.9
Super 66	96°	1.0	1.0
78D	73°/97°	0.9	1.1
90D	69°/89°	0.8	1.3
Superfield NC	116°	0.8	1.3
Super VitreoFundus	124°	0.6	1.8
Contact lens with slit lamp			
Area centralis	84°	1.1	0.9
3Mirror		0.9	1.1
Transequator	132°	0.7	1.4
QuadrAspheric	144°	0.5	2.0

When using lenses with the slit lamp, the overall magnification seen = lens magnification (listed above) × slit lamp magnification (varies from 10 to 25×).

Pupillary examination

Clinical examination

Table 1.13 An approach to examining the pupils

Observe	Check lids, iris color
• *Ask patient to look at a distant target.*	
Measure pupil diameters in ambient **bright** light.	
Measure pupil diameters in ambient **dim** light.	
Check **direct** and **consensual** pupillary response for each side.	
Check for relative afferent pupillary defect (**RAPD**).	
• *Ask patient to look at a near target.*	Check near response

For an approach to diagnosing anisocoria, see p. 659.

Anatomy and physiology

Parasympathetic pathway (Light response)

CN II → **Pretectal** → E-W nuclei → CN III → **ciliary** → short → CONSTRICT
nucleus (bilateral) (inf) **ganglion** ciliary n

Known synapses are marked in bold.

Parasympathetic pathway (Near response)

VACx → FEF → CN III/E-W → Ciliary → Short → CONSTRICT
(area 19) nuclei ganglion ciliary n ACCOMMODATE
↓
→ Medial → CONVERGE
rectus

Light-near dissociation is where dorsal midbrain pathology selectively reduces the response to light while preserving the response to near, and is thought to be due to the near pathway being placed ventral to the more dorsal pretectal nucleus serving the light pathway.

Sympathetic pathway

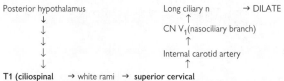

Posterior hypothalamus   Long ciliary n   → DILATE
↓   ↑
↓   CN V$_1$(nasociliary branch)
↓   ↑
↓   Internal carotid artery
↓   ↑
T1 (ciliospinal → white rami → **superior cervical**
center of Budge) communicantes **ganglion**

Pharmacological testing

The diagnosis of anisocoria (p. 659) may in some cases be assisted by pharmacological testing. These tests depend on comparing the response of the abnormal and the normal pupils, thus the agent should be instilled in both eyes and the response measured.

Diagnostic agents for an abnormally large pupil (e.g., for diagnosing Adie's pupil)

Pharmacology

Pilocarpine is a direct muscarinic agonist. A normal pupil will constrict in response to 1% pilocarpine. A response to 0.125% indicates denervation hypersensitivity, as occurs in an Adie's pupil.

Method

Administer a drop of 0.125% pilocarpine to both eyes. At 0 and 30 min measure pupil size when fixing on a distant target in identical dim lighting conditions. In Adie's pupil the affected eye shows a significantly greater response.

Diagnostic agents for an abnormally small pupil (e.g., for diagnosing Horner's pupil)

Pharmacology

Cocaine inhibits norepinephrine reuptake at the neuromuscular junction of the dilator pupillae, thus increasing sympathetic tone. In the presence of a normal sympathetic pathway, cocaine results in dilation. In a Horner's syndrome, the abnormal pupil does not dilate.

Hydroxyamphetamine stimulates release of preformed norepinephrine. In a first or second order Horner's, the post-ganglionic neuron is intact and thus the pupil will dilate in response to hydroxyamphetamine. In a third order Horner's, the pupil will not dilate. This test should not be performed within 48 hours of the cocaine test.

Method

- *Diagnose Horner's pupil:* Administer 4% cocaine to both eyes. Repeat at 1 min. At 0 and 60 min, measure pupil sizes when fixing on a distant target in identical ambient lighting conditions. The test is positive for Horner's if there is no/poor dilation to cocaine.
- *Identify level:* Administer 1% hydroxyamphetamine to both eyes. Measure pupil sizes to distinguish between a first- or second-order neuron lesion (normal dilation) and a third-order neuron lesion (no/poor dilation). This test is not reliable if performed within 48 hours of cocaine test.

Ocular motility examination (1)

Table 1.14 An approach to examining ocular motility

Note visual acuity.	Face turn, head tilt, chin up/
Observe head posture.	down
Hirschberg test	Manifest deviation
Cover/uncover + alternate cover test.	Manifest or latent deviation
• *With/without glasses targets: near (1 foot), distance (20 feet), non-accommodative*	
Examine versions into nine positions of gaze.	Any abnormality: under/ overaction paresis/restriction
• *Ask patient to follow the target (usually a penlight).*	alphabet patterns
• *Perform cover test in each position.*	Lid/head movements
• *Ask patient to report any diplopia in primary position or during test.*	
Examine horizontal and vertical saccades.	Normal/slow
• *Ask patient to look rapidly between widely separated targets.*	Hypo/hypermetric
Examine convergence.	Normal/reduced
• *Assess to both an accommodative and non-accommodative target.*	
Examine horizontal/vertical doll's-eye movements.	Normal/absent
Examine horizontal/vertical optokinetic nystagmus.	Normal/absent/ Convergence retraction
• *Slowly rotate an OKN drum in horizontal and vertical directions.*	nystagmus

Consider prism cover test, Krimsky test, and caloric tests.

General approach

Once a deviation has been detected, try to identify it as
• Manifest or latent.
• Concomitant (constant in all positions of gaze pp. 584, 586) or incomitant (varying p. 588).

For incomitant deviations identify
• Direction of maximum separation.
• Pattern typical of neurogenic (p. 588), mechanical (p. 588), or other (supranuclear, p. 588; myasthenic, p. 588; myopathic, p. 589) pathology.

It is common practice to use a penlight as a target when examining versions and vergences, since the positions of the eyes are highlighted by the corneal reflexes. However, try to ensure that the penlight is not too bright; dazzling the patient is counterproductive.

Corneal reflection tests

Hirschberg test

This test is used to detect or estimate the size of a manifest deviation. Ask the patient to fix his/her gaze on a penlight at 1 foot, and note the corneal reflections. The normal position is just nasal to the center of the cornea. Every 1 mm deviation represents 7° or 15Δ. If the reflection is deflected nasally, the eye is divergent (i.e., exotropic); if deflected temporally, the eye is convergent (i.e., esotropic).

Krimsky test

In the Krimsky test, this deviation is measured by placing a prism bar in front of the deviating eye and finding the prism strength at which the corneal reflexes are symmetrical. The prism should be orientated to "point" in the direction of deviation, i.e., base-out for an esotropia, base-in for an exotropia.

Cover tests

Cover–uncover test

The cover test reveals a manifest deviation. Ask the patient to fix his/her gaze on a target (near, distance, non-accommodative, and some-times far distance). Occlude each eye in turn (starting with the fixing eye) and observe any movement of the uncovered eye. For example, inward movement indicates that the eye was previously divergent (i.e., exotropic), and downward movement that it was previously elevated (i.e., hypertropic).

The uncover test may reveal a latent deviation. Occlude the first eye again for a few seconds. Look for any movement of the covered eye as the occluder is removed. Repeat for the other eye. For example, inward move-ment indicates that the occluded eye has drifted out (i.e., exophoric).

Perform the cover test in the nine positions of gaze to (1) identify the direction of maximum separation (indicates the direction of paretic muscle's action/maximum restriction) and (2) compare ductions and versions.

Ocular motility examination (2)

Cover tests (cont.)

Alternate cover test

This detects the total deviation (latent + manifest) by causing dissociation of binocular single vision (BSV). Ask the patient to fix on a target (near, distance, non-accommodative). Repeatedly cover each eye in turn for 2–3 sec, so that one eye is always covered. Note the direction and amplitude of any deviation elicited. Once BSV is broken down, remove the occluder and note the speed of recovery of each eye in turn. Also look for dissociated vertical deviation (DVD) and manifest latent nystagmus (MLN), which are common in infantile esotropia.

Prism cover test

This measures the angle of deviation. Repeat the alternate cover test but with a prism bar placed in front of one eye, adjusting the prism strength until first neutralization and then reversal of the corrective movement occurs. The prism should be orientated to point in the direction of deviation, i.e., base-out for an esotropia.

Maddox tests

In these dissociative tests, different images are presented to each eye. They are generally used for assessing symptomatic phorias—whether for distance (Maddox rod), for near (Maddox wing), or torsional (two Maddox rods).

Maddox rod

For distance, a single Maddox rod (series of red cylinders) is placed horizontally in front of the right eye and the patient (with distance correction) fixates on a distant spot of white light. The patient will see a vertical red line and a white spot. If there is no phoria, the line will pass straight through the spot. If the image is crossed (i.e., the line is to the left of the light), there is an exophoria; if the line is to the right, there is an esophoria.

   The phoria is then quantified by finding the prism required to neutralize it. The Maddox rod is then orientated vertically and the procedure repeated to identify any vertical phoria. If the line appears below the light, there is a right hyperphoria; if above it, there is a left hyperphoria. This is again quantified by neutralizing with prisms.

Maddox wing

For near, a Maddox wing is used. The patient (wearing his/her usual reading correction) looks through the apertures to view a vertical and horizontal arrow (with the right eye) and corresponding vertical and horizontal scales (with the left eye). The numbers indicated by the arrows (as seen by the patient) indicate the direction and size of the near phoria.

Two Maddox rod test

For torsion, a horizontally orientated Maddox rod is placed in front of each eye (one red, one white). The color of the tilted line is identified by the patient. The corresponding Maddox rod is rotated until the patient reports that it is vertical. The rotation required indicates the size of torsion. The two lines will fuse if there is no residual nontorsional deviation.

Parks–Bielschewsky 3-step test

This is used to identify a single underacting muscle in vertical/torsional deviations. It is particularly useful in superior oblique palsies (see Fig. 1.11, Table 1.15).

1. Perform cover test in primary position: identify higher eye.
2. Perform cover test with gaze to right then left: identify where separation (and diplopia) is greatest. This stage is based on the eye position where greatest vertical action occurs: for the oblique, this is when the eye is adducted; for the vertical recti, this is when the eye is abducted.
3. Perform cover test with head tilting to right then left shoulder: identify where separation (and diplopia) is greatest. This stage is based on the fact that the superior muscles intort the eyes, whereas the inferior muscles extort.

Caloric tests

This tests the vestibular, nuclear, and infranuclear pathways and can be useful in patients with decreased consciousness. Ideally, position the patient with the head inclined backward at 60°. Water placed in either ear causes nystagmus with fast phase as follows: cold–opposite, warm–same (COWS).

Step 1.
Right eye is the higher eye
in the primary position

Step 2.
Disparity is greatest
on gaze to the left

Step 3.
Disparity is greatest on
head tilt to the right

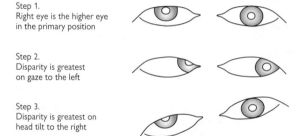

Figure 1.11 Parks–Bielschowsky 3-step test: example of right superior oblique underaction.

Table 1.15 Theoretical manifestations of single muscle underactions

Step 1	Step 2	Step 3	Conclusion
Higher eye	*Worst with gaze to*	*Worst with head tilt to*	*Underaction*
Right eye	Right	Left	RIR
		Right	LIO
	Left	Left	LSR
		Right	RSO
Left eye	Right	Left	LSO
		Right	RSR
	Left	Left	RIO
		Right	LIR

Visual fields examination

Table 1.16 An approach to examining visual fields

Note visual acuity.	Adjust target size if necessary
Observe	Features of stroke, acromegaly, etc.
• Patient with both eyes open and looking at the bridge of your nose.	Gross homonymous defects
• Ask if any part of your face appears to be missing.	
• Patient with nontesting eye occluded	Peripheral defects
• Check whether they can see the white pin. Map out right/left **visual field with the white pin** (coming from unseen to seen, asking the patient to identify when they first see the pin).	
• **Repeat with the red pin** to map right/left central 30° (asking the patient to identify when the pin appears red).	Central defects
• Use red pin to map out right/left **physiological blind spots**.	Enlarged/part of centrocecal scotoma

Any visual field abnormality should be confirmed on formal perimetry (p. 51).

Consider simultaneous presentation of gross targets to elicit inattention (this may occur in the context of stroke syndromes); simultaneous presentation of red targets (e.g., present across the midline to elicit the temporal depression of red perception of early chiasmal disease).

Additional clinical examinations may include pupils, optic discs, ocular motility, cranial nerves, and peripheral nervous system.

Lids/ptosis examination

Table 1.17 An approach to examining the lids

Shake hands	Check for myotonia
Observe	Face, brow, globes, pupils
Measure palpebral aperture.	
Measure upper margin reflex distance.	
Measure position of upper lid crease.	
Measure levator function.	
• *Inhibit frontalis by placing a thumb on the brow.*	
Measure any **lagophthalmos.**	
• *Ask patient to close eyes, gently at first and then squeeze eyes shut.*	
Assess **orbicularis function** and **Bell's phenomenon.**	
• *Try to open patient's eyes against resistance.*	
Assess **fatiguability** over 1 min.	Any worsening of ptosis
• *Ask patient to keep looking upward at a target held superiorly.*	
Examine for Cogan's twitch.	Any overshoot
• *Ask patient to look rapidly from downgaze to a target held in primary position.*	
Assess for jaw-winking.	Any change in ptosis
• *Ask patient to simulate chewing.*	
Check corneal sensation.	Implications for surgery
Examine ocular motility.	Motility abnormality, change in ptosis
Examine pupils.	Anisocoria, hypochromia

Consider examination of fundus, systemic review (myopathy, fatiguability).

Special tests

Fatiguability
The ability to sustain lid elevation is assessed in upgaze. Hold a target superiorly and ask the patient to maintain fixation on it for a minute. Note if either lid drifts down over that time, and reassess palpebral aperture in the primary position at the end of this period. If fatiguability is demonstrated, examine for associated fatiguability of ocular motility and general musculature. This is usually a sign of myasthenia.

Cogan's twitch
Cogan's twitch is an overshoot of the eyelid that occurs on rapid elevation of the eyes from downgaze to the primary position. Ask the patient to look down and then to look at a target held directly in front of him/her. Cogan's twitch may be seen in myasthenia.

Jaw-winking

Synkinesis ("miswiring") may result in a ptosis that varies with use of other facial muscles. This may be seen as jaw-winking, where the lid can be elevated by movement of the jaw (e.g., chewing) (p. 123).

Normal lid measurements

Table 1.18 Normal lid measurements

Palpebral aperture	8–11 mm (female > male)
Upper margin reflex distance	4–5 mm
Upper lid excursion (levator function)	13–16 mm
Upper lid crease position	8–10 mm from margin (female > male)

Orbital examination

Table 1.19 An approach to examining the orbit

Vision	VA, color
Observe	Behavior, body habitus, face, lids
Observe from above.	Globe position
Palpate orbital margins.	Notches, instability, soft tissue signs
Palpate globe (gentle retropulsion).	Pulsation, resistance, pain
Check infraorbital sensation.	Hyposthesia
Perform exophthalmometry.	Globe position
• Document which model was used (e.g., Hertel, Rodenstock).	
If proptosis, assess whether axial or nonaxial	
• Use two clear rulers, one horizontally over the bridge of the nose and one vertically to detect whether axial or nonaxial.	
Auscultate the globe/temporal region.	Bruit
Assess any effect of the Valsalva maneuver.	Increased proptosis
• Use stethoscope bell.	
Check corneal sensation.	Hyposthesia
Proceed to full ophthalmic examination including:	
Pupils	RAPD, anisocoria
Visual fields	
Ocular motility (± forced duction test)	Restriction, paresis
Cranial nerves	
Conjunctiva	Chemosis, injection
Cornea/sclera	Vessels, integrity
Tonometry	Change in upgaze
	Wide pulse pressure
Optic disc	Edema, pallor
	Abnormal vessels
Fundus	Choroidal folds
Consider refraction, neurological, and general systemic examintion, as indicated.	

Special tests

Exophthalmometry

Using the Hertel exophthalmometer, place it level with the orbits and adjust the separation so that the foot plates rest on the lateral orbital rims at the level of the lateral canthi. Close your right eye and ask the patient to fix his/her gaze on your open (left) eye while you align the parallax markers (usually red) and read off where the patient's right corneal apex appears on the scale. Repeat with your right eye and the patient's left eye.

Measurements >20 mm or a difference of >2 mm between globes is suggestive of proptosis. Be aware of patient variables (racial differences, lateral orbitotomy), instrument variability (try to use the same exophthalmometer each time), and operator inconsistency.

Two-ruler test

Horizontal and vertical displacement of the globe may be demonstrated by using two clear plastic rulers. One is placed horizontally over the bridge of the nose at the level of the lateral canthi. Look for horizontal displacement by comparing the distance from the center of the nasal bridge to equivalent points on the globe (e.g., nasal limbus). Look for vertical displacement by measuring vertically (second ruler) to compare the distance from the horizontal meridian (i.e., the first ruler) to equivalent points on the globe (e.g., the inferior limbus).

Nasolacrimal system examination

Table 1.20 An approach to examining the nasolacrimal system

Observe face.	Asymmetry, scars, nasal bridge
Observe/palpate **lacrimal sac**.	Mass, inflammation
• *Check for regurgitation form canaliculi on pressing sac.*	
Observe **lids**.	Contour, position, chronic lid disease
• *Assess with eyes open and closed.*	
Assess **lid laxity**.	
• *Draw lid laterally, medially, and anteriorly.*	
Examine **puncta**.	Position, caliber, discharge
• *Assess with eyes open and closed.*	
Examine **conjunctiva/cornea**.	Inflammation
Measure tear meniscus.	
• *Instill 2% fluorescein in lower fornix.*	
Assess **dye disappearance**.	
Check **dye recovery** from nose.	
• *Use nasendoscope or cotton tip applicator.*	
Cannulate and **probe** puncta/canaliculi.	Patency of puncta, hard or soft stop
• *Use lacrimal cannula attached to a syringe of saline (±fluorescein).*	
Irrigate with saline to estimate flow/ regurgitation.	Upper/lower systems
Consider nasendoscopy, formal Jones testing.	

Dye disappearance test

Instill a drop of fluorescein 2% into each lower fornix. Reassess at 2 min, by which time (almost) complete clearance should have occurred. Prolonged retention indicates inadequate drainage.

Probing

Under topical anesthesia, insert a straight lacrimal cannula into the lower canaliculus and guide it toward the medial wall of the lacrimal sac. Assess whether there is a
• Hard (abrupt) stop, which indicates a patent system as far as the lacrimal sac, or a
• Soft (spongy) stop, which indicates a canalicular block.

Irrigation

Under topical anesthesia, insert a lacrimal cannula into the lower canaliculus and place a finger against the lacrimal sac. Irrigate with saline and assess the following (see also Table 1.21):

- Flow: estimate flow (e.g., in %) conducted (i.e., down nose/back of the throat) vs. regurgitated; if regurgitated, note from which canaliculus.
- Quality of regurgitated fluid: clear or purulent.
- Lacrimal sac distension.

Jones testing

This may be considered in cases of partial obstruction to ascertain the level of block (Table 1.22).

Primary test

Instill fluorescein 2% into the lower fornix. After 5 min, assess for dye recovery with a cotton tip (can be moistened with 4% cocaine) placed at the nasolacrimal duct opening (below the inferior turbinate) or with a nasendoscope.

Secondary test

Wash out the fluorescein from the lower fornix. Under topical anesthesia, insert a lacrimal cannula into the lower canaliculus and irrigate. Assess dye recovery from the nose as before.

Table 1.21 Interpretation of probing and irrigation tests

Level of block	Probing	Irrigation
Punctum	Cannot cannulate	Not possible
Canaliculus (upper/lower)	Soft stop	Regurgitates through same canaliculus only (high pressure)
Common canaliculus	Soft stop	May regurgitate through either canaliculus
Nasolacrimal duct	Hard stop	Lacrimal sac dilates; may regurgitate (± mucus) through either canaliculus

Table 1.22 Interpretation of Jones test

	Result	Interpretation
Primary test		
Dye recovered	Positive	Normal patency
Dye not recovered	Negative	Partial obstruction or lacrimal pump failure
Secondary test		
Dye recovered	Positive	Partial obstruction of nasolacrimal duct
Dye not recovered	Negative	Partial obstruction above the lacrimal sac

Refraction: outline

History

Box 1.4 **Essential history**
- Age; profession; driver; special requirements; Department of Motor Vehicles (DMV)
- Visual symptoms
- Past ophthalmic history
- Family ophthalmic history
- Past medical history
- Drugs/allergies
- Previous eyeglasses/contact lens use

Examination

Box 1.5 **Preparation**
- Focimetry on current eyeglasses (p. 44)   ROOM LIGHTS ON
- VA—unaided + with PH
- Cover/uncover test
- Measure interpupillary distance (IPD) (distance) → set up trial frame

Box 1.6 **Retinoscopy**

ROOM LIGHTS OFF
- Ask patient to look at a nonaccommodative target (e.g., green duochrome).
- Correct for working distance (e.g., if you work at 2/3 m put in +1.5D DS).
- Fog fellow eye with a high PLUS DS lens to prevent accommodation.
- Check retinoscopy reflex.
  - Identify axis of astigmatism.
  - Neutralize reflex in one meridian with DS lenses.
  - If reflex is "with" then add PLUS, if "against," then add MINUS.
  - When point of reversal is reached in one meridian, add cylindrical lenses to neutralize in the other meridian.

Box 1.7 Subjective refraction

- Remove "working-distance" lenses.   ROOM LIGHTS ON
- Occlude eye not being tested.
- Check VA.
- Verify sphere.
  - Ask patient to look at the smallest line that he/she can see clearly.
  - Verify sphere by offering ± DS (usually ± 0.25 DS to fine-tune, but may need ±0.5 DS if poor VA).
  - Ask, "Is the line clearer and easier to read with lens 1 or 2?"
- Verify cylinder axis.
  - Ask patient to look at a round target/easily readable "O."
  - Use cross-cylinder (0.50 D cross-cylinder cf 1.00 D if poor VA).
  - Align handle with axis of trial cylinder.
  - Ask, "Is the circle rounder and clearer with lens 1 or 2?"
  - Rotate trial cylinder toward the preferred cross-cylinder position with respect to its sign ,i.e., a plus trial cylinder is rotated toward the plus sign of the cross-cylinder.
- Verify cylinder power.
  - Repeat the procedure but with the handle at 45° to axis of trial cylinder. This will in effect offer ± 0.25 D cyl (if using the 0.50 cross cylinder).
  - Add 0.25 DS for every 0.5 DC lost.
- Refine best sphere.
  - Plus 1 blur test (should reduce VA by 2 lines).
  - Duochrome test (monocular and binocular; aim for no preference/slight red preference).
- Measure and record back vertex distance (BVD) if >5 DS.
- Check near requirement—at usual reading/working distance.

Box 1.8 Muscle balance, accommodation, and convergence

- Maddox rod (distance muscle balance): place in front of right eye in horizontal then vertical orientation; neutralize with prisms until patient reports that the red line passes through white spot.
- Maddox wing (near muscle balance): ask patient where arrows point.
- RAF rule (perform 3 times for each test).
  - Accommodation amplitude: distance at where text blurs.
  - Near point of convergence: distance where line becomes double.

Refraction: practical hints

Hints on retinoscopy

Positioning yourself

Aim to be as close to the patient's visual axis without obscuring his/her fixation target. If your head gets in the way, they are likely to look at it and start accommodating.

Plus or minus cylinders

Be consistent: either work with **plus** or with **minus** cylindrical lenses.

- If using **plus** cylindrical lenses, you will wish to correct the most **minus** meridian first. This is identified by the following:
  - If both reflexes are *against*, then it is the *slower* reflex.
  - If one is *with* and one *against*, then it is the *against* reflex.
  - If both reflexes are *with*, then it is the *faster* reflex.
- If using **minus** cylindrical lenses, you will wish to correct the most **plus** meridian first. This is identified similarly:
  - If both reflexes are *against*, then it is the *faster* reflex.
  - If one is *with* and one *against*, then it is the *with* reflex.
  - If both reflexes are *with*, then it is the *slower* reflex.

Poor reflex

- Consider media opacity: optimize illumination, check that they are not accommodating on your head.
- Consider high refractive error: use large steps, e.g., ±5 DS, ±10 DS.
- Consider keratoconus if there is swirling reflex or oil-drop sign.

Hints on subjective refraction

Avoiding too much minus

When verifying and refining sphere, check that the patient finds it clearer and easier to read and not just smaller and blacker from the minification effect.

Higher refractive errors

- Put higher power lenses at back of trial frame.
- Measure and document back vertex distance, especially if >5.0 DS.

Prescribing reading add

Estimate requirement on the basis of age and lens status. However, this should be tailored to the individual and their needs (Table 1.23).

Table 1.23 Estimated near corrections

Age 45–50 years	+1.0 DS
Age 50–55 years	+1.5 DS
Age 55–60 years	+2.0 DS
Age > 60 years or pseudophakia	+2.5 DS

Role of muscle balance tests

- These tests depend on binocular vision and are dissociative. They are therefore particularly useful for detecting and quantifying phorias (latent strabismus).
- If the patient has a manifest strabismus but no diplopia, then there is no point in doing the muscle balance tests.
- Do not prescribe prisms unless the patient is symptomatic, and first consider whether further investigation (including orthoptic referral) is necessary.

Causes of spectacle intolerance

The following may lead to asthenopia (refractive discomfort or eyestrain):

- Significant change in axis or size of cylinder.
- Change of lens form.
- Overcorrection, especially of myopes, who will end up permanently accommodating.
- Excessive near correction resulting in an uncomfortably near and narrow reading distance.
- Unsuitable bifocal or progressive lenses—consider occupation, requirements, and general needs of the patient.

Focimetry

The focimeter or lensometer measures the axis and power of eyeglasses and contact lenses. The instrument can also be used to find the optical center, and the power and base direction of any prism in unknown lenses.

Manual focimetry

The vertex power of the lens is measured by taking the inverse of the focal length of the unknown lens. Green light is used to eliminate chromatic aberration.

Components
- Moveable illumination target.
- Viewing telescope.
- Fixed collimating lens (renders light parallel).

Method
- Ensure the eyepiece is focused and target seen sharply focused.
- Insert unknown lens (spectacles mounted with the back surface of the lens against the rest to measure back vertex power).

For simple spherical lenses

Dial (this moves the target backward or forward) until the graticules are sharp and read off the power.

For cylindrical power

The target is rotated, as well as dialed until one set of lines is sharp. The reading is noted. The target is then dialed again until the other lines are sharp. The difference in these two readings is the cylindrical power. The axis of the cylinder is then read from the dialing wheel.

Bifocal addition

Turn the eyeglasses around to measure the front vertex power. The difference between the front vertex power of the distance and near portions is the bifocal add.

Automated focimetry

In principle, four parallel beams of light pass through the unknown lens and strike a photosensitive surface. The deflection of the beams from their original path is measured and used to compute the lens power (Fig. 1.12).

There is a support frame for the spectacles; changing the lever on the unit above the support frame will automatically read either the right or the left lens as required.

The graticules are sharp at two positions

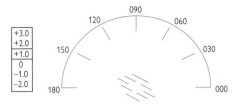

Position 1: the graticules are sharp at an angle of 150° and a power of +1.0D

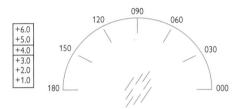

Position 2: the graticules are sharp at an angle of 60° and a power of +4.0D

Result: the lens prescription is therefore +1.0/+3.0 × 060.

Figure 1.12 View through the focimeter.

Chapter 2

47

Diagnostic tests and their interpretation

Visual field testing: general

The visual field is often regarded as "an island of vision surrounded by a sea of darkness" (Traquair's analogy). It is a three-dimensional hill: the peak of the hill is the fovea and at ground level it extends approximately 50° superiorly, 60° nasally, 70° inferiorly, and 90° temporally (Table 2.1).

Indications

Visual field testing aids in diagnosis and in monitoring certain ophthalmic (e.g., glaucoma) and neurological diseases.

Definitions

- A *scotoma* is an area of visual loss or depression surrounded by an area of normal or less depressed vision. An *absolute scotoma* represents a total loss of vision, where no light can be perceived. A *relative scotoma* is an area of partial visual loss, where bright lights or larger targets are seen, whereas smaller and dimmer ones cannot be seen.
- *Homonymous* is when the defects are in the corresponding region of the visual field in both eyes. For example, in a right homonymous hemianopia, there is a defect to the right of the midline in both visual fields.
- *Congruousness* describes the degree to which the field defects match between the two eyes. Generally, the more congruous the field defect the more posterior along the visual pathway the lesion is located.
- *Isopter* is a threshold line joining points of equal sensitivity on a visual field chart.

Caution

Interpretation problems affecting all visual fields can include ptosis or dermatochalasis, miosis, media opacities such as cataracts, incorrect positioning at the machine, poor attention to or incomprehension of the test, tremor, inadequate retinal adaptation, or refractive status (overcorrection by 1 diopter will cause a reduction in sensitivity of 3.6 dB). To compare serial visual fields, background luminance, stimulus size, intensity, and exposure times need to be standardized. Significant changes noted on visual field testing should be confirmed with repeat testing.

Confrontational visual fields (p. 33)

This is a simple qualitative method for gross detection of defects in the peripheral visual field. The use of hat pins (white and red) enables more subtle defects to be plotted. Results should be recorded the way the patient sees them; however, there can be interexaminer variability.

Amsler grid (p. 24)

This is used to assess the central 10° of the visual field. The test is easy to perform and the grid is portable. It is used to detect central and paracentral scotomas. Held at a testing distance of 1 foot, each square subtends 1 degree of visual field.

Table 2.1 Common visual field abnormalities

Altitudinal field defects	Ischemic optic neuropathy Branch retinal artery or vein occlusion Glaucoma Optic nerve or chiasmal lesions Optic nerve coloboma
Arcuate scotoma	Glaucoma Ischemic optic neuropathy Optic disc drusen
Binasal field defect	Glaucoma Bitemporal retinal disease (e.g., retinitis pigmentosa) Bilateral occipital disease Compressive lesion of both optic nerves or chiasm Functional visual loss
Bitemporal hemianopia	Chiasmal lesions Tilted optic discs Sectoral retinitis pigmentosa
Central scotoma	Macular lesions Optic neuritis Optic atrophy Occipital cortex lesions
Homonymous hemianopia	Optic tract or lateral geniculate lesions Temporal, parietal, or occipital lobe lesions
Constriction of peripheral fields	Glaucoma Retinal disease (e.g., retinitis pigmentosa) Bilateral panretinal photocoagulation Central retinal artery occlusion Bilateral occiptal lobe lesions with macular sparing Papilledema Functional visual loss
Blind spot enlargement	Papilledema Glaucoma Optic nerve drusen Optic nerve coloboma Myelinated nerve fibers Myopic discs
Pie in the sky	Temporal lobe lesion
Pie on the floor	Parietal lobe lesion

Kinetic perimetry

This involves presenting a moving stimulus of known luminance from a non-seeing area to a seeing area. The target is then presented at various points around the clock and marked when recognized; these points are then joined, producing a line of equal threshold sensitivity, which is named the *isopter*.

Tangent screen

The tangent screen (Bjerrum screen) is not commonly used in clinical practice.

Indication

It is used for examining the central 30° of visual field at 6.5 feet.

Method

The patient sits 6.5 feet from the screen, wearing a corrective lens for distance, if required. The nontested eye is occluded in turn. The patient fixates on a central spot and informs the operator when he/she sees the target. White or red disc targets are used, either 1 or 2 mm in diameter.

Results

The results are plotted on charts as the patient sees them. The target size and color is the nominator (1 mm white target = 1w), and the denominator is the distance (mm) of the patient from the chart (e.g., 1w/2000).

Goldmann perimetry

This is the most common type of kinetic perimetry in clinical practice (p. 51.)

Static perimetry

Most automated perimetry is based on static on–off stimuli of variable luminance presented throughout the potential field (p. 54).

Goldmann perimetry

- It is usually kinetic (but static perimetry is used for the central field).
- Skilled operators are required.
- It is useful for patients who need significant supervision to produce a reliable visual field.

Method

The machine should be calibrated at the start of each session.

Distance and near add with wide aperture lenses are used during testing (to prevent ring scotoma). Aphakic eyes should, where possible, be corrected with contact lenses.

Seat patient with chin on the chin rest and forehead against rest. Occlude the nontest eye; ask patient to fix gaze on central target and to press the buzzer whenever he/she sees the light stimulus.

From the opposite side of the Goldmann, the examiner directs the stimulus to map out the patient's field of vision to successive stimuli (isopters). The examiner should move the stimulus slowly and steadily from unseen to seen, i.e., inward for periphery and outward for mapping the blind spot/central scotomas. To move the stimulus arm from one side to the other, it must be swung around the bottom of the chart.

Once the peripheral isopters are plotted, the central area is examined for scotoma. The examiner should monitor patient fixation via the viewing telescope. The central 20° with an extension to the nasal 30° is appropriate for picking up early glaucomatous scotomas. The vertical meridian is particularly explored in suspected chiasmal and postchiasmal disease.

Results

Isopters are contours of visual sensitivity. Common isopters plotted are as follows (see also Fig. 2.1):

- I-4e (0.25 mm^2, 1000 asb stimulus).
- I-2e (0.25 mm^2, 100 asb stimulus).
- II-4e (1.0 mm^2, 1000 asb stimulus).
- IV-4e if smaller targets are not seen (16 mm^2, 1000 asb stimulus).

The physiological blind spot should also be mapped.

Interpretation

The target sizes are indicated by Roman numerals (0–V), representing the size of the target in square millimeters, each successive number being equivalent to a 4-fold increase in area.

The intensity of the light is represented by an Arabic numeral (1–4), each successive number being 3.15 times brighter (0.5 log unit steps). It is measured in apostilbs (asb).

A lower-case letter indicates additional minor filters, progressing from *a*, the darkest, to *e*, the brightest. Each progressive letter is an increase of 0.1 log unit.

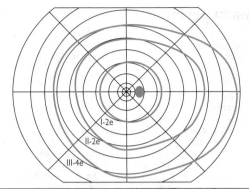

Intensity		dB	Intensity		dB		Object	mm²
1	0.0315	15	a	0.40	4		0	1/16
2	0.100	10	b	0.50	3		I	1/4
3	0.315	5	c	0.63	2		II	1
4	1.00	0	d	0.80	1		III	4
			e	1.00	0		IV	16
							V	64

Figure 2.1 Normal Goldmann visual field of the right eye.

Calibrating the Goldmann perimeter

Setup
- Insert standard test paper, verifying alignment.
- Lock stylus (at 70° on right-hand side), using knob on the pointer arm.

Stimulus calibration
- All levers should be to the right (i.e., V-4e).
- Turn stimulus (or test) light to permanently on.
- Move the white flag (photometer screen; located on left-hand side of machine) to the up position.
- Adjust the stimulus rheostat (knob furthest from examiner on left-hand side) until the light meter reads 1000 asb. If it does not reach 1000 asb, the bulb may need to be rotated or changed.

Background calibration
- Return white flag to down position.
- Set levers to V-1e (stimulus intensity of 32.5 asb).
- Adjust background illumination to match this stimulus intensity. This is achieved by adjusting the lampshade while looking through the notch on one side of the hemisphere to the photometer screen opposite.
- The photometer can be removed and the pointer handle unlocked.

Automated perimetry: performance and interpretation (1)

These machines are usually configured to test static perimetry. The stimulus in this case is stationary but changes its intensity until the sensitivity of the eye at that point is found. It is measured at preselected locations in the visual field. Program selection includes the central 30°, 24°, 10°, or full field.

Suprathreshold tests are quickest to perform and are screening tests. They calculate the threshold adjusted for age by testing a few predefined spots with a 4- to 6-dB step. They may miss subtle variations in a scotoma's contour, as they do not go on to map defects. They should not be used to monitor glaucoma.

Threshold testing steps of 4 dB are used until a visual defect is detected, at which point it is retested in 2-dB steps. This is the gold standard for monitoring glaucoma and requires patient cooperation and concentration; there is a subject learning curve seen in the first few tests.

Humphrey perimetry

- Sensitive and reproducible, but difficult to perform.
- Fixation monitoring (by tracking gaze and retesting the blind spot).

Method of Humphrey visual field (HVF)

The machine automatically calibrates itself on start-up. Selection of programs includes the following:

- Threshold (full threshold or Swedish interactive threshold algorithm [SITA] central 30–2, 24–2, 10–2).
- Suprathreshold testing (screening central 76 point, full-field 120 point, and Esterman).
- Colored stimuli can also be used.

Interpretation of Humphrey perimetry

When analyzing the results of automated perimetry, consider the following:

- Reliability indices (Table 2.2).
- Absolute retinal thresholds.
- Comparison to age-matched controls.
- Overall performance indices (global indices).

Table 2.2 Reliability indices (subject reliability)

Fixation losses	Fixation is plotted; if patient moves and the machine retests and patient sees target in blind spot, then a fixation loss is recorded. Fixation losses above 20% may significantly compromise the test.
False positives	Patient responds to the sound of the machine as if it were about to present a light, but does not present light stimulus. A high false positive occurs in "trigger-happy" patients
False negatives	A brighter light is presented in an area where the threshold has already been determined and the patient does not see it. A high false-negative score occurs in fatigued or inattentive patients.

Automated perimetry: performance and interpretation (2)

Interpretation of Humphrey perimetry (cont.)

Table 2.3 Typical graphical results from automated perimetry (Fig. 2.2)

Gray scale	Decreasing sensitivity is represented by the darker tones. Grayscale tones correspond to 5 dB change in threshold.
Numerical display	Gives the threshold for all points checked (in dB). Bracketed results show the initial test if the sensitivity was 5 dB less sensitive than expected.
Total deviation	Calculated by comparing the patient's measurements with age-matched controls. The upper chart is in decibels and the lower one is in grayscale.
Pattern deviation	Adjusted for any generalized depression in the overall field. This highlights focal depressions in the field, which might be masked by generalized depressions in sensitivity (e.g., cataract and corneal opacities).

Table 2.4 Global indices (a summary of the results as a single number used to monitor change)

Mean deviation (MD)	A measure of overall field loss.
Pattern standard deviation (PSD)	Measure of focal loss or variability within the field, taking into account any generalized depression. An increased PSD is more indicative of glaucomatous field loss than MD.
Short-term fluctuation (SF)	An indication of the consistency of responses. It is assessed by measuring threshold twice at 10 preselected points and calculated on the difference between the first and second measurements.
Corrected pattern standard deviation (CPSD)	A measure of variability within the field after correcting for SF (intratest variability).

Probability values (p)
These values indicate the significance of the defect <5%, <2%, <1%, and <0.5%. The lower the p value, the greater its clinical significance and the less the likelihood of the defect having occurred by chance.

Glaucoma progression analysis
Software available for Humphrey perimetry applies Early Manifest Glaucoma Trial criteria for progression to HVF data. Two visual fields are selected as a baseline for comparison for later exams. Symbols denote points that are worse than baseline on one, two, or three subsequent exams.

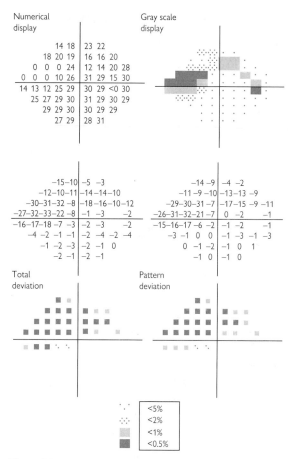

Figure 2.2 Typical graphical results from automated perimetry of the right eye of a patient with glaucoma, demonstrating nasal step and developing superior arcuate field defect.

Automated perimetry: protocols

Swedish interactive threshold algorithm (SITA) (fast or standard)

SITA strategies were created to take 50% less time than conventional algorithms to perform, thus increasing reliability. They are carried out by using prior information and establishing threshold values more quickly.

Esterman grid

Different grids are available for the central field, whole field, and binocular field. Subjects are tested and a percentage score of functional field is given. The binocular field test can be used as a measure of visual disability test for drivers (p. 748).

Short wavelength automated perimetry (SWAP)

SWAP involves standard static threshold testing strategies in which a blue test object is placed on a yellow background, isolating one photoreceptor system (red and green photoreceptors are desensitized by adapting the eye to yellow light). Results suggest that this is more sensitive to early glaucomatous damage than conventional white on white perimetry (SITA-SWAP reduces time comparable to that of SITA HVF).

Caution
• Increased total test time.
• Higher short-term fluctuation.
• Data more affected by nuclear sclerotic cataracts.

Frequency doubling perimetry (FDP)

This measures the function of a subset of specialized retinal ganglion cells (the large magnocellular [M-cell] pathway fibers) by rapid reversal of black and white bars, creating a flickering illusion. These M-fibers are thought to be lost early in glaucoma.

Given its high sensitivity and specificity, FDP may be useful in glaucoma screening. It is a small portable unit that is not sensitive to background illumination levels. It is reported to work independently of refractive errors up to ±7 diopters.

Ophthalmic ultrasonography (1)

This is a relatively inexpensive, reliable diagnostic imaging technique that uses high-frequency ultrasound (US) waves: ocular 8–10 MHz; orbital 4–5 MHz; and anterior segment 50–100 MHz.

Indications

- Measurement of axial length (biometry).
- Assessment of orbital tumors.
- Assessment of orbital disease (thyroid eye disease, measurement of muscles).
- Assessment of anterior chamber configuration (plateau iris configuration).
- Assessment of ocular pathologies such as retinal and choroidal detachments.
- Evaluation of the anterior or posterior segments with opaque ocular media (i.e., cataract or vitreous hemorrhage).
- Location of intraocular foreign bodies.

Method

Suitable electrical stimulation of a piezoelectric crystal results in emitted ultrasound waves. Ultrasound waves reflected backward restimulate the crystal and produce an electric current that can then be converted to a display. Imaging is effectively one-dimensional (A-scan) or two-dimensional (B-scan).

A-scans

These are curves of the amplitude of reflectivity of ocular structures and are used to obtain accurate measurements within the eye. They are mainly used in biometry.

Indications

- Measurement of axial length most commonly for intraocular lens power calculation (biometry).
- Measurement of anterior chamber depth or other intraocular distances.
- Measurement of intraocular mass thickness and characterization of acoustic properties.

Method

A transducer with coupling medium is placed on anesthetized cornea. The ultrasonic wave is emitted and deflections from the ocular tissues are recorded and displayed on a computer. Nonaxial scans are rejected.

Interpretation

This is a one-dimensional time–amplitude display. Corrections need to be made for different media such as silicone (Si) oil in the eye, as the speed of sound varies in different media (slower in oil than in vitreous media). Artifactually low axial lengths may occur in conditions such as asteroid hyalosis or if the eye is compressed during application.

Ophthalmic ultrasonography (2)

B-scans

Cross-sectional images of ocular or orbital tissues are obtained. The acoustic echoes are represented as a two-dimensional image, with their x-y coordinate determined by the echo origin and their brightness by the echo amplitude.

Indications

- Identification of posterior segment pathology in the presence of media opacity preventing fundal view, e.g., identifying retinal break or detachment obscured by vitreous hemorrhage.
- Characterization of intraocular masses by reflectivity and size of lesion.

Method

Ocular (static)

8–10 MHz transducer

- Lubrication agent is applied to closed eyelids.
- The marker on the probe shows one side of the display screen. When the marker is lined horizontally with the lids, it shows horizontal plane. Vertical placement (line to eyebrows) provides a vertical cross-section.
- Scans are captured with the patient's eye in primary position and then sequentially in all four quadrants, horizontally and vertically.

If the probe is moved temporally from the primary position, the scan shows the nasal retina. If the patient moves the left eye nasally while the probe is moved temporally, the nasal retina anterior to the equator can be scanned.

Ocular (dynamic)

Scanning during eye movements can help differentiate between posterior vitreous detachments and retinal detachments.

Orbital

3–5M Hz transducer

- Lubrication agent is applied to closed eyelids.
- Vertical scan planes are used to measure extraocular muscle thickness.
- Horizontal and vertical scans are used for orbital masses.

Anterior-segment or high-frequency scanning

50–100 MHz transducer

- *Indications:* corneal thickness, plateau iris syndrome, pigment dispersion syndrome, iris tumors/masses, position of intraocular lens haptics, assessment of the anterior segment in cases of corneal opacification (e.g., Peters anomaly and sclerocornea).
- *Method:* anesthetized cornea and eyelids open with an immersion bath (water or methylcellulose) as coupling agent or a self-contained water bath probe. High-frequency scans are taken radial and parallel to the limbus at various predetermined positions.
- *Results:* A two-dimensional cross-sectional display of anterior segment structures can be visualized.

Doppler ultrasound

A duplex scanner combines real-time B-scan images with pulsed Doppler images. Vessel patency and flow velocity can be assessed (see Table 2.5). Venous and arterial flows can be distinguished by color Doppler flow mapping. Caution is advised, as distinguishing severe stenosis from complete occlusion is difficult.

Indications
- Assessment of blood flow in central retinal artery, posterior ciliary arteries, ophthalmic artery, and central retinal vein.
- Carotid-cavernous fistulas.
- Vascular lesions.

Table 2.5 Diagnostic features on ultrasound

Posterior vitreous detachment	• Faintly reflective posterior hyaloid face may appear incomplete except on eye movement • Eye movement induces staccato movement with 1 sec after-movement • No blood demonstrated on color flow mapping
Rhegmatogenous retinal detachment	• Highly reflective irregular convex membrane attached at the optic nerve head • Eye movement induces undulating after-movement (unless PVR) • Blood demonstrated on color flow mapping
Tractional retinal detachment	• Highly reflective concave membrane tented into vitreous • Eye movement induces no after-movement of membrane • Blood demonstrated on color flow mapping
Choroidal detachment	• Highly reflective regular dome-shaped membrane • Attached to the vortex ampulla/vein • Blood demonstrated on color flow mapping in retina (6–8 cm/sec) and choroid (8–10 cm/sec)
Vitreous hemorrhage	Reflective particulate matter within the vitreous space (indistinguishable from vitritis)
Vitreous inflammation	Reflective particulate matter within the vitreous space (indistinguishable from hemorrhage)
Choroidal effusion	Acoustically empty suprachoroidal space thickening
Suprachoroidal hemorrhage	Reflective acoustically heterogeneous suprachoroidal space
Posterior scleritis	• Scleral thickness >2.0 mm • Fluid in Tenon's space and optic nerve sheath (T-sign)

Fluorescein angiography (FA)

FA is photography performed in rapid sequence following intravenous (IV) injection of sodium fluorescein ($C_{20}H_{10}O_5Na_2$), an organic water-soluble dye, to image the choroidal and retinal vasculature using spectrally appropriate blue excitation and yellow-green barrier filters. FA is typically used to evaluate the retina and choroid vasculature, but occasionally may be used to assess anterior segment structures.

Sodium fluorescein (wt 376 Da) is 70–85% bound to plasma albumin. Metabolized by the liver and excreted by the kidneys in 24 hours, it has a peak absorption at 490 nm (blue visible spectrum) and emits at 530 nm (yellow visible spectrum). Good photographic results require clear media and dilated pupils.

Indications

- Diagnostic test directly assessing the retinal and choroidal vessels (functional integrity and flow), but indirectly providing information about other retinal structures and pathological features. It is an adjunct to the clinical history and examination findings.
- Evaluation of anterior segment masses or neovascularization.
- Planning of retinal laser procedures.

Contraindications

- Renal impairment (relative contraindication: decreased dose given)
- Known allergy to fluorescein

Side effects

- Skin discoloration
- Nausea and vomiting
- Pruritis
- Urine discoloration (orange)
- Vasovagal syncope (1 in 340)
- Severe anaphylaxis (1 in 1900)
- Fatal anaphylaxis (1 in 220,000)

Method

- Prepare patient: explain the procedure, risks, and benefits and obtain informed consent from the patient. Dilate; check blood pressure (BP); cannulate (medium/large bore vein); ensure that resuscitation facilities (including crash cart) are readily available.
- Seat patient at camera and adjust height for patient comfort and camera alignment. Ask patient to fix their gaze on the fixation target.
- Take color and red-free fundus photographs.
- Inject fluorescein (5 mL 10% IV) and take early rapid-sequence photographs (at around 1-sec intervals for 25–30 sec). Continue less frequent shots, alternating between eyes for up to 5–10 min. Late images may be taken at 10–20 min.

The early shots are critical: it is generally only possible to get a good series of early shots from one eye given the time it takes to move between eyes. It is therefore important that the photographer be informed of which eye takes priority.

Interpretation

FAs should be read sequentially according to their phases: choroidal (prearterial), arterial, capillary, venous, and late. This test should be reported in conjunction with patient history and examination (see also Table 2.6).

Table 2.6 Morphological analysis of fluorescein angiographic (FA) features

Feature	Common causes
Hyperfluorescence	
Window defect	RPE defect (e.g., RPE atrophy, macular hole)
Leakage of dye	• At macula: cystoid macular edema (petalloid appearance), other macular edema
	• At disc: papilledema, ischemic optic neuropathy, inflammation
	• Elsewhere: new retinal vessels, vasculitis, CNV
Pooling of dye	Detachment of the neural retina or RPE (e.g., central serous retinopathy, age-related macular degeneration)
Staining of dye	Drusen, optic disc rim, disciform scars, sclera (seen if overlying chorioretinal atrophy/thinning)
Abnormal vessels	Tumors (hemangiomas, melanomas, etc.)
Autofluorescence (visible without dye)	Disc drusen, large lipofuscin deposits
Hypofluorescence	
Transmission defect	• Preretinal (blocks view of retinal and choroidal circulations): media opacity, especially vitreous opacities (inflammation, hemorrhage, degenerative), preretinal hemorrhage
	• Inner retinal (blocks view of capillary circulation but larger retinal vessels seen): dot and blot hemorrhages (e.g., vein occlusion), intraretinal lipid (e.g., diabetic retinopathy)
	• Prechoroidal (blocks view of choroidal circulation, but retinal circulation seen): subretinal hemorrhage, pigment (e.g., choroidal nevi, congenital hypertrophy of the retinal pigment epithelium [CHRPE], melanoma), lipid, lipofuscin
Filling defects (circulation abnormalities)	• Retinal arteriolar nonperfusion (e.g., arterial occlusion)
	• Retinal capillary nonperfusion (e.g., ischemia secondary to diabetes, vein occlusion)
	• Choroidal nonperfusion (e.g., infarcts secondary to malignant hypertension, etc.)
	• Disc nonperfusion (e.g., ischemic optic neuropathy)

CNV, choroidal neovascularization; RPE, retinal pigment epithelium.

Reporting

Box 2.1 Reporting on FA

1. Report the red-free photo.
2. Specify the phase.
3. Note hyper- and hypofluorescence and any delay in filling (see Table 2.6).
4. Note distinctive features (petalloid, smoke stack, etc.).
5. Note any change in area, intensity, or the fluorescence over time.

Indocyanine green angiography (ICGA)

ICGA is a similar test to FA; however, the contrast agent is indocyanine green, which provides better resolution of the choroidal circulation. ICG is 98% bound to serum proteins that do not pass through the fenestrations of the choriocapillaris. With an excitation peak at 810 nm and emission of 830 nm, the dye is excited by infrared radiation.

Indications

- Suspected choroidal neovascularization (CNV) not clearly visualized on FA (particularly occult-type) or blocked by blood.
- Recurrence of CNV after treatment.
- Consideration of feeder vessel treatment in CNV.
- Suspected idiopathic polypoidal choroid vasculopathy (IPCV).
- Central serous chorioretinopathy (CSCR or CSR).
- Suspected retinal pigment epithelial (RPE) detachments.
- ICG may sometimes be helpful in the assessment of choroidal tumors, choroidal inflammatory disease, or other diseases of the choroidal vasculature.

Method

- ICG powder is mixed with aqueous solvent to make a solution of 40 mg in 2 mL. A red-free photo is taken and the bolus IV injection is given. Frequent images are taken over the first 3 min and then later images at, for example, 5, 10, 15, 20, and 30 min.

Contraindications

- Pregnancy
- Renal impairment
- Iodine allergy (ICG contains 5% iodine)

Side effects

- Nausea and vomiting
- Sneezing and pruritus
- Backache
- Staining of stool
- Vasovagal syncope
- Severe anaphylaxis (1 in 1900)

Interpretation

The angiogram is split into early phase (2–60 sec), early mid-phase (1–3 min), late mid-phase (3–15 min), and late phase (15–30 min) (see also Table 2.7).

Table 2.7 Morphological analysis of ICGA features

Feature	Common causes
Hyperfluorescence	
Window defect	RPE defect
Leakage of dye	Choroidal: choroidal neovascularization (CNV), idiopathic polypoidal chorioidal vasculopathy (IPCV); also leakage from other structures (retina, disc)
Abnormal blood vessels	Choroidal hemangioma
Hypofluorescence	
Transmission defect	RPE detachment (hypofluorescent centrally); blood, pigment, and exudate cause less blockage than in FFA
Filling defects (circulation abnormalities)	Choroidal infarcts secondary to accelerated hypertension, systemic lupus erythematosus (SLE), etc. Choroidal atrophy (e.g., atrophic age-related macular degeneration [AMD], some chorioretinal scars, choroideremia, loss of choriocapillaris)

OCT, HRT, and SLP

The following scanning technologies allow for acquisition of fast, reproducible, high-resolution images of the optic nerve and retina. Given the noncontact, noninvasive nature of these tests and novel cross-sectional imaging information, these diagnostic tests have become commonplace in many ophthalmic practices, assisting in optic nerve head retinal nerve fiber layer (RNFL), foveal, and vitreous macular interface evaluation, and complementing (and occasionally supplanting) FA.

Optical coherence tomography (OCT)

In OCT, light in the near-infrared spectrum (810 nm) from a superluminescent diode is used to create high-resolution cross-sectional images of the retina. A partially reflective mirror is used to split the coherent light beam into a measuring beam and a reference beam. The measuring beam is directed into the eye, where succeeding optical interfaces (e.g., retinal layers, RPE, choriocapillaris) reflect the beam to a variable extent.

The reference beam is directed to a reference mirror, which is adjusted to synchronize the reflected reference beam with the reflected measuring beam returning from the retinal surface. This results in constructive interference. Reflections from deeper structures will be out of phase and cause variable degrees of destructive interference. The interference is interpreted as depth, and amplitude of reflection as brightness.

Early OCT models were based on time-domain OCT technology. More recent models take advantage of spectral-domain (Fourier domain) OCT technology, which circumvents use of a reference beam, enabling faster acquisition of a larger amount of data, ultimately providing higher-resolution images that can yield three-dimensional reconstructed views.

Indications

- Detection and monitoring of macular pathology (e.g., subretinal fluid, macular edema, macular hole, etc.).
- Detection of glaucomatous retinal nerve fiber layer changes.
- Detection of glaucomatous optic disc changes.
- Evaluation of retinal architecture due to underlying tumors (choroidal nevus, choroidal melanoma, choroidal hemangioma).

Method

- A large pupil and clear media ensure accurate measurement.
- Choose the appropriate OCT program for the area to be imaged.
- An 810 nm diode laser measuring beam is directed at the area of interest.

Results

The cross-section indicates layers within the retina that are represented in artificial color: highly reflective (red → white) and poorly reflective (blue → black). Resolution is around 8 μm for time-domain OCT (i.e., OCT3) and around 2–5 μm for spectral-domain OCT.

Interpretation

OCT imaging provides high-resolution images and may be supported by additional analysis software (e.g., for optic disc analysis). RNFL can be compared to a normative database.

Heidelberg retinal tomography (HRT)

The HRT is a type of confocal scanning laser ophthalmoscope (CSLO). It is designed for three-dimensional imaging of the posterior segment of the eye and requires an experienced operator to draw a contour line of the scleral edges of the optic disc.

Indications
- Detection of glaucomatous optic disc damage
- Longitudinal or progressive change detection

Contraindications
- Advanced cataract
- Corneal opacities
- Nystagmus

Method
- A large pupil and clear media ensure accurate measurements.
- A 670 nm diode laser images a series of two-dimensional sections of the optic nerve head (ONH) and the peripapillary retina.
- A three-dimensional topographic image is then built from a series of 16–64 serial optical sections by means of algorithms to find the surface at 384 x 384 (HRT II and III) pixels over a 10° or 15° field of view. The software automatically captures three consecutive 15° images and generates a mean topographic image.

Results

Laser polarimetry can measure RNFL thickness by measuring a change in the rotation of a polarized beam of laser light reflected from the retinal surface. Transverse resolution is around 10 μm, but axial resolution is only around 300 μm.

Interpretation

Pupil size and density of cataracts affect the quality and variability of the results. Measurements are also influenced by the contour line drawn by the operator, acute changes in intraocular pressure (IOP), and possibly the cardiac cycle.

Scanning laser polarimetry (SLP)

The nerve fiber analyzer (GDx) is a scanning laser polarimeter that uses the birefringent properties of the retinal nerve fiber layer. This birefringence arises from the parallel architecture of the axonal microtubules. The change in polarization, called *retardation*, can be quantified by determining the phase shift between polarization of light returning from the eye with that of the illumination laser beam. The degree of retardation is linearly related to the retinal nerve fiber thickness. The nerve fiber analyzer thus estimates the thickness of the peripapillary RNFL on the basis of retardation of polarized light.

GDx is available with a variable corneal compensator (VCC) to adjust for the anterior segment contribution to birefringence. The enhanced corneal compensator (ECC) employs a corneal compensation software technique designed to reduce atypical retardation patterns that can occur during VCC-adjusted scans with poor signal-to-noise ratios.

Indications
- Glaucoma detection

Contraindications
- Nystagmus
- Dense cataracts
- Large amounts of peripapillary atrophy
- Corneal refractive surgery

Method
A polarized laser beam (820 nm) scans the peripapillary retina circumferentially around the scleral canal opening to acquire an image. The backscattered light is captured and analyzed. The edge of the disc is marked by the operator.

Results
The amount of retardation is calculated per pixel and displayed in a retardation map of the scanned area. Note: mild to moderate cataracts do not degrade the result.

Interpretation
RNFL results can be compared to a large normative database that includes Caucasians and patients of African descent.

Corneal imaging techniques

Corneal topography

Corneal imaging techniques are rapidly evolving, given the advances in refractive surgery and the need for accurate measurements of corneal shape, refractive power, and thickness.

Indications

- Assessment of corneal curvature and postoperative corneal changes.
- Detection of macroirregularities, such as astigmatism, keratoconus, and pellucid marginal degeneration.
- Monitoring of contact lens–induced distortion of the cornea and of disease progression.

Methods

Multiple light concentric rings are projected onto the anterior surface of the cornea. The reflected images are captured; computer software is used to analyze the data and generate topographical color-coded maps.

Results

Curvature is expressed as radii of curvature in millimeters (mm) or in keratometric diopters. A color scale is used representing the range of values. The maps are constructed by either comparing the data to itself (relative or normalized scales) or to set ranges (absolute scale). Consequently, different color maps cannot be directly compared and have to be interpreted on the basis of their actual numerical values.

Interpretation

The average adult cornea is steeper in the vertical meridian than in the horizontal one and has with-the-rule astigmatism (a bowtie pattern).

Scanning-slit videokeratography (Orbscan corneal analyzer)

This system uses scanning optical slit technology, combining Placido reflections and direct triangulation.

Indications

- Assessment of anterior and posterior corneal surface elevations (useful for wavefront-guided surgery).
- Indirect measurement of corneal thickness.

Methods

A high-resolution video camera projects numerous light slits at the anterior segment. It captures and analyzes the light reflected using a triangulation system.

Results

The software calculates elevation—i.e., the points per half-slit from both the anterior and posterior surfaces. It then indirectly calculates the corneal thickness.

Interpretation

This is a highly accurate corneal topography system. Although it is reproducible, the main disadvantage is the inability to detect interfaces (e.g., post-LASIK flap).

Corneal ultrasonic pachymetry

This modality is used to measure the thickness of the cornea using a contact 20 Hz ultrasonic probe.

Indications

- Assessment of the appropriateness of refractive surgery (in particular, LASIK, to prevent postoperative corneal ectasia).
- Assessment of accurate applanation IOP (important in normal tension glaucoma and ocular hypertension).
- To measure and monitor corneal edema (such as in Fuchs' dystrophy).

Methods

Instill topical local anesthetic. Hold the ultrasonic probe at 90° to the corneal surface. No coupling agent is required. Pachymetry should be measured centrally, inferonasally, and inferotemporally.

Results

Average central corneal thickness is approximately 540–550 μm.

Interpretation

While this is a simple, portable, and low-cost reproducible method, inaccurate positioning of the probe could result in erroneous results.

Anterior segment OCT (ASOCT)

OCT technology is used to image anterior chamber structures. ASOCT enables noncontact evaluation of anterior segment pathologies.

Indications

- Anatomic narrow angle and anterior chamber depth
- Evaluation of corneal refractive surgical flaps (LASIK flaps)
- Pachymetry
- IOL position

Limitations

Can only image structures that can be penetrated by light, not useful for posterior iris or ciliary body pathology.

Scheimpflug camera (Pentacam)

A rotating Scheimpflug camera acquires up to 50 images a second to generate three-dimensional images and anterior segment biometric calculations.

Indications

- Detailed images of the anterior segment.
- Measurements of anterior chamber angle, chamber volume, chamber depth, pupil diameter.
- Evaluation of corneal characteristics, such as eccentricity, central radius, astigmatism, topography, and pachymetry.
- Accurate measurement of refractive power of the cornea to improved intraocular lens (IOL) calculation for post-LASIK, photorefractive keratectomy (PRK), and refractive keratectomy (RK) patients.

Confocal scanning laser ophthalmoscopy (HRT Rostock)

Cornea module
- Uses HRT technology to image cornea cells and cell layers.

Indications
- In vivo imaging of tissues for evaluation of dystrophies
- Degenerative disorders
- Infectious processes

Electrodiagnostic tests (1)

All electrodiagnostic tests should be performed to the International Society for Clinical Electrophysiology of Vision (ISCEV) standard, as the responses and normal values can still differ between centers because of variation in equipment and technique.

The results of each test is interpreted by the polarity and amplitude of the electrophysical deflections and their latency (implicit time).

Electroretinography (ERG)

ERG is a record of the mass electrical activity from the retina when stimulated by an intense flash of light.

Indications

- Diagnosis of generalized retinal degenerations (such as retinitis pigmentosa [RP], Leber's congenital amaurosis, choroideremia, gyrate atrophy, achromatopsia, congenital stationary night blindness [CSNB], and cone dystrophies).
- Investigation of family members for known hereditary retinal degenerations (such as RP).
- Determining of visual function (pediatric cases).
- Assessment of generalized retinal function in opaque media.
- Evaluation of functional visual loss.

Method

A Ganzfeld or full-field stimulation is created by a bowl perimeter. Electrodes are embedded in a contact lens on the cornea and there is a reference electrode on the forehead.

The scotopic rod-response ERG is measured in dark-adapted eyes (after 30 min in the dark) with a dim white flash 2.5 log units below the standard flash. The maximal response ERG is obtained in dark-adapted eyes using the standard flash. The photopic single-flash cone-response ERG is in light-adapted eyes (after 10 min in the light). The cone-derived flicker response is obtained using a 30 Hz white light flicker stimulus; the rods are unable to respond due to poor temporal resolution.

Results

A single flash-stimulus is followed by an initial negative a-wave and then a positive b-wave, superimposed on oscillatory potentials. This usually takes less than 250 ms. Amplitude (microvolts) and implicit time (milliseconds) of these waves are the two major parameters used to evaluate the ERG response (see Fig. 2.3).

- The a-wave arises from the photoreceptors.
- The b-wave arises from the bipolar and Muller cells.
- The c-wave is an additional waveform seen only in the dark-adapted eye, which reflects RPE activity.

Example: ERG is useful in central retinal vein occlusion (CRVO) to distinguish between nonischemic and ischemic CRVOs. The b wave is affected by large areas of ischemia. This produces a reduced b-wave amplitude, reduced b:a wave ratio, and/or a prolonged b-wave implicit time.

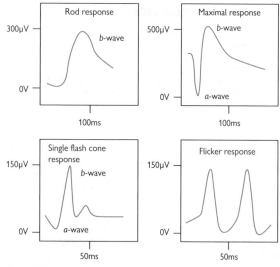

Figure 2.3 Typical ERG in a normal patient.

Interpretation

Table 2.8 Interpreting ERG results

Reduced *a*- and *b*-waves	Retinitis pigmentosa
	Ophthalmic artery occlusion
	Neuroretinitis
	Metallosis
	Total retinal detachment
	Drugs (phenothiazines, chloroquine)
	Cancer- and melanoma-associated retinopathy (CAR and MAR)
Normal *a*-wave and reduced *b*-wave	Congenital stationary night blindness (CSNB)
	X-linked juvenile retinoschisis
	Central retinal vein or artery occlusion
	Myotonic dystrophy
	Oguchi's disease
	Quinine toxicity
Abnormal phototopic and normal scotopic ERGs	Achromatopsia
	Cone dystrophy
Reduced oscillatory potentials	In diabetic patients this can correlate with an increased risk of developing severe proliferative diabetic retinopathy

Electrodiagnostic tests (2)

Pattern electroretinogram (PERG)

Indication

PERG is used for objective assessment of central retinal function.

Method

A reverse checkerboard evokes the small potentials that arise from the inner retina.

Results

A prominent positive component at 50 ms (P50) and a larger negative component at 95 ms (N95) is demonstrated (Fig 2.4).

Interpretation

P50 is driven by macular photoreceptors and can be a key to macular function. N95 appears to identify the retinal ganglion cells.

Electro-oculography (EOG)

This indirectly measures the standing potential of the eye (approx 6 mV). It reflects the activity of the RPE and photoreceptors of the entire retina.

Indications

- Diagnosis of certain macular dystrophies (Best's disease).
- Early detection/screening of individuals at risk (e.g., Best's disease).
- Mild change in patients with adult vitelliform dystrophy.

Method

Electrodes are attached to the medial and lateral canthi. Patients fixate on target lights that move from right to left over 30° horizontal distance. The cornea makes the nearest electrode positive to the other. The potential difference between the two electrodes is amplified and recorded. The test is preformed in the dark- and light-adapted states.

Results

Results are expressed as: Light peak/Dark trough × 100 = Arden index (ratio).

Interpretation

Normally the potential doubles from the dark-adapted to the light-adapted eye: >185% is considered normal; <165%, abnormal.

Visual evoked potentials (VEPs)

VEP measures the electrical response of the visual cortex in response to a changing visual stimulus, such as multiple flash or checkerboard pattern stimuli. VEPs may record generalized cortical response or multifocal response. VEP can be thought of as a limited EEG. It is useful in assessing uncooperative or unconscious patients.

Indications

- Optic nerve disease, particularly subclinical demyelination.
- Chiasmal and retrochiasmal dysfunction.
- Detection of nonorganic visual loss.

Method

A reversing black and white checkerboard or grating is used. The voltage changes vary with time and are plotted as waveforms. Reflecting the central 6–10° of the visual field, the data elicited correspond to cone activity.

Results

A positive deflection occurs at about 100 ms (P100). Negative deflections occur at N75 and N135 (Fig 2.4).

Interpretation

Decreased amplitude and increased latency of P100 in optic nerve dysfunction. However, delays are also common in macular dysfunction; therefore a delayed VEP should not be considered pathognomonic of optic nerve disease.

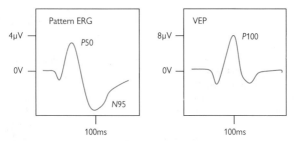

Figure 2.4 Typical waveform of PERG and VEP in a normal patient.

Dark adaptometry

This measures the absolute threshold of photoreceptor activity with time in the dark-adapted eye. It is used in conjunction with the EOG and ERG.

Goldmann–Weekers adaptometry

Indications

- Retinal disorders causing night blindness (RP, congenital stationary night blindness)
- Cone dysfunction
- Evaluation of drugs affecting dark adaption (vitamin A analogues such as isoretinoin)

Method

Subjects are totally light bleached by a bright background light, which is then extinguished. In the dark, they are then presented with a series of dim flashes. The threshold value for which the light is perceived is then plotted against time.

Results

A biphasic curve is plotted. The first curve represents the cone threshold (reached at 5–10 min), the next one represents the rod threshold, which is reached at 30 min. Rhodopsin has now fully regenerated and retinal sensitivity has reached its peak.

Interpretation

Defects in rod metabolism produce abnormally high threshold (higher than 10^2 log units) at 30 min.

Ophthalmic radiology: X-ray, DCG, and CT

X-ray orbits

Indications

Although plain X-rays have been largely superseded by computed tomography (CT) and magnetic resonance imaging (MRI), plain films may be useful in excluding a radio-opaque foreign body (which may preclude an MRI). Other pathology (e.g., orbital fractures) may be identifiable on plain X-ray, but generally it requires further characterization by CT or MRI.

Method

Commonly used views include occipitomental (Water's view), overtilted occipitomental, and lateral. If an intraocular foreign body (IOFB) is suspected, upgaze and downgaze views may show a change in position of a radio-opaque IOFB.

Dacryocystography (DCG)

This requires the injection of radio-opaque contrast medium (oil-based) into the lacrimal drainage system. The technique is similar to cannulation and irrigation of the tear ducts.

Indications

- Aid diagnosis of epiphora
- Plan surgical procedures

Method

The puncta are intubated with polyethylene tubing and a plain film X-ray is taken. A radio-opaque contrast is then injected and further X-ray films taken following the contrast injection.

Results

Contrast is seen in the fornices, canaliculi, common canaliculi, and nasolacrimal ducts if bilateral systems are patent.

Interpretation

A blockage or filling defect at any level will be seen if pathology is present.

Computerized tomography (CT)

CT involves the rotation of a tightly collimated X-ray beam and detector around the patient. From the data gained in different projections, an image of a single plane ("slice") is reconstructed. A series of slices are recorded through the area of interest.

CT is useful for detecting a wide range of orbital and intracranial pathology. A CT head causes a typical effective dose of X-ray irradiation equal to 10 months of natural background radiation.

Patients on metformin may develop lactic acidosis if given radio-opaque contrast media. If the use of contrast is anticipated, indicate on the request form whether the patient is taking metformin. The radiology department can then arrange for the drug to be temporarily stopped around the time of the procedure. Contrast media are relatively contraindicated in patients with renal dysfunction.

Indications
• Orbital cellulitis
• Orbital lesions
• Orbital trauma
• Intracranial lesions
• Cerebrovascular accidents
• Metallic intraocular body

Interpretation
Visualization of the bony orbit and lesions with calcification makes this a good technique for the orbit and globe. The planes that CT can image in are limited; however, additional projections can be reconfigured by computer. True coronal scans are often most useful for evaluating ocular and orbital pathology.

Ophthalmic radiology: MRI and MRA

Magnetic resonance imaging (MRI)

Tissue exposed to a short electromagnetic (EM) pulse undergoes rearrangement of its hydrogen nuclei. When the pulse subsides, the nuclei return to their normal resting state, re-radiating some energy they have absorbed. Sensitive receivers pick up this EM echo. T1 and T2 times are two complex parameters that depend on proton density, tissue components, and their magnetic properties.

Indications

- Optic nerve disease such as glioma, intracranial extension of orbital tumors, suspected compressive optic neuropathy.
- In retrobulbar neuritis, the presence of multiple white matter plaques is predictive of the development of clinical multiple sclerosis (MS).
- Suspected lesions of the chiasm such as pituitary tumors.
- Intracranial aneurysms.

Method

Conventional sequences are T1- and T2-weighted tests determined by the examining radiologist on the basis of clinical situation (see Table 2.9). Additional imaging techniques include specialized fat-suppression techniques, which are useful for optic nerve visualization, usually masked by the high signals from orbital fat, or fluid attenuated inversion recover (FLAIR), which is useful for identifying white matter disease.

Intravenous paramagnetic gadolinium is used as contrast. Gadolinium-enhanced scans are useful in the detection of blood–brain barrier abnormalities, inflammatory changes, and increased vascularity (see Table 2.10). While gadolinium-based contrast media are generally less toxic to the kidneys, patients with renal insufficiency or failure are at high risk for developing nephrogenic systemic fibrosis (NSF).

Interpretation

Always review your own scans in conjunction with the radiology team. It is also important to consider the quality of the scan (e.g., adequate slices, appropriate use of contrast/processing), especially when it is unexpectedly "normal."

Table 2.9 Characteristics of T1- and T2-weighted scans

T1	T2
Excellent anatomical detail	More pathological detail seen
CSF and vitreous have low-intensity signal (black)	CSF and vitreous have high-intensity signal (white)

Table 2.10 Advantages and disadvantages of MRI (compared to CT)

Advantages	Disadvantages
• No ionizing radiation • More sensitive than CT for early tumors • Excellent for surgical planning • Excellent anatomical views • High contrast sensitivity • Multiplanar imaging capability	• Contraindicated in patients with pacemakers, metallic foreign bodies, magnetic aneurysm clips, cochlear implants, and transcutaneous neural stimulators • Bone and calcification appears black and can be missed • Recent hemorrhage not imaged • Requires patient cooperation (steady fixation to prevent ocular movement degrading image) • Noise and claustrophobia • Not approved for the first trimester of pregnancy

Magnetic resonance angiography (MRA)

MRA is a noninvasive method of imaging the intra- and extracranial carotid and vertebrobasilar circulations. The principle of the computerized image construction is based on the hemodynamic properties of flowing blood, rather than on vessel anatomy.

Indications

MRA demonstrates abnormalities such as stenosis, occlusion, arteriovenous malformations, and aneurysms.

Disadvantages

MRA cannot detect aneurysms <5 mm in diameter. Conventional intra-arterial angiography remains the gold standard for accurate diagnosis and surgical planning for berry aneurysms.

Magnetic resonance venography (MRV)

MRV is similar to MRA but the imaging is "gated" to the speed of venous flow. It is useful in identifying venous thromboses (e.g., sagittal sinus thrombosis). It is therefore commonly performed in cases of idiopathic intracranial hypertension.

Trauma

Ocular trauma: assessment

Box 3.1 An approach to assessing ocular trauma

Incident	Date, time, place, witnessing of history (if assault or pediatric case), mechanism of injury, associated head injury (loss of consciousness, nausea, vomiting, seizures), other injuries
Symptoms	↓VA (sudden or gradual), floaters, flashes, field defects, diplopia, pain
POH	Previous/current eye disease
PMH	Any systemic disease, tetanus status
SH	Family support, alcohol or drug abuse
FH	Family history of eye disease
Drug history	Drugs
Allergy history	Allergies
GCS	Conscious level
Visual function	VA, RAPD, color vision, visual fields to confrontation ± formal perimetry
Orbits	Continuity of orbital rim, infraorbital sensation
Soft tissues	Periorbital bruising, edema, surgical emphysema; lid lacerations
Globes	Proptosis, enophthalmos, hypoglobus; pulsatility
Motility	Mechanical restriction or paretic muscle
Conjunctiva	Diffuse or defined subconjunctival hemorrhage, laceration
Cornea	Abrasion or full-thickness laceration (sealed or leaking), FB, rust-ring, infiltrate, edema
AC	Depth, flare, cells (erythrocytes, leukocytes), pigment
Gonioscopy	(May need to be deferred) angle recession/dialysis, FB in angle
Iris	Anisocoria, traumatic mydriasis, iridodialysis, iridodonesis, transillumination defect, FB
Lens	Cataract, FB, phacodonesis, subluxation, Vossius ring (iris pigment imprinted on anterior capsule)
Tonometry	Applanation (may need to be deferred); if ↓IOP consider penetrating injury, retinal detachment
Vitreous	Hemorrhage, pigment, posterior vitreous detachment
Fundus	Retinal edema (commotio retinae), hemorrhage, tear, detachment, dialysis; choroidal rupture; exit wound; optic nerve avulsion

Indirect ophthalmoscopy (indentation may need to be deferred)

AC, anterior chamber; FB, foreign body; FH, family history; GCS, Glasgow Coma Scale; IOP, intraocular pressure; PMH, past medical history; POH, past ophthalmic history; RAPD, relative afferent pupillary defect; SH, social history; VA, visual acuity.

Documentation

Careful assessment and accurate documentation are critical. Legal proceedings often follow trauma cases. Clinical photographs can be very helpful.

Investigations

- If no fundus view is possible because of soft tissue swelling or opaque media, consider B-scan ultrasonography (use water bath) ± CT scan to identify gross intraocular/orbital pathology.
- CT of orbits, face, or head is also valuable in assessing an intraocular foreign body (IOFB), orbital or maxillofacial fractures, and associated cerebral injuries. MRI should be avoided in cases where a ferromagnetic IOFB is suspected. Facial X-rays may assist in diagnosing radio-opaque IOFB (upgaze/downgaze views) and orbital fractures; this modality has largely been replaced by CT.
- If there is suspected globe rupture, manipulation must be kept to a minimum. This includes deferring gonioscopy, scleral indentation, and even tonometry.

Tetanus status and prophylaxis

Current immunization protocol

Tetanus vaccines
- *For children:* Adsorbed tetanus vaccine is given as part of DTP (diphtheria/tetanus/pertussis) at 2 months, 3 months, and 4 months of age, followed by booster doses at school entry (DTP) and school leaving (diphtheria [low dose] and tetanus).
- *For nonimmune adolescents/adults:* Give three doses of 0.5 mL intramuscular (IM) diphtheria (low dose) and tetanus separated by 4 weeks, with a booster after 10 years.

Definitions
- *Immune:* primary immunization is complete (three doses) and within 10 years of a booster dose, or if the patient has received a total of five doses.
- *Tetanus-prone wound:* septic, devitalized, or soil-contaminated; puncture wound; or there is significant delay before surgery (>6 hours).
- *Very high-risk wound:* unusual in ophthalmology but would include injuries such as major facial trauma with soil contamination.

Treatment

Table 3.1 Treatment of open wounds

Patient	Wound	Action
Immune	Clean	Nothing needed
	Tetanus-prone	Clean/debride wound as required. Give tetanus immunoglobulin only if very high risk. Consider antibiotic prophylaxis.
Nonimmune	Clean	Immediate dose of vaccine followed by completion of standard schedule (by PCP).
	Tetanus-prone	Clean/debride wound as required. Immediate dose of vaccine (as above) and tetanus immunoglobulin (at a different site), followed by completion of standard schedule (by PCP). Consider antibiotic prophylaxis.
Uncertain of vaccination status	Clean	As for nonimmune patients with clean wounds. Request PCP to check medical records and complete standard schedule if necessary.
	Tetanus-prone	As for nonimmune patients with tetanus-prone wounds. Request PCP to check medical records and complete standard schedule if necessary.

PCP, primary care physician.

If tetanus vaccine is indicated it should be given immediately (Table 3.2). Immunoglobulin should be given at a different site than that for vaccine.

Table 3.2 Summary of indications for tetanus prophylaxis

Risk		Treatment required		
Patient	Wound	Vaccine	Immunoglobulin	Completion of course by PCP
Immune	Clean	No	No	No
	Tetanus-prone	No	Yes if very high risk	No
Nonimmune	Clean	Yes	No	Yes
	Tetanus-prone	Yes	Yes	Yes
Uncertain of vaccination status	Clean	Yes	No	Yes if needed
	Tetanus-prone	Yes	Yes	Yes if needed

Chemical injury: assessment

Chemical injuries are among the most destructive of all traumatic insults suffered by the eye. They may occur in domestic, industrial, and military settings. Alkalis cause liquefactive necrosis and so penetrate further than acids, which cause coagulative necrosis and so impede their own progress.

Prognostic factors

The severity of a chemical corneal injury is determined by the following:

- *pH:* Alkali agents generally cause more severe injuries than those from acid (see Table 3.3), although very acidic solutions may behave similarly. Most domestic and chemical agents are alkali (or neutral) rather than acid (see Table 3.4).
- *Corneal involvement:* surface area, duration of contact.
- *Limbal involvement:* Corneal re-epithelialization relies on migration of the limbal stem cells.
- *Associated nonchemical injury:* blunt trauma, thermal injury.

Clinical features

These include conjunctival injection or blanching, chemosis, hemorrhage, epithelial defects; corneal epitheliopathy (punctate to complete loss may stain poorly with fluorescein), corneal edema; perilimbal ischemia (blanched vessels with no visible blood flow); anterior chamber activity; and ↑IOP (consider Tonopen rather than Goldmann). Rarely is there necrotic retinopathy.

Complications

- *Conjunctival burns:* cicatricial scarring, symblepharon, and keratoconjunctivitis sicca
- *Significant limbal ischemia:* conjunctivalization, vascularization, and opacification of the cornea
- *Full-thickness burns:* hypotony, iris, ciliary, and lenticular damage; may progress to phthisis bulbi; very poor prognosis
- *Periorbital burns:* first-, second-, or third-degree chemical burns of periorbital tissues

Table 3.3 Alkali injury grading (Roper–Hall classification)

Grade	Corneal appearance	Limbal ischemia	Prognosis
Grade I	Clear cornea	None	Good
Grade II	Hazy cornea: iris details visible	<1/3	Good
Grade III	Opaque cornea: iris details obscured	1/3 to 1/2	Guarded
Grade IV	Opaque cornea: iris details obscured	>1/2	Poor

Table 3.4 Strong acids and alkalis in common use

Substance	Chemical	pH
Common alkalis		
Oven cleaning fluid	Sodium hydroxide	14
Drain cleaning fluid	Sodium (or potassium) hydroxide	14
Plaster	Calcium hydroxide	14
Fertilizers (some)	Ammonium hydroxide	13
Common acids		
Battery fluid	Sulfuric acid	1
Lavatory cleaning fluid	Sulfuric acid	1
Bleach	Sodium hypochlorite	1
Pool cleaning fluid	Sodium (or calcium) hypochlorite	1

Chemical injury: treatment

Immediate

Neutralization of pH by irrigation

Even before a full history or detailed examination is conducted, give copious irrigation until neutral or near-neutral pH (new 7) is confirmed by pH/litmus paper (normal tears may be slightly alkaline). Evert the lids (double-evert the upper lid) to remove retained particulate matter in fornices that may perpetuate alkalinity (e.g., lime, cement).

Acute—all injuries

- *Admit* if injury is severe or there are any other concerns.
- *Topical antibiotics*: prophylaxis.
- *Topical cycloplegia* for comfort/AC activity (e.g., preservative-free cyclopentolate 1% 3×/day).
- *Topical lubricants.*
- *Oral analgesia.*

Topical medication should be preservative-free when possible.

Acute—severe injuries

Admit patient and consider the following:

- Topical steroids (e.g., prednisolone acetate 0.5–1% initially 4–8×/day for <10 days),
- Topical ascorbic acid (e.g., sodium ascorbate 10% up to every 2 hours for <10 days), and
- Oral ascorbic acid (e.g., 2 g 4×/day).

Ascorbic acid is essential for collagen formation and is an effective scavenger of damaging free radicals. It should not be used in acid chemical burns. Less commonly used are topical sodium citrate (reduces neutrophil chemotaxis and inhibits collagenases but is painful) and oral tetracyclines (inhibit collagenases).

Acute—injuries with ↑IOP

Give acetazolamide 250 mg 4×/day ± topical β-blocker (e.g., preservative-free timolol 0.5% 2×/day)

Long-term—complicated cases

Poor corneal healing

Consider surgical treatment to vascularize limbus (conjunctival and tenon capsule advancement), help re-epithelialization (limbal stem cell transplantation), or assist migration (amniotic membrane transplantation).

Corneal opacification

Consider penetrating keratoplasty if there is an adequate ocular surface environment but delay for ≥6 months. Keratoprosthesis remains a surgical option for severely damaged eyes.

Obliterated fornices

Consider division of symblepharon and conjunctival membrane grafting.

Orbital fractures: assessment

Assessment

Table 3.5 Specific features in assessment of potential orbital fractures

History	• Mechanism of injury • Diplopia, areas of numbness, epistaxis, visual symptoms (associated ocular injury)
Physical exam	• Pain, periorbital bruising/edema/hemorrhage, surgical emphysema, globe position, globe pulsation, ocular motility, subconjunctival hemorrhage, discontinuity of orbital rim • Any associated ocular injury • Any potential cervical or head injury (refer to trauma team); collapse may be due to oculocardiac reflex secondary to extraocular muscle (EOM) entrapment
Imaging	• Facial X-rays: droplet sign (soft tissue prolapse in orbital floor fracture); fluid level in maxillary sinus; visible fracture • CT (2 mm coronal slices): identify fractures (bony windows), prolapsed orbital fat/extraocular muscles and hemorrhage • Hess/Lees and fields of binocular vision tests show characteristic mechanical restrictive patterns and allow monitoring of recovery

Clinical features

Orbital floor (maxillary bone)

This is the most common orbital fracture. It usually follows a blow from an object >5 cm (e.g., tennis ball or fist). The force may be transmitted by hydraulic compression of globe or orbital structures ("blow-out") or be directly transmitted along the orbital rim.

• Soft tissue: periorbital bruising, edema, hemorrhage; surgical emphysema.
• Vertical diplopia due to mechanical restriction of upgaze. This may be secondary to tissue entrapment following prolapse through the bony defect (persistent) or soft tissue swelling tenting the extraocular muscle insertion (transient).
• Enophthalmos.
• Infraorbital anesthesia due to nerve damage in infraorbital canal.

Medial wall (ethmoidal)

Medial wall fractures are rare as an isolated feature but they may accompany orbital floor fractures.

• Soft tissue signs as for orbital floor fractures but surgical emphysema may be prominent.
• Horizontal diplopia due to mechanical restriction from medial rectus entrapment.

Orbital roof (frontal)

Orbital roof fractures are very rare as an isolated feature. They are most commonly seen in children following brow trauma.

- Soft tissue signs as for orbital floor fractures but bruising may spread across midline.
- Superior subconjunctival hemorrhage with no distinct posterior limit.
- Inferior or axial globe displacement.
- May have bruit, or pulsation due to communication with cerebrospinal fluid (CSF); carry risk of meningitis.

Lateral wall (zygomatic arch)

The lateral wall is very robust and acts as a protective shield to the globe. Lateral wall fractures are usually only seen following significant maxillo-facial trauma.

Orbital fractures: treatment

All orbital fractures

- Advise patients to refrain from nose blowing, which may contribute to surgical emphysema and herniation.
- Consider antibiotic prophylaxis: commonly anaerobic coverage is prescribed, but there is limited evidence for any benefit.
- Refer to orbital or maxillofacial team for consideration of surgical repair.
- Arrange orthoptic follow-up to monitor recovery and postoperative course.
- Consider oral prednisone to decrease lid and orbital edema.

Fractures of the orbital floor

Table 3.6 Indications for surgical intervention in orbital floor fractures

Immediate	• Persistent oculocardiac reflex
	• Young patient with white-eyed trap-door fracture (orbital floor buckling occurring in children)
	• Significant facial asymmetry
Early (<2 weeks)	• Persistent symptomatic diplopia
	• Significant enophthalmos
	• Hypoglobus
	• Progressive infraorbital hypoesthesia
Observation	• Minimal diplopia (e.g., just in upgaze)
	• Minimal restriction
	• Minimal enophthalmos

Box 3.2 Outline of repair for orbital floor fractures

- Use a subciliary or transconjunctival incision to expose the inferior orbital rim.
- Incise the periosteum 2 mm outside the orbital rim and dissect posteriorly, elevating the periorbita/periosteum off the orbital floor.
- Carefully release all herniated orbital contents, taking care to separate them from the infraorbital nerve and vessels.
- Continue until the whole fracture has been exposed.
- Repair bony defect with an implant (e.g., Teflon, Supramyd) with an overlap of ≥5 mm, which should be fixed in position.
- Close periosteum with absorbable suture (e.g., 4-0 Vicryl).
- Close subciliary/transconjunctival incision.

Lid lacerations

Lacerations involving the eyelid are common, occurring in the context of both blunt and sharp injuries. They carry morbidity in their own right and may be associated with significant injuries of the globe or orbit. Lid lacerations require careful exploration and precise closure, particularly at the lid margin.

Assessment

Table 3.7 Specific features in assessment of lid lacerations

History	Mechanism of injury (and likelihood of associated injuries), likely infective risk (e.g., bites)
Physical exam	Lid laceration (depth, length, tissue viability), lid position, orbicularis function, lagophthalmos, intercanthal distance
	Canalicular involvement, nasolacrimal drainage
	Watch for associated injury of globe or orbit
Imaging	Only indicated if associated globe or orbital injury suspected

Treatment

- *Prophylaxis:* Protect cornea with generous lubrication; administer tetanus vaccine if indicated (p. 82).
- *Surgery:* Assess for surgical repair according to depth, extent of tissue loss, involvement of lid margin, and involvement of canaliculus (see Table 3.8). Complicated lid lacerations should be repaired in the operating room by an experienced surgeon.

Table 3.8 Outline of repair for lid lacerations

Simple superficial, not involving margin	Close with interrupted 6-0 sutures parallel to lid margin; absorbable (e.g., Vicryl) are often preferred (especially for children), but nonabsorbable (e.g., silk) may be used
Partial thickness	Small defect restricted to anterior lamella: consider allowing repair by granulation
	Larger defect requires a reconstructive procedure
Full thickness with tissue loss	*Small defect* (0–25% tissue loss): debride/freshen up wound edges; close with interrupted absorbable (e.g., 6-0 Vicryl) sutures in one layer to tarsus and one layer to skin
	Large defect (25–60% tissue loss): consider lateral cathotomy/cantholysis, Tenzel myocutaneous flap, Mustarde lid-switch (2-stage)
	Very large defect (>60% tissue loss): consider Hughes tarsoconjunctival flap or Mustarde myocutaneous flap
Involving margin	Debride/freshen up wound edges
	Place gray-line suture (nonabsorbable or absorbable, e.g., 6-0 Vicryl), leave long
	Close tarsus with interrupted absorbable suture (e.g., 6-0 Vicryl)
	Place additional marginal suture (lash line) if required, leave long
	Close overlying skin with interrupted absorbable suture (e.g., 6-0 Vicryl); these sutures should also catch the long ends of the marginal sutures to prevent corneal abrasion.
Canalicular laceration	Intubate canalicular system, retrogradely entering the nasolacrimal duct from under the inferior turbinate
	Internally splint the opened duct with silicone tubing
	Close laceration with 6-0 Vicryl
	Leave silicon tubes in situ for 3 months
Postoperative	Topical antibiotic/lubrication for 1 week
	Remove skin sutures at 5–7 days

Blunt trauma: assessment

Traumatic eye injuries account for a significant number of emergency room visits and visual loss in young adults in the United States They are commonly associated with more extensive injuries: ocular involvement occurs in around 10% of all nonfatal casualties. Most ocular trauma is blunt (80%) rather than penetrating (20%), with intraocular foreign bodies (IOFBs) occurring in 1%.

Assessment

Table 3.9 Specific features in assessment of blunt injury

History	Mechanism, associated injuries, tetanus status
Physical exam	• Globe: look for anterior or posterior rupture • Cornea: check fluorescein staining, clarity • AC: check for cells or flare, and depth (compare with other eye) • Iris/ciliary body: note abnormalities of pupil and examine iris root and angle by gonioscopy (if stable) • Lens: opacity, position, stability • Vitreous: posterior vitreous detachment (PVD), hemorrhage • Fundus: note commotio retinae (usually temporal); check macular pathology (e.g., hole); examine equator/periphery for retinal tears/dialysis; consider choroidal rupture (often masked by blood) • Optic nerve: check function and disc appearance • IOP • Watch for "occult" posterior rupture; check for associated orbital or adnexal injuries
Imaging	Consider orbital/facial X-ray, B-scan US, CT orbits/brain (assess extent of damage, particularly when clinical assessment is limited)

Clinical features

Globe
• Anterior rupture is usually obvious with herniation of uveal tissue, lens and vitreous and other signs of injury (e.g., severe subconjunctival hemorrhage, hyphema, etc.).
• Posterior rupture: suspect this if there is deep AC and low IOP (compare with contralateral eye).

Anterior segment
• Corneal abrasion (epithelial defect; p. 99), corneal edema (transient endothelial decompensation, spontaneously resolves).
• Hyphema: red blood cells in the AC (p. 100).
• Iris: miosis (usually transient), mydriasis (often permanent), and sphincter rupture (irregular pupil; permanent); iris root abnormalities include iridodialysis (dehiscence from ciliary body) and angle recession (late risk of glaucoma; p. 316).
• Lens: Vossius ring (imprint of iris pigment on anterior capsule), cataract (anterior or posterior subcapsular); subluxation/luxation of the lens.

Posterior segment

- Vitreous: posterior vitreous detachment (PVD), vitreous hemorrhage.
- Commotio retinae: retinal edema; gray-white appearance ± intraretinal hemorrhage if severe. This usually completely resolves, but it may result in macular hole or pigmentary change.
- Retinal dialysis: full-thickness circumferential break at the ora serrata; commonly superonasal (when traumatic). It is not related to PVD and thus progression to any retinal detachment is slow (several months). Irregular retinal tear(s) may occur at the equator (p. 420).
- Macular holes: acute or late (p. 436).
- Choroidal rupture: rupture through choroid, Bruch's membrane, or retinal pigment epithelium (RPE) but sclera is intact; the rupture is usually concentric to the optic disc. It is usually obscured initially by overlying subretinal blood. Later a white streak of sclera may be visible. CNV is a late complication.
- Traumatic optic neuropathy: acutely ↓optic nerve function (including RAPD) in presence of normal disc and retina appearance; later, disc pallor.
- Optic nerve avulsion: ↓/absent optic nerve function depending on completeness of avulsion; defect in place of optic disc. Confirm by B-scan ultrasound if dense vitreous hemorrhage prevents clinical view.
- Retinitis sclopetaria: full-thickness rupture of the retina, RPE, Bruch's membrane, and choroid after high-velocity injuries (usually due to shock wave of high-velocity impact passing close to sclera).

Blunt trauma: treatment

Primary repair of globe rupture

- Admit patient and prepare for general anesthesia (GA): NPO, determine last meal/drink, coordinate with anesthesiologist, obtain electrocardiogram (ECG) and blood tests (if indicated).
- Prophylaxis: protect globe with clear plastic-shield systemic antibiotic (e.g., ciprofloxacin PO 750 mg bid) ± topical antibiotic; administer tetanus vaccine if indicated (p. 82).
- Surgery: assess and proceed with primary repair (see Table 3.12, p. 97).

Secondary repair

- Iris: most injuries involving the iris (other than herniation through a ruptured globe) do not require surgical intervention.
- Lens: significant lens injuries resulting in ↓VA (opacity, subluxation), ↑IOP (lens-related glaucoma; p. 314), or inflammation (breached capsule) warrant removal of the lens; some cases may require a vitreoretinal approach.
- Vitreoretinal: retinal tears or retinal dialysis require urgent referral for vitreoretinal assessment and repair; macular holes should also be referred but can generally be treated electively.

Other

- Commotio retinae: no treatment is usually indicated, since most cases spontaneously recover. Some have persistent or late ↓VA due to macular hole or pigmentary change.
- Choroidal rupture: no treatment is indicated; however if a CNV develops, this can be treated in the conventional manner.
- Traumatic optic neuropathy: coordinate care with a neuro-ophthalmologist. Megadose systemic corticosteroids are sometimes given, which, while of proven benefit in spinal injuries, are unproven in traumatic optic neuropathy.

Penetrating trauma/IOFBs: assessment

Small (<2 mm) foreign bodies may leave a sealed wound and minimal clinical signs. Penetrating trauma should be excluded following injury from sharp objects and projectiles with high mass and/or velocity. An intraocular foreign body (IOFB) must be excluded in all cases of penetration.

Double perforation (through-and-through injury) should be considered even if the IOFB is now within the globe. Posterior rupture following significant blunt trauma should always be considered.

Infective and toxic complications of IOFBs may have a more severe impact on visual outcome than the initial physical injury.

Assessment

Table 3.10 Specific features in assessment of penetrating injury and IOFBs

History	Source (hammer on steel, machinery, explosive), probable IOFB material, likely toxicity and infective risk, tetanus status
Ophthalmic examination	*Entry site:* identify location and integrity (leak) of wound
	Low or asymmetric IOP
	Trajectory: look for iris hole (transillumination), focal cataract and lens tract, retinal hemorrhage
	Location: include gonioscopy and dilated funduscopy
	Watch for occult IOFB in angle, ciliary body, pars plana
Investigation	Orbital X-ray (upgaze/downgaze), ultrasound, CT, ERG (chronic retained IOFB: flat *b*-wave)

Clinical features

Mechanical injury

- Globe: penetration, perforation or double perforation (through and through) of corneosclera and uvea.
- Anterior segment: angle recession (late risk of glaucoma; p. 317), iridodialysis, hyphema (p. 100); lens capsule injury, cataract formation, zonular dehiscence, subluxation.
- Posterior segment: vitreous liquefaction, vitreous hemorrhage, abnormal vitreoretinal traction, retinal hemorrhage, retinal tear, retinal detachment.

Introduction of infection

- Endophthalmitis, panophthalmitis.

Toxicity

- Siderosis, chalcosis (see Table 3.11).

Siderosis (ferrous foreign body)

Dissociated iron has a predilection for deposition in epithelial tissue (lens, RPE) causing metabolic toxicity and cellular death. RPE toxicity results in ↓VA, constricted visual field, and RAPD.

Clinical features include injection, heterochromia (iris reddish brown), ↑IOP (secondary glaucoma), anterior capsular cataract, reddish ferrous deposits at lens epithelium, coarse degenerative pigment dispersion, and retinal detachment.

VEP testing shows *b*-wave attenuation. ERG shows a flat *b*-wave.

Chalcosis (copper foreign body)

Pure copper IOFBs result in rapid fulminant endophtahlmitis. Chalcosis results from FB of alloys (brass, bronze) of copper and mirror the ocular signs of Wilson's disease: Kayser–Fleischer ring, anterior "sunflower" cataract, and yellow retinal plaques.

Table 3.11 Toxicity and intraocular foreign bodies

Inert ← - → Toxic			
Platinum	Aluminum	Iron	Copper
Silver	Zinc		Organic Material
Gold	Nickel		Soil
Lead	Mercury		
Glass			
Plastic			
Stone			
Carbon			

Penetrating trauma/IOFBs: treatment

With penetrating injuries, the urgent priority is to repair the integrity of the globe. If present, IOFBs are ideally removed at the time of primary repair. While additional procedures may be carried out at the time of primary repair (e.g., lensectomy, vitrectomy, retinal detachment repair), these are commonly deferred to a planned secondary rehabilitative procedure. Occasionally, iatrogenic penetrating injuries occur, e.g., in up to 1 in 1000 peribulbar injections.

General

- Admit and prepare patient for GA: NPO, determine last meal or drink, coordinate care with anesthesiologist, obtain ECG and/or blood tests (if indicated).
- Prophylaxis: protect globe with clear plastic-shield systemic antibiotic (e.g., ciprofloxacin PO 750 mg bid) ± topical antibiotic; administer tetanus vaccine if indicated (p. 82).
- Surgery: assess and proceed with primary repair, IOFB removal, and any additional procedures required (Table 3.12).

Primary repair

Table 3.12 Management of penetrating injuries

All wounds	• Debride contaminated nonviable tissue.
	• Carefully maintain the anterior chamber to avoid expulsion of ocular contents.
Small self-sealing corneal wound	• Shelved corneal laceration with formed anterior chamber may not require formal closure.
	• Observe until healed; consider bandage contact lens (BCL) and treat with adequate antibiotic coverage.
Corneal wound	• This may require anterior chamber deepening or stabilization with viscoelastic.
	• Return exposed viable iris tissue through perforation; excise exposed tissue if nonviable.
	• Directly close corneal wound with perpendicular deep 10-0 nylon sutures and rotate them to bury knots.
	• Remove viscoelastic.
Involving limbus	• Expose adjacent sclera to determine full posterior extent of wound.
	• Start closure at limbus and proceed posteriorly.
Scleral	• Conjunctival peritomy, expose and explore sclera
	• Return exposed viable uveal tissue through perforation.
	• Cut prolapsed vitreous flush to wound, taking care not to induce vitreous traction.
	• Direct scleral closure

IOFB removal

Table 3.13 IOFB removal

Anterior chamber IOFB	Corneal approach; removal with fine forceps
Angle IOFB	Scleral trap-door approach
Lenticular IOFB	If in clear lens matter, consider leaving in situ or remove with lens at time of cautious cataract surgery (potential capsular and zonular instability)
Ciliary body IOFB	Cannot be directly visualized, so consider using an electroacoustic locator and electromagnetic removal through scleral trap-door approach
Posterior segment IOFB	Plan secondary vitrectomy after formation of PVD (7–10 days) unless significant toxic or infection risk.
	Use an intraocular magnet or vitrectomy IOFB forceps.
	Reserve direct trans-scleral delivery for those IOFBs that are easily accessible.

Secondary procedures

Planned secondary repair of posterior segment trauma is usually performed 4–10 days after the initial injury after formation of PVD. Secondary repair may be performed earlier in the presence of an IOFB (not removed at the primary repair), retinal detachment or endophthalmitis.

Secondary repair may include vitrectomy, membrane dissection (if PVR), encircling buckle (if breaks), lensectomy (if cataract; IOL commonly deferred), intravitreal antibiotics (if endophthalmitis), and tamponade (usually C3F8 or silicone oil).

Sympathetic ophthalmia

Sympathetic ophthalmia is a rare bilateral granulomatous panuveitis in which trauma to one eye may cause sight-threatening inflammation in the untraumatized "sympathizing" eye. Its nature, clinical features, prophylaxis, and treatment are discussed in the uveitis section (p. 378).

Corneal foreign bodies and abrasions

Corneal foreign bodies

Most corneal foreign bodies (FBs) are metallic. They are effectively sterilized by air friction during projection to the eye. Microbial keratitis more commonly follows stone, ceramic, and organic FBs. Remember to exclude a second intraocular or subtarsal FB.

Clinical features

- Photophobia, pain, injection, lacrimation, blurred vision; history of projectile striking eye; failure to wear protective eyewear while working, welding, hammering.
- Metallic FB associated rust ring (forms within 48 hours) or infiltrate; ± anterior uveitis.

Treatment

For removal, explain to the patient what you are about to do and give him/her a target to stare at. Instill topical anesthetic (e.g., proparacine 1%) and remove FB and rust ring under slit-lamp visualization (e.g., with 26 gauge needle).

Give topical antibiotic (e.g., ofloxacin 0.3% 4x/day for 5 days) and consider short-term cycloplegic (for comfort/AC activity) and nonsteroidal anti-inflammatory (NSAID) preparations.

Warn the patient that the eye will feel uncomfortable once the anesthetic has worn off.

Corneal abrasions

Corneal abrasions are superficial corneal wounds. Corneal abrasions are common and often innocuous, but they may cause severe pain and distress. Epithelial denuding exposes the stromal receptors, triggering pain, photophobia, and lacrimation and increasing the risk of bacterial invasion.

Clinical features

- *Superficial/partial-thickness corneal laceration:* Differentiate from deeper partial- or full-thickness lacerations through careful oblique illumination of the wound tract and the Seidel's test (identifies leaking full-thickness wounds). Note depth and dimensions.
- *Complications* include microbial keratitis (p. 186) and recurrent erosions (especially if abrasion is large, ragged, involving the basement membrane, and in a predisposed patient) (p. 201).

Treatment

Give topical antibiotic (e.g., ofloxacin 0.3% 4x/day for 3 days); if there is associated infiltration, treat as a microbial keratitis. Debride any rough devitalized (gray) tissue that may hamper re-epithelialization from ingrowth of neighboring epithelium.

For supportive treatment consider short-term topical cycloplegic (for comfort/AC activity) and topical NSAIDs. Patching is not advisable for most abrasions since it has been shown to delay closure for abrasions <10 mm. However, patching may help make larger abrasions feel more comfortable.

Hyphema

Blood in the anterior chamber is most commonly seen in the context of blunt trauma. It ranges from a relatively mild microhyphema (erythrocytes suspended in the aqueous) to a total "8-ball" hyphema where the anterior chamber fill is complete.

Table 3.14 Specific features in assessment of hyphema

History	Mechanism of injury (potential for IOFB, globe rupture), ↓VA (stable, worsening may suggest rebleed), sickle cell status, risk factors, drug history (e.g., aspirin, NSAIDs, warfarin, etc.)
Physical exam	Measure and record depth and distribution of hyphema, IOP, iris trauma or abnormality (defer gonioscopy where possible).
	Dilated funduscopy: rule out any posterior segment injury.
Imaging	Sickle cell status
	Consider B-scan US and CT to rule out additional globe or orbital injuries (particularly if adequate clinical assessment is not possible).

Causes
- Trauma: blunt or penetrating.
- Surgery: e.g., trabeculectomy, iris manipulation procedures.
- Spontaneous: iris/angle neovascularization, hematological disease, tumor (e.g., juvenile xanthogranuloma), IOL erosion of iris, herpetic anterior uveitis.

Clinical features
- Erythrocytes in the anterior chamber: in minor bleeds, most erythrocytes fail to settle and are only visible with the slit lamp (microhyphema); larger bleeds result in a macroscopically visible layer (hyphema).
- Complications: rebleeds, corneal staining (especially if ↑IOP), red cell glaucoma.

Treatment
- Admit high-risk cases (Box 3.3).
- Strict bed rest and globe protection (e.g., shield, glasses).
- Avoid aspirin and antiplatelet agents, NSAIDs, and warfarin if possible (communicate with prescribing physician).
- Give topical steroid (e.g., dexamethasone 0.1% or prednisolone acetate 1% 4×/day) and consider cycloplegia (e.g., atropine 1% 2×/day, but is controversial).

Monitoring and follow-up
- Daily review (inpatient or outpatient) for IOP check and to rule out rebleeds while hyphema is resolving. As condition improves, the patient can be discharged (if hospitalized) and follow-up extended.

- From 2 weeks the patient can usually return to normal levels of activity and gonioscopy ± indented indirect ophthalmoscopy can be performed.
- Annual IOP checks (risk of angle recession glaucoma).

Red cell glaucoma

Hyphema (usually traumatic) leads to blockage of the trabecular meshwork by red blood cells. In 10% cases a rebleed may occur, usually at around 5 days. Patients with sickle cell disease/trait do worse and are harder to treat (e.g., sickling may be worsened by the acidosis from carbonic anhydrase inhibitors).

Treatment

- Of hyphema: as above.
- Of IOP: topical (e.g., β-blocker, α_2-agonist, carbonic anhydrase inhibitor) or systemic (e.g., acetazolamide) agents as required but avoid topical and systemic carbonic anyhdrase inhibitors in sickle cell disease/trait.

If medical treatment fails, consider AC paracentesis ± AC washout.

Box 3.3 High-risk features in hyphema

- Children and others with increased risk of noncompliance
- Rebleed
- Large hyphema (>1/3)
- Sickle cell disease/trait
- On antiplatelets (e.g., aspirin) or anticoagulants (e.g., warfarin)
- Significant associated injury

Lids

Anatomy and physiology (1)

The eyelids are vital to the maintenance of ocular surface integrity. Their functions include a mechanical barrier to a variety of insults, a sweeping mechanism to remove debris from the cornea (e.g., blink reflex), and a vital contribution to the production and drainage of the tear film. They also contribute to facial expression, and even minor aberrations or asymmetry may affect cosmesis.

General

At their simplest, the lids comprise a layered structure of skin, orbicularis oculi, tarsal plates/septum, and conjunctiva (Fig. 4.1). The orbital portion is more complex with preaponeurotic fat and retractors lying deep to the septum. The interpalpebral fissure is usually 30 mm wide and 10 mm high (slightly higher in females).

The resting position of the upper lid is 2 mm below the superior limbus (higher in children); for the lower lid, the resting position is level with or just above the inferior limbus.

Skin and eyelashes

The skin of eyelids is very thin and has loose connective tissue but no subcutaneous fat. It contains eccrine sweat glands and sebaceous glands.

The lashes are arranged in 2–3 rows along the lid margins and number approximately 150 on the upper and 75 on the lower lid. They are replaced every 4–6 months but can grow back faster if cut.

The lash follicles have apocrine sweat glands (of Moll) and modified sebaceous glands (of Zeis).

Orbicularis oculi

This sheet of striated muscle is divided into orbital and palpebral portions; the latter is further subdivided into preseptal and pretarsal parts. Innervation is by temporal and zygomatic branches of facial nerve (CN VII) for the orbicularis overlying the upper lid, and by the zygomatic branch alone for the lower lid.

The *orbital* portion forms a ring of muscle arising from the medial canthal tendon and parts of the orbital rim.

The *preseptal* part of each lid runs from the medial canthal tendon, arches over the anterior surface of the orbital septum, and inserts into the lateral horizontal raphe. Similarly, each *pretarsal* part arises from the medial canthal tendon, arches over the tarsal plates, and inserts into the lateral canthal tendon and horizontal raphe.

Horner's muscle is formed by deep pretarsal fibers running medially to insert onto the lacrimal crest. Functions of the orbicularis oculi include lid closure and the lacrimal pump mechanism.

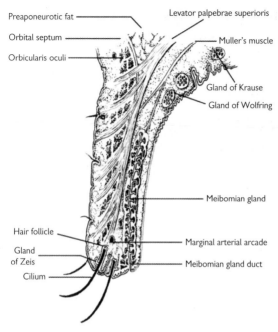

Figure 4.1 Anatomical section of the lid.

Anatomy and physiology (2)

Orbital septum and tarsal plates

The *septum* is a sheet of tissue that arises from the orbital rim at the arcus marginalis, where it is continuous with orbital fascia and periosteum. Toward the palpebral margin, it is thickened, forming the tarsal plates, which maintain the shape of the lid. These are 25 mm long, 1 mm thick, and of variable height: around 10 mm high for the upper lid, 5 mm for the lower lid in Caucasians; these measurements are lower in Asians. They also contain the meibomian glands (numbering around 35 in the upper lid, 25 in the lower lid), which secrete the lipid component of the tear film.

Canthal tendons

At each end, the tarsal plates are stabilized by a horizontal canthal tendon. The medial canthal tendon is well developed with an anterior limb arising from the anterior lacrimal crest, and a posterior limb from the posterior lacrimal crest; the two limbs envelope the lacrimal sac.

The lateral canthal tendon lies just posterior to the horizontal raphe and inserts into the zygomatic bone (Whitnall's tubercle) and merges posteriorly with the lateral check ligament (from the sheath of lateral rectus).

Fat pads

The preaponeurotic fat pads are extensions of orbital fat lying just posterior to the orbital septum. In the upper eyelid, there are two fat pads, the central or preaponeurotic fat pad and the medial fat pad, whereas in the lower eyelid, there are three fat pads—the medial, central, and lateral fat pads.

Lid retractors

The upper lid retractors comprise levator palpebrae superioris (LPS) and Muller's muscle. LPS originates from the orbital apex and runs forward over superior rectus to the orbital rim. At this point, it is stabilized by the superior transverse ligament of Whitnall (a fascial bridge running between the trochlea and the lacrimal gland fascia) permitting the distal LPS to run steeply downward and insert as an aponeurosis into septum, tarsus, and orbicularis. Innervation is via oculomotor nerve (CN III).

Muller's muscle is an accessory retractor muscle supplied by the sympathetic system. Overaction is demonstrated in sympathetic overdrive and thyroid eye disease; underaction is seen in Horner's syndrome.

The lower lid retractors are more rudimentary but are similarly divided into voluntary and sympathetic groups.

Conjunctiva (p. 154)

The *conjunctiva* is a mucous membrane comprising nonkeratinized epithelium, basement membrane, and stroma. The epithelium of the palpebral conjunctiva is of stratified squamous form. It contains mucin-secreting goblet cells and crypts of Henle.

Nerves, arteries, veins, lymphatics

Nerves

Sensation to the lower lid is mainly via infraorbital nerve (CN V_2), with the infratrochlear branch of nasociliary nerve (CN V_1) innervating the medial canthal area. Sensation to the upper lid is via lacrimal, supraorbital, and supratrochlear nerve (CN V_1). Orbicularis oculi is innervated by CN VII, LPS by CN III, and Muller's muscle by the sympathetic system.

Arteries

Arterial supply is provided by three arcades that form anastamoses between the medial palpebral artery (from the terminal ophthalmic artery) and the lateral palpebral artery (from the lacrimal artery). In the upper lid there is a marginal arcade 2 mm above the margin and a peripheral arcade at the top of the tarsal plate. In the lower lid, the arcade lies 4 mm below the margin.

Veins

Venous drainage is to superficial temporal vein laterally and to the ophthalmic and angular veins medially.

Lymphatics

Lymphatic drainage is to the parotid glands laterally, the submandibular glands inferiorly, and the anterior cervical chain inferomedially.

Eyelash disorders

Misdirected lashes

Misdirection of the eyelashes is a common source of ocular irritation. Corneal changes range from mild punctate epitheliopathy to ulceration, secondary infection, and scarring.

Treatment options include epilation, electrolysis, cryotherapy (double freeze-thaw technique), photoablation, and surgery. In pseudotrichiasis, surgical correction of the entropion or epiblepharon is curative. In other forms of misdirection, surgical excision is usually reserved for resistant cases.

Trichiasis

Lashes arise from their normal position but are posteriorly directed.

Distichiasis

Lashes arise from an abnormal position (e.g., from or slightly posterior to the meibomian glands). It is an uncommon congenital abnormality that may be sporadic or autosomal dominant.

Metaplastic lashes

Lashes arise from an abnormal position secondary to chronic injury, e.g., cicatrizing conjunctivitis (p. 168).

Pseudotrichiasis

Lashes arise from normal position but are posteriorly directed because of lid entropion or epiblepharon.

Lash infestations

Infestation of the lashes by lice causes itching, blepharitis, and a follicular conjunctivitis. The lice and nits (eggs) are easily identified on slit-lamp examination.

Treatment options include mechanical removal or destruction (e.g., cryotherapy) for localized cases and chemical treatment for generalized cases. Chemical options (e.g., malathion or permethrin) require a 12-hour application to the whole body repeated 7 days later; aqueous malathion is effective in treating lash phthiarisis (unlicensed use), but ocular contact is contraindicated with all these agents. Generalized infestation also requires laundry of all clothes and linen to >50°C.

Phthiriasis

This is infestation by *Phthirus pubis* (crab louse) and is most commonly seen in adults. It is usually acquired as a sexually transmitted infection.

Pediculosis

This is infestation by *Pediculus humanus corporis*, or *capitis* (head louse). If the patient is heavily infested, the lice may spread to involve the lashes.

Madarosis

This is partial or complete loss of lashes. It may be a purely local phenomenon, or associated with systemic disease (Table 4.1).

Lash poliosis

This is whitening of the lashes. It may be associated with premature graying of the hair, a purely local phenomenon, or systemic pathology (Table 4.2).

Table 4.1 Causes of madarosis

Local	Cicatrizing conjunctivitis (p. 168)
	Iatrogenic (cryotherapy, radiotherapy, surgery)
Systemic	Alopecia (patchy, totalis, universalis)
	Psoriasis
	Hypothyroidism
	Leprosy

Table 4.2 Causes of poliosis

Local	Chronic lid margin disease
Systemic	Sympathetic ophthalmia
	Vogt–Koyanagi–Harada syndrome
	Waardenburg syndrome

Blepharitis

In general ophthalmology, the term *blepharitis* is often used as shorthand for chronic lid margin disease. However, blepharitis refers to any inflammation of the lid and thus includes a wide range of disease, such as preseptal cellulitis, internal and external hordeola, and herpes simplex (HSV) and varicella zoster virus (VZV) infections.

The diagnosis of blepharitis therefore lacks precision but is often used given the considerable overlap between the main causes of chronic lid margin inflammation, discussed below. The descriptive terms *anterior* and *posterior* blepharitis are sometimes used to indicate the distribution of disease.

Unilateral blepharitis (and recurrent chalazia) in an elderly patient should be treated with extreme suspicion since lid tumors (e.g., sebaceous cell carcinoma) may present in this way.

Bacterial blepharitis

This results in a mainly anterior blepharitis. It is usually due to lid commensals, most commonly staphylococci, but may also arise from streptococci, *Propionibacterium acnes*, and *Moraxella*.

Clinical features
- Burning, gritty, crusted.
- Injected lid margins, scales at lash bases, external hordeolum (abscess of lash follicle and associated glands), preseptal cellulitis.

Treatment
- Lid hygiene: regular lid-margin cleaning (e.g., by cotton tip applicator dipped in dilute baby shampoo).
- Ocular lubricants: tear film instability is common.
- Antibiotics: topical antibiotics may be required for acute exacerbations; external hordeola and preseptal cellulitis also require oral antibiotics.
- Topical steroids (weak) may be required in severe cases with corneal involvement.
- Oral doxycycline is given for severe recalcitrant disease.

Meibomianitis

This is a mainly posterior blepharitis arising from inflammation of the meibomian glands. It is often associated with facial rosacea.

Clinical features
- Burning, worse in mornings.
- Inflamed meibomian gland openings, thickened secretions, glands may become obstructed ± chalazia (lipogranulomatous inflammation within meibomian gland) ± internal hordeolum (acute abscess formation within meibomian gland).

Treatment
Give oral tetracyclines (contraindicated in children under age 12, in breast-feeding or pregnant women, or in those with hepatic or renal impairment).

Consider lid hygiene and topical therapies as for bacterial blepharitis.

Seborrheic blepharitis

This results in a mixed anterior–posterior blepharitis arising from excessive meibomian secretions. It is commonly associated with seborrheic dermatitis of the scalp.

Clinical features
- Burning, gritty, crusted.
- Lashes stuck together by soft scales, oily lid margin, foamy tear film.

Treatment
Treatment is as for meibomianitis, with tetracyclines, lid hygiene, and topical therapies as needed.

Lid lumps: cysts, abscesses, and others

Anterior lamella

External hordeolum (stye)

This is an acute abscess within a lash follicle and its associated glands of Zeis and Moll. It results in a tender lump with associated inflammation. It is usually Staphylococcal in origin.

Treatment is with warm compresses; if associated with preseptal cellulitis, consider appropriate oral antibiotics.

Cyst of Moll

These chronic cysts (or apocrine hidrocystomas) are markedly translucent and arise from blockage of the apocrine duct of the gland of Moll. They may be incised under local anesthesia. Similar lesions may arise from blockage of the eccrine ducts of sweat glands of the eyelid skin.

Cyst of Zeis

These chronic cysts are poorly translucent and arise from blockage of the gland of Zeis. Similar sebaceous cysts may arise in the periorbital skin but rarely from the lids.

Xanthelasma

These common lesions result from the deposition of lipids within perivascular xanthoid cells and may be a sign of hyperlipidemia. Clinically, they appear as yellowish subcutaneous deposits located on the medial aspect of the lids and periorbit.

Molluscum contagiosum

These pearly, umbilicated nodules are common in children and young adults. They are caused by a dsDNA virus of the pox virus group; profuse lesions are seen with HIV infection. Transmission is by close contact. If at the lid margin, they may cause a persistent follicular conjunctivitis (p. 162).

Treatment: if troublesome, the lesions may be removed by cryotherapy, cauterization, shave excision or expression.

Posterior lamella

Internal hordeolum

This is an acute abscess within a meibomian gland. It results in a tender lump with associated inflammation. It is usually staphylococcal in origin.

Treatment for acute cases is with warm compresses; for acute with preseptal cellulitis, add in oral antibiotics (p. 472). For chronic cases (or large acute lesion) also perform incision and curettage.

Chalazion

This is the most common of all lid lumps. They arise from chronic lipogranulomatous inflammation of blocked meibomian glands. They are usually located on the upper lid and are more common in patients with chronic marginal blepharitis, rosacea, or seborrhoeic dermatitis.

Treatment: small chalazia are often ignored by the patient and resolve with time. Persistent or symptomatic lesions may be treated surgically by incision and curettage. Steroid injection of triamcinolone into the lesion is often effective. Any recurrence of the lesion should be regarded as suspicious and a biopsy sent for histology.

Box 4.1 Outline of incision and curettage of a chalazion

- Consent: discuss what the procedure involves, the likelihood of further chalazia recurrence, and risks, including bruising, bleeding, and infection.
- Identify location of chalazion (it will be less obvious after instillation of anesthetic).
- Instill topical anesthesia in the fornix of the affected eye.
- Prep surgical area with 5% povidone iodine.
- Inject local anesthetic (e.g., 1–2% lidocaine with epinephrine 1 in 200,000) subcutaneously to the affected lid.
- Evert lid with guarded lid clamp.
- Incise chalazion vertically with surgical blade (e.g., No. 11) from the conjunctival surface.
- Curette to remove the chalazion contents and to break down any loculations.
- Instill topical antibiotic.
- Remove clamp and apply pressure to ensure hemostasis.
- Apply eye patch; this can be removed prior to leaving the department.
- Post-procedure: apply topical antibiotic. If atypical or recurrent chalazion, curettings or biopsy should be sent for histology.

Lid lumps: benign and premalignant tumors

Benign tumors

Anterior lamella

Papillomas

Skin papillomas are very common. They are derived from squamous cells. They may be nonspecific or related to human papilloma virus (viral wart or verruca vulgaris). They are either broad-based (sessile) or narrow-based (pedunculated) protrusions with irregular surfaces formed from finger-like extensions.

Seborrheic keratosis (basal cell papilloma)

These are common, especially in the elderly. They are derived from basal cells. They are broad-based protrusions, usually brown in color, with a greasy irregular surface.

Keratoacanthoma

These are uncommon tumors that grow rapidly for 2–6 weeks and then spontaneously involute over a few months. They are nonpigmented protrusions with a keratin-filled central crater. Some cases cannot be distinguished clinically from a squamous cell carcinoma (SCC). In these cases, complete excision is necessary, since an incomplete specimen may again be indistinguishable from an SCC on histological examination.

Nevi

These are common cutaneous lesions that are classified according to depth. They arise from arrested epidermal melanocytes.

Junctional nevi are flat, brown, and located at the epidermis–dermis junction. Dermal nevi are elevated, may not be visibly pigmented, and are located within the dermis. Compound nevi are slightly elevated and share features of junctional and dermal types.

Overall, there is a low risk of transformation, which is slightly higher for the more superficial nevi.

Vascular

Congenital vascular anomalies such as capillary hemangioma (strawberry nevi) and port wine stain may involve the lids.

Posterior lamella

Pyogenic granuloma

This is an abnormal response to injury, such as trauma or, less commonly, inflammation. It is a red, highly vascular mass that appears to be a hemangioma with associated granulation tissue.

Premalignant tumors

Actinic keratosis

This common lesion of sun-exposed skin is relatively uncommon on the lids. Clinically, it is a flat, scaly lesion with hyperkeratosis and may have a keratin horn. Histologically, it shows parakeratosis and cellular atypia but no invasion.

Lid lumps: malignant tumors

Basal cell carcinoma (BCC)

This is the most common lid malignancy (90% of lid malignancies in Caucasians). It preferentially affects the lower lid, followed by medial canthus, upper lid, and then lateral canthus.

Risk factors include increasing age, white skin, sun exposure, and some cutaneous syndromes (xeroderma pigmentosa, basal cell nevus syndrome). It is locally invasive but very rarely metastasizes.

Clinical features

- *Nodular type:* firm nodule, rolled pearly edges, fine telangiectasia, surface ulceration.
- *Morpheaform (sclerosing) type:* often minimal surface changes overlying extensive infiltration, so may mimic chronic inflammation or scarring (e.g., chronic marginal blepharitis).

Treatment

Wide local excision may be achieved with Mohs micrographic technique (especially for morpheaform type) or excisional biopsy, ideally with frozen-section control. A 3–4 mm margin is recommended.

Squamous cell carcinoma (SCC)

This is much less common (2–5% of lid malignancies in Caucasians, but most common in Asians) but has a much higher risk of malignant spread. It preferentially affects the lower lid. Risk factors include increasing age, white skin, sun exposure, and xeroderma pigmentosa.

Clinical features

- *Nodular type:* hyperkeratotic, with irregular margins; resembles BCC.
- *Plaque type:* erythematous, scaly, hyperkeratotic plaque.

Both types may ulcerate, show lymphatic and perineural spread, and metastasize.

Treatment

Wide local excision may be achieved with Mohs micrographic technique or excisional biopsy, ideally with frozen-section control. This is usually curative for early lesions. Orbital involvement may require exenteration.

Sebaceous gland carcinoma

This uncommon tumor (1–2% of lid malignancies in Caucasians, second most common tumor in Asians) usually arises from the meibomian glands or, occasionally, the glands of Zeis. It is aggressive and carries a significant mortality rate (10% overall mortality rate, but up to 67% 5-year mortality rate if it metastases). It is more common in the upper lid.

Risk factors include increasing age and female sex.

Clinical features

- *Nodular type:* firm nodule resembling chalazion (so biopsy recurrent chalazion).
- *Spreading type:* diffuse infiltration may involve the conjunctiva and resemble chronic blepharoconjunctivitis.

Treatment

Confirm diagnosis with full-thickness lid biopsy (alert histopathologist and send fresh tissue to assist with fat staining). Map biopsies of the conjunctival surface help determine the extent of tumor, including possible skip lesions. Wide local excision is essential but may be difficult to achieve because of pagetoid and multicentric spread.

Cryotherapy of the surgical conjunctival margins is helpful to limit local recurrence. Diffuse local disease can respond to topical mitomycin C chemotherapy. Regional lymph node clearance and exenteration may be performed depending on tumor extent.

Malignant melanoma

Melanoma only rarely affects the lids (<1% lid malignancies in Caucasians). However, it must be considered when assessing pigmented lesions, since it can be fatal.

Risk factors include increasing age, white skin, sun exposure and sunburn, and some cutaneous syndromes (dysplastic nevus syndrome, xeroderma pigmentosa). It has a noninvasive horizontal growth phase followed by an invasive vertical growth phase.

Clinical features

- *Lentigo maligna type:* initially flat pigmented lesion with well-defined margins (lentigo maligna), but that starts to show elevation as it invades dermis (malignant transformation).
- *Superficial spreading type:* smaller pigmented lesion with irregular margins and mild elevation, ± nodules, induration; more aggressive.
- *Nodular type:* nodule (may not be visibly pigmented) with rapid growth, ulceration and bleeding.

Treatment

Wide local excision with 10 mm margins (confirmed on histology) is recommended but not always possible. Some clinicians recommend regional lymph node dissection for tumors >1.5 mm thick or with evidence of hematogenous or lymphatic spread.

Prognosis

Poor prognosis correlates with histological depth of invasion (by Clark's levels) and thickness (by the Breslow system). Thus, the 5-year survival rate post-excision is 100% for tumors ≤0.75 mm thick but only 50% for those >1.5 mm thick.

Kaposi's sarcoma

This is a rare tumor arising from human herpes virus 8 (HHV8) in the general population but is relatively common in HIV patients with AIDS. Clinically, it is a vascular purple-red nodule that may also affect the conjunctiva. Treatment for symptomatic lesions is usually radiotherapy; it is not curative.

Merkel cell carcinoma

This is a very rare tumor that is more common in the elderly. It shows rapid growth and is highly malignant. Clinically, it is a nontender purple nodule, usually on the upper lid.

Ectropion

Ectropion is abnormal eversion of the eyelid (usually the lower) away from the globe. This disruption frequently causes irritation and may threaten the integrity of the ocular surface. It may occasionally be congenital but is usually acquired as a result of involutional, cicatricial, mechanical, or paralytic processes.

Involutional ectropion

This is the most common form and results from age-related tissue laxity.

Clinical features (nonspecific)

The following features are present in most ectropia:

• Variable irritation, epiphora, recurrent infections
• Everted lid (varies from slightly everted punctum to eversion of the whole lid), conjunctival irritation (± keratization)

Clinical features (specific)

Test for lid laxity (pull away from globe; >10 mm is abnormal), medial canthal tendon laxity (pull lid laterally; >2 mm movement of punctum is abnormal), lateral canthal tendon laxity (pull lid medially; >2 mm movement of canthal angle is abnormal; lateral canthus also has rounded appearance), and inferior retractor weakness.

Treatment

Surgery is directed toward the specific defect. Most commonly, this requires lid shortening for horizontal laxity, but the procedure of choice will depend on the relative contribution of the lid, tendons, canthal position, etc. (Table 4.3).

Cicatricial ectropion

This is uncommon. It occurs when scarring vertically shortens the anterior lamella. Causes include trauma, burns, radiotherapy, and dermatitis.

Clinical features (specific)

• Scarring, no skin laxity, tension lines in skin when lid put into position; features of underlying disease.

Treatment

Medical: the cicatrizing process should be controlled as best possible
Surgical: skin-gaining procedures (Table 4.3)

Mechanical ectropion

This is uncommon. It occurs when masses (e.g., tumors) displace the lid away from the globe.

Clinical features (specific)

• Visible/palpable mass, e.g., tumor, cyst, edema.

Treatment

Removal of the cause may lead to complete resolution; if there is residual lid laxity, treat as for involutional ectropion (Table 4.3).

Paralytic ectropion
This is uncommon. It occurs when CN VII palsy causes orbicularis weakness.

Clinical features (specific)
There is weakness of the orbicularis and other facial muscles, as well as lagophthalmos; corneal exposure is likely. Corneal sensation may be compromised by underlying disease. These patients must be taught that their only warning of exposure-related problems might be redness of the eye or ↓VA.

Treatment
Surgical treatment depends on the severity and associated laxity. Options include medial canthoplasty, lateral tarsorrhaphy, lid-shortening procedures, and botulinum toxin to the upper lid.

Congenital ectropion
This condition is rare, but may be seen in Down syndrome and blepharophimosis syndrome. It may occur in both lower and upper lids and is due to a shortage of skin.

Table 4.3 Overview of common ectropion surgical procedures

Operation	Indication	Procedure
Horizontal lid shortening		
Wedge excision	Lid laxity, no tendon laxity	Full-thickness pentagon excised
Kuhnt–Symanowski	As above + excess skin	Wedge excision + lower lid blepharoplasty
Lateral tarsal strip	Lateral/generalized laxity	Lid shortened laterally and tightened ± elevated at lateral canthus
Medial canthal resection	Medial laxity only	Lid shortened laterally and tightened at medial canthus
Vertical lid shortening		
Diamond excision	Mild medial ectropiont	Diamond of tarsoconjunctiva excised just inferior to punctum
Combined shortening procedures		
Lazy-T procedure	Medial ectropion with lid laxity	Diamond excision + wedge excision
Skin-gaining procedures		
Z-plasty	Focal scars	Z-incision with middle stroke excising scar gains vertical height
Skin flap/graft	Congenital/cicatricial skin loss	Transposition flap with pedicle or distant graft
Horizontal fissure shortening		
Lateral tarsorrhaphy	Cornea threatened by lagophthalmos	Fuses the lids at lateral aspect

Entropion

Entropion is abnormal inversion of the eyelid (usually the lower) toward the globe. Abrasion of the cornea by the inwardly directed lashes can result in ulceration and secondary infection. It may occasionally be congenital, but is usually acquired as a result of involutional or cicatricial processes.

Involutional entropion

This is the most common form and results from inferior retractor dysfunction tissue laxity and possibly override of preseptal orbicularis over pretarsal orbicularis.

Clinical features (nonspecific)

The following features are present in most entropion:
- FB sensation, photophobia, blepharospasm, epiphora.
- Inverted lid (transient/permanent), pseudotrichiasis, keratopathy, pannus formation.

Clinical features (specific)

Test for inferior retractor weakness or dehiscence (reduced movement of lower lid in downgaze), lid laxity (pull away from globe; >10 mm is abnormal), medial canthal tendon laxity (pull lid laterally; >2 mm movement of punctum is abnormal), and lateral canthal tendon laxity (pull lid medially; >2 mm movement of canthal angle is abnormal; lateral canthus also has rounded appearance).

Treatment

Surgery is directed toward the specific defect. Most commonly, this requires reattachment of the retractors and lid shortening for horizontal laxity (Table 4.4).

Cicatricial entropion

This condition is uncommon. It occurs when scarring vertically shortens the posterior lamella. It is caused by cicatrizing conjunctivitis, most commonly due to trachoma, ocular cicatricial pemphigoid and other bullous diseases, chemical injuries, radiotherapy, and trauma (p. 168).

Clinical features (specific)

- *Chronic:* loss of plica semilunaris, loss of forniceal depth, formation of symblepharon/ankyloblepharon, dry-eye signs.
- *Acute:* papillary conjunctivitis, subconjunctival vesicles, evolving picture.

Treatment

- *Medical:* the cicatrizing process should be optimally controlled, especially before surgical intervention (p. 168).
- *Surgical:* retractor reattachment may suffice in mild cases. Transverse tarsotomy (tarsal fracture) or mucosal graft is needed if there is moderate or severe loss of posterior lamella (Table 4.4).

Congenital entropion

This condition is very rare and often resolves with time, without the need for intervention. Pretarsal orbicularis is hypertrophied, forming a marked ridge. The lashes do not usually damage the cornea, but recurrent infections are common.

Upper lid entropion

This is most commonly seen in cicatricial disease, notably trachoma. As with lower lid entropion, it may threaten corneal integrity. Treatment depends on the underlying disease and severity of entropion.

Table 4.4 Overview of common entropion surgical procedures

Operation	Indication	Procedure
Retractor reattachment		
Jones plication (modified)	Retractor dehiscence	Reattachment/tightening of the retractors via subciliary incision
Horizontal lid shortening		
Wedge excision	Lid laxity, no tendon laxity	Full-thickness pentagon excised
Kuhnt–Symanowski	As above + excess skin	Wedge excision + lower lid blepharoplasty
Lateral tarsal strip	Lateral/ generalized laxity	Lid shortened laterally and tightened ± elevated at lateral canthus
Medial canthal resection	Medial laxity only	Lid shortened laterally and tightened at medial canthus
Posterior lamella reconstruction		
Transverse tarsotomy	Moderate loss of posterior lamella	Tarsal fracture and eversion of distal tarsus
Hard palate mucosal graft	Severe loss of posterior lamella	As above + limited separation of lamellae + graft to posterior lamella
Limitation of orbicularis override		
Wies procedure	Orbicularis override	Everting sutures and full-thickness lid split
Quickert procedure	As above + lid laxity	As above + wedge excision to shorten lid

Ptosis: acquired

Ptosis is an abnormal low position of the upper lid. Normal lid position and thus lid measurements vary slightly according to age, gender, and ethnicity. The average values are presented in Table 4.5.

An appearance of ptosis may be simulated by a number of conditions (pseudoptosis). True ptosis may be congenital (either isolated or syndromic) but is most commonly acquired as an involutional degeneration. However, ptosis may also be the presenting feature of a number of serious conditions.

Involutional ptosis

This very common condition arises from disinsertion of the levator palpebrae superioris (LPS). It increases with age and is more common after ophthalmic surgery (occurs in 6% post cataract extraction), trauma, or chronic contact lens use.

Clinical features

These include uni- or bilateral ptosis, high upper lid crease, compensatory brow lift, normal levator function, and deep upper sulcus.

Treatment

Surgery involves anterior levator advancement (Box 4.2).

Neurogenic ptosis

Third nerve palsy

Ptosis may arise as part of a third-nerve palsy, a potential ophthalmic emergency (p. 547). It is classically a complete ptosis due to loss of levator function, usually associated with ocular motility abnormalities and sometimes with mydriasis. Aberrant regeneration is common in chronic compressive lesions.

Surgery (frontalis suspension) is delayed for at least 6 months (spontaneous improvement is common) and until any motility disturbance has been successfully corrected.

Horner's syndrome

This syndrome causes a partial ptosis with preservation of levator function (p. 554). It may be associated with ipsilateral miosis, lower lid elevation, and, in some cases, anhydrosis.

Surgery for persistent and significant ptosis is by Fasanella–Servat procedure (posterior mullerectomy) or anterior levator resection.

Table 4.5 Normal lid measurements

Palpebral aperture	8–11 mm (female > male)
Upper margin reflex distance	4–5 mm
Upper lid excursion (levator function)	13–16 mm
Upper lid crease position	8–10 mm from margin (female > male)

Myasthenic ptosis

Myasthenia gravis may cause variable and fatiguable uni- or bilateral ptosis and ocular motility disturbance (p. 562). Surgical repair should be avoided except in refractory disease causing severe visual disability.

Myopathic ptosis

The chronic progressive external ophthalmoplegia (CPEO) group causes a bilateral, usually symmetric ptosis, associated with restricted ocular motility.

Surgical repair (usually frontalis suspension) requires caution, since lid closure is also abnormal. It is therefore delayed until ptosis is visually significant.

Mechanical ptosis

Masses, infiltrations, or edema of the upper lid may cause ptosis. The ptosis often resolves with correction of the underlying disease.

Pseudoptosis

- *Brow ptosis* is a lowering of the eyebrow due to frontalis dysfunction.
- *Dermatochalasis* is a common condition in which upper eyelid skin hangs in folds from the lid. It is more common in the elderly.
- *Blepharochalasis*: abnormal lid elastic tissue permits recurrent episodes of lid edema that lead to abnormal redundant skin folds.

Other simulators of ptosis are listed in Table 4.6.

Table 4.6 Causes of pseudoptosis

Ipsilateral pathology	Excessive skin	Brow ptosis
		Dermatochalasis
	Inadequate globe size	Microphthalmos
		Phthisis bulbi
		Prosthesis
	Incorrect globe position	Enophthalmos
		Hypotropia
Contralateral pathology		Contralateral lid retraction

Ptosis: congenital

Isolated congenital ptosis

This is a developmental myopathy of the levator. It is usually unilateral, with absent skin crease and reduced levator function, and the lid fails to drop normally in downgaze.

Treatment

Surgery: if levator function is reasonable, then anterior levator resection should be sufficient. For poor levator function, frontalis suspension should be performed. To optimize symmetry, this should be bilateral with excision of the uninvolved levator.

Blepharophimosis syndrome

This autosomal dominant condition is characterized by horizontally shortened palpebral fissures, telecanthus, severe bilateral ptosis with poor levator function, and commonly epicanthus inversus and ectropia.

Treatment

Surgery is first directed toward correcting the telecanthus and epicanthus. Bilateral frontalis slings are performed later.

Marcus Gunn jaw winking syndrome

This is a synkinesis in which innervation of the ipsilateral pterygoids causes elevation of the ptotic lid during chewing.

Treatment

Surgery requires levator resection (mild) or bilateral levator excision with frontalis suspension (severe).

Box 4.2 Outline of anterior levator advancement

- Administer subcutaneous local anesthetic (unless GA).
- Mark level of desired postoperative lid crease and make skin incision at this level.
- Divide orbicularis and septum and retract the preaponeurotic fat pads up to expose LPS.
- Free LPS from any remaining attachments to the tarsus and from the underlying Muller muscle.
- Advance the aponeurosis and suture to tarsus (partial thickness—evert lid to check; e.g., 6–0 Mersilene).
- In the awake patient, the resultant position should be observed and adjusted accordingly.
- Reform the lid crease by suturing the subcutaneous tissues and orbicularis to the tarsus (e.g., 7–0 Vicryl).
- Close skin incision (e.g., 7–0 polypropylene—remove at 1 week).

Miscellaneous lid disorders

Congenital

Epiblepharon

This is a common horizontal fold of skin running just below the lower lid, caused by the lack of a lower eyelid crease and overriding of the orbicularis. It is more common in Asians or patients with Down syndrome. It may cause the lid to invert with pseudotrichiasis. It is rarely significant and usually resolves as the midface develops.

If keratopathy develops, surgical intervention involving reforming of an inferior lid crease is necessary.

Epicanthic folds

These are common folds of skin that may arise in one of four patterns around the medial canthus:

- *Epicanthus palpebraris:* medial vertical fold between upper and lower lids; present in 20% normal children, usually resolves.
- *Epicanthus tarsalis:* primarily upper lid fold typical of Asian races.
- *Epicanthus inversus:* primarily lower lid fold seen in blepharophimosis and Down syndrome.
- *Epicanthus superciliaris:* fold arising above the brow; rare.

Telecanthus

This is wide separation of the medial canthi despite normally positioned orbits (i.e., normal interpupillary distance), in contrast to hypertelorism, where the whole orbits are widely separated. It may be isolated, secondary to trauma (most common), or syndromic (e.g., blepharophimosis).

Cryptophthalmos

This is a failure of lid development so that the surface ectoderm remains continuous over the surface of an often poorly developed eye. Even with cosmetic improvement, visual prognosis is often poor. It is sometimes autosomal dominantly inherited.

Ankyloblepharon

These are abnormal areas of upper and lower lid fusion and are of variable severity. They may be isolated or syndromic.

Coloboma

These are focal lid defects arising from failure of lid development or interference of amniotic bands. They are usually located medially in the upper lid and laterally in the lower lid.

Acquired

Floppy eyelid syndrome

In this uncommon condition, an excessively lax upper lid can spontaneously evert during sleep, resulting in exposure and chronic papillary conjunctivitis. It is more common in obese patients and may be associated with sleep apnea (with risk of pulmonary hypertension and other cardiovascular complications). Sleep studies are therefore recommended. Severe lid disease may be cured by lid-shortening procedures.

Lid retraction

Table 4.7 Causes of lid retraction

Congenital		Isolated
		Down syndrome
		Duane syndrome
Acquired	Systemic	Thyroid eye disease
		Uremia
	Neurological	CN VII palsy
		CN III misdirection
		Marcus Gunn syndrome
		Parinaud syndrome
		Hydrocephalus
		Sympathetic drive (including medication)
	Mechanical	Cicatricial
		Surgical
		Globe (buphthalmos/myopia/proptosis)

Lacrimal

Anatomy and physiology

The lacrimal system comprises a secretory component (tear production by the lacrimal gland) and an excretory component (tear drainage by the nasolacrimal system).

Anatomy

Lacrimal gland

This almond-shaped bilobar gland is located in the shallow lacrimal fossa of the superolateral orbit. It is held in place by fascial septa and divided into palpebral (smaller superficial part) and orbital (larger deeper part) lobes by the levator palpebrae superioris aponeurosis. Around 12 ducts run from the orbital lobe through the aponeurosis and palpebral lobe to open into the superolateral fornix.

The gland is of serous type, but also contains mucopolysaccharide granules. It is innervated by the parasympathetic system: superior salivary nucleus (pons) → greater petrosal nerve → synapse at pterygopalatine ganglion → zygomatic nerve (V_2) → lacrimal nerve (V_1) → lacrimal gland.

Nasolacrimal system

Tear drainage starts with the upper and lower lacrimal puncta (0.3 mm diameter), which are located around 6 mm lateral to the medial canthus. These are angled backward and are located within the slightly elevated lacrimal papilla.

The superior and inferior canaliculi comprise a vertical part (the ampulla: 2 mm long, up to 3 mm wide) and a horizontal part (8 mm long, up to 2 mm wide). The terminal canaliculi usually fuse to form the common canaliculus, on average 2 mm before entering the lacrimal sac. The sac is around 12 mm in length and lies within the lacrimal fossa. The lacrimal fossa lies posterior to the medial canthal tendon and lateral to the ethmoid sinus (although this is variable).

The nasolacrimal duct is around 18 mm long and runs parallel to the nasojugal fold (i.e., inferolaterally). The first 12 mm lies in the bony nasolacrimal canal and the last 6 mm within the mucous membrane of the lateral wall of the nose. It opens into the inferior meatus via the ostium lacrimale just beneath the inferior turbinate.

There are a number of valves along the system, the most important ones being the valves of Rosenmuller (entry into the lacrimal sac) and Hasner (exit from the nasolacrimal duct).

Physiology

Production (secretion) of tears may be basic or reflex.

Basic secretion

- *Lid:* meibomian glands (number around 60) → outer lipid layer, which reduces evaporation.
- *Conjunctiva:* glands of Krause (number around 28) and glands of Wolfring (number around 3) → middle aqueous layer, which has washing and antimicrobial functions; and goblet cells → inner mucin layer, which helps stabilize the tear film.
- *Lacrimal gland* may also contribute to basal secretion.

Reflex secretion

The lacrimal gland is innervated by the parasympathetic system.

Excretion

Tears flow along the marginal tear strips and are drained into the distensible ampulla. This is probably both passive (70% is drained via the inferior canaliculus vs. 30% via the superior) and active (i.e., suction). From the ampulla, an active lacrimal pump then drives the tears first into the sac and then down the nasolacrimal duct into the nose.

Contraction of the pretarsal orbicularis oculi (superficial and deep heads) compresses the loaded ampulla, while contraction of the preseptal orbicularis (deep head which inserts onto lacrimal fascia) forcibly expands the sac, creating a wave of suction toward the sac. With relaxation of orbicularis, the ampulla reopen and the sac collapses, expelling the tears down the nasolacrimal duct.

The watery eye: assessment

This is a common complaint, particularly in the elderly population. It ranges from the transient and trivial (e.g., associated with a local irritant) to the permanent and disabling. Objective quantification is difficult, but the main issue is how much of a problem it is for the patient.

Box 5.1 A systemic approach to assessing the watery eye

Symptoms	Episodic or permanent, frequency of wiping eyes, exacerbating factors, site where tears spill over (laterally or medially)
POH	Previous surgery or trauma; concurrent eye disease; herpes simplex blepharoconjunctivitis
PMH	Previous ENT problems (e.g., sinusitis); surgery or nasal fracture
Drug history	Prosecretory drugs (e.g., pilocarpine)
Allergy history	Allergies or relevant drug contraindications
Visual acuity	Best-corrected/pinhole
Face	Scars (previous trauma or surgery), asymmetry, prominent nasal bridge
Lacrimal sac	Swelling, any punctal regurgitation on palpation
Lids	Position (ectropion, entropion, or low lateral canthus), laxity (lid or canthal tendons)
Puncta	Position, scarring, concretions, patency
Conjunctiva	Irritation (e.g., chronic conjunctivitis)
Cornea	Inflammation, chronic corneal disease
Tear film	Meniscus high/low
Dye disappearance test	
Dye recovery	Cotton tip applicator or, ideally, nasendoscope
Cannulation	Patency of puncta
Probing	Hard/soft stop
Irrigation	Flow, regurgitation

Perform nasendoscopy when possible. Consider formal Jones testing and imaging (contrast dacryocystography, lacrimal scintillography) if required. For specific tests, see Chapter 1 (p. 38).

Table 5.1 Causes of the watery eye (common causes in bold)

Increased production	Basal	Autonomic disturbance
		Prosecretory drugs
	Reflex	Local irritant (e.g., FB, trichiasis)
		Systemic disease (e.g., TED)
		Chronic lid disease (e.g., blepharitis)
		Chronic conjunctival disease (e.g., OCP)
		Chronic corneal disease (e.g., KCS)
Lacrimal pump failure	Lid tone	**Lid laxity**
		Orbicularis weakness (e.g., CN VII palsy)
	Lid position	Ectropion
Decreased drainage	Punctal obstruction	Congenital: punctal atresia
		Idiopathic stenosis (elderly)
		HSV infection
		Post-irradiation
		Trachoma
		Cicatricial conjunctivitis
		Secondary to punctal eversion
	Canalicular obstruction	**Idiopathic fibrosis**
		HSV infection
		Chronic dacrocystitis
		Cicatricial conjunctivitis
		5-FU administration (systemic)
	Nasolacrimal duct obstruction	Congenital: **delayed canalization**
		Idiopathic stenosis
		Trauma (nasal or orbital fracture)
		Post-irradiation
		Wegener's granulomatosis
		Tumors (e.g., nasopharyngeal carcinoma)
		Nasal pathology (chronic inflammation polyps)

FB, foreign body; 5-FU, 5-fluorouracil; HSV, herpes simplex virus; KCS, keratoconjunctivitis sicca; OCP, ocular cicatricial pemphigold; TED, thyroid eye disease.

The watery eye: treatment

Increased production

This is usually due to reflex tearing in response to a chronic irritant or disease. Treatment is directed toward controlling the disease process, e.g., ocular lubricants for keratoconjunctivitis sicca (KCS). It is important to explain this to the patient, since it will seem counterintuitive to be treating a watery eye with drops.

Lacrimal pump failure

This is usually a function of lid laxity and ectropion causing punctal eversion. This often leads to secondary punctal stenosis. Treatment is directed toward restoring the position of lid and punctum, often with a lid-shortening procedure (see Table 5.2 and p. 118).

Table 5.2 Surgical procedures to improve nasolacrimal drainage

Operation	Indication	Procedure
Punctal position		
Ziegler cautery	Very mild medial ectropion	Cauterize tissue 5 mm inferior to punctum; causes scarring and inversion
Diamond excision	Mild medial ectropion	Diamond of tarsoconjunctiva excised just inferior to punctum
Lazy-T procedure	Medial ectropion with lid laxity	Diamond excision + wedge excision
Lateral tarsal strip	Ectropion with generalized laxity	Lid shortened laterally and tightened + elevated at lateral canthus
Punctal obstruction		
1- or 3-snip procedure	Isolated punctal stenosis	Vertical and small medial cut in the punctal ampulla enlarges opening
Canalicular obstruction		
Silastic tube insertion	Partial obstruction	Canaliculi intubated with silastic tube secured at nasal end; left for 6 months
DCR with Jones tube	Complete obstruction	DCR with a Jones (Pyrex) tube from sac to medial canthus
Nasolacrimal duct obstruction		
DCR	Most nasolacrimal duct obstructions	The lacimal sac is opened directly to nasal mucosa by a rhinostomy

DCR, dacryocystorhinostomy.

Decreased drainage

Obstruction may arise at the level of the punctum, the canaliculi, the sac, or the nasolacrimal duct. The extent of surgery required will depend on the level of blockage, but most cases arising distal to the puncta require a dacryocystorhinostomy (Table 5.2).

Dacryocystorhinostomy (DCR)

The aim of a dacryocystorhinostomy is to create an epithelium-lined tract from the lacrimal sac to the nasal mucosa. The conventional external route has a success rate of around 90%.

Endonasal DCR has the advantage of no external scar but is less effective. Laser-assisted endonasal DCR has the lowest success rates, possibly because of the smaller ostium created.

Indication

DCR is used for acquired nasolacrimal duct obstruction or congenital nasolacrimal obstruction in which a probe cannot be passed.

Method

Box 5.2 Outline of external DCR

1. Make cutaneous incision on lateral aspect of nose and inferior to medial canthal tendon (around 8–10 mm long).
2. Dissect down to bone, reflect periosteum from anterior lacrimal crest, and divide the superficial limb of the medial canthal tendon.
3. Reflect the lacrimal sac laterally.
4. Use Kerrison punches to create an opening through the bone of the sac fossa to the nasal cavity.
5. Divide the lacrimal sac and the exposed nasal mucosa vertically to form anterior and posterior flaps.
6. Anastamose mucosa of the sac and the nose by suturing the posterior and then the anterior flaps together.
7. Silastic tubes can be inserted to keep the ostium open if there is concern about premature closure by granulation tissue.
8. Close skin incision.

Postoperative care

If the nose has been packed at the end of the operation, the packing can usually be removed on the first day after surgery. Prophylactic oral antibiotics are commonly prescribed.

Complications

Hemorrhage with epistaxis may occur early (within 24 hours) or late (4–7 days) when clot retraction occurs. Treat with nasal packing (± thrombin-soaked packs). If hemostasis is still not achieved, the vessel may need embolization.

Other complications include failure (closure of the ostium), scar formation, infection, and, very rarely, orbital hemorrhage.

Lacrimal system infections

Canaliculitis

This uncommon chronic condition usually arises from the gram-positive bacteria *Actinomyces israelii* (streptothrix), but may be due to *Nocardia*, fungi (*Candidia, Aspergillus*) or viruses (HSV, VZV).

Clinical features
- Unilateral epiphora, recurrent "nasal" conjunctivitis, inflammation of the punctum and canaliculus, expression of discharge, or concretions from the canaliculi.
- In *Actinomyces* infection, these are bright yellow concretions ("sulfur granules"). The lacrimal sac is not swollen, and both sac and nasolacrimal duct are patent.

Investigation and treatment
Remove concretions (send for microbiological analysis) and consider irrigation (e.g., with penicillin G 100,000 U/mL or iodine 1%—ensure drainage out through nose, not nasopharynx) and topical antibiotics.

Acute dacryocystitis

This condition is relatively common in patients with complete or partial nasolacrimal duct obstruction. It is usually due to staphylococci or streptococci. Acute dacryocystitis is easily identified and requires urgent treatment to prevent a spreading cellulitis.

Clinical features
- Pain around sac, worsening epiphora.
- Tender, erythematous lump just inferior to medial canthus, may express pus from puncta on palpation, + preseptal cellulitis.

Investigation and treatment
Send discharge to microbiology.
- *Antibiotics:* systemic (e.g., cephalexin 500 mg 4×/day for 7 days). Consider warm compresses, gentle massage (encourages expression), and incision and drainage if pointing (but may not heal until DCR is performed).
- *Surgery:* most cases have associated nasolacrimal duct obstruction requiring DCR.

Chronic dacryocystitis

In chronic dacryocystitis, there may be recurrent ipsilateral conjunctivitis, epiphora, and a mucocele. It may be identified by demonstration of nasolacrimal duct obstruction and expression of the contents of the mucocele. Surgical treatment is with DCR.

Conjunctiva

Anatomy and physiology

The *conjunctiva* is a mucous membrane that is essential for a healthy eye. At the histological level, it comprises epithelium, basement membrane, and stroma. At the macroscopic clinical level, it is divided into palpebral, forniceal, and bulbar parts.

Microscopic

Epithelium

This is a 2- to 5-layered, nonkeratinized epithelium that may be stratified squamous (palpebral and limbal) or stratified columnar (bulbar conjunctiva). It contains goblet cells.

Epithelial basement membrane

Stroma

This is vascular connective tissue containing lymphoid tissue and accessory lacrimal glands.

Macroscopic

Palpebral

This is firmly adherent to the posterior lamella of the lid; it contains the crypts of Henle and goblet cells (both secrete mucin).

Forniceal

This is loose and relatively mobile with redundant tissue. It contains accessory lacrimal glands of Krause and Wolfring (secrete aqueous component of tears) and goblet cells.

Bulbar

This is loosely attached to Tenon's layer, but firmly attached at the limbus. It contains glands of Manz (secrete mucin) and goblet cells.

The tear film

Although conventionally described as a defined trilaminar structure, it is becoming apparent that the tear film is more complex. It appears that the layers blend together, forming a sponge-like material on the surface of the eye. The aqueous component is supported by lipid (which resists evaporative loss of aqueous) and mucin (which helps stabilize the aqueous against the otherwise hydrophobic epithelium) (see Fig. 6.1).

	Lipid	Meibomian glands Glands of Zeis
	Aqueous	Lacrimal gland Glands of Krause Glands of Wolfring
	Mucin	Goblet cells Glands of Manz Crypts of Henle
‖‖‖‖‖‖‖‖‖‖‖‖	*Epithelium*	

Figure 6.1 Tear film components and their origins.

Conjunctival signs

Table 6.1 Conjunctival signs and their pathophysiology

Sign	Pathology	Causes
Hyperemia	Dilated blood vessels, nonspecific sign of inflammation	• *Generalized*—e.g., conjunctivitis, dry eye, drug hypersensitivity, contact lens wear, scleritis • *Localized*—e.g., episcleritis, scleritis, marginal keratitis, superior limbic keratitis, corneal abrasion, FB • *Circumcorneal*—e.g., anterior uveitis, keratitis
Discharge	Inflammatory exudate	• Purulent—bacterial conjunctivitis • Mucopurulent—bacterial or chlamydial conjunctivitis • Mucoid—vernal conjunctivitis, atopic keratoconjunctivitis, dry eye syndrome • Watery—viral or allergic conjunctivitis
Papillae	Vascular response: projections of a core of vessels, surrounded by edematous stroma and hyperplastic epithelium; also chronic inflammatory cells	• Bacterial conjunctivitis • Allergic conjunctivitis (perennial or seasonal) • Atopic keratoconjunctivitis • Vernal keratoconjunctivitis • Blepharitis • Floppy eyelid syndrome • Superior limbic keratoconjunctivitis • Contact lens
Giant papillae	Papillae that with chronic inflammation have lost the normal fibrous septa that divide them	• Vernal keratoconjunctivitis • Atopic keratoconjunctivitis • Contact lens–related giant papillary conjunctivitis • Exposed suture • Prosthesis • Floppy eyelid syndrome
Follicles	Lymphoid hyperplasia with each follicle comprising an active germinal center	• Viral conjunctivitis • Chlamydial conjunctivitis • Drug hypersensitivity • Parinaud oculoglandular syndrome
Lymphadenopathy	Temporal 2/3 drains to the preauricular nodes, nasal 1/3 to the submandibular nodes	• Viral conjunctivitis • Chlamydial conjunctivitis • Gonococcal conjunctivitis • Parinaud oculoglandular syndrome

Table 6.1 *Continued*

Sign	Pathology	Causes

Pseudo-membrane	Exudate of fibrin and cellular debris; loosely attached to the underlying epithelium; easily removed without the epithelium and without bleeding	• Infective conjunctivitis
		  • Adenovirus
		  • *Streptococcus pyogenes*
		  • *Corynebacterium diphtheriae*
		  • *Neisseria gonorrhoeae*
		• Stevens–Johnson syndrome (acute)
		• Graft-versus-host disease
		• Vernal conjunctivitis
		• Ligneous conjunctivitis

Membrane	Exudate of fibrin and cellular debris; firmly attached to the underlying epithelium; attempted removal strips off the epithelium, causing bleeding	• Infective conjunctivitis
		  • Adenovirus
		  • *Streptococcus pneumoniae*
		  • *Staphylococcus aureus*
		  • *Corynebacterium diphtheriae*
		• Stevens–Johnson syndrome (acute)
		• Ligneous conjunctivitis

Cicatrization	Scarring	• Trachoma • Atopic keratoconjunctivitis • Topical medication • Chemical injury (acid/alkali) • Ocular mucous membrane pemphigoid (OMMP, formerly OCP) • Erythema multiforme, Stevens–Johnson syndrome, toxic epidermal necrolysis • Other bullous disease (e.g., linear IgA disease, epidermolysis bullosa) • Sjögren syndrome • Graft-versus-host disease

Hemorrhagic conjunctivitis	Subconjunctival hemorrhages	• Infective conjunctivitis
		  • Adenovirus
		  • Enterovirus 70
		  • Coxsackie virus A24
		  • *Streptococcus pneumoniae*
		  • *Haemophilus aegyptius*

Table 6.2 Conjunctivitis: an outline of clinical features

Etiology	Main symptoms	Onset	Visual acuity	History	Discharge	Chemosis	Lids	Preauricular lymphadenopathy
Bacterial	Red Sticky Gritty	Acute/ hyperacute	Should be normal/near normal when discharge blinked away. Reduced acuity and photophobia suggests additional involvement, such as keratitis.	±Known contact	Purulent	Mild	Papillae	Occasional
Viral	Red Watery Gritty	Acute		±Known contact	Watery	Moderate	Follicles	Common
Chlamydial	Red Persistent discharge	Subacute		Sexual history	Mucopurulent	Mild	Follicles	Common
Allergic	Red Itchy Swelling	Acute/subacute/ recurrent		Atopy	Watery	Severe	Papillae	No
Toxic (drops)	Discomfort + redness worse with drop instillation	Acute		Medication	Minimal	Mild	Follicles	No

Bacterial conjunctivitis

Acute bacterial conjunctivitis

Common conjunctival bacterial pathogens are *Staphylococcus epidermidis*, *Staphylococcus aureus*, *Streptococcus pneumoniae*, *Haemophilus influenzae*, and *Moraxella lacunata*. There is some variation according to climate (*Haemophilus aegyptius* in warm climates, *H. influenzae* and *Streptococcus* in cool climates) and age (traditionally, *H. influenzae* occurs in children).

Bacteria have to overcome the protective mechanisms of the eye: lids (physical barrier, blink reflex), tears (flushing effect, lysozyme, β-lysin, lactoferrin, IgG, IgA), and conjunctiva (physical barrier, conjunctiva-associated lymphoid tissue).

Clinical features
• Acute, red, gritty, sticky eye; usually bilateral but may be sequential.
• Purulent discharge, crusted lids, diffusely injected conjunctiva with papillae; may have mild chemosis.

Investigation
Reserve microbiological investigation for cases that are severe, recurrent, resistant, or atypical or occur in vulnerable populations (e.g., immunosuppressed, neonates). For these patients, take conjunctival swabs for culture sensitivities.

Treatment
• Topical antibiotics (e.g., ofloxacin 4×/day or trimethoprim/polymyxin B 4×/day for 1 week). Patients may find drops easier than ointment (more frequent administration is required). The frequency is reduced as the infection is controlled, and continued for 48 hours after healing.
• Advise patients to follow up if the condition worsens or persists after treatment. They should practice measures to reduce spread, such as frequent hand washing, minimal touching of eyes, not sharing towels or sheets, not shaking hands, etc. You need to wash your hands and clean the equipment before treating the next patient.

Gonococcus (adult)

Gram-negative diplococcus is found in adults (via sexual transmission) and neonates (born to infected mothers). The incubation period is 3–5 days in adults and 1–3 days in neonates. Gonococcus (*Neisseria gonorrhoea*) may penetrate the cornea in the absence of an epithelial defect.

Clinical features
• Hyperacute onset (<24 hours) with severe purulent discharge, marked lid swelling and chemosis, papillae, preauricular lymphadenopathy, ± pseudomembrane, ± keratitis.
• Keratitis: marginal ulceration may progress rapidly, resulting in a ring ulcer, perforation, and endophthalmitis.
• Systemic: history of (unprotected) sexual activity, urethritis, proctitis, vaginitis. Although often asymptomatic in women, it is a significant cause of infertility.

Investigation
- Conjunctival scrapings/swabs for immediate Gram stain, culture, and sensitivities.
- After appropriate explanation to the patient, refer to a urogenital clinic for assessment, treatment, and contact tracing.

Treatment
- Local microbiological/infectious disease consultation is vital.
- Topical antibiotic (e.g., ofloxacin 0.3% 2 hourly), saline irrigation of discharge 4×/day.
- With keratitis consider admission, ceftriaxone 1 g IV 2×/day for 3 days, topical antibiotic (e.g., ofloxacin 0.3% hourly), and saline irrigation; treat chlamydial coinfection.
- Systemic treatment, usually by a urogenital physician, may include ceftriaxone 1 g IM stat and cotreatment for possible chlamydial coinfection (e.g., tetracycline 250 mg PO 4×/day 6 weeks).

Gonococcus (neonate)
See Chapter 18, Ophthalmia neonatorum (p. 680).

Viral conjunctivitis

Adenovirus

Over 40 serotypes of this dsDNA virus have been identified. The incubation period is approximately 1 week, and virus shedding continues for a further 2 weeks. The spectrum of presentation may be generalized into two distinct syndromes:

- *Pharyngoconjunctival fever*—serotypes 3, 4, 7, and many others; aerosol transmission; common in children and young adults. Systemic upset (typically upper respiratory tract infection) is common. Keratitis is only present in up to 30% and is usually mild.
- *Epidemic keratoconjunctivitis*—serotypes 8, 19, 37; transmission by contact (fingers, instruments). Keratitis may occur in up to 80% and can be severe; systemic features are rare.

Clinical features

- Acute onset (7–10 days), watering, burning, itching, ± photophobia or blurred vision (if keratitis).
- Watery discharge, lid edema, moderate chemosis, follicles (inferior > superior), tender preauricular lymphadenopathy, ± subconjunctival petechial hemorrhage, ± pseudomembrane, ± symblepharon, ± keratitis.
- Keratitis: first diffuse epithelial keratitis (days 1–7; fluorescein staining), then focal epithelial keratitis (days 7–30; fluorescein staining), and finally subepithelial opacities (from day 11 on, may last years; nonstaining).

Investigation

- Conjunctival swabs (viral transport medium) for viral antigen determination or polymerase chain reaction (PCR).

Treatment

- Supportive (cool compresses and artificial tears) ± topical antibiotics (supposedly to prevent secondary bacterial infection). When subepithelial opacities significantly affect vision, some clinicians advocate low-dose topical steroids. However, the opacities recur on cessation of steroids, thereby encouraging long-term steroid dependency.
- Advise patient to follow up if condition worsens or persists after treatment. Measures to reduce spread include frequent hand washing, minimal touching of eyes, not sharing towels or sheets, not shaking hands, etc.
- Wash hands and clean equipment before the next patient.

Molluscum contagiosum

This dsDNA virus of the pox virus group is common in children and young adults; profuse lesions are seen with HIV infection. Transmission is by close contact. The lesions may be missed if buried in the lash margin, causing a persistent follicular conjunctivitis.

Clinical features
These include chronic history, a pearly, umbilicated nodule at the lid margin, mucoid discharge, and follicles.

Treatment
Remove the lid lesion (e.g., cryotherapy, cauterization, shave excision, expression).

Herpes simplex (type 1)
Blepharokeratoconjunctivitis usually occurs as a primary infection of this dsDNA virus.

Clinical features
These include burning, foreign body sensation; unilateral follicular conjunctivitis, preauricular lymphadenopathy, ± lid vesicles, ± keratitis (p. 194).

Treatment
Give oral acyclovir. If there is keratitis, then treat accordingly (p. 194).

Other viruses
Other viruses causing follicular conjunctivitis include other members of the herpes group, enterovirus 70, coxsackie A24, influenza A, and the Newcastle disease virus.

Chlamydial conjunctivitis

Chlamydia are gram-negative bacteria that exist in two forms: a spore-like infectious particle (elementary body) and the obligate intracellular reproductive stage (reticular body) that replicates within the host cell (seen as an inclusion body).

Adult inclusion conjunctivitis

This disease of *Chlamydia trachomatis* serotypes D to K is almost always sexually transmitted, although occasional eye-to-eye infection is reported. It is most common in young adults. It may be associated with keratitis.

Clinical features

- Subacute onset (2–3 weeks), unilateral or bilateral, mucopurulent discharge, lid edema ± ptosis, follicles (papillae initially), nontender lymphadenopathy, superior pannus (late sign).
- Keratitis: punctate epithelial erosions, subepithelial opacities, marginal infiltrates.
- Systemic (common, but often asymptomatic): cervicitis (females), urethritis (males).

Investigation

- Conjunctival swabs are taken usually for immunofluorescent staining, but cell culture, PCR, and ELISA may be used.
- After appropriate explanation to the patient, refer to a urogenital clinic for assessment, treatment, and contact tracing.

Treatment

First-line treatment is erythromycin ointment 4×/day. Systemic (oral) treatment is usually best administered at the urogenital clinic (after appropriate investigation). Options include oral azithromycin 1 g stat or doxycycline 100 mg 2×/day for 1 week. If the patient is pregnant, erythromycin (e.g., 500mg 2×/day for 2 weeks) is usually given.

Neonatal chlamydial conjunctivitis

See Chapter 18, Ophthalmia neonatorum (p. 680).

Trachoma

Trachoma accounts for 10–15% of global blindness and is the leading preventable cause. It is caused by *Chlamydia trachomatis* serotypes A, B, Ba, and C, in conditions of crowding and poor hygiene in which the common fly acts as the vector. In endemic areas, it may start in infancy; in nonendemic areas (such as the United States), patients usually present with the complications of chronic scarring. Disease classification is presented in Table 6.3.

The World Health Organization (WHO) is aiming to eliminate trachoma as a blinding disease by 2020. A useful strategy is the SAFE strategy: **S**urgery for in-turned eyelashes, **A**ntibiotics for active disease, **F**ace washing (or promotion of facial cleanliness), and **E**nvironmental improvement to reduce transmission.

Clinical features
- Distinctive follicular reaction (more marked in the upper, rather than lower lid), conjunctival scarring (with ensuing Arlt lines on the superior tarsus, trichiasis, entropion, dry eyes), limbal follicles (which may scar to form Herbert pits).
- Keratitis: superficial, subepithelial, ulceration, secondary microbial keratitis, pannus formation.

Investigation (if acute)
Swabs are usually for immunofluorescent staining, but cell culture, PCR, and ELISA may be used.

Treatment
- Azithromycin 1 g PO stat (nonapproved indication, but now standard practice for prevention and eradication)
- Ocular lubricants, surgical correction of lid position

Table 6.3 World Health Organization (WHO) classification

TF	Trachomatous inflammation: follicular	>5 follicles on upper tarsus
TI	Trachomatous inflammation: intense	Tarsal inflammation sufficient to obscure >50% of the tarsal vessels
TS	Trachomatous scarring	Conjunctival scarring
TT	Trachomatous trichiasis	Trichiasis
CO	Corneal opacity	Corneal opacity involving at least part of the pupillary margin

Allergic conjunctivitis

Seasonal and perennial allergic rhinoconjunctivitis

These extremely common ocular disorders arise from type I hypersensitivity reactions to airborne allergens. These may be seasonal (grass, tree, weed pollens, ragweed) or perennial (animal dander, house dust mite).

Clinical features
• Itching, watery discharge; history of atopy
• Chemosis, lid edema, papillae, mild diffuse injection

Investigation
Consider conjunctival swabs (microbiology), skin prick testing, serum IgE, and radioallergosorbent test (RAST)

Treatment
• Identify and eliminate allergen where possible (e.g., change bedding, reduce pet contact, introduce air conditioning).
• If mild: artificial tears (dilutes allergen).
• If moderate: mast cell stabilizer (e.g., sodium cromoglycate 2% 4×/day, lodoxamide 0.1% 4×/day) or topical antihistamine (azelastine 0.05% 2–4×/day for 6 weeks maximum, levocabastine 0.05% 2–4×/day), and oral antihistamine (e.g., chlorphenamine 4 mg 3–6×/day).
• If case is severe, include a short course of an additional mild topical steroid (e.g., fluorometholone 0.1% 4×/day for 1 week).

Vernal keratoconjunctivitis (VKC)

This is an uncommon but serious condition of children and young adults (onset age 5–15 years; duration 5–10 years). Before puberty, it is more common in males but subsequently shows no gender bias.

Although its incidence is decreasing among the white population, it is increasing in Asians. Caucasians more commonly exhibit the tarsal/palpebral form, whereas the limbal form is more common in darker-skinned races; however, a mixed picture is often seen. It is more common in warm climates and is usually seasonal (spring to summer).

Over 80% of patients have an atopic history. Although there is type I hypersensitivity involvement, there is also a cell-mediated role with a predominantly Th2 cell type.

Clinical features
• Itching, thick mucous discharge; typically young male, presenting in spring with history of atopy.
• Tarsal signs: flat-topped giant ("cobblestone") papillae on superior tarsus.
• Limbal signs: limbal papillae, white Trantas dots (eosinophil aggregates).
• Keratitis: superior punctate epithelial erosions, vernal ulcer with adherent mucus plaque (may result in subepithelial scar), pseudogerontoxon (corneal lesion resembling segment of arcus senilis).

Treatment

- Topical: mast cell stabilizer (e.g., sodium cromoglycate 2% g 4×/day), ± topical steroid ± cyclosporine (either 2% drops or 0.2% oinment 3–4×/day); consider mucolytic (e.g., acetylcysteine 5% 4×/day).
- Acute exacerbations may require intensive treatment with topical steroids (e.g., dexamethasone 0.1% PF hourly) but then titrate down to the minimum potency and frequency required to control exacerbations (e.g., fluorometholone 0.1% 1–2×/day). Cyclosporine may be used as an adjunct with a steroid-sparing role.
- Systemic: consider an antiviral (e.g., acyclovir 200 mg 4×/day) if using immunosuppressants since these patients are vulnerable to herpes simplex keratitis.
- Surgical: consider debridement or superficial lamellar keratectomy to remove plaques.

Atopic keratoconjunctivitis

This is a rare but serious condition of adults (onset 25–30 years). Patients are usually atopic, commonly with eczema of the lids and staphylococcal lid disease. Control of lid disease is an important aspect of treatment.

This is a mixed type I and IV hypersensitivity response, but with a higher Th1-cell type component than that in vernal disease.

Clinical features

- Itching, redness; photophobia ± blurred vision (if keratitis); history of atopy.
- Lid eczema, staphylococcal lid disease (anterior blepharitis), small tightly packed papillae, otherwise featureless tarsal conjunctiva (due to inflammation); chemosis + limbal hyperemia (acute exacerbations); may cicatrize (chronic) with forniceal shortening.
- Keratitis: inferior punctate epithelial erosions, shield ulcers, pannus, corneal vascularization, herpes simplex, or microbial keratitis.
- Associations: keratoconus, cataract.

Treatment

- Topical: treat as for VKC, including ocular lubricants + mast cell stabilizer (usually less effective than in VKC) ± topical steroid (e.g., initially dexamethasone 0.1% PF hourly) ± cyclosporine (2% drops or 0.2% ointment 3–4×/day).
- Oral: consider antihistamines (they may help with itching) and corticosteroids (for severe acute exacerbations). If using immuno-suppressants, consider an antiviral (e.g., acyclovir 200 mg 4×/day), since these patients are vulnerable to herpes simplex keratitis.
- Surgical: consider debridement or superficial lamellar keratectomy to remove plaques.
- For lid disease: consider topical (e.g., erythromycin ointment 4×/day) and oral (e.g., doxycycline 100 mg 1×/day 3 months) antibiotics.
- For secondary infective keratitis, give topical antivirals and antibiotics.

Cicatricial conjunctivitis

In this potentially blinding condition, conjunctival inflammation with scarring leads to the loss of conjunctival function (such as goblet cells) and architecture. Onset may be insidious, delaying diagnosis. Although there are many causes, cicatrization has broadly similar ocular features, and similar treatment modalities may be considered.

Primary

Ocular mucous membrane pemphigoid (OMMP)

Mucous membrane pemphigoid is more common in women, usually >60 years of age but may occur in adolescents. It is thought to be a type II hypersensitivity reaction with linear deposition of immunoglobulin (Ig) and complement at the basement membrane of mucosal surfaces, leading to loss of adhesion and bulla formation and subsequent cicatrization.

Oral mucosa and conjunctiva are most commonly affected, although skin and other mucous membranes may be involved. Ocular mucous membrane pemphigoid (OMMP) was formerly known as ocular cicatricial pemphigoid (OCP).

Clinical features
- Irritation.
- Chronic papillary conjunctivitis, subconjunctival vesicles →ulcerate, progressive subconjunctival fibrosis and cicatrization (loss of plica semilunaris and fornices, formation of symblepharon/ankyloblepharon), dry eye signs, trichiasis, secondary microbial keratitis, corneal neovascularization, corneal melt, perforation.

Treatment
- Topical: tear substitutes, corticosteroids and antibiotics (preservative-free).
- Systemic immunosuppression (for acute phase of disease): dapsone if mild or moderate; corticosteroids, methotrexate, azathioprine or cyclophosphamide if severe (consult with a rheumatologist; all patients need monitoring). Systemic immunosuppression is generally required for >1 year.
- Consider silicone contact lenses and surgery (for correction of lid and lash position; punctal occlusion or tarsorrhaphy to upper lid; botulinum toxin is of limited use given the mechanical restriction; corneal transplant or surface reconstruction procedures; keratoprosthesis).

Erythema muliforme, Stevens–Johnson syndrome, and toxic epidermal necrolysis (TEN, Lyell disease)

These are acute vasculitides of the mucous membranes and skin that are associated with drug hypersensitivity (sulfonamides, anticonvulsants, allopurinol) or infections (e.g., mycoplasma, HSV). They are thought to result from a type III hypersensitivity response and may represent different variants of the same disease.

Clinical features
- Acute fever/malaise and skin rash (e.g., target lesions or bullae) and hemorrhagic inflammation of ≥2 mucous membranes.
- Papillary or pseudomembranous conjunctivitis → cicatrization (as for OMMP but is classically nonprogressive once acute illness subsides).

Other bullous diseases in which cicatricial conjunctivitis is common include linear IgA disease (linear IgA at the dermoepidermal junction) and epidermolysis bullosa.

Secondary

Injury
Thermal, radiation, chemical (especially alkali), and surgical injuries may all cause cicatrization.

Anterior blepharitis (staphylococcal)
Limited cicatrization and keratinization of the lid margin with reduced tear film quality may cause chronic irritation.

Infective conjunctivitis
Cicatrization is most common with *Chlamydia* trachomatis, but may also occur after membranous and pseudomembranous conjunctivitis.

Drugs
Reactions may vary from mild irritation to drug-induced cicatricial conjunctivitis (DICC), which is clinically indistinguishable from OMMP. Drugs implicated may be systemic (practolol, penicillamine) and topical (propine, pilocarpine, timolol, idoxuridine, gentamicin (particularly 1.5%), guanethidine).

Inherited
Consider ectodermal dysplasia if there are associated abnormalities of hair and teeth.

Systemic
Consider rosacea, Sjögren syndrome, and graft-versus-host disease (GVHD). GVHD occurs in some bone marrow transplant patients where the donor's leukocytes attack the immunosuppressed recipient. In the acute response, there is toxic epidermal necrolysis, which may include a pseudomembranous conjunctivitis. In chronic GVHD, there are scleroderma-like changes of the skin and Sjögren-like changes of the glands to cause keratoconjunctivitis sicca.

Neoplastic
Unilateral cicatrizing conjunctivitis may be due to sebaceous cell carcinoma, conjunctival intraepithelial neoplasia (CIN), or squamous cell carcinoma.

Keratoconjunctivitis sicca

Although patients report dry eyes commonly, most often they are describing mild tear film instability associated with blepharitis. While some symptomatic relief will be obtained from artificial tears, in these cases the blepharitis itself should be the focus of treatment. However, true keratoconjunctivitis sicca may be severe and very painful and threaten vision.

Keratoconjunctivitis sicca

Clinical features

- Burning (may be very painful) ± blurred vision (due to corneal involvement).
- Mucus strands; small or absent concave tear meniscus; punctate epitheliopathy; filaments; mucus plaques; tear film breakup time <10 sec; rose bengal and/or lissamine green staining pattern; Schirmer test <5 mm over 5 min (without topical anesthetic).

Treatment

Artificial tears (Table 6.4)

- *Consider viscosity:* low-viscosity drops require frequent administration (sometimes more than hourly) but have minimal effect on vision; more viscous gels will transiently blur the vision but are longer lasting and may be effective when used only 4–6×/day. Highly viscous paraffin-based ointments significantly blur vision and may only be suitable for night-time use.
- *Consider preservative-free preparations* to reduce risk of epithelial toxicity if frequent administration is required.
- *Consider physiological tear substitutes:* hyaluronic acid (HA) is a natural component of tears. It is now becoming commercially available for topical application. These preparations are classified as devices rather than as medications. It improves the symptoms of dry eye and appears to have a protective effect on the epithelium. In extreme cases, autologous serum may be used.

Table 6.4 Artificial tears and lubricants

Viscosity	Frequency	Preserved-form examples	Preservative-free examples
Low Hypromellose/ polyvinyl alcohol	q4h–q6h	Hypromellose Hypotears	Liquifilm (PF) Refresh
Medium Carbomer/ cellulose	1–6×/day	Viscotears GelTears	Celluvisc Viscotears PF
High Paraffins	1–4×/day		Lacri-lube Lubri-Tears Simple eye ointment

- Treat blepharitis: lid hygiene ± oral antibiotic (e.g., doxycycline 100 mg 1×/day 3 months).
- Treat active inflammation: consider topical or systemic corticosteroids; if responsive, these patients may benefit from topical cyclosporine (e.g., Restasis).
- Increase secretion: pilocarpine hydrochloride 5 mg 1–4×/day (increase slowly from 5 mg/day to try to reduce anticholinergic side effects). Pilocarpine is approved for dry mouth and dry eyes in Sjögren syndrome but is only effective if there is some residual lacrimal gland function.
- Mucolytic (if filaments, mucus plaques): acetylcysteine 5% 4×/day (warn that it stings).
- Environmental—lower room temperature, moist chamber goggles, room humidifier (limited success).
- Punctal occlusion—temporary or permanent.

Causes of dry eye

Table 6.5 Causes of dry eyes

Lacrimal gland inflammation	Isolated	Keratoconjunctivitis sicca (KCS)
	Primary Sjögren syndrome	KCS with xerostomia (dry mouth)
	Secondary Sjögren syndrome	KCS with xerostomia associated with connective tissue disease, such as rheumatoid arthritis, SLE, systemic sclerosis, GVHD
Lacrimal gland destruction		Tumor
		Idiopathic orbital inflammatory disease
		Thyroid eye disease
		Sarcoid
Lacrimal gland absence		Congenital
		Acquired
Lacrimal gland duct scarring		Cicatrizing conjunctivitis (any) (p. 148)
Meibomian gland dysfunction		Blepharitis
Neurological		Familial dysautonomia (Riley–Day syndrome)
Superior limbic keratoconjunctivitis		Idiopathic superior limbic keratoconjunctivitis (SLK)
		Thyroid eye disease

Miscellaneous conjunctivitis and conjunctival degenerations

Toxic conjunctivitis

Topical medication (e.g., aminoglycosides, antivirals, glaucoma treatments, preservatives, and contact lens solutions) may result in an inferior papillary reaction. With chronic usage, topical medication (e.g., glaucoma treatments, antibiotics, and antivirals) may cause a follicular reaction and conjunctival cicatrization. Inferior punctate epitheliopathy may be seen.

Treatment is to discontinue the offending agent and consider a preservative-free ocular lubricant (e.g., Celluvisc).

Parinaud's oculoglandular syndrome

This is a rare unilateral conjunctivitis with granulomatous nodules (+ follicles) on the palpebral conjunctiva, ipsilateral lymphadenopathy (preauricular/submandibular), and systemic upset (malaise, fever). It is most commonly due to cat-scratch disease (*Bartonella henselae*), but also consider tularemia, mycobacteria (e.g., tuberculosis), sarcoid, syphilis, lymphoproliferative disorders, infectious mononucleosis, or fungi.

Investigations will be dictated by history but consider getting conjunctival biopsy, conjunctival swabs, full blood count (FBC), VDRL, chest X-ray, Mantoux testing, and serology (for cat-scratch disease and tularemia).

Ligneous conjunctivitis

This is a rare idiopathic chronic conjunctivitis of children (especially girls) that is characterized by recurrent pseudomembranes or membranes of the "wood-like" tarsal conjunctiva and often of other mucous membranes (e.g., oropharynx, trachea). Histologically, these comprise fibrin, albumin, IgG, and T and B cells. Treat with topical cyclosporine.

Pinguecula

A yellow-white patch of interpalpebral bulbar conjunctiva is located just nasal or temporal to the limbus. It represents elastotic degeneration of collagen. Reassurance and occasionally ocular lubrication are usually all that is required.

Pterygium

This occurs in patients exposed to dry climates and high ultraviolet (UV) light. It usually arises from the nasal limbus and grows slowly across the cornea. Histologically, it is akin to pinguecula with elastotic degeneration of collagen, but with additional destruction of Bowman's layer.

It is adherent to underlying tissue for the whole length; unlike pseudopterygium, which is a fold of conjunctiva, only attached at the base and apex, usually resulting from inflammation of the corneal ulceration with adherence of local conjunctiva.

Clinical features
- Cosmetic issues, astigmatism; it may encroach on visual axis, with foreign body sensation.
- Triangular pink-white fibrovascular band. Signs of activity include rapid growth, engorged vessels, gray leading edge in the cornea, and punctate epitheliopathy. Signs of stability include an iron line (Stocker line) just anterior to the margin.

Treatment
Reserve the following treatment for progressive, vision-threatening lesions, since recurrence is common and may be aggressive.

Excise with conjunctival autograft; amniotic membrane graft or mitomycin C (MMC) may be used when removing recurrent pterygia. If the visual axis is involved, lamellar keratoplasty may also be required.

Concretions
Seen in the elderly and those with chronic blepharitis, these yellow-white deposits may erode through the palpebral conjunctiva, causing a foreign body sensation. If troublesome, they can be removed with a needle (at the slit lamp under topical anesthetic).

Retention cyst
This very common, thin-walled, fluid-filled conjunctival cyst occasionally causes symptoms if it disturbs the corneal tear film. It can be punctured with a needle (at the slit lamp under topical anesthetic) but may recur, in which case, consider excision.

Pigmented conjunctival lesions

Benign

Congenital

- *Conjunctival epithelial melanosis:* often bilateral, flat, and patchy freely moving brown pigmentation, which may be diffuse (usually denser around the limbus and anterior ciliary nerves) or focal, e.g., around an intrascleral nerve (Axenfeld loop).
- *Conjunctival freckle:* common, tiny flat freely moving pigmented area.
- *Melanocytoma:* rare, black pigmentation, fixed, slowly growing.

Acquired

- Deposits, e.g., mascara in the inferior fornix, adrenochrome on forniceal/palpebral conjunctiva (from chronic adrenaline administration).

Premalignant

Primary acquired melanosis (PAM)

This is rare in African Americans. Histological differentiation is vital, since PAM without atypia is a benign melanocytic proliferation, whereas PAM wth atypia has a 50% risk of transformation to melanoma by 5 years.

Clinical

- Unilateral, single or multifocal flat freely moving area of irregular brown pigmentation. Pigmentation and size of the lesion may increase, decrease, or remain constant over time.
- Nodules within PAM suggest malignant transfromation to melanoma.

Treatment

For PAM with atypia use excision + cryotherapy, radiotherapy, and antimetabolite.

Conjunctival nevus

These lesions have a low risk of transformation.

Clinical

These single, defined, freely moving brown-pigmentation cysts occur most commonly at the limbus, followed by the caruncle/plica. They may increase in pigmentation or size at puberty.

Congenital ocular melanocytosis

Oculodermal melanocytosis (nevus of Ota) is the most common variant, followed by the limited dermal and ocular forms. Oculodermal melanocytosis is more common in females and Asians.

Clinical

There is unilateral hyperpigmentation of the face (most commonly in a CN V_1/CN V_2 distributions; ipsilateral iris hyperchromia, glaucoma [10%] associated with trabecular hyperpigmentation), and melanoma (ocular, dermal, or central nervous system).

Malignant

Melanoma

Consider this first when confronted with abnormal conjunctival pigmentation.
Although rare, it may be fatal (more common in middle age). Melanoma most commonly arises from atypical primary acquired melanosis, but may arise from a nevus or de novo.

Clinical

- Solitary gray, black, or nonpigmented vascularized nodule fixed to episclera; most commonly at the limbus.
- It may metastasize to draining lymph nodes, lung, liver, or brain.

Prognosis

Five-year mortality is 13%. Poor prognostic factors include a multifocal lesion; caruncle, fornix, or palpebral location; thickness >1 mm; recurrence; and lymphatic or orbital spread.

Treatment

Treatment is with wide local excision + double freeze-thaw cryotherapy to excised margins. Consider adjunctive radiotherapy and antimetabolite if incomplete excision or diffuse. Exenteration may be necessary if the lesion is unresectable.

Key points

- Congenital pigmented lesions that are stable, regular, flat, and asymptomatic (i.e., not bleeding, discharging, inflamed, or affecting vision) are likely to be benign.
- Acquired pigmented lesions that are growing, irregular, elevated, or symptomatic (e.g., bleeding, itchy, painful, inflamed) are more likely to be malignant.
- Specialist consultation and advice should be sought for all potentially malignant and premalignant lesions.

Nonpigmented conjunctival lesions

Benign

Papilloma

Pedunculated form

This form is common from teenage years onward, associated with human papilloma virus (HPV) 6 and HPV 11. Papillomas most commonly arise from palebral, forniceal, or caruncular conjunctiva and are often bilateral and multiple.

They often resolve spontaneously, but cryotherapy may be used for large or persistent lesions.

Sessile form

This form is common in middle age. Lesions most commonly arise from bulbar or limbal conjunctiva and are usually unilateral and solitary.

Treatment is with excision.

Epibulbar choristoma

Dermoids

This is an uncommon choristoma of childhood; it is associated with Goldenhar syndrome. This is a soft yellow limbal mass, which is usually unilateral; it may encircle the limbus.

Dermoids can be excised with a lamellar graft if they are limbal but if forniceal they require a CT scan to rule out intraorbital and intracranial extension.

Lipodermoid

This uncommon choristoma of adults is a soft white mass at the lateral canthus.

Pyogenic granuloma

Typically, a rapidly growing red vascular mass occurs after previous trauma or surgery.

Premalignant

Conjunctival intraepithelial neoplasia (carcinoma in situ, dysplasia)

These lesions are rare; they are more common over age 50 years. They may transform into squamous cell carcinoma. They appear as a fleshy, freely moving mass with tufted vessels located at the limbus.

Treatment is with excision + MMC ± cryotherapy to affected limbus.

Malignant

Conjunctival squamous cell carcinoma

This is the most common malignant conjunctival tumor worldwide but is rare in temperate climates. It is more common over 50 years of age. UV light and HPV are risk factors, and it may be associated with HIV in younger patients. It may arise from intraepithelial hyperplasia or de novo.

Clinical

There is persistent unilateral keratoconjunctivitis, atypical "dysplastic" epithelium, and a limbal gelatinous mass, which may infiltrate the cornea and sclera and penetrate the globe. It rarely metastasizes.

Treatment

Treatment is with excision (2–3 mm clear margins) + MMC and double freeze-thaw cryotherapy to margins or enucleation or exenteration (if very advanced).

Conjunctival Kaposi sarcoma

This is typically a bright red mass, usually in the inferior fornix, which may mimic a persistent subconjunctival hemorrhage. It may be caused by HHV8 (commonly in the presence of HIV).

Treatment is with focal radiotherapy if it is large or aggressive.

Conjunctival lymphoma

This is typically a salmon-pink subconjunctival infiltrate, often bilateral. Histology is essential as it may be benign or malignant. Most commonly, it represents extranodal non-Hodgkin's lymphoma, although it may also arise in the orbit (anterior spread) or in mucosal associated lymphoid tissue (MALToma).

Treatment is with excision ± local radiotherapy.

Mucoepidermoid carcinoma

This is a very rare, aggressive tumor that may mimic a pterygium. It arises from conjunctival mucus-secreting cells and squamous cells.

Infiltration from lid tumors

Sebaceous cell carcinoma of the lid may spread to involve the conjunctiva, thus it presents as a unilateral cicatrizing conjunctivitis (lid tumors, p. 115).

Key point
- Specialist consultation and advice should be sought for all potentially malignant and premalignant lesions.

Cornea

Anatomy and physiology

The cornea acts as a clear refractive surface and a protective barrier to infection and trauma. Its anterior surface is elliptical (11.7 mm horizontally, 10.6 mm vertically), whereas its posterior surface is circular (11.7 mm). It is thinnest centrally (520 μm) and thicker peripherally (660 μm).

Anatomy

The cornea consists of five layers. From anterior to posterior, these are as follows:

Epithelium

This is a nonkeratinized stratified squamous epithelium (5–7 cell layers thick), which accounts for around 10% of the thickness of the adult cornea. It is of ectodermal origin. Only the columnar basal cells are capable of the cell division required to replenish the continual desquamation of superficial cells from the anterior surface.

Basement membrane zone

The basement membrane (BM) zone consists of the epithelial BM and Bowman's layer, which is a thin, avascular, superficial stromal layer of collagen fibrils. It is also of ectodermal origin. It is unable to regenerate and thus heals by scarring.

Stroma

The stroma accounts for around 80% of corneal thickness. Despite active deturgence, its main component is water (75%). Of its dry weight, 70% is collagen (types I, IV, V, VI), and the remainder is proteogylcan ground substance (chrondroitin sulfate and keratan sulfate).

Keratocytes are a resident population of modified fibroblasts involved in remodeling after injury. The stroma is of mesodermal origin.

Descemet's membrane

Descemet's membrane consists of a fetal anterior banded zone (present at birth) and a posterior nonbanded zone (produced later by the endothelium). It is of mesodermal origin. It is not capable of regeneration.

Endothelium

This is a monolayer of hexagonal cells forming a continuous mosaic that is best seen with spectral microscopy. It is of mesodermal origin. It is unable to regenerate. Cell loss with age is compensated by enlargement (polymegathism) and migration of neighboring cells.

Physiology

Corneal transparency

Corneal transparency is dependent on the following:

- Active deturgence. The *endothelium* is relatively permeable. A passive flow of water and nutrients from the aqueous is drawn across into the stroma ("stromal swelling pressure"). To prevent overload (edema) and maintain its transparency, the endothelium pumps Na^+ back out into the aqueous by active $Na^+K^+ATPase$, together with a passive movement of water. Water may also pass through hormonally

mediated aquaporins. The *epithelium* is relatively impermeable because of the presence of apical tight junctions.
- Regular orientation and spacing of stromal collagen fibers. This reduces diffractive scatter of light. After injury, loss of architecture may result in opacity and scarring.

Refraction
The cornea acts as a biconcave lens accounting for 70% of the eye's total dioptric power. The radii of curvature of the anterior surface is 7.68 mm, the posterior surface is 6.8 mm. The cornea is a robust elastic surface. Its shape is maintained by structural rigidity and intraocular pressure.

Nutrition and nerve supply
The cornea is avascular and relies on diffusion from the limbus and aqueous for nutrition. Langerhans cells (antigen-presenting cells) are present in the epithelium but are usually restricted to the outer third. The first division of the trigeminal nerve forms stromal and subepithelial plexi, responsible for corneal sensation.

Corneal signs

Table 7.1 Epithelial signs and their pathophysiology

Sign	Pathology	Causes
Punctate epithelial erosions	Multiple fine areas of epithelial loss; stain well with fluorescein, poorly with RB	• *Superior*—e.g., vernal keratoconjunctivitis, superior limbic keratitis, floppy eyelid syndrome, poor contact lens fit • Interpalpebral—e.g., keratoconjunctivitis sicca, ultraviolet exposure, corneal anesthesia • Inferior—e.g., blepharitis, exposure keratopathy, ectropion, poor blink, poor Bell's phenomenon, rosacea, drop toxicity
Corneal filaments	Mucus strands coated with epithelial cells adherent to cornea; stain poorly with fluorescein, well with RB	Keratoconjunctivitis sicca, recurrent erosion syndrome, corneal anesthesia, exposure keratopathy, herpes zoster ophthalmicus
Punctate epithelial keratitis	Tiny white spots of epithelial and inflammatory cells; stains poorly with fluorescein, well with RB	• Viral keratitis (adenovirus, HSV, molluscum contagiosum) • Thygeson's superficial punctate keratopathy
Epithelial edema	Loss of luster + translucency; microvesicles and bullae	↑IOP, postoperative, contact lens over wear, aphakic/pseudophakic bullous keratopathy, Fuchs' endothelial dystrophy, trauma, acute hydrops, herpetic keratitis, congenital corneal clouding

RB, rose bengal.

Table 7.2 Iron lines (best visualized with cobalt blue light on slit lamp)

Line	Location	Causes
Ferry's	At trabeculectomy margin, so usually superior	Trabeculectomy
Stocker's	At pterygium margin, so usually lateral	Pterygium
Hudson–Stahli	Usually horizontal inferior 1/3 of cornea	Dry eye syndrome (common in elderly)
Fleischer	Ring around base of cone, so usually inferocentral	Keratoconus

Table 7.3 Stromal signs and their pathophysiology

Sign	Pathology	Causes
Pannus	Subepithelial fibrovascular in-growth	Trachoma, tight contact lens, phlyctenule, herpetic keratitis, rosacea keratitis, chemical keratopathy, marginal keratitis, vernal keratoconjunctivitis, atopic keratoconjunctivitis, superior limbal keratoconjunctivitis
Stromal infiltrate	Focal opacification due to leukocyte aggregations (sterile) or microbial colonization	*Sterile*—marginal keratitis, contact lens related *Infective*—bacteria, fungi, viruses, protozoa
Stromal edema	Thickened, gray opaque stroma	Postoperative, keratoconus, Fuchs' endothelial dystrophy, herpetic disciform keratitis
Cornea farinata	Deep stromal faint flour-like opacities	Idiopathic (innocuous)
Crocodile shagreen	Reticular polygonal network of stromal opacity	Idiopathic (innocuous)

Table 7.4 Endothelial signs and their pathophysiology

Sign	Pathology	Causes
Descemet's folds	Folds in intact DM	Postoperative, ↓IOP, disciform keratitis, congenital syphilis
Descemet's breaks	Breaks through DM with associated edema of overlying stroma	Birth trauma (vertical), keratoconus/keratoglobus (hydrops), infantile glaucoma (Haab's striae—horizontal)
Guttata	Wart-like protuberances at endothelium	*Peripheral:* Hassell–Henle bodies (physiological in the elderly) *Central:* Fuchs' endothelial dystrophy
Pigment on endothelium	Dusting of pigment from iris on endothelium	Pigment dispersion syndrome (Krukenberg spindle), pseudoexfoliation syndrome, postoperative, trauma
Keratic precipitates	Aggregates of inflammatory cells on endothelium	Keratitis (e.g., disciform, microbial, marginal) Anterior uveitis (e.g., idiopathic, HLA-B27, Fuchs' heterochromic cyclitis, sarcoidosis, etc.)

DM, Descemet's membrane.

Corneal diagrams

Accurate documentation of corneal disease is important for assessing disease progression and response to treatment. Pictorial representation is generally easiest. Note height, width, and depth of any lesions and any areas of corneal thickening or thinning.

Using standardized shading schemes can be useful (Fig. 7.1), but since a number of different schemes have been described, include additional identifying labels to prevent any misunderstanding.

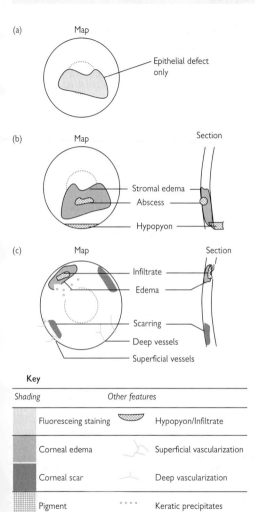

Figure 7.1 a) Corneal abrasion, b) microbial keratitis, and c) marginal keratitis.

Microbial keratitis: assessment

This is a common sight-threatening treatable ophthalmic emergency. Common pitfalls include delay in diagnosis, inappropriate sample collection for Gram stain and culture, injudicious or inadequate therapy, drug toxicity, and delayed follow-up, all of which may result in a suboptimal visual outcome.

Table 7.5 Risk factors for microbial keratitis

Ocular	Trauma	Corneal abrasion
	Contact lens	Extended wear > soft > daily disposable > rigid gas permeable; poor hygiene
	Iatrogenic	Corneal surgery (e.g., LASIK) Removal of suture Loose suture Long-term topical steroids and antibiotics
	Ocular surface disease	Dry eyes Bullous keratopathy Chronic blepharoconjunctivitis Corneal anesthesia Chronic keratitis (e.g., HSV) Cicatricial disease
	Lid disease	Entropion Lagophthalmos Trichiasis
	Nasolacrimal disease	Chronic dacryocystitis
Systemic	Immunosuppression	Drugs Immunodeficiency syndromes Diabetes Rheumatoid arthritis
	Nutritional	Vitamin A deficiency

Clinical features
- Pain, FB sensation, redness, photophobia, tearing, discharge (may be purulent), ↓VA.
- Circumlimbal/diffuse injection, single, or multiple foci of white opacity within stroma ± edema, usually associated epithelial defect and anterior uveitis.
- *Complications:* limbal and scleral extension, corneal perforation, endophthalmitis, panophthalmitis.

Investigations
Perform early and adequate corneal scraping for Gram stain and culture. (Box 7.1).

If the patient wears contact lenses, send lenses, solutions, and cases for culture, and inform patient that these items will likely be destroyed.

Consult with a microbiologist, especially regarding length of incubation and antibiotic sensitivities required, and if there are unusual clinical features.

Box 7.1 How to perform a corneal infiltrate culture

- Instill preservative-free topical anesthesia (and perform scrape prior to use of fluorescein).
- Use a Kimura spatula, No. 15 blade or 25-gauge needle.
- Scrape both the base and leading edge of the ulcer (from uninvolved to involved cornea).
- Place material onto glass slide for microscopy and staining (Gram stain, Ziehl–Neelsen, methenamine silver, etc.)
- Plate onto blood agar (aerobes), chocolate agar (*Neisseria, Hemophilus*), and Sabouraud agar (fungi), and consider non-nutrient *E. coli*–enriched agar (if acanthamoeba suspected). When plating small samples, rows of C-streaks are more effective than the traditional technique.
- Consider also culture in thioglycolate (anaerobes) and enrichment (bacteria) broths.

Table 7.6 Microbiological processing of corneal scrapes

Routine stains	Gram stain	B	F	A
Additional stains	Giemsa stain	B	F	A
	Gomori/methenamine silver		F	A
	PAS		F	A
	Calcofluor white		F	A
	Ziehl–Neelson				M N
Routine media	Blood agar	B		
	Chocolate agar	B		
	Sabouraud's dextrose agar		F	
	Thioglycolate broth	B (an)		
Additional media	Lowenstein–Jensen				M N
	Non-nutrient *E. coli*–enriched agar			A

B, bacteria; B(an), anaerobic bacteria; F, fungi; A, acanthamoeba; M, mycobacteria; N, nocardia.

Table 7.7 Common bacterial causes of keratitis

		Frequency	Penetration of intact epithelium	Virulence
Gram positive	*Staphylococcus aureus*	Common	−	+
	Staphylococcus epidermis	Common	−	+/−
	Streptococcus pneumonia	Common	−	++
Gram negative	*Pseudomonas aeruginosa*	↑ in contact lens wearers	−	+++
	Neisseria gonorrhoea	↑ in neonates	+	+++
	Haemophilus	↑ in children	+	+

Microbial keratitis: treatment

The treatment of microbial keratitis can be divided into a sterilization phase followed by a healing phase. During the sterilization phase, appropriate topical antibiotics are administered intensively. Once the ulcer is thought to be sterile, topical corticosteroids may be added to reduce scarring.

Initial treatment

- Stop contact lens wear.
- Admit patient if there is severe infection, poor compliance, or other concerns.

> **Box 7.2 Indications for admission**
>
> - Severe infection: >1.5 mm diameter infiltrate, hypopyon, purulent exudate, or complicated disease.
> - Poor compliance likely: either with administering drops or returning for daily review.
> - Other concerns: monocular, failing to improve, etc.

> **Box 7.3 Dual therapy vs. monotherapy in empirical treatment of microbial keratitis**
>
> - *Dual therapy*: commonly "fortified" preparations of a cephalosporin (cefuroxime 5%) with an aminoglycoside (e.g., gentamicin 1.5%—beware of toxicity) or a fluoroquinolones (e.g., ofloxacin). Penicillin 0.3% may be substituted for the cephalosporin if streptococcal infection is suspected.
> - *Monotherapy* with fluoroquinolones (e.g., ofloxacin) may be adequate for most cases of microbial keratitis but is insufficient for resistant species of *Staphylococcus aureus* and *Pseudomonas aeruginosa*.

- Consider oral antibiotics: if there is a limbal lesion or corneal perforation, then add in systemic fluoroquinolone therapy (e.g., oral ciprofloxacin 750 mg 2×/day).
- Cycloplegia (e.g., cyclopentolate 1% 2×/day) for photophobia and ciliary spasm and oral analgesia if the patient has severe pain.

Ongoing treatment

- Monitor response and progression daily (inpatient and outpatient) by degree of injection, size of epithelial defect (measure on slit lamp), size of infiltrate, extent of corneal edema, and degree of anterior uveitis. Taper frequency and switch to nonfortified preparations with clinical improvement.
- If initial culture results show no growth and current regimen proves clinically ineffective, consider withholding treatment for 24 hours

before rescraping and biopsying the cornea. The original slides can be restained to identify less common organisms (e.g., mycobacteria, fungi).
• Consider topical steroids. Use carefully following re-epithelialization, and in the presence of sterile culture, to reduce stromal scarring and possibly improve visual outcome. Steroid initiation requires frequent (often inpatient) follow-up.

Treatment of complications

Persistent epithelial defect

If epithelial defect persists for >2 weeks, then consider switching to preservative-free preparations of topical medication, reducing frequency of topical medication, prescribe ocular lubrication, and assisting lid closure.

Resistant or progressive keratitis

Seek specialist consultation and advice. In threatened scleral extension, consider oral ciprofloxacin, which has high bioavailability at the limbus. In patients with threatened corneal perforation, consider oral ciprofloxacin, bandage contact lens (± cyanoacrylate glue), or emergency penetrating keratoplasty (PK).

Endophthalmitis

Perform diagnostic vitrectomy and administer intravitreal antibiotics (p. 282).

Microbial keratitis: acanthamoeba

Isolated from soil, dust, sea, fresh and chlorinated water, acanthamoeba are ubiquitous free-living protozoa. Capable of encystment in unfavorable conditions, the organism can survive extreme temperatures, desiccation, and pH.

Acanthamoeba keratitis remains rare (0.1–0.2 per million persons in the United States), but its incidence is rising with increased contact lens use. It is largely resistant to normal first-line broad-spectrum antibiotics, and late suspicion and diagnosis can lead to devastating and irrevocable corneal scarring.

Risk factors

- *Contact lens (CL) wear:* especially with extended-wear CL, poor CL hygiene (e.g., rinsing in tap water), or after swimming with CL (ponds, hot tubs, swimming pools).
- *Corneal trauma:* notably in a rural or agricultural setting.

Clinical features

- *Variable:* ranges from asymptomatic, FB sensation, ↓VA, or tearing to severe pain (disproportionate to often relatively mild clinical findings).
- Epithelial ridges, pseudo- and true dendrites; stromal infiltrates (may progress circumferentially to form a ring); perineural infiltrates; ↓ corneal sensation.
- *Complications:* limbal and scleral extension, corneal perforation, intractable scleritis.

Investigation

- Perform early and adequate corneal cultures (Box 7.1). The epithelium is often fairly loose, and some clinicians deliberately debride all affected epithelium.

If the patient wears contact lenses, send lenses, solutions, and cases for culture, and inform patient that they will be destroyed.

- *Stains:* Gram (stains organisms), Giemsa (stains the organism and cysts), Calcofluor white (stains cysts visualized under UV light); also send a sample to histology (in formalin).
- *Culture:* non-nutrient agar with *E. coli* overlay, at 25° and 37°C, may require up to 14 days.

If there is strong clinical suspicion but there are negative cultures, consider immunofluorescent assay, electron microscopy, or PCR. Also consider stopping treatment for 24–48 hours and performing corneal biopsy.

Treatment

Initial treatment

- Consider inpatient admission.
- Stop contact lens wear (culture lenses, solutions, cases).
- Intensive topical antiamoebic agents, commonly a biguanide (PHMB 0.02% or chlorhexidine) and an aromatic diamidine (e.g., propamidine isethionate 0.1% or hexamidine) administered hourly. Aminoglycosides or imidazoles may give additional benefit.
- Oral analgesia and cycloplegia.

Ongoing treatment
- Taper treatment according to clinical improvement. Clinical relapse is common and may signify incomplete sterilization of active acanthamoeba trophozites or reactivation of resistant intrastromal cysts. Treatment is prolonged (20–40 weeks).
- Consider cautious use of topical steroids (while continuing anti-amoebic agents) to reduce corneal scarring.

Treatment of complications
- If scleritis: consider aggressive scleral resection and prolonged treatment of the infection.
- If poor visual outcome: consider PK once treatment is completed and cornea is sterile.
- If severe, intractable pain: patients may occasionally require enucleation for severe pain.

Prevention
Patient education can reduce or eliminate risk factors identified in more than 90% of cases of acanthomoeba keratitis.

Table 7.8 Antiamoebic agents

Class	Mechanism	Examples
Aminoglycosides	Inhibit protein synthesis	Neomycin; paramonycin
Aromatic diamidines	Inhibit DNA synthesis	Propamidine isethionate (brolene); hexamidine
Biguanide	Inhibit function of membrane	Polyhexamethylene biguanide (PHMB); chlorhexidine
Imidazoles	Destabilize cell wall	Clotrimazole; fluconazole; ketoconazole

Fungal keratitis

The most common pathogens are *Fusarium* and *Aspergillus* (filamentous fungi) in warmer climates and *Candida* (a yeast) in cooler climates.

Risk factors

Risk factors include trauma (including LASIK), immunosuppression (e.g., topical corticosteroids, alcoholism, diabetes), ocular surface disease, and contamination with organic matter.

Clinical features

- Variable: onset ranges from insidious to rapid; pain, photophobia, tearing.
- Gray elevated infiltrate with feathery edges ± satellite lesions ± epithelial defect.
- *Complications:* limbal and scleral extension, corneal perforation, endophthalmitis (p. 404).

Investigation

- Perform early and adequate corneal culture (Box 7.1).
- *Stains:* Gram (stains fungal walls), Giemsa (stains walls and cytoplasm); Grocott's methenamine silver (GMS), periodic acid–Schiff (PAS), and Calcofluor white may also be used.
- *Culture:* Sabouraud's dextrose agar (for most fungi) and blood agar (for *Fusarium*); may require up to 14 days. In vitro sensitivities are poorly predictive of in vivo sensitivity and so is little used clinically.

If there is strong clinical suspicion but there are negative investigations, consider corneal biopsy.

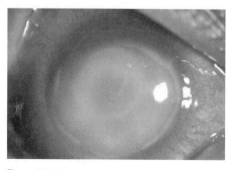

Figure 7.2 Fungal corneal ulcer with central necrotic infected corneal tissue with peripheral stromal infiltration. See insert for color version.

Treatment

Initial treatment

- Consider inpatient admission.
- Intensive topical broad-spectrum antifungal agents (e.g., econazole 1% or natamycin 5% hourly). For severe or unresponsive disease, add a second agent (e.g., amphotericin 0.15% for *Candida*, clotrimazole 1% for *Aspergillus*). Where a systemic antifungal is required, oral administration of either fluconazole and itraconazole will reach therapeutic levels in the cornea.
- Avoid corticosteroids (reduce or stop them if patient is already on them).
- Oral analgesia and cycloplegia.

Ongoing treatment

- Taper treatment according to clinical improvement. Clinical relapse is common and may signify incomplete sterilization or reactivation.
- Consider PK for progressive disease (to remove fungus or prevent perforation) or in the quiet but visually compromised eye.

Table 7.9 Antifungal agents

Class	Mechanism	Examples
Polyene	Destabilize cell wall	Natamycin, amphotericin
Imidazole	Destabilize cell wall	Clotrimazole, econazole
Triazole	Destabilize cell wall	Itraconazole, voriconazole
Pyrimidine	Cytotoxic	Flucytosine

Herpes simplex keratitis

The herpes simplex virus (HSV) is a double-stranded DNA virus with two serotypes. Herpes simplex virus 1 (HSV1) shows airborne transmission and classically causes infection of the eyes, face, and trunk; herpes simplex virus 2 (HSV2) infection is sexually transmitted and usually causes genital herpes with rare ophthalmic involvement.

Primary infection is usually blepharoconjunctivitis, occasionally with corneal involvement (Fig. 7.3). Following this, the virus ascends the sensory nerve axon to reside in latency in the trigeminal ganglion.

Viral reactivation, replication, and retrograde migration to the cornea results in recurrent keratitis, which may be epithelial, stromal, endothelial (discoid), or neurotrophic. Potential intraocular involvement includes anterior uveitis, retinal vasculitis and retinitis.

Blepharoconjunctivitis

HSV1 infection is common (90% of the population are seropositive). Primary infection occurs in childhood with generalized viral malaise and is usually ophthalmologically silent. The most common ocular manifestation is a self-limiting blepharoconjunctivitis characterized by periorbital vesicular rash, follicular conjunctivitis, and preauricular lymphadenopathy.

HSV keratitis in primary infection is rare. Prophylactic topical acyclovir ointment 5×/day or oral acyclovir prophylaxis may be considered.

Epithelial keratitis

Clinical features

- FB sensation, pain, blurred vision, lacrimation.
- Superficial punctate keratitis → stellate erosion → dendritic ulcer (branching morphology with terminal bulbs cf. pseudodendrites) → geographic ulcer (large amoeboid ulcer with dendritic advancing edges; more common with immunosuppression or topical steroids). Ulcer base stains with fluorescein (de-epithelized); ulcer margins stain with rose bengal (devitalized viral-infected epithelial cells); ↓ corneal sensation.
- Systemic: may have associated orofacial or genital ulceration.

Investigation

This is usually a clinical diagnosis but when there is diagnostic uncertainty, investigate both for viral and other microbial (p. 166) causes.

- Conjunctival and corneal swabs (viral transport medium): culture, PCR and ELISA.
- Corneal scrapings: Giemsa stain (multinuclear giant cells).

Treatment

- *Topical antiviral:* trifluridine 1% 8×/day (watch for epithelial toxicity after 1 week fo therapy), acyclovir 3% drops initially 5×/day gradually tapering down but continued for at least 3 days after complete healing; if resistant, consider ganciclovir 0.15% gel initially 5×/day.
- Consider cycloplegia (e.g., cyclopentolate 1% 2×/day) for comfort and AC activity.

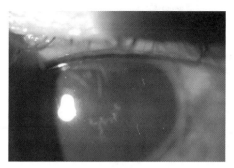

Figure 7.3 Herpetic keratitis with corneal dendrites and superficial fluorescein staining. See insert for color version.

The Herpetic Eye Disease Study (HEDS) findings showed that treatment of patients with epithelial keratitis with oral acyclovir does not reduce the rate of stromal disease or iritis. If the patient is on topical steroids for coexistent ocular disease, reduce steroid dose (potency and frequency) when possible but do not stop until epithelium has healed.

When HSV keratitis is occurring in a corneal graft, reduction of topical steroids may increase the risk of graft rejection. If there are recurrent attacks, consider prophylactic treatment with oral antivirals (e.g., acyclovir 400 mg PO 2×/day), since long-term suppressive therapy reduces the rate of recurrent HSV epithelial keratits and stromal kerattis.

Stromal keratitis

Stromal keratitis occurs in a relatively superficial form or rare but much more severe necrotizing interstitial keratitis. It may occur with or without epithelial ulceration. Future recurrences may be more likely than epithelial disease.

Clinical features
- Multiple or diffuse opacities → corneal vascularization, lipid exudation, and scarring; or may → thinning; AC activity.
- Complications: ↑IOP; rarely perforation.

Treatment
- *Topical steroid:* defer until epithelium is intact; aim for minimum effective dose (e.g., prednisolone 0.1–1% 1–4×/day titrating down in frequency and strength).
- *Antiviral:* acyclovir, either systemic (initially 400 mg 5×/day, then reduce; prophylactic dose is 400 mg 2×/day) or topical (3% drops 5×/day); systemic acyclovir is preferred, especially with atopic keratoconjunctivitis, ocular surface disease, or frequent recurrences.
- Cycloplegia (e.g., cyclopentolate 1% 2×/day) for comfort or AC activity.

- Monitor IOP and treat as necessary.
- Surgery may be indicated acutely for perforation (tectonic graft) or in the long term for scarring (usually PK).

Disciform keratitis (endotheliitis)

Disciform keratitis probably results from viral antigen hypersensitivity rather than reactivation.

Clinical features

- Painless ↓VA, halo.
- Central/paracentral disc of corneal edema, Descemet's folds, mild AC activity, fine keratic precipitates (KP); Wessely ring (stromal halo of precipitated viral antigen/host antibody).
- *Complications:* ↑IOP, chronic anterior uveitis.

Treatment

- *Topical steroid:* defer (when possible) until epithelium is intact; aim for minimum effective dose (e.g., prednisolone acetate 0.1–1% 1–4×/day titrating down in frequency and strength); some patients may require low dose (e.g., prednisolone 0.1% alt −1×/day) for months or even maintenance.
- *Antiviral:* acyclovir either systemic (as above) or topical (3% drops 5×/day until ≥3 days after complete healing); continue as prophylaxis (can ↓ frequency) until on low frequency or low-strength topical steroid.
- Cycloplegia (e.g., cyclopentolate 1% 2×/day) for comfort/AC activity.
- Monitor IOP and treat as necessary (p. 380).

Herpes zoster ophthalmicus

The varicella zoster virus (VZV) is a double-stranded DNA virus of the herpes group. Primary infection of VZV results in chicken pox (varicella). Reactivation of virus dormant in the sensory ganglion results in shingles (herpes zoster) of the innervated dermatome. Involvement of the ophthalmic branch of the trigeminal nerve occurs in 15% of shingles cases and results in herpes zoster ophthalmicus (HZO).

Transmission is by direct contact or droplet spread. Those never previously infected with VZV may contract chicken pox from contact with shingles. VZV infection may be more severe in the immunosuppressed, the elderly, pregnant women, and neonates. Maternal infection may also cause fetal malformations (3% risk in first trimester).

Systemic and cutaneous disease

Clinical features

These include viral prodrome, preherpetic neuralgia (mild intermittent tingling to severe constant electric pain), rash (papules → vesicles → pustules → scabs) predominantly within the V1 dermatome; Hutchinson's sign (cutaneous involvement of tip of the nose, indicating nasociliary nerve involvement and likelihood of ocular complications). They may be disseminated in the immunocompromised.

Treatment

• *Systemic antiviral:* start as soon as rash appears either acyclovir PO 800 mg 5×/day for 7–10 days, valacyclovir PO 1 g 3×/day for 7 days, or famciclovir PO 500 mg 3×/day for 7 days. If immunosuppressed, then give acyclovir IV 10 mg/kg q8h.

Postherpetic neuralgia may cause depression (even suicide); treatments include amitriptyline, gabapentin, and topical capsaicin cream.

Keratitis

Clinical features

• *Epithelial:* superficial punctate keratitis + pseudodendrites often with anterior stromal infiltrates; acute (onset 2–3 days after rash; resolve in few weeks); common.
• *Stromal:* nummular keratitis with anterior stromal granular deposits is uncommon and occurs early. Necrotizing interstitial keratitis with stromal infiltrates, thinning, and even perforation (cf. HSV) is rare and occurs late.
• *Disciform:* endotheliitis with disc of corneal edema, Descemet's folds, mild AC activity, fine KPs (cf HSV); late onset; chronic; uncommon.
• *Neurotrophic:* corneal nerve damage causes persistent epithelial defect, thinning, and even perforation; late onset; chronic; uncommon.
• *Mucus plaques:* linear gray elevations loosely adherent to underlying diseased epithelium/stroma; late onset; chronic.

Treatment

Ensure adequate systemic antiviral treatment.

- *Epithelial:* topical lubricants, usually preservative free (e.g., Celluvisc 8×/day).
- *Stromal and disciform:* topical steroid treatment (e.g., prednisolone acetate 0.1–1% 1–4×/day titrating down in frequency and strength); some patients may require low dose (e.g., prednisolone 0.1% alt –1×/ day) for months or even maintenance. Threatened perforation may require gluing, bandage contact lens, or tectonic grafting.
- *Neurotrophic:* preservative-free topical lubricants (e.g., Celluvisc 8×/day + Lacrilube nightly) and consider tarsorrhaphy (surgical or with botulinum toxin–induced ptosis), amniotic membrane graft, or conjunctival flap.
- Mucus plaques require mucolytics (e.g., acetylcysteine g 3×/day).
- Anterior uveitis: topical steroid treatment and cycloplegia (e.g., cyclopentolate 1% 2×/day) for comfort and AC activity.
- Monitor IOP. Assess whether it is due to inflammation or steroids and treat accordingly.
- Corneal scarring: axial scarring may require PK.

Other complications associated with HZO

Ocular complications include conjunctivitis, glaucoma, anterior uveitis, necrotizing retinitis (ARN, PORN), episcleritis, scleritis, optic neuritis, and cranial nerve palsies.

Systemic complications include strokes (cerebral vasculitis) and neuralgia.

Thygeson's superficial punctate keratopathy

This is a rare condition, most commonly arising in young adulthood. It may last anywhere from 1 month to years. The etiology is idiopathic, but a viral cause is suspected. It is bilateral but often asymmetric.

Clinical features
- Bilateral recurrent FB sensation, photophobia, and tearing.
- Coarse, stellate gray-white epithelial opacities in a white quiet eye. The opacities appear slightly elevated but are classically nonstaining with fluorescein or rose bengal. There may be a slight epithelial haze.

Treatment
Give topical corticosteroids (e.g., fluorometholone [FML] 0.1%), which can be rapidly tapered; sometimes a mild maintenance dose (even 1×/week) is required to prevent further episodes.

Consider therapeutic contact lens for vision and comfort.

Recurrent erosion syndrome

As clinical features may have resolved by the time the patient sees an ophthalmologist, a provisional diagnosis of recurrent erosion syndrome (RES) may be made on history alone. RES is indicative of failure of epithelial to basement membrane adhesion.

Risk factors
- Trauma.
- Corneal dystrophy: anterior (especially epithelial basement membrane dystrophy and Reis–Buckler dystrophy) or stromal dystrophies.
- Post-keratoplasty.
- Diabetes.

Clinical features
- Recurrent episodes of severe pain and photophobia usually upon opening eyes after sleep; aggravated by blinking; history of corneal trauma (often forgotten). Patients may be extremely distressed and may become obsessive about it.
- Variable degree of epithelial irregularities or defects. Patients may also have signs of underlying disease, e.g., microcysts, maps, dots, fingerprints, or stromal changes.

Treatment

Acute erosion

Give supportive therapy with topical lubricants. Consider epithelial debridement if heaped up, devitalized epithelium: anesthetize cornea, gently break away nonadherent gray epithelium with moistened cotton tip applicator, or sponge. Use post-procedure topical antibiotic.

Prophylaxis

Give topical lubricants (e.g., carbomer gel 4×/day with lacrilube nightly for 3 months). Stress importance of continuation of treatment after symptomatic resolution.

In refractory or severe cases, consider extended-wear therapeutic contact lens (for ≥2 months), anterior stromal micropuncture, or excimer laser epithelial keratectomy. Anterior stromal micropuncture aims to induce epithelial adhesion through scarring. Consider its use in resistant, symptomatic RES outside the visual axis. It is performed at the slit lamp (if cooperative patient) or in minor procedure room with topical anesthesia, and using a bent 25 gauge needle to cover the defective area with closely packed micropunctures through epithelium and Bowmans layer.

Tetracyclines (e.g., doxycycline 100 mg 1×/day for 3 months) with topical steroids may be beneficial, since they inhibit matrix metalloproteinase activity and promote epithelial stability. Tetracyclines are, however, contraindicated in children under age 12, in pregnant or breast-feeding women, or in patients with hepatic or renal impairment.

Corneal degenerative disease (1)

Arcus

This is a common, bilateral, degeneration secondary to progressive deposition of lipid in the peripheral stroma. It is usually age related but may be associated with hyperlipidemia.

Causes

Most bilateral cases have no systemic association, but hyperlipidemia (notably type II) should be ruled out in those presenting at a young age (arcus juvenilis). Unilateral arcus is rare and may signify contralateral carotid compromise or previous ocular hypotony.

Clinical features

Progressive peripheral opacity starts (and remains thickest) at 3 o'clock and 9 o'clock but spreads circumferentially to form a complete ring of around 1 mm thickness. Typically the central margin is blurred but the peripheral margin is sharp, thereby leaving a zone of clear perilimbal cornea (which may show thinning: a senile furrow).

Cornea farinata

This is a bilateral symmetrical degeneration of deep stromal, faint flour-like opacities that are prominent centrally but remain visually insignificant.

Crocodile shagreen

A faint reticular polygonal network of stromal opacities resembles crocodile skin. Anterior stromal shagreen is more common than posterior but both forms are innocuous and asymptomatic.

Vogt's limbal girdle

This is a common bilateral degeneration. There is chalky white peripheral corneal deposition at 3 o'clock and 9 o'clock. It may be separated from the limbus by a clear perilimbal zone (type I) or it may extend to the limbus (type II). Both types are innocuous and asymptomatic.

Primary lipid keratopathy

A rare, idiopathic corneal deposition of cholesterol, fat, and phospholipids appears as yellow-white stromal deposits with no associated vascularization. This condition is usually innocuous and nonprogressive and requires no treatment.

Secondary lipid keratopathy

Causes

This may accompany corneal vascularization following ocular injury or inflammation. Common causes include previous herpetic (simplex or zoster disciform) keratitis, trauma, uveitis, and interstitial keratitis.

Clinical features

Corneal vascularization has associated yellow-white stromal deposition.

Treatment

Treat underlying cause of ocular inflammation. Long-term mild cortico-steroid (e.g., fluorometholone) is occasionally useful. Consider feeder vessel occlusion or PK.

- Occlusion of the feeder vessel may be done by argon laser photocoagulation or direct needle point cautery under the operating microscope. Anterior segment fluorescein angiography may help identify the feeder vessel.
- Penetrating keratoplasty is performed if the disease is severe or persistent and once the eye is quiet. However, prognosis is guarded given the poor condition of host tissue and preoperative vascularization.

Corneal degenerative disease (2)

Band keratopathy

This is a common progressive subepithelial deposition of calcium phosphate salts that may be due to ocular or systemic causes (Table 7.10).

Causes

Table 7.10 Causes of band keratopathy

Ocular	Anterior segment inflammation	Chronic anterior uveitis
		Chronic keratitis
		Chronic corneal edema
		Silicone oil in AC
	Phthisis bulbi	
Systemic		Primary (familial)
		Senile
		Ichthyosis
		Hypercalcemia
		Hyperphosphatemia
		Hyperuricemia
		Chronic renal failure

Clinical features
- Often asymptomatic; FB sensation, pain, ↓VA.
- White opacities starting at 3 and 9 o'clock progressing centrally to coalesce to form a band.

Treatment
- Identify and treat underlying cause as appropriate.
- Consider therapeutic contact lens for comfort (often as a temporary measure).
- Remove calcium salts by chemical chelation (disodium ethylenediamine tetra-acetic acid) followed by mechanical debridement (e.g., gentle scraping with No. 15 blade); or excimer laser keratectomy.

Salzmann nodular degeneration

This uncommon slowly progressive degeneration is usually seen as a complication of chronic keratitis. It arises from replacement of Bowman's layer by eosinophilic material.

Causes

These include trauma, chronic keratitis including trachoma, phlyctenular keratitis, vernal keratitis, interstitial keratitis; post–corneal surgery; and idiopathic causes.

Clinical features
- Glare, ↓VA, astigmatism, pain (if loss of overlying epithelium).
- Well-defined gray-white elevated nodules; iron lines (indicate chronicity). There may be associated epithelial breakthrough or discomfort.

Treatment
Identify and treat underlying keratitis. Consider lubrication, bandage contact lens, or excimer laser keratectomy.

Corneal dystrophies: anterior

Epithelial basement membrane dystrophy (map-dot-fingerprint dystrophy, Cogan's microcystic dystrophy)

This is the most common corneal dystrophy, with a prevalence of around 2.5%. Although there are pedigrees demonstrating autosomal dominant inheritance, most clinical presentations appear to be nonfamilial. There is a slight female predilection. It usually presents in early adulthood.

Pathophysiology

The basic defect appears to lie in epithelium–basement membrane interaction. In the absence of normal desmosomes and anchoring fibrils, there is continued secretion and intraepithelial extension of basement membrane (maps), degeneration of sequestered epithelial cells (dots or microcysts), and deposition of fibrillar material (fingerprints).

Clinical features

- Bilateral, asymmetrical; may be asymptomatic; but recurrent erosions in 10–33% (pain, lacrimation, photophobia).
- Epithelial maps (faint opacities), dots/microcysts, fingerprints (curvilinear ridges).

Treatment

Treatment is the same as for recurrent erosion syndrome (RES) (p. 180).

Reis–Buckler dystrophy

This is a relatively common autosomal dominant, progressive dystrophy. It usually presents with recurrent erosions in early childhood. With age these become less painful (because of ↓ corneal sensation) but central opacity may lead to ↓VA.

Pathophysiology

This is caused by a mutation in the keratoepithilin gene *BIGH3* (Ch5q). There is progressive degeneration of Bowman's layer with subepithelial collagen deposition (stains blue with Masson trichome). Thiel–Behnke (honeycomb dystrophy) is a similar but milder condition arising from a different mutation in *BIGH3*.

Clinical features

- Bilateral recurrent erosions (pain, lacrimation, photophobia); later ↓VA.
- Multiple subepithelial gray reticular opacities usually starting centrally.

Treatment

Treatment is as for RES (p. 180).

Consider excimer laser superficial keratectomy, or lamellar/penetrating keratoplasty if there is ↓VA.

Meesman's dystrophy

This rare autosomal dominant dystrophy usually presents in adulthood.

Pathophysiology

This is caused by mutations in the genes for keratins K3 (Ch12) and K12 (Ch17), which normally form the cytoskeleton of the epithelial cell.

Clinical features
- Initially asymptomatic; mild ocular irritation, photophobia, and mild decrease VA in adulthood.
- Discrete clear epithelial vesicles; initially central but spread peripherally (sparing the limbus).

Treatment
Treatment is not usually required; however, rarely, lamellar keratoplasty may be considered in patients with significant photophobia or visual impairment.

Corneal dystrophies: stromal (1)

Lattice dystrophy types I, II, III

These are rare autosomal dominant dystrophies involving the progressive deposition of amyloid in the corneal stroma and sometimes elsewhere in the body.

Type I is the most common form and is isolated to the eye. Type II forms part of familial systemic amyloidosis (Meretoja's syndrome). Type III is rare, isolated to the eye, and is seen in patients of Japanese origin.

Pathophysiology

Type I lattice dystrophy is caused by a mutation in the keratoepithilin gene *BIGH3* (Ch5q). Type II results from a mutation in the gene for the plasma protein gelsolin (Ch9q).

In all types, amyloid is deposited in the stroma, but in types I and II it may also disrupt the basement membrane and epithelium. Amyloid stains with Congo red and demonstrates birefringence and dichroism at polarizing microscopy.

Clinical features

- ↓VA, recurrent erosions (pain, lacrimation, photophobia).
- Bilateral (often asymmetric) criss-cross refractile lines; later these may be obscured by a progressive central corneal haze (types I and II).
  In type III the lines are thicker and more prominent. The peripheral cornea is usually spared.

Systemic features

In type II there is lattice dystrophy with familial amyloidosis (Meretoja's syndrome): mask-like facies, skin laxity, cranial nerve palsies (commonly CN VII with additional risk of corneal exposure), peripheral neuropathy, renal failure, and cardiac failure.

Treatment

Treatment is as for recurrent erosion syndrome (RES) (p. 180).

Consider PK or excimer laser keratectomy if decrease A. Recurrence after either procedure is common. If type II disease is suspected, refer to physician for assessment of systemic involvement.

Granular dystrophy

This is a rare autosomal dominant dystrophy involving deposition of hyaline material in the corneal stroma. It presents in adulthood.

Pathophysiology

Granular dystrophy is caused by a mutation in the keratoepithilin gene *BIGH3* (Ch5q). Hyaline material (probably phospholipids) deposited in the stroma stains red with Masson trichrome.

Clinical features

- ↓VA; occasionally recurrent erosions
- Bilateral (often asymmetric) white crumb-like opacities in otherwise clear stroma; initially central but progressively coalesce

Treatment

Treatment is as for recurrent erosion syndrome (RES) (p. 180).

If there is ↓VA, consider PK, or lamellar keratoplasty for relatively superficial disease. Recurrence is common.

Avellino dystrophy

This is a very rare autosomal dominant dystrophy with some features of both granular and lattice dystrophies. It is usually seen in those originating from Avellino, Italy.

Pathophysiology

Avellino dystrophy is caused by a mutation in the keratoepithilin gene *BIGH3* (Ch5q). The stromal deposit stains both for hyaline (Masson trichrome) and amyloid (Congo red; birefringence and dichroism by polarizing light microscope).

Clinical features

- ↓VA; recurrent erosions (pain, lacrimation, photophobia).
- Bilateral (often asymmetric) granular-type opacities in anterior stroma, and lattice-type lines in deeper stroma; may have a central subepithelial haze later.

Treatment

Treatment is as for recurrent erosion syndrome (RES) (p. 180).

Consider PK for ↓VA. Recurrence is common.

Corneal dystrophies: stromal (2)

Macular dystrophy

This is a rare autosomal recessive dystrophy involving deposition of a glycosaminoglycan in the stroma. Abnormal stromal collagen packing causes loss of corneal translucency, usually from early adulthood.

Pathophysiology

This is effectively an ocular-specific mucopolysaccharidosis, arising from mutations in the gene for carbohydrate sulfotransferase (*CHST6;* Ch 16q). Abnormal glycosaminoglycans similar to keratan sulfate accumulate. These stain with Alcian blue or colloidal iron. Macular dystrophy may be subclassified as type I (no keratan sulfate) and type II (low keratan sulfate).

Clinical features

- Gradual painless ↓VA; this is often an incidental finding.
- Bilateral (often asymmetric) focal ill-defined gray-white stromal opacities superimposed on diffuse clouding. It may involve the whole cornea being superficial centrally, but potentially involving full stromal thickness peripherally. The cornea may be thinned.

Treatment

If ↓VA, consider PK, or lamellar keratoplasty for relatively superficial disease. Recurrence is rare.

Schnyder's crystalline dystrophy

This is a rare progressive dystrophy presenting in childhood with an autosomal dominant inheritance pattern. Stromal crystals contain cholesterol and neutral fat (stains red with oil red O). It may be associated with systemic hypercholesterolemia.

Clinical features

- ↓VA, glare.
- Central anterior stromal yellow-white (often scintillating) crystals with associated corneal haze and arcus.

Treatment

Consider excimer laser keratectomy or PK if there is ↓VA. Recurrence may occur. Check fasting lipids.

Congenital hereditary stromal dystrophy (CHSD)

This is a very rare autosomal dystrophy that presents at birth with bilateral corneal clouding without edema. It is nonprogressive. It appears to arise from abnormalities of stromal collagen but with normal anterior and posterior corneal layers. Corneal thickness is normal.

Treatment requires penetrating keratoplasty.

Other dystrophies of the corneal stroma
- Central cloudy dystrophy: autosomal dominant, similar changes to posterior crocodile shagreen, visually insignificant.
- Fleck dystrophy: autosomal dominant, white flecks throughout stroma, visually insignificant.
- Posterior amorphous corneal dystrophy: autosomal dominant, gray sheets in deep stroma, nonprogressive, rarely visually significant.

Corneal dystrophies: posterior

Fuchs' endothelial dystrophy (FED)

This common corneal dystrophy may be autosomal dominant or sporadic. It is more commonly seen in females (F:M 4:1) and with increasing age. Presentation is usually gradual with ↓VA from middle age but may be acute after endothelial injury (e.g., intraocular surgery). There appears to be an increased incidence of primary open-angle glaucoma (POAG).

Pathogenesis

Primary endothelial dysfunction associated with $Na^+K^+ATPase$ pump failure allows the accumulation of fluid. Mutation in the gene for the collagen VIII α_2 chain has been seen in patients with FED and with posterior polymorphous corneal dystrophy (PPMD). Microscopically, there is irregular thickening of Descemet's membrane, protuberances (guttata), and flattening, irregularity in size, and loss of endothelial cells.

Clinical features

- Gradual ↓VA (often worse in morning); this may arise after intraocular surgery.
- Stage 1: corneal guttata (appear centrally cf. the peripheral Hassall–Henle bodies, which are normal with age); may extend to give beaten-metal appearance; pigment on endothelium.
- Stage 2: stromal edema → Descemet's folds and epithelial bullae.
- Stage 3: recurrent corneal erosions → subepithelial vascular pannus and stromal haze.

Investigations

Specular microscopy can show ↓cell count, ↑average cell diameter, ↓hexagons, and ↑variation in cell size.

Treatment

Relieve corneal edema and improve comfort.
- Topical hypertonic agents: 5% NaCl.
- Treat ocular hypertension.
- Warm air blown on the eyes (e.g., hair dryer) in the morning.
- Bandage contact lens for bullous change.

Visual rehabilitation

Persistent corneal opacity may require PK. In the presence of coexisting cataract, a triple procedure is performed (i.e., combined PK, lens extraction, and posterior chamber intraocular lens [PCIOL] insertion). In the absence of any stromal scarring, Descemet's stripping endothelial keratoplasty (DSEK) is an option.

Prevention

Corneal decompensation may be inadvertently accelerated by the ophthalmologist:
- *Cataract surgery:* consider 1) protecting the endothelium with additional heavy viscoelastic (soft shell technique) and minimizing phaco-time, and 2) referral of more severe cases to a corneal

specialist for elective simultaneous PK, cataract extraction, and IOL (a triple procedure). Careful patient counseling regarding risk of decompensation is essential prior to surgery.

- *Ocular hypertension/glaucoma:* topical β-blocker is preferred; topical carbonic anhydrase inhibitors may induce endothelial failure.

Congenital hereditary endothelial dystrophy (CHED)

CHED is an important cause of bilateral corneal edema in otherwise healthy term neonates (p. 617). It is usually autosomal recessive. An autosomal dominant variant has been linked to the same region (Ch20q) as posterior polymorphous dystrophy (PPMD). It appears to be a dysgenesis in which neural crest cells fail to complete differentiation into normal endothelium.

Clinical features

Autosomal recessive type

Bilateral marked corneal edema occurs from birth. Stroma is up to 3× normal thickness. There is severe ↓VA, amblyopia, and nystagmus; it is not usually painful.

Autosomal dominant type

Bilateral mild corneal edema occurs from infancy with tearing and photophobia. This type has milder ↓VA and no nystagmus; it is gradually progressive.

Treatment

Treatment is with PK; visual outcome is often limited by amblyopia.

Posterior polymorphous dystrophy (PPMD)

PPMD is usually autosomal dominant but has a very variable expression. It shares features with iridocorneal endothelial (ICE) syndrome and the anterior segment dysgenesis, all of which may form part of a continuum of failed neural crest terminal differentiation.

Clinical features

Clusters or lines of vesicles, irregular broad bands or diffuse haze of the posterior cornea ± iridocorneal adhesion, corectopia, glaucoma (closed or open angle).

Treatment

Treatment is not usually necessary. Consider penetrating keratoplasty if there is significant ↓VA.

Corneal ectasias

Keratoconus

This is a common corneal ectasia characterized by progressive *conical* distortion of the cornea with irregular astigmatism, axial stromal thinning, apical protrusion, and increasing myopia. Prevalence estimates vary widely (0.05–5%) according to the population studied, the techniques used, and the definition adopted.

The etiology is unclear but may be a combination of repeated trauma (e.g., eye-rubbing) and abnormalities of corneal stroma (e.g., in connective tissue disorders). Previously, only 10% cases were thought to be familial. However, analysis by videokeratography suggests a high prevalence among asymptomatic family members that is consistent with autosomal dominant inheritance with variable penetrance.

Keratoconus usually presents in early adulthood; an earlier presentation is associated with a worse prognosis.

Risk factors

Table 7.11 Associations of keratoconus

Ocular		Leber's congenital amaurosis
		Vernal keratoconjunctivitis
		Floppy eyelid syndrome
		Retinitis pigmentosa
		Retinopathy of prematurity
Systemic	Atopy	Asthma
		Eczema
		Hayfever
	Connective tissue	Ehlers–Danlos syndrome
		Marfan syndrome
		Osteogenesis imperfecta
	Other	Down syndrome
		Crouzon syndrome
		Apert syndrome

Clinical features

- Usually bilateral (but asymmetric) progressive irregular astigmatism with ↓VA. Progression continues into early adulthood but usually stabilizes by mid-30s.
- Corneal steepening/thinning (cone), Vogt's striae (vertical lines in the stroma that may disappear upon pressure), Fleischer ring (iron deposition at base of cone), conical distortion of lower lid on downward gaze (Munson's sign), abnormal focusing of a slit-lamp beam orientated obliquely across the cone from the temporal side (Rizutti's sign), scissoring reflex on retinoscopy, oil droplet reflex on ophthalmoscopy.
- *Complications*: acute hydrops (Descemet's membrane rupture with acute corneal edema, may result in scarring); corneal scar.

Investigations
- *Videokeratography*: This has largely replaced manual keratometry. It is used for diagnosis and monitoring of disease. It may also classify keratoconic changes according to:
  Severity: mild (<48D), moderate (48–54D), and severe (>54D).
  Morphology: cone, nipple, oval, bowtie, and globus.

Treatment
Counsel patient on the progressive nature of the disease, frequent changes in refractive error, and the potential impact on lifestyle (notably driving) and career. Since disease usually stabilizes by the mid-30s, a patient with good VA at age 35 is unlikely to need a keratoplasty.
- *Mild astigmatism*: spectacle or contact lens correction.
- *Moderate astigmatism*: rigid gas permeable lens (8.7–14.5 mm), scleral lens (PMMA).
- *Severe astigmatism*: deep lamellar keratoplasty (if normal Descemet's membrane) or penetrating keratoplasty. 90% of patients with keratoconus achieve clear grafts, but postoperative astigmatism ± anisometropia often necessitate additional contact lens use.

Keratoglobus

This is a very rare bilateral ectasia characterized by global corneal thinning and significant risk of rupture at minor trauma. It may be acquired (probably as an end-stage keratoconus) or congenital (autosomal recessive associated with Ehlers–Danlos type VI and brittle cornea syndrome).

Treatment includes protection from trauma, scleral contact lenses, and sometimes lamellar epikeratoplasty.

Pellucid marginal degeneration

This is a rare bilateral progressive corneal ectasia of the peripheral cornea. It results in crescenteric thinning inferiorly and marked against-the-rule astigmatism. It presents in the third to fifth decade with non-inflammatory, painless visual distortion. Hydrops is rare.

Treatment is with hard contact lenses; it is usually uncorrectable with eyeglasses. Surgical intervention is usually disappointing. Surgical techniques include eccentric penetrating keratoplasty, wedge resection, and lamellar keratoplasty.

Posterior keratoconus

This is a rare nonprogressive congenital abnormality of the cornea in which there is abnormal steepening of the posterior cornea in the presence of normal anterior corneal surface. It is usually an isolated unilateral finding, but may be associated with ocular (e.g., anterior lenticonus, anterior polar cataract) or systemic abnormalities.

Treatment is not usually necessary, but requires penetrating keratoplasty if there is significant ↓VA.

Peripheral ulcerative keratitis

Peripheral ulcerative keratitis (PUK)

PUK is an aggressive sight-threatening form of keratitis that is sometimes associated with underlying systemic disease (Box 7.4). The etiology is uncertain, although the rheumatoid model suggests that immune complex deposition at the limbus causes an obliterative vasculitis with subsequent corneal inflammation and stromal melt (see Table 7.12).

Causes

Box 7.4 Causes of peripheral ulcerative keratitis

- Idiopathic.
- Rheumatoid arthritis (RA).
- Wegener's granulomatosis.
- Systemic lupus erythematosus (SLE).
- Relapsing polychondritis.
- Polyarteritis nodosa.
- Microscopic polyangiitis.
- Churg–Strauss syndrome.

Clinical features

- Variable pain and redness (may be none); ↓VA.
- Uni- or bilateral peripheral ulceration with epithelial defect and stromal thinning; associated inflammation at the limbus (elevated, injected) associated scleritis.
- *Systemic features* (if associated disease) include degenerative joints (rheumatoid arthritis), saddle nose (Wegener's granulomatosis), skin changes (psoriasis, scleroderma, systemic lupus erythematosus), and degenerative pinna cartilage (relapsing polychondritis).

Investigations

These are as directed by systemic review. Consider blood pressure (BP); complete blood count (CBC), erythrocyte sedimentation rate (ESR), urinalysis, liver function tests, Glu, C-reactive protein (CRP), vasculitis screen (including rheumatoid factor [RF], antinuclear antibody [ANA], antineutrophil cytoplasmic antibody [ANCA], dsDNA), cryoglobulins, hepatitis C serology; and chest X-ray.

Treatment

- Emergency referral to corneal specialist and involve patient's physician and rheumatologist.
- Systemic immunosuppression (coordinate with rheumatologist) may include corticosteroids, methotrexate, mycophenolate, azathioprine, or cyclophosphamide.
- Topical immunosuppression: steroids (but use with caution in rheumatoid arthritis or if there is significant thinning since keratolysis may be accelerated) or cyclosporine.

Table 7.12 Corneal complications of rheumatoid arthritis

Marginal furrow	Peripheral thinning without inflammation or loss of epithelium; contact lens cornea; does not perforate
Peripheral ulcerative keratitis	Peripheral inflammation, epithelial loss, infiltrate and stromal loss; may perforate
Acute stromal keratitis	Acute-onset inflammation with stromal infiltrates but epithelium often preserved
Sclerosing keratitis	Gradual juxtalimbal opacification of corneal stroma bordering an area of scleritis
Keratolysis	Stromal thinning ("corneal melt") due to associated inflammation

- Ocular lubricants, topical antibiotics to prevent secondary infection and cycloplegic (for pain and AC activity).
- Globe protection (e.g., glasses by day, shield at night).
- Consider bandage contact lens + cyanoacrylate glue for pending or actual perforation. Surgical options include amniotic membrane grafts, lamellar keratoplasty, patch grafts, and, rarely, conjunctival flaps.

Mooren's ulcer

This is a rare form of peripheral ulcerative keratitis that appears to be autoimmune. It is rarely associated with hepatitis C. It exists in two forms. The limited form is typically seen in middle-aged and elderly Caucasians and presents with unilateral disease that is fairly responsive to treatment. The more aggressive form is typically seen in young Africans with bilateral disease that may relentlessly progress despite treatment.

Clinical features
- Pain, photophobia, ↓VA.
- Uni- or bilateral progressive peripheral ulceration; leading edge undermines epithelium; gray infiltrate at advancing margin; ulcer advances centrally and circumferentially; underlying stromal melt. There is no perilimbal clear zone and no associated scleritis (but conjunctival and episcleral inflammation).
- *Complications:* perforation; uveitis; cataract; at end stage the cornea is thinned and conjunctivalized (Fig. 7.4).

Investigations
Conduct systemic workup to rule out hepatitis C or any of the diseases associated with PUK (Box 7.5).

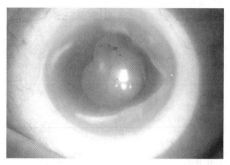

Figure 7.4 Rheumatoid arthritis–associated peripheral ulcerative keratitis with extensive area of cornea thinning. See insert for color version.

Box 7.5 Systemic work up PUK

ESR
ANA
Rheumatoid factor
ANCA
dsDNA
Cryoglobulin
Hepatitis B/C

Treatment
- Topical steroids (e.g., medroxyprogesterone reduces collagenolytic activity).
- Systemic immunosuppression: corticosteroids, cyclophosphamide, or cyclosporine (consult with physician or rheumatologist); interferon if coexistent hepatitis C (as directed by a hepatologist).
- Also topical antibiotics, cycloplegia, globe protection, bandage contact lens ± glue, and surgical options as for peripheral ulcerative keratitis with systemic disease.

Other peripheral corneal diseases

Marginal keratitis

This is a common inflammatory reaction due to hypersensitivity to staphylococcal exotoxin. It is often seen in patients with atopy, rosacea, or chronic blepharitis.

Clinical features

- Pain, FB sensation, redness (may be sectoral or adjacent to lid margins), photophobia, tearing, ↓VA.
- Sterile, white, subepithelial peripheral corneal infiltrate; most commonly at 2, 4, 8, and 10 o'clock but may spread circumferentially to coalesce. A perilimbal clear zone of cornea is preserved; epithelial ulceration (stain with fluorescein) and vascularization may occur.

Treatment

- Topical steroid/antibiotic is commonly used to hasten resolution.
- Treat associated blepharitis or rosacea (p. 110).

Rosacea associated keratitis

Acne rosacea is a chronic progressive disorder characterized by cutaneous telangectasia and sebaceous hyperplasia. Affecting the face and eyes, rosacea presents in middle age, shows a female bias, and is more common in fair-skinned individuals.

Clinical features

There is telangiectasias at the lids, meibomianitis, and keratitis (ranges from inferior punctate epithelial erosions to marginal infiltrates to significant corneal thinning and perforation). Facial flushing is characteristically worse with consumption of alcohol or spicy food.

Treatment

- Oral antibiotics, either a tetracycline (e.g., doxycycline 100 mg 1×/day for 3 months; tetracyclines are contraindicated in children under 12, in pregnant or breast-feeding women, and in hepatic or renal impairment) or a macrolide (e.g., erythromycin 500 mg 2×/day).
- Treat associated blepharitis with lid hygiene, ocular lubricants, and topical antibiotics or ointment (for acute exacerbations).
- If moderately severe, consider topical steroids ± antibiotics (e.g., dexamethasone 0.1% ± topical azithromycin). Use with caution if significant stromal thinning occurs as keratolysis may be accelerated.
- If very severe (threatened corneal perforation), systemic immunosuppression is usually necessary (e.g., azathioprine, cyclosporine, or mycophenolate).

Phlyctenulosis

Children are more commonly affected than adults. Phlyctens appear to be a hypersensitivity response, most commonly to staphylococcal or mycobacterial proteins, and rarely to adenovirus, fungi, *Neisseria*, lymphogranuloma venereum, and leishmaniasis. They may be located at the conjunctiva or the cornea.

Conjunctival phlyctens are inflamed nodules, which may stain with fluorescein. They often resolve spontaneously. Corneal phlyctens are gray nodules with associated superficial vascularization that may gradually move from limbus to central cornea.

Treatment is with topical steroid (e.g., prednisolone acetate 1% 4×/day).

Dellen

This is nonulcerative corneal thinning seen adjacent to raised limbal lesions due to local drying and tear film instability. It is usually asymptomatic. Scarring and vascularization are rare.

Treatment is with lubrication and removal of the precipitant (e.g., cessation of contact lens wear; removal of limbal mass).

Terrien's marginal degeneration

This is a rare cause of bilateral asymmetrical peripheral thinning, most commonly seen in young to middle-aged males (M:F 3:1). It is noninflammatory and is thus sometimes considered an ectasia or degeneration.

Clinical features

- Initially asymptomatic; painless ↓VA (against the rule astigmatism).
- Initially there is yellow lipid deposition with fine vascularization at the superior marginal cornea. Thinning occurs on the limbal side of the lipid line with a fairly steep leading edge; overlying epithelium is intact. A perilimbal clear zone of cornea is preserved.
- *Complications*: opacification may spread circumferentially and rarely centrally. Rarely, there may be associated inflammation (usually in younger men).

Treatment

- Eyeglasses or contact lenses for astigmatism.
- If there is severe thinning or risk of perforation, consider surgical options, including crescentic or eccentric lamellar/PUK.

Neurotrophic keratopathy

The ophthalmic branch of the trigeminal nerve (CN V) is responsible for corneal sensation. Reduction of corneal sensation leads to the following:
- Loss of the normal feedback responsible for maintaining a healthy epithelium
- Predisposition to inadvertent trauma and opportunistic infection
- Impairment of epithelial repair
- Delayed clinical presentation

Causes

Table 7.13 Causes of corneal hyposthesia/anesthesia

Congenital	Familial dysautonomia (Riley–Day syndrome)
	Anhydrotic ectodermal dysplasia
Acquired	Herpes simplex keratitis
	Herpes zoster keratitis
	Corneal scarring
	Traumatic/surgical section of CN V
	Irradiation
	Compressive/infiltrative (e.g., acoustic neuroma)

Clinical features
- Painless red eye, ↓VA.
- ↓Corneal sensation; interpalpebral punctate epithelial erosions → larger defects with heaped gray edges, epithelial edema; opportunistic microbial keratitis; perforation.

Investigation
If the cause of corneal anesthesia is not yet established, the patient will need full assessment (e.g., neurological referral, CT/MRI head scan, etc.).

Treatment
- Ensure adequate lubrication: consider ↑frequency or ↑viscosity; consider preservative-free preparations.
- Treat any secondary microbial keratitis (p. 166).
- For significant ulcerative thinning, consider admission, protective measures such as globe protection (e.g., glasses by day, shield at night), bandage contact lens, or tectonic grafting with amniotic membrane and measures to promote corneal healing, such as tarsorrhaphy (surgical or botulinum toxin induced) and topical application of autologous serum.

Prevention
- Assess corneal protective mechanisms: check corneal sensation, tear film, lid closure (CN VII), Bell's phenomenon; correct where possible.
- Warn patient of risk of corneal disease and that a red eye or ↓VA requires urgent ophthalmic assessment.

Exposure keratopathy

In exposure keratopathy, there is failure of the lids' normal wetting mechanism, with consequent drying and damage to the corneal epithelium.

Causes

Table 7.14 Causes of exposure keratopathy

VIIn palsy	Idiopathic (Bell's palsy)
	Stroke
	Tumor (e.g., acoustic neuroma, meningioma, choleastoma, parotid, nasopharyngeal)
	Demyelination
	Sarcoidosis
	Trauma (temporal bone fracture)
	Surgical section
	Otitis
	Ramsay Hunt syndrome (Herpes zoster)
	Guillan–Barré syndrome
	Lyme disease
Lid abnormality	Nocturnal lagophthalmos
	Ectropion
	Traumatic defect in lid margin
	Surgical (e.g., overcorrection of ptosis)
	Floppy eyelid syndrome
Orbital disease	Proptosis
	Thyroid eye disease

Clinical features
- Irritable, red eye(s); may be worse in the mornings.
- Punctate epithelial erosions (usually inferior if underlying lagophthalmos; central if due to proptosis); → larger defects; opportunistic microbial keratitis; perforation.

Investigation
If the cause of exposure keratopathy is not yet established, the patient will need further investigation as directed by full ophthalmic and systemic assessment.

Treatment
- Ensure adequate lubrication: consider ↑frequency or ↑viscosity; preservative-free preparations may be preferred if >6×/day.
- Ensure adequate lid closure: use temporary measures if early resolution is anticipated (tape lids shut at night), intermediate (temporary lateral/central tarsorrhaphy; botulinum toxin–induced ptosis) vs. permanent surgical procedures (e.g., lid weights or permanent tarsorrhaphy for lagophthalmos; orbital decompression if proptosis).
- Treat secondary microbial keratitis (p. 201).

- If there is significant ulcerative thinning, consider admission, globe protection (e.g., glasses by day, shield at night), gluing, bandage contact lens, or lamellar grafting.

Prevention

- Assess corneal protective mechanisms: check corneal sensation, tear film, lid closure (CN VII), Bell's phenomenon; correct where possible.
- Warn patient of risk of corneal disease and that pain, photophobia, or ↓VA requires urgent ophthalmic assessment.

Deposition keratopathies

Wilson's disease (hepatolenticular degeneration)

This rare autosomal recessive condition arises from deficiency in a copper-binding protein, leading to low levels of ceruloplasmin and copper deposition throughout the tissues including the cornea.

Clinical features

- Kayser–Fleischer ring (brownish peripheral ring at level of Descemet's membrane); starts superiorly and usually continuous with limbus; sunflower cataract (anterior and posterior subcapsular opacities).
- Systemic: liver failure, choreoathetosis (basal ganglia deposition), and psychiatric problems

Vortex keratopathy

A number of drugs may result in deposits at the corneal epithelium. Similar appearances occur in Fabry's disease.

Causes

These include amiodarone, chloroquine, suramin, indomethacin, tamoxifen, chlorpromazine, atovaquone, and Fabry's disease.

Clinical features

- Asymptomatic; not an indication for withdrawing treatment.
- Swirling gray lines radiating from infracentral cornea.

Crystalline keratopathies

Infectious crystalline keratopathy presents as feathery stromal opacities in the absence of significant inflammation. These are biofilms (i.e., slime) arising from the presence of *Streptococcus viridans* or, rarely, *Staphylococcus epidermidis*, *Pseudomonas aeruginosa*, or *Candida* species. Most commonly seen in graft tissue after a penetrating keratoplasty, they also occur in the presence of ocular surface disease (e.g., ocular mucous membrane pemphigoid, Stevens–Johnson syndrome).

Noninfectious crystalline keratopathy includes deposition of gold (chrysiasis due to systemic treatment in rheumatoid arthritis), immunoglobulin (multiple myeloma, Waldenstrom's macroglobulinaemia, lymphoma), urate (gout), cysteine (cystinosis), and lipids (lipid keratopathy, Schnyder's crystalline dystrophy).

Mucopolysaccharidosis keratopathy

The mucopolysaccharidoses are a group of inherited enzyme deficiencies (usually autosomal recessive) in which there is an accumulation and deposition of glycosaminoglycans. This may be widespread, causing skeletal abnormalities, organomegaly, and mental retardation (e.g., Hurler's syndrome, MPS1) (Table 7.15), or limited (e.g., corneal deposition in macular dystrophy) (p. 189).

Table 7.15 Mucopolysaccharidoses associated with corneal clouding

Systemic		
	MPSI	Hurler, Scheie, Hurler–Scheie
	MPSIV	Morquio
	MPSVI	Maroteaux-Lamy
	MPSVII	Sly
Limited		Macular dystrophy

Keratoplasty: principles

Corneal grafting has been performed for over 100 years. It may be performed as an elective procedure to improve vision or as an emergency procedure for corneal perforation. It may involve full-thickness replacement of a button of corneal tissue (penetrating keratoplasty) or partial-thickness replacement (lamellar keratoplasty).

Penetrating keratoplasty (PK)

Indications

- *Visual:* keratoconus, pseudophakic/aphakic bullous keratopathy, Fuchs' endothelial dystrophy, other corneal dystrophies, scarring secondary to trauma, chemical injury, or keratitis.
- *Tectonic:* corneal thinning, threatened perforation, or actual perforation.

Cautions

Poor prognostic factors include corneal vascularization, reduced corneal sensation, active inflammation, peripheral corneal thinning, herpetic disease, ocular surface disease, severe dry eye diseases, and uncontrolled glaucoma.

Method

- *Consent:* Explain what the operation does, the need for frequent postoperative visits and long-term follow-up, and the importance of immediate attention if there are problems. Explain the nature of organ donation, that the donors are screened but that there is still a small risk of transmission of infectious agents. Explain the delay in visual rehabilitation and possible complications, including failure, graft rejection, infection, hemorrhage, worsened vision, and need for correction of astigmatism (contact lenses ± refractive surgery).
- *Preoperative:* miotic (e.g., pilocarpine 1%).
- *Prep:* with 5% povidone iodine and drape.
- *Check donor material:* healthy looking corneoscleral ring in clear media.
- *Determine button sizes:* depends on corneal morphology and pathology, but commonly 7.5 mm for the host, and 0.25–0.5 mm larger for the donor.
- *Mark cornea:* measure height and width of cornea with calipers and mark center with ink; consider marking periphery with radial keratotomy marker to assist with suture placement.
- *Perform paracentesis* and fill AC with viscoelastic.
- *Excise donor button:* cut from endothelial side using a trephine (types include hand-held, gravity, and vacuum-driven).
- *Excise host button:* cutting with the trephine (numerous designs) may be full thickness or stopped at the first release of aqueous to perform a slower decompression with the blade or corneal scissors.
- *Place cardinal sutures:* use 4 to 8 10–0 nylon sutures to secure the donor button in position.
- *Complete suturing:* use either additional interrupted sutures (often 16 in total) or a continuous running suture. Aim for 90% suture depth. Ensure that suture tension is even and attempt to minimize astigmatism.
- Refill AC with balanced salt solution.

- *Postoperative:* give topical steroid and antibiotic; if there is a low risk of rejection, then a combined preparation (e.g., maxitrol 4×/day) may be sufficient; if higher risk, consider preservative-free dexamethasone 0.1% q2h and antibiotic drops. Also consider oral acetazolamide in the immediate postoperative period (especially if there is coexistent glaucoma), and oral acyclovir (if HSV disease).
- *Follow-up* is as clinically indicated but commonly at 1 day, 1 week, 1 month, and then every 2–3 months. Regular refraction/autorefraction and corneal topography permits adjustment and removal of sutures to minimize astigmatism. Use antibiotic/steroid coverage to reduce risk of infection and rejection and check for wound leaks. A continuous running suture should not usually be removed for at least a year.

Deep lamellar keratoplasty (DLK)

Indications
DLK is suitable for diseases in which the host endothelium/Descemet's membrane is healthy, e.g., most keratoconus, stromal dystrophies, scarring. Although DLK requires a longer surgical time than that for penetrating keratoplasty, there is a reduced risk of rejection.

Method
A deep stromal pocket is formed from a superior scleral (or corneal) incision and filled with viscoelastic, thus permitting a trephine to excise a deep but partial-thickness button. Visualization of depth may be assisted by filling the AC with air.

Superficial lamellar keratoplasty

Indications
Tectonic: reinforce thinned cornea in threatened perforation or post-pterygium excision

Visual (uncommon): anterior stromal scarring

Method
A trephine is used to cut to the desired depth before using a blade or microkeratome to separate the button at the base.

Triple procedure

Indications
This includes visually significant cataract with disease that requires penetrating keratoplasty, most commonly Fuchs' endothelial dystrophy.

Method
A penetrating keratoplasty is performed with cataract extraction (usually by extracapsular "open sky" rather than phacoemulsification) and IOL implantation.

Descemet's stripping endothelial keratoplasty (DSEK) or deep lamellar endothelial keratoplasty (DLEK)
The aim of DSEK and DLEK is to selectively replace the endothelial layer. They are both useful in endothelial dystrophies such as Fuchs' endothelial dystrophy or pseudophakic/aphakic bullous keratopathy.

Keratoplasty: complications

Early postoperative complications (see Table 7.16)

Wound leak—Seidel positive leak, shallow AC, soft eye
- Consider lubricants, bandage contact lens, patching, or resuturing.

↑*IOP*—causes include retained viscoelastic, malignant glaucoma, choroidal effusion, choroidal hemorrhage, wound leak
- Identify and treat cause.

Persistent epithelial defect (>2 weeks duration)—causes include ocular surface disease such as dry eye, blepharitis, rosacea, exposure, or systemic disease such as diabetes or rheumatoid arthritis
- Identify and treat cause; ensure generous lubrication and that all drops are preservative free; consider taping lid shut or tarsorrhaphy.

Endophthalmitis—rare, but sight-threatening ophthalmic emergency
- Recognize and treat urgently (p. 254).

Primary graft failure—endothelial failure causes persistent graft edema from day 1 in a quiet eye.
- Observe for 2–4 weeks; consider regraft if edema persists.

Early graft rejection (see below)

Urrets–Zavalia syndrome—a fixed dilated pupil may occur after either PK or DLK; it is presumed to be due to iris ischemia.

Late postoperative complications

Astigmatism
- Monitor with corneal topography; adjust running suture or remove interrupted sutures (at steepest axes), but ensure that wound is secure. It can be improved with hard contact lens ± arcuate keratotomies.

Microbial keratitis—risk is increased by epithelial disturbance, sutures, and chronic steroid use.
- Recognize and treat urgently (p. 168).

Suture-related problems
- Remove loose or broken sutures and check for wound leaks; use antibiotic/steroid cover to reduce risk of infection and rejection. If there is wound leak it may require resuturing. A continuous running suture should not usually be removed for at least a year.

Disease recurrence in graft
This is common with viral keratitis (e.g., HSV) and some corneal dystrophies (e.g., macular dystrophy).
- Identify and treat if possible (e.g., acyclovir for HSV); the patient may require another graft.

Late graft rejection (p. 208).

Graft rejection

This is the most common cause of graft failure. This complication is usually due to endothelial rejection, which occurs in about 20% of grafts.

Have a low threshold for patient admission—prompt and adequate treatment may save the graft. Anterior uveitis occurring in a patient with a corneal graft should be considered graft rejection until proven otherwise. Although for most cases topical steroid drops are sufficient, in severe rejection episodes or high-risk grafts, consider oral prednisolone and/or pulsed IV methylprednisolone.

Epithelial rejection

Graft epithelium is replaced by host epithelium, resulting in an epithelial demarcation line.
- Increased topical steroids to at least double current regimen (e.g., prednisolone acetate 1%, up to hourly).

Stromal/subepithelial rejection

This is indicated by subepithelial infiltrates.
- Increased topical steroids to at least double current regimen (e.g., prednisolone acetate 1%, up to hourly).

Endothelial rejection

This is indicated by corneal edema, keratic precipitates, Khodadoust line (inflammatory cell–graft endothelial demarcation line), and AC activity.
- Intensive topical steroids (e.g., prednisolone acetate 1% hourly day and night/steroid ointment at bedtime); consider subconjunctival or systemic corticosteroids if patient fails to improve; cycloplegia (e.g., cyclopentolate 1% 3×/day).

Table 7.16 Summary of complications in keratoplasty

Early	Wound leak
	↑IOP
	Flat anterior chamber
	Iris prolapse
	Persistent epithelial defect
	Endophthalmitis
	Primary graft failure
	Early graft rejection
	Urrets–Zavalia syndrome
Late	Astigmatism
	Graft rejection
	Microbial keratitis
	Suture-related problems (loose, abscess, endophthalmitis)
	Disease recurrence in graft
	Glaucoma

Refractive surgery: outline

Photorefractive keratectomy (PRK)

Indications
There are good results for +3D to −6D. Advantages over LASIK include no issues of flap stability (military, contact sports).

Method
Remove epithelium surgically and selectively ablate stroma with excimer laser.

Complications
These include under- or overcorrection, visual aberrations, corneal haze, corneal scarring, decentration, central corneal islands (elevations), microbial keratitis, and recurrent erosions.

Laser stromal in situ keratomilieusis (LASIK)

Indications
There are good results for +4D to −8D and up to 4D astigmatism. Advantages over PRK include less pain and faster visual rehabilitation.

Method
Form partial-thickness flap with microkeratome, selectively ablate stroma with excimer laser, and reposition flap.

Complications
Diffuse lamellar keratitis
- Stage 1 white granular haze (2%); stage 2 "shifting sands" white infiltrate (0.5%); stage 3 white clumped central infiltrate (0.2%); stage 4 stromal melt (0.02%).

Treat with intensive topical steroids and consider surgical flap manipulation (i.e., lifting and irrigation).

Flap complications
- Incomplete flap (≤1.2%), buttonhole flap (≤0.6%), thin flap (≤0.4%), irregular flap (≤0.1%), flap wrinkles or malposition (≤4%), lost flap.

Treat lost flap as epithelial erosion (p. 210); consider surgical repositioning of malpositioned flaps.

Other complications
These include under- or overcorrection, visual aberrations, corneal haze, corneal scarring, central corneal islands, microbial keratitis, epithelial ingrowth, keratectasia (in undiagnosed keratoconus), and dry eye syndrome.

Laser subepithelial keratomilieusis (LASEK)

Indications
There are good results for low myopia. Advantages over PRK include less pain, less haze, and faster visual rehabilitation. Advantages over LASIK include no issues of flap stability (military, contact sports).

Method
Create epithelial flap, selectively ablate stroma with excimer laser, and reposition flap.

Complications
These include under- or overcorrection, visual aberrations, corneal haze, epithelial defects, pain, and lamellar keratitis.

Table 7.17 Refractive procedures

Procedure	Mechanism
CORNEAL	
Central	
PRK	Remove epithelium surgically, selectively ablate stroma with excimer laser
LASIK	Form partial-thickness flap with microkeratome, selectively ablate stroma with excimer laser, replace flap
LASEK	Loosen epithelium sheet with alcohol, lift epithelial flap, selectively ablate stroma with excimer laser, reposition epithelial sheet
Keratomileusis	Remove partial-thickness corneal button and reshape the button (keratomileusis) or corneal bed (in situ keratomileusis)
Epikeratophakia	Remove epithelium, perform annular keratectomy, suture on shaped donor lenticule of Bowman's layer/anterior stroma
Keratophakia	Form partial-thickness flap with microkeratome, place intrastromal donor lenticule of corneal stroma, replace flap
Intracorneal lens	Form partial-thickness flap with microkeratome, place intrastromal synthetic lens (e.g., hydrogel), replace flap
Peripheral	
Radial keratotomy	Deep radial corneal incisions flatten central cornea
Thermakeratoplasty	Laser shrinkage of peripheral stromal collagen in a radial pattern flattens periphery and steepens central cornea
Intracorneal ring	Thread synthetic ring into mid-stromal tunnel
LENS	
Clear lens extraction	Remove crystalline lens and replace with synthetic PCIOL
Phakic intraocular lens	Leave crystalline lens intact and place synthetic PCIOL in angle or sulcus

Contact lenses: outline

Contact lenses (CL) are optical devices that rest on the surface of the cornea. They are usually refractive but may also be used to improve cosmesis (e.g., therapeutic CL for scarred cornea or novelty CL) or provide protection (bandage CL).

Material

The ideal CL must not only have excellent optical properties but also be inert, well tolerated by the ocular surface, comfortable to wear, and have good oxygen transmissability. Oxygen transmissibility (Dk/L) depends on oxygen permeability (Dk) and lens thickness (L). Oxygen permeability itself (Dk) depends on diffusion (D) and solubility (k).

Hard lenses

Originally made of glass and later of polymethyl methacrylate (PMMA), these have excellent optical properties but are minimally oxygen permeable (Dk = 0), thus compromising epithelial metabolism with risk of overwear. They were of 23–25 mm in size ("scleral").

Currently available scleral lenses are usually made of rigid gas-permeable (RGP) materials and may be suitable for severe keratoconus, severe irregular astigmatism, and some ocular surface disorders.

Rigid gas permeable (RGP)

Made of complex polymers (which may include silicone, PMMA, and others), these lenses permit excellent diffusion of oxygen (D) with resultant good permeability (Dk from 15 to >100). They are usually 8.5–9.5 mm in size ("corneal").

RGP CLs vary in their permeability (Dk), their wetting angle (a low value equates to good tear film spread and improved comfort), and their refractive index.

Given their rigidity, the space behind the RGP CLs becomes filled in by the lacrimal lens. This effectively neutralizes corneal astigmatism and makes them the treatment of choice for conditions where this is an issue (e.g., keratoconus).

Hydrogel (soft)

Made of polymers of hydroxethyl methylacrylate, these CLs absorb much more fluid (high water content) than the RGP lenses. This makes them softer, more comfortable, and more quickly tolerated but also reduces their effectiveness in correcting astigmatism. They are usually 13.5–14.5 mm in size so as to just cover the limbus ("semiscleral").

In hydrogel lenses, a higher water content results in greater solubility (k) and therefore better permeability (Dk from 10 to around 40). However, it also increases the minimum central thickness of the lens (L). This means that the overall oxygen transmissibility (Dk/L) is fairly constant, whatever the water content.

Hydrogel CLs do not vault over the cornea and thus there is no significant lacrimal lens to neutralize corneal astigmatism. However, toric CLs can treat astigmatism provided the lens is stabilized (e.g., prism, thin zones).

Silicone hydrogel

The new silicone hydrogel CLs combine some of the advantages of RGP materials with hydrogel lenses and have excellent Dk values (up to 140).

Wearing schedule

Duration of wear: daily wear vs. extended wear

In daily wear, there is a regular CL-free period. The lens is cleaned and disinfected (conventional CL) or discarded (disposable CL).

Extended wear has a role in certain patients (e.g., aphakes) but is discouraged for the general population. The Dk values for soft hydrogels and many RGP materials are sufficient for daily wear but are inadequate for extended wear and result in corneal compromise. For those requiring extended wear, certain silicone hydrogel lenses have been approved for continuous wear of up to 1 month.

Duration of lens: conventional vs. disposable

Conventional lenses are usually replaced annually. They are more expensive (per lens) and of superior optical quality but are more vulnerable to damage or loss because of their long life span.

Disposable lenses are commonly replaced daily, biweekly, or monthly. They are cheaper and of slightly poorer quality but are less likely to be damaged or lost during their life span.

Lens notation

CL parameters are noted as follows: base curve, diameter, and power.

Contact lenses: fitting

Refractive contact lenses

- Measure corneal curvature (keratometry), pupil diameter, vertical palpebral aperture, and corneal/visible iris diameter.
- Either:
  1. Predict the lens parameters required (from nomograms incorporating the above measurements and known refractive error) and order the lens on a sale-or-return basis; or
  2. Use a trial lens set to determine the best fit.

Rigid gas permeable

Estimate CL parameters

The base curve is dictated by the flattest K reading and may be "on K" (i.e., the same curvature), steeper than K, or flatter than K. If on K, the lacrimal lens formed by the tear film is plano. If steeper or flatter, it confers a plus or minus power of around 0.25D per 0.05 mm difference of curvature.

The lens diameter may be influenced by the diameters of the cornea and pupil, and even lid position. A large lens may cause discomfort as it encroaches on the limbus and a small lens may cause flare if its edge impinges on the pupil.

The lens power is determined by either calculation (from the back vertex distance and spectacle correction) or over-refraction with a trial lens in place.

Assess fit after 20 min

The CL should be centered horizontally, with its lower edge >2 mm above the lower lid but with its upper edge just under (superior positioning) or just below the upper lid (interpalpebral positioning). The lens should move 1–2 mm with blinking and allow tear flow between the cornea and the contact lens. Less movement implies that the CL is too tight or steep; more movement implies the lens is too loose or flat. Fluorescein is used to assess the fit.

Good alignment results in shallow central clearance (little fluorescence seen) with intermediate touch (black ring) and free tear movement in the periphery (bright fluorescence). If it is too steep, there is high central clearance (bright fluorescence); if too flat, there is central touch (black).

Hydrogel (soft)

Estimate CL parameters

The base curve is estimated from the flattest K and adjusted according to type of lens (e.g., add 1 mm for low–water content lenses) and the individual patient.

The lens diameter should exceed the corneal diameter covering the limbus by ≥1 mm. The lens power is calculated as above.

Assess fit after 20 min

The CL should be comfortable, fully cover the cornea, be fairly centered, and move 1–2 mm with blinking (<1 mm implies that CL is too tight or steep; ≥3 mm is probably too loose or flat).

Follow-up

Ensure that patients understand how to care for their lenses (including hygiene). Discuss potential complications (e.g., microbial keratitis) and how they present, and the need for lens removal and urgent review in such circumstances.

Follow-up should be fairly frequent initially. For long-standing uncomplicated CL wear, it may be reduced to an annual visit.

Nonrefractive contact lenses

Therapeutic ("bandage") and cosmetic contact lenses are plano (or even opaque) (Table 7.18). They usually come in a few standard sizes and are fitted according to size and base curve.

Table 7.18 Commonly used therapeutic contact lenses (CL)

Hydrogel	Very thin hydrogel CL; drapes well on the cornea; good for patients with dry eyes
Silicone hydrogel	High oxygen permeability; good for bandage CL.
Intralimbal	Rigid gas-permeable CL of large diameter; useful for postsurgical and irregular corneas

Contact lenses: complications

Painful red eye in the contact lens wearer
First rule out microbial keratitis. Then consider alternative diagnoses.

Microbial keratitis (p. 166)
There is white infiltrate ± epithelial defect, mucopurulent infiltrate, and AC inflammation.
- Ophthalmic emergency: treat aggressively (p. 168). Consider pseudomonas and acanthamoeba (more commonly seen in contact lens wearers).

Sterile keratitis
There are small multiple anterior stromal infiltrates, usually nonstaining; they may be only mildly symptomatic.
- Differentiate from microbial keratitis. Consider temporarily stopping (if severe) or reducing (if mild) CL wear; increase and improve CL care, using preservative-free solutions or change to alternative CL.

Giant papillary conjunctivitis
Itching + mucoid discharge occurs in the presence of giant papillae of the upper lid. Reduce daily wearing time.
- Mast-cell stabilizer (e.g., cromolyn sodium 4×/day). Consider temporarily stopping (if severe) or reducing (if mild) CL wear; improve CL care, using preservative-free solutions or change to alternative CL.

Tight lens syndrome
This characterized by tight, nonmoving lens with anterior corneal edema and AC reaction.
- Remove lens; use topical cycloplegic if there is severe AC reaction; replace with flatter lens when patient has recovered.

Toxic keratopathy
Disinfectant or enzyme is inadvertently introduced into the eye, resulting in diffuse punctate epithelial erosions ± subepithelial infitrates.
- Remove lens; rinse eye well; use preservative-free artificial tears; educate patient about CL care.

Preservative keratopathy
Preservative (e.g., thiomersal) exposure occurs with punctate epithelial erosions (may be superior limbic pattern) ± subepithelial infiltrates.
- Remove lens; use preservative-free artificial tears; educate patient about CL care and change to preservative-free cleaning solutions.

Tear film disturbance
Poor blink response or ill-fitting lens result in punctate staining at 3 or 9 o'clock with interpalpebral hyperemia.
- Use preservative-free artificial tears; check CL fit.

Painless red eye

Neovascularization

Superficial neovascularization at 3 and 9 o'clock is common. It usually does not extend >2–3 mm.

- Remove lens; if severe, consider a short course of topical steroid; replace with a lens with high oxygen permeability (Dk).

Other complications

Other complications include abnormalities of the epithelium, including microcysts, endothelial polymegathism, loss of lens, and corneal abrasion.

Optical effects include spectacle blur (one's spectacle correction is transiently incorrect after CL wear), flexure (refractive change due to flexing of CL), visual flare (edge effect), accommodative effects (e.g., a myopic person has to accommodate more when switching from glasses to CL), and aberrations (spherical and chromatic).

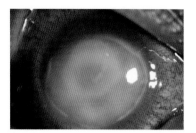

Plate 1, see Fig. 7.2

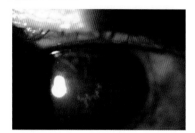

Plate 2, see Fig. 7.3

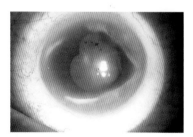

Plate 3, see Fig. 7.4

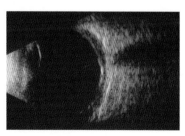

Plate 4, see Fig. 8.1

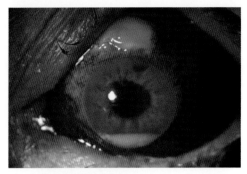

Plate 5, see Fig. 10.1

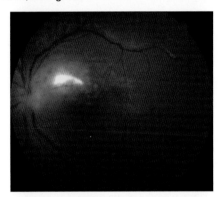

Plate 6, see Fig. 11.1

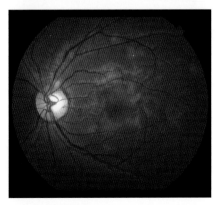

Plate 7, see Fig. 11.2

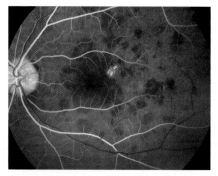

Plate 8, see Fig. 11.3

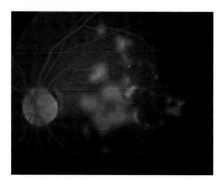

Plate 9, see Fig. 11.4

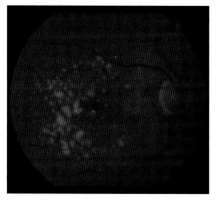

Plate 10, see Fig. 13.1

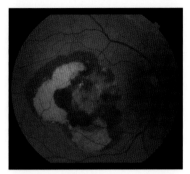

Plate 11, see Fig. 13.2

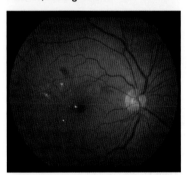

Plate 12, see Fig. 13.5

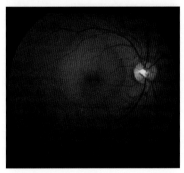

Plate 13, see Fig. 13.6

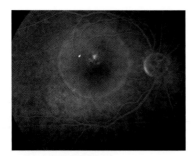

Plate 14, see Fig. 13.7

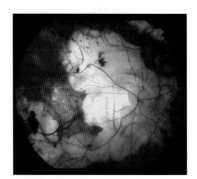

Plate 15, see Fig. 13.9

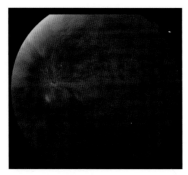

Plate 16, see Fig. 13.10

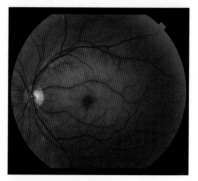

Plate 17, see Fig. 13.11

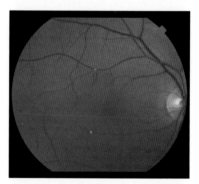

Plate 18, see Fig. 13.12

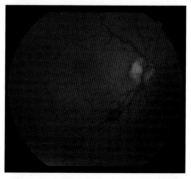

Plate 19, see Fig. 13.13

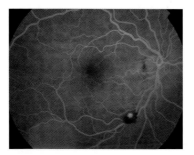

Plate 20, see Fig. 13.14

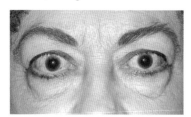

Plate 21, see Fig. 14.2

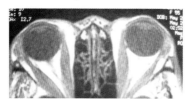

Plate 22, see Fig. 14.3

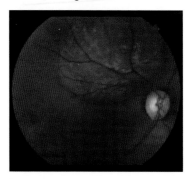

Plate 23, see Fig. 15.1

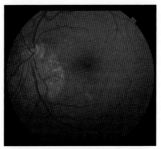

Plate 24, see Fig. 15.2

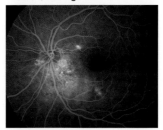

Plate 25, see Fig. 15.3

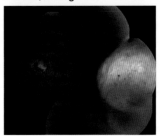

Plate 26, see Fig. 15.4

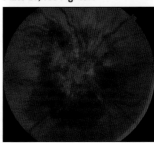

Plate 27 Papillitis with severe optic nerve edema, with associated nerve fiber layer hemorrhage and Paton's line in the peripapillary region.

Sclera

Anatomy and physiology

The *sclera* is the tough outer coat of the globe covered by a loose connective tissue layer, the *episclera*. The sclera develops from a condensation of mesenchymal tissue situated at the anterior rim of the optic cup. This forms first at the limbus at around week 7 and proceeds posteriorly to surround the optic nerve and form a rudimentary lamina cribrosa at week 12.

Sclera

Anatomy

The sclera is almost a complete sphere of 22 mm diameter. Anteriorly it is continuous with the cornea, and posteriorly with the optic nerve. It is thickest around the optic nerve (1.0 mm) and thinnest just posterior to the rectus muscle insertions (0.3 mm).

Sclera consists of collagen (mainly types I, III, and V, but also IV, VI, and VIII), elastin, proteoglycans, and glycoproteins. The stroma consists of a roughly criss-cross arrangement of collagen bundles of varying sizes (10–15 μm thick, 100–150 μm long). This renders it opaque but strong. The inner layer (lamina fusca) blends with the uveal tract, separated by the potential suprachoroidal space.

The sclera itself is effectively avascular but is pierced by a number of vessels. It is innervated by the long and short ciliary nerves.

Physiology

The sclera provides a tough, protective coat that is rigid enough to prevent loss of shape (with its refractive implications) but can tolerate some fluctuation in intraocular pressure (IOP). Scleral opacity is due to the irregularity of collagen and its relative hydration. The limited metabolic demands are supported by episcleral and choroidal vasculature.

Inflammation of the sclera leads to engorgement of mainly the deep vascular plexus. This is relatively unaffected by the administration of topical vasoconstrictors (e.g., phenylephrine).

Episclera

Anatomy

This layer of connective tissue comprises an inner layer apposed to the sclera, intermediate loose connective tissue, and an outer layer that fuses with the muscle sheaths and the conjunctiva juxtalimbally. It is heavily vascularized with a superficial and deep anterior plexus (which underlie and anastamose with the conjunctival plexus) and a posterior episcleral plexus supplied by the short posterior ciliary vessels.

Physiology

The episclera gives nutrition to the sclera and provides a low-friction surface assisting the free movement of the globe within the orbit. Inflammation of the episclera leads to engorgement of the conjunctival and superficial vascular plexus. These blanch with administration of topical vasoconstrictors (e.g., phenylephrine), leading to visible whitening.

Table 8.1 Scleral perforations

Location	Transmits
Anterior	Anterior ciliary arteries
Middle	Vortex veins
Posterior	Long + short ciliary nerves
	Long + short posterior ciliary arteries
Lamina cribrosa	Optic nerve

Episcleritis

This common condition is a benign, recurrent inflammation of the episclera; it is most common in young women. Episcleritis is usually self-limiting and may require little or no treatment. It is not usually associated
with any systemic disease, although around 10% may have a connective
tissue disease.

Simple episcleritis

Clinical features

- Sudden onset of mild discomfort, tearing ± photophobia; may be
  recurrent.
- Sectoral (occasionally diffuse) redness that blanches with topical
  vasoconstrictor (e.g., phenylephrine 10%); globe nontender;
  spontaneous resolution 1–2 weeks.

Investigation

Investigations are not usually required unless there is a history suggestive
of systemic disease.

Treatment

- *Supportive:* reassurance ± cold compresses.
- *Topical:* consider lubricants ± NSAID (e.g., ketorolac 0.3% 3×/day;
  uncertain benefit). Although disease improves with topical steroids,
  there may be rebound inflammation on withdrawal.
- *Systemic:* if severe or recurrent disease, consider oral NSAID
  (e.g., flurbiprofen 100 mg 3×/day for acute disease).

Nodular episcleritis

Clinical features

- Sudden onset of FB sensation, discomfort, tearing ± photophobia. It
  may be recurrent.
- Red nodule arising from the episclera; can be moved separately
  from the sclera (cf. nodular scleritis) and conjunctiva (cf. conjunctival
  phlycten); blanches with topical vasoconstrictor (e.g., phenylephrine
  10%); does not stain with fluorescein; globe nontender (cf. scleritis).
  Spontaneous resolution occurs in 5–6 weeks.

Investigation

Investigations are not usually required unless there is persistent inflammation or a history suggestive of systemic disease.

Treatment

Treat as for simple episcleritis, but there is a greater role for ocular
lubricants.

Anterior scleritis (1)

This uncommon condition is a sight-threatening inflammation of the sclera. It is associated with systemic disease in around 50% of patients, most cases being of a connective tissue disease.

The condition is most common in middle-aged women and is bilateral in 50% of the condition cases.

Classification

Table 8.2 Classification of scleritis and approximate frequency

Anterior	Non-necrotizing	Diffuse	50%
		Nodular	25%
	Necrotizing	With inflammation	10%
		Without inflammation	5%
Posterior			10%

Risk factors

- *Associated diseases:* rheumatoid arthritis, Wegener's granulomatosis, relapsing polychondritis, systemic lupus erythematosus, polyarteritis nodosa, inflammatory bowel disease, psoriatic arthritis, ankylosing spondylitis, Cogan's syndrome, rosacea, atopy, gout, infection (e.g., syphilis, tuberculosis, bacterial, fungal, and herpes zoster).
- *Local:* trauma, surgery (including surgery-induced necrotizing scleritis [SINS]).

Diffuse non-necrotizing anterior scleritis

Clinical features

- Subacute onset (over 1 week) of moderate or severe pain, redness, tearing ± photophobia.
- Diffuse injection of deep vascular plexus that does not blanch with vasoconstrictors (e.g., phenylephrine 10%), edema; globe tender; usually nonprogressive but may last for several months if untreated.

Investigations

- CBC, ESR, RF, ANA, ANCA, CRP, ACE, uric acid, syphilis serology, chest X-ray, urinalysis.
- Anterior segment fluorescein angiography (ASFA): rapid arteriovenous transit time, rapid intense leakage from capillaries and venules.

Treatment

- *Oral:* NSAID (e.g., flurbiprofen 100 mg 3×/day; can be tapered down once disease is controlled).
- If not controlled, consider systemic immunosuppression: commonly corticosteroids (e.g., prednisone 1 mg/kg/day) ± other immuno-suppressants (coordinate with a PCP or rheumatologist).
- Topical corticosteroids are usually an adjunct to systemic therapy.
- Periocular corticosteroids (e.g., subtenons or transseptal triamcinolone acetonide) can be given in patients with no evidence of scleral thinning.

Nodular non-necrotizing anterior scleritis

Clinical features

- Subacute onset (over 1 week) moderate to severe pain, FB sensation, redness, tearing ± photophobia.
- Red nodule arising from the sclera; cannot be moved separately from underlying tissue (cf. nodular episcleritis); does not blanch with topical vasoconstrictor (e.g., phenylephrine 10%); globe tender.

Investigations

These are as for diffuse anterior scleritis.

Treatment

Treat as for diffuse anterior scleritis, but add topical lubricants.

Anterior scleritis (2)

Necrotizing anterior scleritis with inflammation

Clinical features
- Subacute-onset (3–4 days) severe pain, redness, tearing ± photophobia.
- White avascular areas surrounded by injected edematous sclera; scleral necrosis → translucency revealing blue-black uveal tissue. Anterior uveitis suggests very advanced disease.

Scleral thinning and degree of scleral injection may be best appreciated under natural or room light. Necrotizing scleritis in general has a greater association with a systemic autoimmune condition than non-necrotizing scleritis.

Complications include peripheral ulcerative keratitis, acute stromal keratitis, sclerosing keratitis, uveitis, cataract, astigmatism, glaucoma, and perforation.

Investigations
- CBC, ESR, RF, ANA, ANCA, CRP, ACE, uric acid, syphilis serology, chest X-ray, urinalysis.
- ASFA: arteriovenous shunts with perfusion of veins before capillaries, and islands of no blood flow.

Treatment
- Systemic immunosuppression commonly involves corticosteroids (e.g., prednisone 1 mg/kg/day tapering down) ± immunosuppressants such as cyclophosphamide, methotrexate, cyclosporine, or azathioprine; coordinate with a PCP or rheumatologist.
- Intravenous infliximab in recalcitrant cases for rapid control of inflammation.
- Scleral biopsy for patients completely unresponsive to immunosuppressive therapy.
- Scleral patching or reinforcement for areas of significant thinning
- If there is risk of perforation, protect globe (e.g., glasses by day, shield at night) and consider scleral patch graft.

Necrotizing anterior scleritis without inflammation (scleromalacia perforans)

Scleromalacia perforans is usually seen in severe chronic seropositive rheumatoid arthritis.

Clinical features
- Asymptomatic
- Small yellow areas of necrotic sclera coalesce to reveal large areas of underlying uvea in a quiet eye.
- *Complications:* although this does not usually result in ocular perforation, this situation may arise after minor trauma.

Investigations
- As for necrotizing anterior scleritis with inflammation.

Treatment
- Systemic immunosuppression commonly involves corticosteroids and/or other immunosuppressants (as discussed above); coordinate with PCP or rheumatologist.
- Topical: generous lubrication.
- If there is risk of perforation, protect globe (e.g., glasses by day, shield at night) and consider scleral patch graft.
- Systemic treatment is crucial since the scleritis is an indicator of poor rheumatoid control with mortality of 50% over 10 years due to systemic vasculitis.

Posterior scleritis

Posterior scleritis is uncommon but is probably underdiagnosed. The condition may be overlooked on account of more obvious anterior scleral inflammation or because there is isolated posterior disease, and thus the eye appears white and quiet (often despite severe symptoms). It is associated with systemic disease (usually rheumatoid arthritis or vasculitis) in up to one- third of cases.

Clinical features
- Mild–severe deep pain (may be referred to brow or jaw region), ↓VA, diplopia, photopsia, hypermetropic shift.
- White eye (unless anterior involvement), lid edema, proptosis, lid retraction, restricted motility; choroidal folds, annular choroidal detachment, exudative retinal detachments, macular edema, disc edema.

Investigation
B-scan ultrasonography: scleral thickening with fluid in Tenon's space (T-sign).

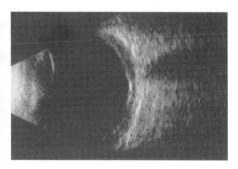

Figure 8.1 B-scan ultrasound of a patient with posterior scleritis with scleral and choroidal thickening forming a "T sign." See insert for color version.

Treatment
- Oral: NSAID (e.g., flurbiprofen 100 mg 3×/day; can be tapered down once disease controlled).
- If not controlled, consider systemic immunosuppression: commonly corticosteroids (e.g., prednisone 1 mg/kg/day) ± other immuno-suppressants (coordinate with PCP or rheumatologist); these may include methotrexate, azathioprine, cyclosporine, and cyclophosphamide.
- The response to therapy may be monitored by measuring the posterior scleral thickness on serial B-scan ultrasound, FA for presence of choroidal leakage or OCT for presence of subretinal fluid.

Lens

Related pages:
Congenital cataracts 📖 p. 625–627

Anatomy and physiology

The *lens* is a transparent, biconvex structure with an outer acellular capsule. It provides one-third of the refractive power of the eye. In the unaccommodated state, the lens is around 4 mm thick, with a 10 mm anterior radius of curvature, a 6 mm posterior radius of curvature, a refractive index of 1.386 (1.406 centrally), and an overall diopter power of 18D.

Anatomy

Embryologically derived from surface ectoderm

Capsule

This unusually thick basement membrane is rich in type IV collagen; the anterior capsule arises from the epithelium, while the posterior capsule arises from the elongating fiber cells. The capsule is thicker at the equator than centrally and thicker anteriorly (8–14 µm, increasing with age) than posteriorly (2–3 µm).

Epithelium

The lens epithelium lies just deep to the anterior capsule. Centrally, the epithelium is cuboidal and nonmitotic; peripherally, the epithelium is columnar and mitotic, producing almost 2 million transparent lens fibers over an adult's life.

Fibers

As the cells elongate (up to 10 mm long), transparency is attained by loss of organelles, a tight regular arrangement, and a 90% crystallin composition. The nucleus (comprising embryonic and fetal parts) consists of the fibers laid down before birth; however, the clinical "nucleus" observed at the slit lamp also includes deep cortex.

Lens sutures are formed by interdigitation of the ends of the fibers. The most visible example are the two Y-shaped sutures of the fetal nucleus—anterior Y, posterior λ. The cortex contains the more recently formed fibers and the nucleus contains the older nondividing cells.

Zonules

These comprise sheets of suspensory fibers composed of fibrillin (Ch15q) that arise at the ciliary body and attach to the lens pre-equatorially, equatorially, and post-equatorially.

Physiology

The lens has a low water (65%) and high protein (35%) content. It has a resting pH of 6.9 and a relatively low temperature and is relatively hypoxic. Most energy production and active transport occurs at the epithelium, but peripheral lens fibers demonstrate significant protein synthesis (mainly of crystallins), and even central lens fibers show limited carbohydrate metabolism.

Although oxidative phosphorylation occurs at the epithelium, most energy production is anaerobic (via glycolysis, pentose–phosphate pathway, and the α-glycerophosphate shuttle). Most glucose is thus converted to glucose-6-phosphate and, to a lesser degree, sorbitol.

The high refractive index of the lens results from the crystallin content of its fibers. These proteins, compromised mostly of crystallin, are extremely stable and provide good short-range order (predominantly β-sheet secondary structure).

Clarity of the lens is attained by minimizing lens fiber scatter with narrow lens fiber membranes, small interfiber spaces, tightly packed regular contents (crystallin), absence of blood vessels, and loss of organelles.

Detoxification of free radicals is achieved by glutathione, supported by ascorbic acid (cf. hydrogen-peroxide catalase elsewhere in the body). In the process, glutathione is oxidized to GSSG, which would potentially form disulfide bonds with lens proteins were it not returned to its reduced state by glutathione reductase.

Cataract: introduction

Cataracts account for around 50% of global blindness, representing around 18 million people. While cataracts are ubiquitous, occurring in almost every aging population, the inequity of eye care means that 99% of bilateral blindness due to cataracts is seen in developing countries. Cataracts account for 50% of cases of reversible low vision in the United States.

Risk factors

The prevalence of cataract increases markedly with age. In the United States, a visually significant cataract (VA <20/40) is present in approximately 2.5% of those aged 40–49, 6.8% of those aged 50–59, 20% of those aged 60–69, 42.8% of those aged 70–79, and 68.3% of those aged >80.

Other risk factors include exposure to sunlight, smoking, alcohol, dehydration, radiation, corticosteroid use, and diabetes mellitus. Nutritional or vitamin supplementation has not consistently been shown to be useful in preventing cataract formation.

Pathogenesis

The way in which these factors cause cataracts is unclear, although a common pathway appears to be protein denaturation (e.g., by oxidative stress). Metabolic disturbance (hyperglycemia in diabetes mellitus or hyperuremia in dehydration or renal failure), toxins (e.g., smoking, alcohol), loss of anti-oxidant enzymes (e.g., superoxide dismutase), membrane disruption, reduced metabolism, failure of active transport, and loss of ionic–osmotic balance may all contribute to this process.

Clinical presentations

Common

- Change in vision—reduced acuity, contrast sensitivity, or color appreciation, glare, monocular diplopia, or ghosting.
- Change in refraction—typically a myopic shift due to nuclear sclerosis.
- Change in fundus view—clinicians may have difficulty "looking in" long before the patients feel they have difficulties "looking out." This may be a problem when trying to monitor or treat posterior segment disease such as diabetic retinopathy or macular degeneration.

Uncommon

Phacomorphic glaucoma

The large cataractous lens may cause anterior bowing of the iris with secondary angle closure. Presentation may occur as acute angle closure with high IOP, shallow AC, and fixed semidilated pupil.

Phacomorphic glaucoma can be distinguished from *primary* angle closure glaucoma by the presence of an ipsilateral swollen cataractous lens and contralateral open angle with deep AC.

Phacolytic glaucoma

The hypermature cataract loses soluble lens proteins through the anterior capsule, causing trabecular obstruction and subsequent secondary open-angle glaucoma. Note raised IOP, lens protein in a deep AC (may form a pseudohypopyon), open angles, and hypermature cataract.

Phacoanaphylactic uveitis (i.e., phacoantigenic, lens-induced granulomatous uveitis)

Phacoanaphylactic uveitis is a misnomer, as the inflammatory response is not a type I phacoanyphylactic response but a granulomatous inflammatory response to lens proteins. This condition usually follows traumatic capsular rupture or postoperative retention of lens material (it must be distinguished from endophthalmitis). The IOP may be high, normal, or low.

Cataract: types

Cataracts may be classified according to age of onset, morphology, grade of opacification, and maturity.

Age of onset

Cataracts may be congenital (p. 625), juvenile or presenile (p. 626), or age related (senile) (p. 234).

Morphology

Cataract morphology may be divided into fiber based (pattern relates to anatomical structure of the lens) or nonfiber based (a more random distribution). Fiber-based cataracts may be divided into sutural (pattern relates to lens sutures) and nonsutural types (Table 9.1).

Grade

Grading systems have been designed that aim to quantify the degree of opacification. These vary from simple assessment by direct ophthalmoscopy to more sophisticated methods such as the Lens Opacities Classification System III (LOCS III), where slit-lamp examination is compared to a standard set of photographs (separate set for nuclear, cortical, and posterior subcapsular).

Maturity of cataract

- *Immature:* opacification is incomplete.
- *Mature:* opacification is total.
- *Hypermature:* lysis of cortex results in shrinkage, seen clinically as wrinkling of the capsule.
- *Morgagnian:* liquefaction of cortex allows the harder nucleus to drop inferiorly (but remaining still within the capsule).

Table 9.1 Classification of cataract morphology

Fiber based	Sutural	Congenital sutural
		Concussion
		Storage disorder
		Deposition
	Nonsutural	Lamellar
		Nuclear
		Cortical
Nonfiber based		Subcapsular
		Lamellar
		Coronary
		Blue dot
		Christmas tree

Type	Cause	Properties
Sutural 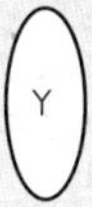	Congenital	Non-progressive
	Concussion	Often flower-shaped (lens fiber separation and fluid entry); anterior and posterior
	Storage disorder	Usually start posteriorly; • Fabry's disease, mannosidosis
	Deposition	Usually start anteriorly; • Copper, gold, silver, iron, chlorpromazine
Nuclear 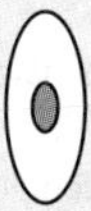	Congenital	Nonprogressive; limited to embryonic nucleus (cataracta centralis pulverulenta) or more extensive
	Age-related	Increased white scatter (light scattering) and brunescence (brown chromophores)
Lamellar 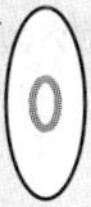	Congenital/infantile	Localized to a particular lamella (layer) ± extensions (riders) • Inherited, rubella, diabetes, glactosemia, hypocalcemia
Coronary 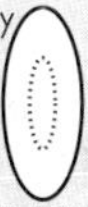	Sporadic	Round opacities in the deep cortex forming a "crown" • Occasionally inherited
Cortical 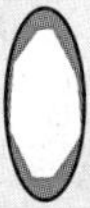	Age-related	Spoke-like opacities in the superficial cortex, spreading aling fibers at an unpredictable rate
Subcapsular 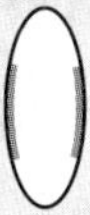	Age-related/presenile	Granular material just beneath capsule, posterior (more common and visually significant) or anterior • Diabetes, corticosteroids, uveitis, radiation
Polar 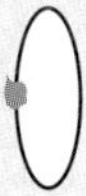	Congenital	Anterior—with abnormalities of capsule ± anterior segment (persistent pupillary membrane, anterior lenticonus, Peters anomaly) Posterior—with abnormalities of capsule ± posterior segment (persistent hyperplastic primary vitreous, Mittendorf dots, posterior lenticonus)
Diffuse 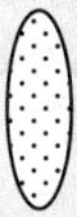	Congenital	Focal blue dot opacities are common and visually insiginificant Also present in Lowe syndrome carriers
	Age-related	Christmas tree cataracts are highly reflective crystalline opacities

Figure 9.1 Cataract types.

Cataract surgery: assessment

Surgical removal of cataracts is effective and safe. In the United States, 85 to 95% of patients attain best-corrected visual acuity (BCVA) ≥20/40 within 3 months of surgery, 58% had BCVA of 20/25 or better, and 75% are within 1D of predicted refraction. Sight-threatening complications are rare. However, this is in part due to careful preoperative preparation and postoperative assessment.

1) Referral

Referrals may be made by the PCP, optometrist, or ophthalmologist.

Appropriate referral
- The cataract is likely responsible for the patient's visual complaint.
- The cataract is compromising the patient's lifestyle.
- The risks and benefits of cataract surgery have been discussed with the patient.
- The patient wishes to have the operation.

2) Outpatient appointment

Table 9.2 Initial assessment for cataract surgery

Visual symptoms	Blur at distance/near, glare, distortion, color perception, "second sight" (myopic shift)
POH	Previous acuity; history of amblyopia, strabismus, previous surgery or trauma; concurrent eye disease; refraction
PMH	Diabetes, hypertension; ability to lie flat and still for 20–30min; anesthetic history (if GA considered)
SH	Occupation, driving, hobbies, daily tasks
Meds	Warfarin, antiplatelet agents; topical medication
Visual acuity	Distance/near, unaided/best-corrected/pinhole/glare testing
Pupils	Check for relative afferent papillary defect (RAPD)
Cataract	Morphology, density, maturity, zonular stability
Other factors	Globe (deep-set, small/large), lids (blepharitis, entropion, ectropion), nasolacrimal (mucocele), cornea (scarring, guttata), anterior chamber depth, IOP, iris (pseudoexfoliation syndrome, iridodonesis, posterior synechiae, inducible mydriasis), lens (pseudoexfoliation syndrome [PXF], phacodonesis, lens–vitreous interface) optic disc (e.g., glaucoma, neuropathy), macula (e.g., AMD), fundus

Appropriate scheduling for cataract surgery

- There is a visually significant cataract responsible for the patient's complaint and compromising his/her lifestyle.
- There is no coexisting ocular disease precluding surgery. Any disease that may affect surgery (e.g., PXF) or outcome (e.g., AMD) has been discussed with the patient and an appropriately guarded prognosis given.
- The patient wants to proceed and understands the risks.
- Informed consent is taken and a surgical plan is formulated (p. 236).

The younger patient

In the younger patients, also consider why they might have developed pre-senile cataracts (e.g., trauma, steroids, etc., p. 626).

3) Preoperative assessment

For patient convenience, this is often on the same day as the initial assessment. Aspects of the workup may be performed by a suitably trained assistant or technician according to local protocol.

History

- General health—past medical history, drugs, allergies.
- Social history—support, telephone, ability to manage topical medication.
- Education—surgery, postoperative care, information leaflet.

Investigation

- Biometry/IOL power calculations.

Treatment

- Prescription of preoperative treatments—e.g., topical antibiotics for blepharitis, or atropine for poor dilation.

Cataract surgery: consent and planning

Nature of the operation

Explain what a cataract is: "The clear lens in your eye has become cloudy," and what the operation does: "The operation is real surgery where an incision is made on the eye to remove the cataract and replace it with a new plastic lens."

General risk

For all patients, warn of sight-threatening risks, notably corneal edema, glaucoma, retinal detachment or tear (0.1%), endophthalmitis (0.1%), and choroidal hemorrhage (0.1%). Advise of the possibility of requiring a second operation ± GA (dropped nucleus or dislocated IOL [0.5%]).

The most common intraoperative complication is posterior capsule rupture with vitreous loss (1–4%), which may have a significant effect on outcome. The most common postoperative complication is posterior capsular opacification (PCO) (10–50% in 2 years). Discuss with the patient postoperative refractive needs (e.g., the need for glasses for near or intermediate vision).

Anesthetic options include topical, local (peribulbar or retrobulbar), or general (GA) (p. 690). The risk of a GA will depend on the general health of the patient and, if necessary, should be discussed with the anesthesiologist before the day of surgery. Risks of retrobulbar anesthesia include globe rupture (0.006–0.1%) and life-threatening events such as brainstem anesthesia or the oculocardiac reflex (0.03%).

Specific risk

Assess and warn patient of any additional risk, such as technical difficulties, guarded visual prognosis, and any increased risk of sight-threatening complications. Consider whether subspecialist review is indicated (e.g., for posterior polar cataracts, the presence of endothelial dystrophies, or retinopathy).

Common technical issues

Table 9.3 Common technical issues

Feature	Risk	Strategy
Positional		
Cervical spondylosis	Head-up posture	Tilt feet up
Deep-set eye	Poor access	Temporal approach
View		
Oily tear film	Aberrant reflexes	External methylcellulose
Poor red reflex	Difficult capsulorhexis	Vision Blue (trypan blue)
Access		
Short axial length	Crowded AC	High viscosity viscoelastic
Poor dilation	Inadequate access	Iris hooks or iris stretch techniques

Table 9.3 (Contd.)

Feature	Risk	Strategy
Zonular integrity		
Age >90 years	Zonular dehiscence	Minimize lens movement
Pseudoexfoliation	Zonular dehiscence	Minimize lens movement
Pre-op phacodonesis	Zonular dehiscence	Vitreoretinal approach
White cataract	Zonular dehiscence	Consider ECCE/chopping
PC integrity		
Shallow AC depth	Iris/PC trauma	High-viscosity viscoelastic
Posterior polar	PC rupture	Viscodissection or vitreoretinal approach

Guarded visual prognosis
Note history of amblyopia or evidence of pre-existing corneal opacity, vitreous opacities, or macular or optic nerve disease.

Increased risk of sight-threatening complications
- *Endophthalmitis*—note lid disease (blepharitis, trichiasis, entropion, ectropion), conjunctivitis, nasolacrimal disease (obstruction, mucocele, etc.), diabetes. Pretreat when possible, e.g., lid hygiene and antibiotics for blepharitis and conjunctivitis, surgery for lid malposition or nasolacrimal obstruction.
- *Retinal detachment*—note high myopia, lattice degeneration, previous retinal detachment, and retinal tear.
- *Choroidal hemorrhage*—possibly uncontrolled hypertension, age, arteriosclerosis, high intraocular pressure.
- *Corneal decompensation*—note endothelial dystrophy (e.g., Fuchs').

Desired outcome
Consider the refractive needs of the patients. When aiming for emmetropia (most patients), explain that while they may need no or weak glasses for distance, they will need reading glasses. Patients with significant ametropia or astigmatism are more complex.

High ametropia
Complications include anisometropia, which may lead to aniseikonia.

Preoperatively, with bilateral cataracts, discuss options: (1) aim for emmetropia and do the second eye shortly thereafter; (2) aim for leaving ametropic (but up to 3D nearer emmetropia than the other eye), with less immediate need for a second operation; (3) if there is unilateral cataract, particularly where the second eye has good acuity and accommodative function, consider aiming for emmetropia and using a contact lens on the second eye until surgery is indicated.

Astigmatism
Pre-existing astigmatism can usually be reduced by choosing to operate "on-meridian." For higher degrees of astigmatism, additional refractive incisions can be placed at the time of cataract surgery or toric IOLs can be placed (p. 239).

Presbyopia correcting strategies

Discuss with all patients options regarding presbyopia correction, including monovision (one eye set for distance and one for near) as well as premium lenses (ReSTOR, ReZoom, Crystalens), despite assumptions of the patient's ability to afford the out-of-pocket expense. Questionnaires can be useful to screen for patients who are good candidates for premium lenses.

In general, patients should be highly motivated to reduce postoperative dependence on eyeglasses, have reasonable postoperative expectations regarding results, and have no significant ocular comorbidities.

Multifocal lenses (e.g., ReSTOR, ReZoom)

Divide light into multiple planes such that at any given moment near and far objects are in focus. Patients report decreased need for glasses for near vision (50–80% reporting spectacle independence for near work after bilateral implantation). Complications include subjective loss of contrast and visual phenomena such as glare and haloes.

Accomodative lens (Crystalens)

Design of the IOL allows for shift of the lens during accommodation. This improves near and intermediate unaided vision compared to that with monofocal lenses set for emmetropia.

Accomodative IOLs have lower rates of spectacle independence for near when compared with multifocal lenses, but improved visual acuity at intermediate distances and lower rates of glare and haloes. Outcomes are more dependent than multifocal lenses on the healing response of the capsular bag and ability of the ciliary body to accommodate.

Cataract surgery: perioperative

Preoperative check (on the day of surgery)

Patient preparation

- Ensure mydriasis—e.g., cyclopentolate 1% + phenylephrine 2.5% + diclofenac 0.1%. In the presence of a poorly dilated pupil or if there is a history of tamsulosin (i.e., flomax) or other systemic α_1-blockers associated with intraoperative floppy iris syndrome (IFIS), consider the use of intracameral epinephrine, mechanical dilators such as iris hooks, and/or a highly cohesive viscoelastic (e.g., Healon 5).
- Topical antibiotics reduce bacterial load of conjunctiva.
- Assess the red reflex and consider the use of trypan blue (Vision Blue) or other capsule-staining dye.
- Check that consent form has been completed.
- Check for any new ophthalmic problems, especially evidence of active infection.
- Mark side of operation.
- Operating surgeon should confirm IOL type and power, and axis and operating position.

IOL selection

- Check that the biometry does indeed belong to the patient.
- Check for *intraocular* consistency in axial length and K values (i.e., that they are similar and the standard deviation is low).
- Check for *interocular* consistency in axial length and K values. If axial length difference >0.3 mm, confirm by B-scan and if the difference in K readings >1D, then consider corneal topography.
- Check appropriate formula used (Table 9.4).
- Select appropriate lens power as discussed with patient and consistent with postoperative expectations (usually, but not always, aiming for emmetropia).

Astigmatic targeting

If operating on-meridian, a clear corneal incision is placed on the steep corneal meridian. This should be based on keratometry as the refractive astigmatism may include a lenticular component that will be dealt with by lens removal.

The astigmatic effect of the incision increases with depth and length of the wound. It can be enhanced by an opposite refractive incision (on-meridian surgery) or by single or paired incisions at another meridian (off-meridian surgery).

Table 9.4 IOL formula recommendations

<22 mm	Hoffer Q or SRK/T
22–24.5 mm	SRK/T, Holladay, Haigis
>24.6 mm	SRK/T

Previous cornea refractive surgery commonly alters the refractive power of the central cornea, thereby reducing the accuracy of the paracentral measurements obtained by traditional keratometry. Patients who received myopia-correcting refractive ablation tend to have hyperopic shifts in their refractive outcomes, whereas the opposite is true for patients who have hyperopic correction.

Multiple strategies exist to overcome the limitations of traditional keratometry. Patients should be aware of limitations of biometry, the higher frequency of less accurate refractive outcomes, and the potential need for further surgery to obtain spectacle independence.

Box 9.1 IOL selection after refractive surgery

No one method for assessment of corneal refractive power stands out as superior. Many surgeons seek a consensus from a variety of techniques.

Formulas
- Difference in prerefractive and postrefractive K values.
- Postrefractive surgical corneal topographic data (Pentacam, EyeSys, Galilei, Tomey).
- Biometric data (IOL master).
- A postrefractive IOL calculator is available on the American Society of Cataract and Refractive Surgery Web site (www.ascrs.org).

Keratometric measurements performed after refractive surgery are unreliable in traditional biometric formulas. Methods to correct the keratometry readings include the following:
- Clinical history method

   Corrected K = pre-laser K − change in refractive error at
   6 months

- Contact lens method
- Measure refraction with and without a 40D hard contact lens

   Corrected K = 40 + (refraction with contact lens − refraction
   without contact lens)

These corrected K values are entered into SRK-T, Haigis, Hoffer Q, and Holladay 2 formulas and the highest IOL power is selected.

Cataract surgery: postoperative

Postoperative check (on the next day)

Examination

- Cornea — Wounds sealed (Seidel test negative), clarity
- AC — Formed, activity
- Pupil — Round
- PCIOL — Centered and in the bag
- IOP — Check and lower as necessary

Give clear instructions regarding use of postoperative drops, use of a clear shield when sleeping, limitations on activities (e.g., avoid eye make-up, swimming, activities that will injure or contaminate the eye), what to expect (1–2 days of discomfort, watering), what to worry about (increasing pain or redness, worsening vision), and where to get help (including telephone number).

Use acronym **RSVP**: **R**edness (increased), **S**ensitivity (light), **V**ision (decreased), **P**ain (increased).

Refractive review (usually 2–4 weeks later)

Examination

- VA — Unaided, pinhole, BCVA (best-corrected vision acuity)
- Cornea — Wounds sealed (Seidel test negative), clarity
- AC — Depth and activity
- Pupil — Round
- PCIOL — Centered and in the bag
- IOP
- Fundus — No CME, no retinal holes, breaks, or tears.

Either prepare to operate on second eye and discharge patient to referring physician, or schedule for routine follow-up in 3–6 months. If there is unexpectedly poor unaided or BCVA, perform refraction to look for "refractive surprise" and dilated funduscopy to check for subtle cystoid macular edema (CME) (especially if VA [pin hole] < VA [unaided]) or other ocular pathology (e.g., PCO).

Phacoemulsification (1)

Preparation

Instill povidone iodine 5% aqueous solution in fornix, and 10% aqueous solution to clean the lashes and skin to reduce bacterial load and risk of endophthalmitis. Careful draping maximizes surgical view, keeps lashes out of the surgical field, and prevents pooling of fluid.

Incision

Wound construction is critical. The wound needs to be large enough to allow easy access of instruments, but small enough to permit a stable AC and reduce risk of iris prolapse (e.g., 2.8 mm).

Wound construction options include clear corneal incisions (which may be tri-, bi-, or uniplanar) and scleral tunnels. Scleral tunnels are fairly astigmatically neutral, whereas corneal incisions tend to cause flattening. This can be made use of by operating on-meridian to reduce any pre-existing corneal astigmatism.

At the end of the operation, the wound must seal to become watertight at physiological pressures or a suture should be placed. Suture placement should also be considered in patients with a history of eye-rubbing, dementia, or other mental handicaps, or in whom concurrent or subsequent surgery is planned (e.g., combined with glaucoma surgery, retinal surgery or injections).

Introduction and movement of instrumentation should respect the shape of the wound to reduce the risk of stripping off Descemet's membrane or stretching of the tissue.

Ophthalmic viscosurgical devices (OVDs; viscoelastics)

OVDs are solutions of long-chain polymers with a range of viscosity and cohesive properties. Higher-viscosity cohesive OVDs are used for stabilizing the AC and opening the bag prior to IOL insertion. Lower-viscosity dispersive OVDs are used to isolate part of the surgical field (e.g., protecting a vulnerable cornea in the soft-shell technique, keeping the iris or vitreous out of the way).

Viscoadaptives are more advanced OVDs that can behave like a higher-viscosity cohesive OVD or like a dispersive according to AC fluid dynamics (see Table 9.5).

Continuous curvilinear capsulorhexis

The aim is to achieve a 5–6 mm continuous central anterior capsulectomy via cystotome and/or forceps under viscoelastic. This is large enough to assist lens removal (and reduce risk of postoperative capsular phimosis) and small enough to stabilize the lens (and reduce risk of post-operative capsular opacification).

In the presence of poor red reflex or significant cortical opacities, visibility may be assisted by the use of trypan blue (often injected under air and washed out after 1 minute). Intumescent cataracts can be decompressed by puncturing the AC and aspirating lens matter.

A capsulorhexis running out to the periphery may be rescued by deepening the AC or pushing the iris back with more or higher-viscosity viscolelastic, e.g., Healon 5. If unable to bring the capsulorhexis back in, consider tearing in the opposite direction from the start position; capsulorhexis scissors or forceps or a can-opener capsulotomy. Review whether to continue with cautious phacoemulsification or convert to extracapsular cataract extraction (ECCE).

A small capsulorhexis can be extended after insertion of the posterior chamber intraocular lens (PCIOL) by making a nick (e.g., with a cystotome) and then tearing with forceps as usual.

Hydrodissection

Injection of balanced salt solution under the anterior capsular rim separates the nucleus from the cortex and is seen as a fluid wave passing posteriorly. If successful, it permits rotation of the nucleus. If overly aggressive, this may cause posterior capsule rupture or prolapse of the lens into the anterior chamber (although this is a desired event for some surgical techniques).

Table 9.5 Ophthalmic viscosurgical devices

Group	Subgroup	Content	Example	Molecular weight
Viscoadaptive		Hyaluronic acid	Healon 5	4000–8000 kDa
Higher viscosity	Superviscous	Hyaluronic acid	Healon GV	4000–8000 kDa
	Viscous	Hyaluronic acid	Healon Provisc	1000–2000 kDa
Lower viscositys	Medium viscosity	Hyaluronic acid	Viscoat	100–500 kDa
	Very low viscosity	HPMC	Occucoat	80–90 kDa

Phacoemulsification (2)

Phacoemulsification

Rotate the probe to enter wound with minimal trauma.

Technique

Many variations to disassemble the nucleus exist; techniques should be selected on the basis of nuclear density, zonular pathology, and surgeon comfort.

Divide and conquer

The groove should be about 1.5 phaco tips wide and as deep as safely possible (this is usually around 3 mm deep centrally). An improving red reflex may assist in judging depth. Use a second instrument to rotate nucleus 90° to form the next groove, and continue until a cruciate configuration is formed. Insert both instruments deep into each groove, gently pulling apart to crack the nucleus into four segments. Use a higher vacuum setting to bring each segment centrally to be emulsified.

Horizontal chop

Use high vacuum and sufficient phaco power to bury the phaco tip into the nucleus just proximal to the center while aiming steeply posterior. The second instrument is inserted under the anterior capsule and chopped horizontally through the stabilized nucleus against the phaco probe. This is repeated to generate wedges that can then be emulsified as described above section (Divide and conquer).

Vertical chop

This is similar to the horizontal chop, except the second instrument is directed posteriorly then peripherally to cleave the nucleus.

Chip and flip

Sculpt to form a bowl and then flip it anteriorly to complete emulsification safely.

Pumps and fluidics

The traditional distinction between a vacuum pump (e.g., Venturi system) and a peristaltic pump has become blurred by hybrids such as the scroll pump.

Vacuum systems

Use a Venturi or a diaphragm pump to generate a low pressure relative to the anterior chamber. Flow is dependent on this pressure difference and thus cannot be altered independently of vacuum.

Peristaltic systems

The pressure gradient is generated by milking fluid along compressible tubing by a series of rollers. Flow and vacuum can be set separately. A low flow setting results in a more gradual, gentler response, thus aiding cautious manipulation. This may be helpful in training. Higher flow results in a faster (but more aggressive) response from the phaco probe.

Adjusting the vacuum level limits the maximum vacuum that will be generated once the tip is occluded.

Phaco-power modulation

Phaco power can be delivered as continuous or intermittent. Intermittent modes are all directed at using phaco power more efficiently, reducing the effective phaco time (EPT = phaco time × percentage phaco power used). These modes include pulse (usually linear control of energy with fixed or varying pulse rate), burst mode (fixed phaco power with variable duration and interval), and assorted modifications such as sonolase (Whitestar), and "no burn" and "cool" phaco.

Torsional or transversal phacoemulsification (Alcon OZil, AMO Ellips) directs ultrasonic movements and energy at the phaco needle tip laterally. This results in less repulsion of the nuclear material and improved "followability" with lower energy within the eye. It can be alternated with or without linear phaco movements.

Dual linear

This method permits simultaneous foot control of both phaco power (pitch, i.e., vertical pedal détente) and aspiration (yaw, i.e., lateral pedal movements). It is particularly useful for the phaco chop technique.

Irrigation and aspiration (IA)

IA is usually automated (straight/curved/45°/90° tips) and can be combined or split (bimanual). Manual IA is an alternative (Simcoe). Cortex is engaged peripherally and dragged centrally where the vacuum can be increased under direct view.

Intraocular lens (IOL)

Most IOLs are designed to be injected through small incisions and do not require wound enlargement. Occasionally, it is necessary to enlarge the wound enough to allow the introduction of the lens (e.g., 3.0 mm for a foldable IOL) before introducing it with either a special forceps or an injector.

Fill the capsular bag with viscoelastic before implanting the lens, placing the lead haptic directly into the bag before dropping and dialing in the second haptic. The choice of lens is typically based on capsular integrity and desired postoperative refraction (p. 251).

Wound closure

Well-constructed wounds sized for foldable lenses are usually self-sealing but may be assisted by stromal hydration. If in any doubt of wound stability, suture the wound closed.

ECCE and ICCE

Extracapsular cataract extraction (ECCE)

ECCE is en bloc removal of the lens while retaining the lens capsule and integrity of the anterior vitreous face (see Table 9.6). The operation typically requires a superior 9–10 mm biplanar corneal (or limbal) incision, injection of viscoelastic to form the AC, anterior capsulotomy (usually can-opener technique), hydrodissection, nucleus expression (gentle digital pressure or irrigating vectis), aspiration of cortex, and lens implantation (usually rigid PMMA lens into the bag).

A small-incision ECCE can be performed by creating a larger internal wound opening that narrows at its external limit (like a funnel).

Intracapsular cataract extraction (ICCE)

This is removal of the whole lens, including the capsule, and was widely practiced during the 1960s and 1970s. The operation requires a 150° corneal (or limbal) incision, a peripheral iridectomy (PI), zonular digestion (α-chymotrypsin), forceps or cryoprobe removal of the lens, and insertion of an ACIOL (angle or iris-supported), a sutured lens, or aphakic correction (eyeglasses or contact lenses).

Table 9.6 Types of cataract extraction

Technique	Advantages	Disadvantages
Intracapsular (ICCE)	• No PCO • Can deal with zonular dialysis	• Higher rates of CME and retinal detachment • Higher rate of rubeosis in diabetic eyes • ACIOL, sutured lens or aphakia • Sutures required
Extracapsular (ECCE)	• PCIOL • Lower rate of CME and retinal detachment than with ICCE • Useful in setting of zonule or capsule compromise	• PCO • Sutures required
Phacoemulsification	• More stable AC/IOP • PCIOL • Lower rate of CME, retinal detachment, and expulsive hemorrhage • Sutureless wound • Reduced astigmatism • Faster visual rehabilitation • Reduced postoperative inflammation • Topical anesthesia possible	• PCO • Expensive equipment • Dropped lens fragments

Intraocular lenses

Choice of lens

Phacoemulsification with an intact posterior capsule and anterior capsulorhexis permits the use of a foldable PCIOL (smaller wound, usually sutureless) that can be placed in the bag (preferable optically and physiologically).

In the presence of a small tear in the anterior or posterior capsule, it may still be possible to implant the lens in the capsular bag. If there is a significant PC tear but an intact anterior capsule, consider sulcus fixation with capture of the IOL optic under the anterior capsulorhexis. If there is anterior and posterior capsular damage or zonular instability, consider an ACIOL or suture-fixated PCIOL.

For extracapsular cataract extraction, the larger incision is sufficient for implantation of a rigid PMMA lens into the bag or sulcus.

Posterior chamber intraocular lens (PCIOL)

IOLs may be classified according to their material (silicone, acrylic, PMMA) (see Tables 9.7 and 9.8), interaction with water (hydrophilic or hydrophobic), and design (one piece or three piece; spherical or toric; rounded or square-edged). Lens behavior therefore arises from a number of contributing factors.

For example, hydrophilic acrylic lenses appear to be the most biocompatible with little attachment of inflammatory cells. However, the hydrophobic acrylic IOLs appear to have the lowest PCO rates, but this may be due to their square-edge design rather than the material.

Material

Table 9.7 Types of PCIOL

Material	Advantages	Disadvantages
Rigid		
PMMA	• Follow-up >50 years • Stable	• Large incision needed • Higher rate of PCO
Foldable		
Silicone	• Follow-up >15 years • Folds easily	• Rapid unfolding • Poor handling when wet • Adherence to silicone oil
Hydrophobic acrylic	• Higher n allows thinner lenses • Slow unfolding • Low PCO rate (some designs)	• Glistenings in optic (some lenses)
Hydrophilic acrylic	• Slow unfolding • Low inflammatory cell attachment • Resistant to Nd:YAG laser damage	• Calcium deposition on or in optic (some lenses)

Table 9.8 PCIOL materials

Lens type	Material	Refractive index (n)
Rigid		
PMMA	Polymethyl methacrylate	1.49
Flexible		
Silicone	Silicone polymers	1.41–1.46
Hydrophobic acrylic	Acrylate + methacrylate	1.54
Hydrophilic acrylic	Polyhydroxyethyl-methylacrylate + hydrophilic acrylic monomer	1.47

Design
- *Square-edged vs. rounded:* IOL optics with square posterior edges appear to reduce posterior capsular opacification by reducing migration of lens epithelial cells.
- *Toric vs. spherical:* toric IOLs can correct for preoperative astigmatism but may cause problems or be ineffective if not perfectly positioned.
- *Short-wavelength filtration:* some recent IOLs filter out short-wavelength blue light as this may be linked to accelerated age-related macular changes in pseudophakic patients.
- *Pseudoaccommodative lenses* are multifocals that may be diffractive or refractive in nature. They are attended by a loss of contrast sensitivity and are not always tolerated.
- *Accommodative IOLs* alter their focal length by anteroposterior movement within the capsular bag.

Anterior chamber intraocular lens (ACIOL)

ACIOL use is mainly associated with intracapsular cataract extraction but may still be of use where there is innate or acquired loss of capsular support. These may be angle supported or iris supported. Angle-supported lenses are sized to the anterior chamber (measure "white to white").

In earlier designs, sizing was critical: too large and they would cause inflammation and local destruction; too small and they would be unstable and again cause irritation.

Modern one-piece lenses with three- or four-point fixation are much better tolerated and sizing is less critical. ACIOLs may be introduced by means of a glide. A peripheral iridectomy should be performed at the time of surgery to avoid iris bombe from pupillary block.

Cataract surgery and concurrent eye disease

Intraoperative floppy iris syndrome (IFIS)

Hypotonic iris smooth muscle results from ischemia, inflammation, or most commonly use of tamsulosin (i.e., Flomax) or other systemic α_1-blocker.

Iris smooth muscle atrophy results in varying degrees of IFIS, most commonly manifesting as mild to severe miosis and iris prolapse through corneal incisions. Consider use of a combination of preoperative mydriatics, intracameral epinephrine, mechanical dilators such as iris hooks or the Malyugin ring, and/or a highly cohesive viscoelastic (Healon 5).

Pupil stretching can exacerbate iris floppiness and should be avoided.

Diabetes

- *Complications:* fibrinous anterior uveitis, posterior capsular opacification (PCO), progression of retinopathy, and macular edema. Risk of complications increases with degree of retinopathy.
- *Preoperative:* if severe nonproliferative (NPDR) or proliferative diabetic retinopathy (PDR), treat patient (PRP or anti-VEGF agent, i.e., bevacizumab) prior to surgery when possible. Treat CSME (focal, grid laser, bevacizumab, triamcinolone) before surgery.
- *Postoperative:* consider topical NSAID (e.g., ketorolac 0.3% 3×/day for 1 month). An extended course of topical steroids may be required. See patient at 1 day, 1 week, and then 6 weeks to monitor for CME or anterior segment neovascularization.

Glaucoma

- *Complications:* postoperative pressure spike, progression of field loss, failure of previous trabeculectomy
- *Preoperative:* stabilize IOP control, identify degree of vision loss due to glaucomatous field loss, consider combining cataract surgery with IOP-lowering procedure (e.g., trabeculectomy).
- Consider clear corneal wound to prevent scarring of conjunctiva, thereby facilitating future drainage surgery. Meticulous removal of viscoelastic is needed to prevent postoperative IOP spike.
- *Postoperative:* consider extended use of postoperative acetazolamide or topical IOP-lowering agents to minimize postoperative pressure spikes (and risk of "wipe-out" to a vulnerable optic nerve). Although there have been concerns about CME, the continuation of prostaglandin analogues postoperatively is probably safe. In the short eye, watch for aqueous misdirection syndrome. See patient at 1 day, 1 week, and then 6 weeks.

Uveitis

- *Complications:* exacerbation of inflammation, fibrinous anterior uveitis, synechiae, raised IOP, CME, PCO.
- *Preoperative:* control inflammation and IOP as much as possible. In well-controlled anterior uveitis, consider intensive topical steroids for 2 weeks prior to surgery (e.g., dexamethasone 0.1% q2h). In patients with chronic uveitis, consider 500 mg IV methylprednisolone 1 hour before surgery, or prednisolone 40 mg PO for 1 week prior to surgery.
- *Intraoperative:* ensure adequate pupillary access (synechialysis, iris hooks, iris stretching) but avoid unnecessary iris manipulation. Ensure meticulous cortical clearance. Perform a well-centered 5–6 mm capsulorhexis (to reduce postoperative capsular phimosis, iris-capsule synechiae). Give subconjunctival or intravitreal steroid (e.g., betamethasone 4 mg).
- *Postoperative:* frequent potent topical steroids (e.g., dexamethasone 0.1% q2h) and taper slowly; if oral steroids were started or increased preoperatively, these should be tapered slowly to zero or maintenance dose. Consider mydriatic (e.g., cyclopentolate 1%). In persistent fibrinous uveitis, consider intracameral recombinant tissue plasminogen activator (rtPA). See patient at 1 day, 1 week, and as necessary.

Postvitrectomy

- *Complications:* PCO, retinal (re)detachment, vitreous hemorrhage.
- *Preoperative:* silicone oil slows sound transmission (estimated at 987 m/sec), and this must be incorporated when calculating axial length from an A-scan. Additionally, the axial length may not be stable within a year of scleral buckling procedures and may be unpredictable after macular surgery.
- *Intraoperative:* use clear corneal incision (rather than scleral tunnel). Poor mydriasis may require iris hooks or stretching. Fluctuation of AC depth and the risk to the flaccid PC may be minimized by well-constructed wounds, lower bottle height, reduced vacuum, and lifting of the iris with a second instrument. Minimize nucleus manipulation to protect damaged zonules. Use acrylic or PMMA lenses (*not* silicone), placing in the bag or sulcus.
- *Postoperative:* warn patient about retinal detachment, dilate at follow-up review.

Cataract surgery: complications

Intraoperative

Posterior capsule rupture without vitreous loss (approximately 3% of surgeries)

The main goals when confronted with a PC tear (without vitreous loss) are to avoid vitreous traction or loss and maintain as much capsule and zonular support as possible. To prevent vitreous prolapse, the anterior chamber should remain pressurized by maintaining irrigation and using a viscoelastic to tamponade the vitreous posteriorly prior to withdrawing instruments.

If the PC tear is small and well defined, a PCIOL may still be placed in the bag either at the time of surgery or as a secondary procedure. However, with larger, poorly defined PC tears, it is safer to place the lens in the sulcus provided that sufficient anterior capsule remains to stabilize the IOC.

Assuming equal A-constants, a sulcus-fixated lens should be about 0.5D lower power than that calculated for placement in the capsular bag.

Posterior capsule rupture with vitreous loss (approximately 1% of surgeries)

Clear the wound and AC of vitreous with manual (sponge or scissors) and/or automated vitrectomy while maintaining as much posterior capsule as possible. Dilute triamcinolone in the anterior chamber can stain vitreous, thereby enabling more efficient and complete vitreous removal.

If sufficient anterior capsule remains, place the lens in the sulcus (see note above); otherwise, consider an ACIOL with a peripheral iridotomy or suture fixate a PCIOL.

Anterior capsule problems

The capsulorhexis has a tendency to run out in a number of situations: shallow AC, positive posterior pressure, young patients, and intumescent cataracts. Stabilize the AC with a more cohesive viscolelastic (e.g., Healon 5). Decompress intumescent cataracts by puncturing the AC and aspirating lens matter.

If unable to bring the capsulorhexis back in, options include returning to the start and attempting a second tear in the opposite direction with use of capsulorhexis scissors and switching to a can-opener technique. Depending on the security of the resulting capsulorhexis, either continue with cautious phacoemulsification or convert to ECCE.

Zonular dehiscence

Consider stabilizing the capsule with iris hooks (secure the capsule in the area of dialysis) or a capsular tension ring (stabilizes the bag and redistributes forces away from individual zonules). Partially subluxed lenses may be more safely removed via phacoemulsification with the use of capsular tension rings with or without fixation loops (FDA approved) or with capsular tension segments (not FDA approved, but available through compassionate use).

If zonular dehiscence is associated with vitreous loss, an anterior or posterior vitrectomy will be required (consider co-surgery with a vitreoretinal surgeon).

Loss of nuclear fragment posteriorly (0.3%)

Nuclear material is inflammatory. Very small fragments can be observed but may require prolonged topical steroids. Larger fragments require removal via a pars plana vitrectomy, ideally within 1–2 weeks. Refer patient immediately to a vitreoretinal surgeon.

Start on their preferred regime to control inflammation, reduce risk of infection, and prevent increased IOP (partly to preserve corneal clarity). One therapeutic example is dexamethasone 0.1% q2h, gatifloxacin q6h, and acetazolamide SR 250 mg bid.

Choroidal hemorrhage (0.1%)

Suspect this if there is a sudden increase in IOP with AC shallowing, iris prolapse, loss of vitreous, and loss or darkening of the red reflex. This is often associated with the patient complaining of severe pain. Immediately suture all wounds closed, give IV pressure-lowering treatment (e.g., acetazolamide or mannitol), and start intensive topical steroids.

Prognosis is poor, with only 45% of patients achieving VA ≥20/40 in that eye.

Postoperative—early

Corneal edema (10%)

Control IOP and inflammation with topical IOP-lowering treatment (avoid carbonic anhydrase inhibitors, which can suppress endothelial cell function).

Elevated IOP (2–8%)

Control with topical treatment or acetazolamide. In extreme cases, consider releasing aqueous fluid from the paracentesis wound under sterile conditions.

Increased anterior inflammation (2–6%)

If there is greater than expected inflammation, increase topical steroids, maintaining normal antibiotic coverage (e.g., moxifloxacin 4x/day), but always have a low threshold of suspicion for endophthalmitis.

Wound leak (1%)

Observe, use a bandage contact lens, or hydrate wound with BSS and 27 gauge needle in exam room under sterile conditions. Return patient to operating room and suture wound closed if there is persistent or severe AC shallowing (with iris prolapse or iridocorneal touch).

Iris prolapse (0.7%)

Return patient to operating room, assess vitality of extruded iris (may require excision), reform AC, and suture wound closed.

Endophthalmitis (0.1%) (p. 253)

Postoperative—late

Posterior capsule opacification (10–50% by 2 years)

Consider YAG posterior capsulotomy if capsule opacification is causing reduced vision or monocular diplopia or is preventing assessment or treatment of fundal pathology.

In uveitic patients, defer until opacification is causing VA ≤20/40 or preventing fundus view *and* 6 months post-surgery *and* 2 months since last exacerbation.

Cystoid macular edema (1–12%) (p. 257)

Retinal detachment (0.7%)

Risk is increased in axial myopes, patients with lattice degeneration, or retinal detachment (RD) in the previous eye. Risks are increased if there has been vitreous loss. Refer immediately to vitreoretinal surgeon.

Corneal decompensation

Risk is increased if there is pre-existing endothelial dystrophy, diabetes, intraoperative endothelial trauma or phaco-burn, long phaco time or power or long irrigation time, or ACIOL. Control IOP and inflammation. Consider hypertonic drops (e.g., sodium chloride 5%), bandage contact lens (for comfort in bullous keratopathy), endothelial keratoplasty (DSEK), or penetrating keratoplasty.

Chronic endophthalmitis (p. 255)

Postoperative endophthalmitis

Acute postoperative endophthalmitis

This is a sight-threatening emergency requiring rapid assessment and treatment. Onset is usually 1–7 days after surgery. The most common organisms are *Staphylococcus epidermidis*, *Staphylococcus aureus*, and *Streptococcus* species.

Historically, acute postoperative endophthalmitis after cataract surgery occurred at a rate of 1.79 per 1000 cases, but recent reports suggest the rate has increased to 2.47 per 1000 cases, possibly because of poorly constructed clear corneal and temporal corneal incisions.

Suspect

Suspect this if the patient has pain, worsening vision, disproportionate or increasing postoperative inflammation (including hypopyon), posterior segment inflammation, and lid swelling. An RAPD and inaccurate light projection suggest a poor prognosis.

Risk factors include patient flora (blepharitis, conjunctivitis, nasolacrimal disease), comorbidity (diabetes), and complicated surgery (PC rupture with vitreous loss, ACIOL, prolonged surgery).

Diagnosis

Perform an AC tap and vitreous biopsy (with simultaneous intravitreal antibiotics); use automated vitrector to perform a vitreous biopsy. Consider B-scan ultrasound to indicate the degree of vitritis and integrity of retina.

Treatment

Consider hospital admission if the patient is incapacitated by the condition.

- *Intravitreal antibiotics:* consider vancomycin 1 mg in 0.1 mL (gram-positive coverage) combined with either amikacin 0.4 mg in 0.1 mL or ceftazidime 2 mg in 0.1 mL (gram-negative coverage). Ceftazidime can precipitate with vancomycin and so requires a different syringe.
- *Vitrectomy:* if VA is LP or worse (the Early Vitrectomy Study found a significant, threefold improvement in attaining 20/40 for this group; in diabetics, there was a trend toward benefit whatever the baseline VA).

Consider

- Oral moxifloxacin or gatifloxacin have broad antibiotic coverage and excellent intraocular penetration.
- *Topical antibiotics:* possibilities include hourly fourth-generation fluoroquinolones (moxifloxacin or gatifloxacin) or fortified vancomycin (50 mg/mL), amikacin (20 mg/mL), or ceftazidime (100 mg/mL) with a view to increasing anterior-segment concentration of the intravitreal drugs. There is no evidence of clinical benefit.
- *Corticosteroids* may be topical (e.g., dexamethasone 0.1% hourly), intravitreal (dexamethasone 0.4 mg in 0.1 mL), or systemic (prednisone PO 1 week). While steroids reduce inflammation and some sequelae of endophthalmitis, there is no evidence that it improves VA.

If failure to respond at 24 hours
Consider repeating AC tap, vitreous biopsy, and intravitreal antibiotics.

Chronic postoperative endophthalmitis

Onset is usually 1 week to several months after surgery. The most common organisms are *Propionobacterium acnes*, partially treated *S. epidermidis*, and fungi.

Suspect

Suspect this if there is chronic postoperative inflammation, which flares up whenever steroid treatment is reduced. A white plaque on the posterior capsule suggests *P. acnes* infection.

Diagnosis

Perform an AC tap and vitreous biopsy and consider removal of posterior capsule. Send sample for smears (Gram, Giemsa, and methenamine-silver stain) and culture (blood, chocolate, Sabouraud's, thioglycolate broth, and solid anaerobic medium; the last is especially important for *P. acnes*). PCR may also be helpful.

Treatment

For *P. acnes* or low-grade *S. epidermidis*, consider vitrectomy and posterior capsulectomy, intravitreal vancomycin, and, if necessary, IOL removal. For suspected fungal infection, consider vitrectomy with or without IOL removal, intravitreal amphotericin B (5–10 µg), and subsequent systemic antifungals according to sensitivity (see also Box 9.2).

American Academy of Ophthalmology recommendations for endophthalmitis prophylaxis

- Preoperative treatment of blepharitis and other lid pathology.
- 5% povidine iodine prep in the conjunctival fornices and 10% povidine iodine prep of the lids.
- Special attention to achieving a watertight closure of incisions.
- Other measures, including preoperative antibiotics, intracameral antibiotics, or subconjunctival antibiotics, are left to the surgeon's preference.

Box 9.2 Recommendations for prophylaxis and treatment of endophthalmitis

Prophylaxis

Perform skin and conjunctival sac preparation with 5% aqueous povidone iodine at least 5 min before surgery. It is safe and effective in significantly reducing ocular surface flora. Additional benefit may be gained by postoperative instillation into the sac.

Identifying and treating risk factors such as blepharitis, conjunctivitis, or mucocoele is probably more useful than universal antibiotic prophylaxis. The use of antibiotics in irrigating solutions is controversial.

Treatment

- *VA > LP:* single-port vitreous biopsy via the pars plana should be performed using a vitreous cutting-suction device. The specimens are directly smeared for Gram stain etc. and plated for culture. Directly inject amikacin and vancomycin (or gentamicin and ceftazidime).
- *VA < LP:* three port pars plan vitrectomy and intravitreal antibiotics. High-dose systemic prednisone may be given (e.g., 60–80 mg daily), rapidly reducing dose to none over a week to 10 days. Steroids are contraindicated if there is a fungal infection.

If the clinical course warrants it, the biopsy and intravitreal antibiotic injection may be repeated after 48–72 hours.

Postoperative cystoid macular edema

Irvine–Gass syndrome

Suspect

Suspect this if there is worsening vision (may decrease with pinhole), perifoveal retinal thickening and optic nerve leakage, ± cystoid spaces. There is increased risk in patients with diabetes mellitus, complicated surgery, postoperative uveitis, or previous CME (in the other eye post-routine surgery).

Diagnosis

Clinical appearance ± FA (typically dye leakage from both the optic disc as well as the parafovea into the cystoid spaces in a petalloid pattern) ± OCT demonstrates intraretinal cystic changes and thickening.

Prophylaxis

Consider adding a topical NSAID (e.g., ketorolac 0.3% 3x/day for 1 month) to the usual postoperative steroid regime for high-risk groups (patients with diabetes mellitus, uveitis, previous CME, or complicated surgery with vitreous loss).

Treatment

A step-wise approach is recommended. Review the diagnosis (e.g., OCT, FA) if atypical or slow to respond. One approach is as follows:

1. Topical: steroid (e.g., dexamethasone 0.1% 4x/day) + NSAID (e.g., ketorolac 0.3% 3x/day).

Review in 4–6 weeks. If CME is persistent, then continue as follows:

2. Periocular steroid (e.g., orbital floor/subtenons; methylprednisolone/triamcinolone) and continue topical treatment.

Review in 4–6 weeks. If persistent, then continue as follows:

3. Consider repeating periocular or giving intravitreal steroid.
4. Anti–vascular endothelial growth factor (VEGF) agents (e.g., bevacizumab) or pars plana vitrectomy with peeling of internal limiting membrane may be necessary for recalcitrant cases.

Abnormalities of lens size, shape, and position

Abnormalities of size, shape, and position (Table 9.9) may both affect the refractive power of the lens and increase optical aberration. In addition, most of these abnormalities are associated with lens opacity. Most common among this group are disorders of lens position (i.e., ectopia lentis).

Ectopia lentis

This may be complete (dislocation or luxation) or partial (displacement or subluxation). Do not neglect possible acquired causes of ectopia lentis.

Complications
- Refractive (edge effect, lenticular astigmatism, lenticular myopia, aphakic hypermetropia, diplopia).
- Anterior dislocation can cause glaucoma, corneal decompensation, or uveitis.

Treatment
- *Refractive:* contact lenses, eyeglasses.
- *Dislocation* into the posterior segment (followed by aphakic correction) by either 1) YAG zonulolysis or 2) mydriatics + lay the patient on his/her back if lens is already dislocated anteriorly.
- *Lensectomy* (followed by aphakic correction, ACIOL, or suture-fixated PCIOL). Partially subluxed lenses may be more safely removed via phacoemulsification with the use of capsular tension rings with or without fixation loops (FDA approved) or with capsular tension segments (not FDA approved, but available through compassionate use).

Causes
Congenital
- *Familal ectopa lentis* (AD): uni- or bilateral superotemporal lens subluxation; no systemic abnormality.
- *Ectopia lentis et pupillae* (AR): superotemporal dislocation with pupil displacement in the opposite direction; no systemic abnormality.
- *Marfan syndrome* (AD, Ch15, fibrillin): bilateral superotemporal lens subluxation with some preservation of accommodation, lattice degeneration, retinal detachment, anomalous angles, glaucoma, keratoconus, blue sclera, axial myopia; musculoskeletal (arachnodactyly, disproportionately long-limbed, joint laxity, pectus excavatum, kyphoscoliosis, high arched palate, herniae); cardiovascular (aortic dilatation, aortic regurgiation, aortic dissection, mitral valve prolapse).
- *Weill–Marchesani syndrome* (AR): bilateral anteroinferior lens subluxation, microspherophakia, retinal detachment, anomalous angles; musculoskeletal (short stature, brachydactyly); neurological (reduced IQ).

Table 9.9 Abnormalities of lens size, shape, and position

Abnormality	Condition	Associations
Size	Microphakia (small lens)	Lowe syndrome
	Microspherophakia (small spherical lens)	Familial microspherophakia (AD) Peters anomaly Marfan syndrome (AD) Weill–Marchesani syndrome (AR) Hyperlysinemia (AR) Alport syndrome (XD) Congenital rubella
Shape	Coloboma (inferior notch)	Iris/choroid colobomata Giant retinal tears
	Anterior lenticonus (bulge in anterior lens)	Alport syndrome
	Posterior lenticonus (bulge in posterior lens)	Unilateral—usually sporadic Bilateral—familial (AD/AR/X) Lowe syndrome (X)
	Lentiglobus (extreme lenticonus)	Posterior polar cataract
Position	Ectopia lentis (congenital)	Familial ectopia lentis (AD) Marfan syndrome (AD) Weill–Marchesani syndrome (AR) Homocystinuria (AR) Familial microspherophakia (AD) Hyperlysinemia (AR) Sulphite oxidase deficiency (AR) Stickler syndrome (AD) Sturge–Weber syndrome (sproradic) Crouzon syndrome (sporadic) Ehlers–Danlos syndrome (AD/AR) Aniridia
	Ectopia lentis (acquired)	Trauma High myopia Buphthalmos Ciliary body tumor Hypermature cataract Pseudoexfoliation

AD, autosomal dominant; AR, autosomal recessive; X, X-linked; XD, X-linked dominant.

- *Homocystinuria* (AR, cystathionine synthetase abnormality →
  homocysteine and methionine accumulation): bilateral inferonasal
  lens subluxation, myopia, glaucoma; skeletal (knock-kneed, marfanoid
  habitus, osteoporosis); hematological (thromboses, especially
  associated with general anesthesia); characteristic facies (fine, fair hair);
  neurological (low IQ).
- *Hyperlysinemia* (AR, lysine α-ketogluatarate reductase): lens
  subluxation, microspherophakia; musculoskeletal (joint laxity,
  hypotonia); neurological (epilepsy, low IQ).
- *Sulphite oxidase deficiency* (AR): lens subluxation; neurological
  (hypertonia, low IQ); life expectancy less than 5 years.

Acquired

These include trauma, high myopia (hyper)mature cataract, pseudoexfoliation, buphthalmos, and ciliary body tumor.

Glaucoma

Related pages:

Anatomy and physiology

Glaucoma has classically been described as a progressive optic neuropathy with characteristic changes in the optic nerve head and corresponding loss of visual field. In many cases, optic nerve damage is identified clinically or with imaging technologies prior to visual field loss.

In some cases of "glaucoma," the optic nerve and visual fields are normal but the intraocular pressure (IOP) is at such a high level that glaucomatous damage is considered imminent or inevitable. Glaucoma represents a final common pathway for a number of conditions, for most of which raised IOP is the most important risk factor.

In Western countries, glaucoma is present in 1% of those over 40 and 3% in those over 70 years old. It is the second leading cause of irreversible blindness worldwide. In the United States, glaucoma is estimated to affect nearly 3 million individuals and will increase to 3.6 million by 2020. African Americans are three times more likely than white Americans to have glaucoma.

Anatomy

- *Anterior chamber angle* extends from Schwalbe's line (the termination of Descemet's membrane on the peripheral cornea) posteriorly to the trabecular meshwork (TM), scleral spur, or ciliary body (depending on the angle configuration) where an acute angle is formed with the peripheral iris.
- *Trabecular meshwork* is a reticulated band of fibrocellular sheets, with a triangular cross-section and base toward the scleral spur.
- *Schlemm's canal* is a circumferential septate drain with an inner wall of endothelium containing giant vacuoles and an outer wall obliquely punctuated by collector channels that drain into the episcleral veins.
- *Scleral spur* is a firm fibrous projection from the sclera, with Schlemm's canal at its base and the longitudinal portion of the ciliary muscle inserting into its posterior surface.
- *Ciliary body* comprises the ciliary muscle and ciliary epithelium, arranged anatomically as the pars plana and pars plicata (containing the ciliary processes). Contraction of the ciliary muscle permits accommodation and increases trabecular outflow. The ciliary epithelium is a cuboidal bilayer arranged apex to apex with numerous gap junctions. The inner layer is nonpigmented, with high metabolic activity, and posteriorly is continuous with the neural retina. The outer layer is pigmented and posteriorly is continuous with the RPE.

Physiology

Aqueous production

Aqueous humor is a clear, colorless, plasma-like balanced salt solution produced by the ciliary body. It is a structurally supportive medium providing nutrients to the lens and cornea. It differs from plasma in having lower glucose (80% of plasma levels), low protein (assuming an intact blood aqueous barrier), and high ascorbate.

It is formed at around 2.5 µL/min by a combination of active secretion (70%), ultrafiltration (20%), and osmosis (10%). Active secretion is complex, involving the maintenance of a transepithelial potential by the Na^+K^+ pump, ion transport by symports and antiports (including the important $Na^+/K^+/2Cl^-$ symport), calcium- and voltage-gated ion channels, and carbonic anhydrase.

Aqueous outflow

While the trabecular route is the major outflow, the uveoscleral contribution may be as much as 30%. The outflow capacity through the trabecular route and uveoscleral route varies and has been demonstrated to decrease with age.

Trabecular (conventional) route

Most aqueous humor leaves the eye by this passive, pressure-sensitive route. Around 75% of outflow resistance is due to the trabecular meshwork itself, the major component being the outermost (juxtacanalicular) portion of the trabecular meshwork. This comprises several layers of endothelial cells embedded in ground substance that appears to act as a filter, which is continually cleaned by endothelial cell phagocytosis.

Further transport into Schlemm's canal is achieved via pressure-dependent transcellular channels (seen as giant vacuoles of fluid crossing the endothelium) and paracellular pores. Aqueous is then transported via collector channels to the episcleral veins and on to the general venous circulation.

Uveoscleral (unconventional) route

The aqueous passes across the iris root and ciliary body into the supraciliary and suprachoroidal spaces from where it escapes via the choroidal circulation.

Intraocular pressure (IOP)

$$\text{Flow in} = \text{Flow out} = C\,(\text{IOP} - Pv) + U$$

where C is the pressure-sensitive outflow facility (via trabecular meshwork), U is the pressure-independent outflow (via uveoscleral route), and Pv is the episcleral venous pressure.

Typical values are as follows:

$$\text{Flow in} = C\,(\text{IOP} - Pv) + U$$

2.5 μL/min = **0.3** μL/min/mmHg (16 − 9 mmHg) + **0.4** μL/min

Variation in IOP

Within the population

Based on population studies, normal IOP is generally taken to be mean IOP (16 mmHg) ± 2 SD (2 × 2.5 mmHg), i.e., a range of 11–21 mmHg. However, there is a positive skew to this distribution.

Within the individual

Mean diurnal variation is approximately 5 mmHg in normal patients but may fluctuate from 10 to 15 mmHg in primary open-angle glaucoma (POAG). In most individuals, IOP tends to peak early morning upon awakening. Pulse pressure, respiration, extremes of blood pressure, and season also have an effect on IOP variation.

Glaucoma: assessment

At initial consultation (Table 10.1) consider 1) evidence for glaucoma (Table 10.2) vs. normal variation or alternative pathology (Table 10.3); 2) evidence for underlying cause (i.e., type of glaucoma—steroid responsive, pigmentary); 3) factors influencing treatment (age, vision, comorbidities).

Be cautious of interpreting any one abnormality in isolation—e.g., apparent field defects may be artifactual and disappear with repeated testing because of the "learning effect"; a patient with a normal IOP one day may have a high IOP another day.

Table 10.1 An approach to assessing possible glaucoma

Visual symptoms	Asymptomatic; halos, eye pain, headache, precipitants (dim light, exercise); subjective loss of vision/field
POH	Previous surgery or trauma; concurrent eye disease; refractive error; use of topical steroids; history of ocular inflammation.
PMH	Diabetes, hypertension, smoking; migraine, Raynaud's phenomenon; vascular disease; asthma or COPD, renal disease
FH	Family members with glaucoma and their outcome
Medication	Current or previous topical medications, current drugs (interactions), systemic β-blockers, current or previous use of steroids (any route)
All	Allergies or relevant drug contraindications
Visual acuity	Best-corrected
Visual function	Check for RAPD, color vision
Cornea	Pigment deposition; consider pachymetry, endothelial cell abnormalities
AC	Peripheral or central depth, cells, pigment
Gonioscopy	Angle configuration, iris approach, abnormal pigmentation, PAS, neovascularization
Tonometry	IOP (Goldmann applanation preferred)
Iris	Transillumination defects, PXF, heterochromia, rubeosis
Lens	Cataract (swollen, hypermature), ACIOL
Optic disc	Size, vertical cup–disc ratio; color; flat, elevated, or tilted; neuroretinal rim (including contour, notches, hemorrhages); pits, colobomata, drusen; peripapillary atrophy
Disc vessels	Baring, bayonetting
Peripapillary area	Hemorrhages, atrophy, pigmentation, retinal nerve fiber layer defects
Fundus	Chorioretinal scarring, retinoschisis, retinal detachment (can cause field loss)

Table 10.2 The glaucoma triad

Evidence for glaucoma	Features
Raised IOP	>21 mmHg
Abnormal optic disc	Cup–disc ratio asymmetry Large cup–disc ratio for disc size Neuroretinal rim notch or thinning (ISNT rule: Inferior-Superior-Nasal-Temporal rule) Disc hemorrhage Vessel bayoneting/nasally displaced Peripapillary atrophy (B-zone)
Visual field defect	Nasal step Arcuate scotoma Altitudinal scotoma Residual temporal or central island of vision

The ISNT rule describes the normal contour of the disc rim, being thickest inferiorly, followed by the superior and nasal quadrants, with the temporal region being thinnest.

Table 10.3 A short differential diagnosis of the glaucoma triad

IOP	Optic discs	Visual field	Consider
Raised IOP	Normal	Normal	Ocular hypertension
	Borderline	Normal	Glaucoma suspect
	Borderline	Consistent defect	Highly suspicious: treat as early-stage glaucoma
	Abnormal	Consistent defect	Glaucoma
Normal IOP	Normal	Normal	Normal
	Borderline	Normal	Physiological cupping/glaucoma suspect
	Stable abnormality	Stable defect	Congenital disc anomaly Previous optic disc insult
	Evolving abnormality	Evolving defect	Normal-tension glaucoma, other optic neuropathy

Box 10.1 Obtaining history of presenting illness (HPI)—an example

Patient presenting with loss of vision
- Did the event occur suddenly or gradually?

Sudden loss of vision is commonly associated with a vascular occlusion (e.g., anterior ischemic optic neuropathy [AION], central retinal arterial [CRAO] or vein [CRVO] occlusion, or bleeding (e.g., vitreous hemorrhage, 'wet' macular degeneration). Gradual loss of vision is commonly associated with degenerations or depositions (e.g., cataract, macular dystrophies, or "dry" macular degeneration, corneal dystrophies).

- Is the vision loss associated with pain?

Painful blurring of vision is most commonly associated with anterior ocular processes (e.g., keratitis, anterior uveitis), although orbital disease, optic neuritis, and giant cell arteritis may also cause painful loss of vision.

- Is the problem transient or persistent?

Transient loss of vision is commonly due to temporary or subcritical vascular insufficiency (e.g., giant cell arteritis, amaurosis fugax, vertebrobasilar artery insufficiency), whereas persistent loss of vision suggests structural or irreversible damage (e.g., vitreous hemorrhage, macular degeneration).

- Does the problem affect one or both eyes?

Unilateral disease may suggest a local (or ipsilateral) cause. Bilateral disease may suggest a more widespread or systemic process.

- Is the vision blurred, dimmed or distorted?

Blurring or dimming of vision may be due to pathology anywhere in the visual pathway from cornea to cortex; common problems include refractive error, cataract, and macular disease. Distortion is commonly associated with macular pathology, but again may arise from high refractive error (high ametropia/astigmatism) or other ocular disease.

- Where is the problem with their vision?

A superior or inferior hemispheric field loss suggests a corresponding inferior or superior vascular event involving the retina (e.g., retinal vein occlusion) or optic disc (e.g., segmental AION). Peripheral field loss may indicate retinal detachment (usually rapidly evolving from far periphery), optic nerve disease, chiasmal compression (typically bitemporal loss), or cortical pathology (homonymous hemianopic defects). Central blurring of vision suggests diseases of the macula (positive scotoma: a "seen" spot) or optic nerve (negative scotoma: an unseen defect).

- When is there a problem?

For example, glare from headlights or bright sunlight is commonly due to posterior subcapsular lens opacities.

Ocular hypertension (OHT)

Ocular hypertension describes a condition of IOP >21 mmHg (representing 2 SD above the population mean) in the presence of a healthy optic disc and normal visual field. This population is positively skewed, with 5–7% of those aged >40 having an IOP >21 mmHg.

In the absence of glaucomatous damage, it is difficult to differentiate those in whom such an IOP elevation is physiological from those in whom it is pathological (i.e., will convert to POAG).

Risk of conversion to POAG

In the Ocular Hypertension Treatment Study (OHTS), the conversion rate was found to be 9.5% over 5 years (untreated). If treated with topical medication (to reduce IOP by >20% and to achieve ≤24 mmHg), this conversion rate was reduced to 4.4%.

Risk factors (and their hazard ratios [HR]) demonstrated in the OHTS trial include the following:
- Older age: HR 1.2 per decade.
- Higher IOP: HR 1.1 per mmHg.
- Larger cup–disc (C/D) ratio: HR 1.2 per 0.1.
- Greater pattern standard deviation (PSD): HR 1.3 per 0.2dB.
- Thinner central corneal thickness (CCT): HR 1.7 per 40 μm.

While thin CCT is an independent risk factor for glaucoma, thinner CCT also leads to underestimation of IOP; thus the true IOP may be higher than the recognized IOP. Patients who have had corneal refractive procedures may also have thin corneas and artificially low IOPs. Relatively thin corneas (CCT < 555 μm) were associated with a three-fold greater risk of conversion to POAG than that of thick corneas (>588 μm).

Some practitioners use a pachymeter routinely and correct the IOP for corneal thickness. One estimate is that for every 20 μm that the CCT is <550 μm (mean population CCT), the IOP is underestimated by 1 mmHg (though the change is not truly a linear relationship). Interestingly, this calculation reclassifies many normal-tension glaucoma (NTG) patients as high-tension POAG, and OHT patients as normal.

Other possible risk factors include abnormalities in corneal hysteresis, African-Caribbean race, FH, myopia, and other suspicious disc or peripapillary changes.

Whom to treat?

There is considerable variation in practice. Some practitioners treat all patients >21 mmHg. Consider treating the following:
- Isolated OHT if IOP >30 mmHg.
- OHT and suspicious disc if IOP >21 mmHg.
- OHT and thin cornea if IOP >21 mmHg.

Other factors that may suggest a lower threshold for treatment include

- OHT and only eye.
- OHT and CRVO in either eye.
- OHT and an accumulation of risk factors, including thin CCT, FH of blindness, African or Hispanic heritage, large optic nerve head (ONH) cupping, diabetes, age, and RNFL thinning on disc imaging.

There are calculators available that attempt to quantify a patient's risks on the basis of OHTS criteria.

Monitoring

For those not requiring treatment, follow up in 6–12 months (IOP, disc appearance, RNFL analysis) and perform perimetry every 12 months.

For those requiring treatment, follow up as per POAG (p. 269).

Primary open-angle glaucoma (POAG)

This is an adult-onset optic neuropathy with glaucomatous disc and/or field changes, open angles, and no other identifiable cause for glaucoma (cf. secondary open-angle glaucomas). The term is usually reserved for those with high-tension glaucoma, i.e., IOP >21 mmHg (cf. normal tension glaucoma, NTG). POAG is present in 1% of the population over age 40.

Risk factors

- *Age*: increasing age (uncommon <40 years).
- Race: African Caribbean: more frequent, younger onset, more vision loss
- *FH*: first-degree relative confers 1 in 8 risk; higher in siblings.
- Steroid-induced IOP elevation is more common in POAG and those with a FH of POAG.

Other possible risk factors include diseases that reduce oxygen delivery to the optic nerve, such as respiratory (COPD or sleep apnea) and vascular disease (e.g., diabetes and hypertension), and myopia (the disc is believed to be more vulnerable because of the scleral canal morphology).

Clinical features

- Usually asymptomatic (rarely eye ache and halos—transient corneal edema if very high IOP). Decreased vision with central scotoma.
- IOP >21 mmHg, often with high diurnal variability.
- Disc changes: C/D asymmetry, high C/D for disc size, vertical elongation of the cup, neuroretinal rim notch/thinning (does not follow ISNT rule; p. 265), disc hemorrhage, vessel bayoneting/nasally displaced, peripapillary atropy (B-zone). B-zone peripapillary atrophy describes choroidal atrophy immediately adjacent to the disc; it may correspond to areas of ganglion cell loss and field defects. The α-zone is more peripheral, irregularly pigmented, and less specific for glaucoma.
- Retinal nerve fiber layer loss is clinically identified or detected by imaging analysis.
- Visual field defects: 1) focal defects respecting the horizontal meridian including nasal step, baring of the blind spot, arcuate defects, and altitudinal defects; 2) generalized depression.

Treatment

The Early Manifest Glaucoma Trial (EMGT) evaluated the role of intervention in early glaucoma and found that IOP lowering decreases the progression of glaucoma damage.

- Counseling (see Box 10.2).
- Medical: topical—prostaglandin analogue, β-blocker, α-agonist, carbonic anhydrase inhibitor; all have contraindications and side effects.
- Argon (ALT) or selective (SLT) laser trabeculoplasty may be appropriate first-line treatment for those who are frail or in whom medication adherence is likely to be an issue. ALT may be effective in those with moderate trabecular pigmentation (e.g., in PXF, PDS). IOP control fails with time following ALT, with 50% failure rate at 5 years.
- Trabeculectomy (antimetabolite augmented) may be appropriate first-line treatment for those who hope to be drop-free or have a high risk of progression. Otherwise consider surgery if maximal medical therapy fails (p. 299).

- Newer surgical techniques to enhance outflow (canaloplasty, trabectome, iStent, Express shunt, suprachoroidal shunt) may also be effective, although long-term clinical evidence is lacking compared with that for more established surgical procedures.
- While more surgeons are using aqueous shunts (Ahmed, Baerveldt, Molteno) for primary glaucoma surgical intervention, tube shunts have historically been reserved for patients who failed standard filtration surgery.
- Cyclodestructive procedures (ciliary body ablation) (cyclodiode, cyclocryotherapy) is typically reserved for the most recalcitrant glaucoma in patients with limited visual potential (p. 298).

Box 10.2 An approach to medical treatment of glaucoma

1) Counsel patient
Provide education on the nature and natural history of the condition; implications for driving; effect of drop therapy; important medication side effects; importance of medication adherence and compliance; probability of lifelong treatment; treatment of asymptomatic disease (patient unlikely to notice day-to-day benefit).

2) Define target IOP
There is usually ≥20% reduction initially; the target IOP should be lower if there is already advanced disease damage, disease continues to progress, or other risk factors are present.

3) Select drug
For first-line medication consider a prostaglandin agonist or β-blocker. Note contraindications (see p. 702).

4) Teach how to administer drops correctly and effectively

5) Review treatment (e.g., 1–2 months later)
- *Effects*—is there significant IOP reduction and has the target IOP been reached? Some advocate a treatment trial of one eye so that therapeutic efficacy and side effects can be gauged against the other eye (which theoretically controls for diurnal variation).
- *Side effects*—local (e.g., allergic) and systemic (e.g., lethargy, dizziness, wheezing, etc.).

6) Decide about further treatment
- If there is no significant reduction in IOP, stop drops and try another first-line agent; check adherence and compliance.
- If there is a significant reduction but target IOP is not met, augment with another agent (another first-line drug or second-line agent such as topical carbonic anhydrase inhibitor).
- If target IOP is achieved, continue; review (e.g., 3 months).
- If target IOP is achieved BUT disc or field continues to progress, then target IOP level may need to be lowered even further. Consider other risk factors such as pressure spikes (may need to measure IOP diurnal curve), systemic hypotension, or poor compliance.
- Diurnal curves involve regular IOP checks (e.g., every 1–2 hours) over an extended period of the day (e.g., 0800–1800 or later; less commonly for a full 24-hour period).

Normal-tension glaucoma (NTG)

NTG, also known as normal-pressure glaucoma and low-tension glaucoma, is generally regarded as a subcategory of POAG, although some have suggested a distinct pathogenesis, such as vascular anomalies, systemic hypotension, and inherited abnormalities of the optic nerve.

NTG is present in at least one-third or more of all patients with open-angle glaucoma.

Risk factors

- Age: NTG is more common in the elderly, but up to one-third of patients may be <50 years.
- Race: NTG is more common in Japan (may constitute >50% of all OAG).
- Sex: possible female preponderance.

Clinical features

- Usually asymptomatic.
- IOP <21 mmHg.
- Disc changes are as for POAG, although disc hemorrhages and acquired pits may be more common and the cup may be larger and shallower.
- Visual field defects are similar to those in POAG, although 1) focal defects occur more often in the superior hemifield (especially superonasal) and are said to be deeper, steeper, and closer to fixation; 2) generalized depression is less marked than in high-tension POAG.
- NTG may be more common in patients with history of vasospasm (Raynaud's), migraine, hypotension, systemic ischemia (vasculopathy, respiratory disease), and autoimmune disease.

Differential diagnosis and Investigations

- POAG—perform diurnal curve to assess IOP range.
- Secondary glaucoma—clinical assessment.
- Compressive optic neuropathy—consider MRI optic nerves/chiasm if disc and field defects do not correlate, if there is an atypical field defect, or if VA or color vision is affected.
- Other optic neuropathies—consider sending blood for CBC, B_{12}, folate, ESR, VDRL, TPHA, ACE, ANA, ANCA, CRP, Lebers Hereditary Optic Neuropathy; get CXR (p. 338).
- Previous history of OHT that caused optic nerve damage, with subsequent normal IOP and no progressive glaucoma damage (postoperative IOP spikes, steroid-responsive glaucoma).

Whom to treat?

The Collaborative Normal Tension Glaucoma Study (CNTGS) demonstrated that in patients with diagnosed NTG, an IOP reduction of >30% slows the rate of field loss, but that even without treatment, 50% of NTG patients actually show no progression of field defects at 5 years.

Risk factors for progression were the following:

- Female sex.
- Migraine.
- Disc hemorrhage at diagnosis.

Medical treatment

Generally, as for POAG, some clinicians emphasize the role of ONH perfusion and the possible role of nocturnal dips in blood pressure. On this basis, consider using once-daily prostaglandin analogues (better IOP control at night) instead of nonselective β-blockers (may reduce blood flow at night) or other class agents (carbonic anhydrase inhibitors or α-agonists).

Primary angle-closure glaucoma (PACG)

PACG is a condition of elevated IOP resulting from partial or complete occlusion of the angle by the iris. It is present in approximately 0.1% of the general population over 40 years old, but up to 1.5% of the Chinese population over 50.

Risk factors

Epidemiological

- Age: >40 years old; mean age of diagnosis ± 60 years.
- Female sex.
- Race: Chinese, South East Asians, Inuits (i.e., Eskimos).

Anatomical

Pupillary block mechanism

- Narrow angle, shallow AC, relatively anterior iris–lens diaphragm, large lens (older, cataractous), small corneal diameter, short axial length (usually hyeropic).

In pupillary block, apposition of the iris to the lens impedes aqueous flow from the posterior chamber to the anterior chamber, causing a relative buildup of pressure behind the iris, anterior bowing of the peripheral iris, and subsequent angle closure.

Plateau iris mechanism

- Plateau iris configuration (anteriorly rotated ciliary body that apposes the peripheral iris to the TM; AC depth normal centrally, shallow peripherally with flat iris plane).

Mild forms of plateau iris configuration are vulnerable to pupillary block, but greater plateau iris configurations may result in plateau iris syndrome, where the peripheral iris bunches up and blocks the TM directly. This means that acute or chronic angle closure can occur despite a patent peripheral iridotomy (PI).

Acute angle-closure glaucoma (AACG)

Clinical features

- Pain (periocular, headache, abdominal), blurred vision, halos, nausea, vomiting.
- *Ipsilateral:* red eye, raised IOP (usually 40–80 mmHg), corneal edema, angle closed, fixed semidilated pupil; glaucomflecken; contralateral narrow angle; bilateral shallow AC.

Differential diagnosis

Consider secondary angle closure (e.g., phacomorphic, inflammatory, neovascular) or acute glaucoma syndromes such as Posner–Schlossman syndrome (glaucomatocyclitic crisis) or pigment dispersion syndrome (Table 10.2).

If there is no view to the posterior chamber, perform a B-scan ultrasound to rule out pathologies that shift the lens–iris diaphragm forward (e.g., tumor, hemorrhagic choroidal).

Subacute and chronic angle closure glaucoma

Subacute

Incomplete closure of the angle may result in episodes of increased IOP (causing blurred vision, halos, and red eye) that spontaneously resolve. Treat with prophylactic Nd-YAG PI.

Chronic

This may occur from 1) synechial closure, which is either asymptomatic ("creeping") or follows repeated episodes of acute or subacute angle closure, or 2) a POAG-like mechanism of trabecular dysfunction in narrow but clinically open angles. Treat with Nd-YAG PI plus medical therapy, goniosynechiolysis, and/or drainage surgery, as required (Box 10.3).

Box 10.3 An approach to treatment of AACG

Immediate

Systemic: acetazolamide 500 mg IV stat, then 250 mg PO 4×/day

Ipsilateral eye

- β-blocker   e.g., timolol 0.5% stat, then 2/day
- Sympathomimetic   e.g., apraclonidine 1% stat
- Steroid   e.g., prednisolone 1% stat, then q30–60 min
- Pilocarpine 2%   Once IOP <50 mmHg; e.g., twice in first hour then 4×/day
- Consider corneal indentation with a 4-mirror goniolens, which may help relieve pupillary block. Laying the patient supine may allow the lens to fall back away from the iris. Analgesics and anti-emetics may be necessary.
- Promptly assess and treat contralateral eye with laser PI (LPI).

Intermediate

- Check IOP hourly until there is adequate control.
- If IOP is not improving, consider systemic hyperosmotics (e.g., glycerol PO 1 g/kg of 50% solution in lemon juice or mannitol 20% solution IV 1–1.5 g/kg).
- If IOP is still not improving, consider acute LPI (can use topical glycerine to temporarily reduce the corneal edema).
- If IOP is still not improving, review the diagnosis (e.g., could this be aqueous misdirection syndrome or neovascular glaucoma?), consider repeating LPI, or proceeding to surgical PI or even emergency trabeculectomy.

Definitive

- Bilateral laser (e.g., Nd-YAG) or surgical PI

Some eyes may develop chronically elevated IOP from either synechial closure or a POAG-like mechanism and will require long-term medical or surgical treatment.

Pseudoexfoliation (PXF) syndrome

This is a common but easily missed cause of secondary glaucoma. It is a systemic condition in which a whitish dandruff-like material is deposited over the anterior segment of the eye and other organs such as skin, heart, lungs, kidneys, and meninges (see Table 10.4).

Although the PXF material's exact nature is unclear, it appears to include abnormal elastic microfibrils, basement membrane material, and glycosaminoglycans. In some parts of Scandinavia, PXF is present in up to 20% of the general population and up to 90% of the glaucoma population.

Risk factors

- Age: >40 years old; increases with age.
- Female sex.
- Race: Northern European (e.g., Finnish, Icelandic); Mediterranean (Cretan); possibly any population in which it is carefully evaluated.
- Family ocular history: the *LOXL1* gene variant has been shown to have a strong association with pseudoexfoliation syndrome and glaucoma.

Clinical features

- Dandruff-like material on pupillary border and anterior lens capsule (centrally and peripherally with a clear intermediate zone), peripupillary transillumination defects, poor mydriasis, iridodonesis or phacodonesis (there is risk of dialysis during cataract surgery), pigment in the AC.
- Gonioscopy: irregular pigment deposition in the TM and anterior to Schwalbe's line (Sampaolesi's line), PXF material in the angle; angle is usually open but may be narrow.

PXF glaucoma

Glaucoma occurs in up to 10% of patients with PXF (i.e., up to 10-fold increased risk). Although the disease presents similarly to POAG, the disease course is more severe, with poorer response to medication and more frequent need for surgery.

Mechanism of glaucoma

- *Open angle:* deposition of PXF material and pigment in the trabecular meshwork.
- *Narrow angle* (rare): weak zonules with anterior movement of the lens–iris diaphragm; posterior synechiae (PS).

Clinical features

- Features of PXF (see above), increased IOP, optic disc changes, and visual field defects as for POAG (p. 269).
- IOPs tend to increase over time and become more resistant to IOP-lowering therapy.

Treatment of PXF glaucoma (open-angle type)

- Medical: as for POAG, but generally less effective; there is a greater role for miotics (e.g., pilocarpine).
- ALT is particularly effective early on; >50% failure rate by 5 years
- Trabeculectomy has a higher complication rate but similar overall success to trabeculectomy in POAG.

Table 10.4 Chronic glaucoma diseases

Glaucoma type	Critical features	Additional features
Open angle		
Primary open angle	Increased IOP; optic disc cupping; visual field defect; normal open angle	Other glaucomatous disc changes
Normal tension	Normal IOP; disc cupping; visual field defect; normal open angle; disc hemorrhage	Other glaucomatous disc changes
Pseudoexfoliation	Dandruff-like material on pupil margin and lens surface	Unevenly pigmented TM; peripupillary iris TI defects
Pigment dispersion	Mid-peripheral spoke-like iris TI defects; trabecular pigmentation	Pigment in AC, on cornea, lens, iris, male myopes aged 20–45
Steroid-induced	Increased IOP associated with steroid use (but may be lag of weeks or months)	Signs of underlying pathology, e.g., uveitis, eczema
Angle recession	Recessed iris and angle	Other signs of trauma
Intraocular tumor	Posterior segment tumor	Cataract; mass seen on US
Closed angle		
Chronic angle closure	Peripheral anterior synechiae (PAS)	May have had subacute attacks of angle closure
Angle pulled shut (anterior pathology)		
Neovascular	Rubeosis causing angle to zip shut	Signs of underlying pathology e.g., diabetes, CRVO
Inflammatory closed angle	Angle zipped shut by PAS	Signs of uveitis
ICE syndrome	Abnormal endothelial growth over angle	Iris distortion/atrophy; corneal hammered-metal appearance
Epithelial down-growth	Epithelial down-growth through wound to spread over angle	Surgical or traumatic wound
Angle pushed shut (posterior pathology)		
Phacomorphic	Ipsilateral intumescent lens	Appositional closure; contralateral open angle
Aqueous misdirection	Shallow AC despite patent PI; no iris bombé	Usually post-surgery in hyperopia

Consider delayed presentation of glaucoma syndromes that present acutely or subacutely, e.g., Posner–Schlossman syndrome (PSS), inflammatory open angle, steroid-induced, red cell, Ghost cell, lens-induced.

Pigment dispersion syndrome (PDS)

This describes the release of pigment from the mid-peripheral posterior surface of the iris, from where it is distributed around the anterior segment. Pigment release is thought to occur as a result of posterior bowing of the mid-peripheral iris rubbing against the zonules.

This unusual iris configuration may be due to reverse pupillary block in which there is a transient increased IOP in the AC relative to the posterior chamber. This theory is supported by an observed improvement in the condition when treated with miotics or YAG PI.

Risk factors

- Myopia.
- Age: 20–40.
- Male sex.
- Race: Caucasian.

Clinical features

- Pigment on the corneal endothelium (sometimes in a vertical line—Krukenberg spindle), pigment elsewhere (e.g., in the AC), mid-peripheral spoke-like transillumination defects; increased rate of lattice degeneration (see Table 10.5).
- Gonioscopy: open angle, concave peripheral iris, 360° dense homogeneous pigmentation of the TM, and may be anterior to Schwalbe's line inferiorly.
- Pigment in the anterior vitreous (Scheie's line).

Pigmentary glaucoma

Glaucoma may develop in 10–35% of patients with PDS. Often OHT will resolve with age, as less pigment is available to be released and obstruct the TM.

Clinical features

- Usually asymptomatic, but blurred vision, halos, and red eye(s) may occur after acute pigment shedding following mydriasis or exercise (pigment storm).
- Increased IOP ± corneal edema (if acute); features of PDS (see above); optic disc changes and visual field defects as for POAG (p. 269).

Treatment

Topical: as for POAG; miotics have theoretical benefits (minimize iridozonular contact) but tend to be poorly tolerated in this age group and carry a small risk of inducing retinal detachment (myopia, lattice degeneration).

ALT or SLT particularly effective early on; >50% failure rate by 5 years

Trabeculectomy: similar success rate to that for surgery in POAG, but increased risk of hypotony maculopathy (especially if augmented with antimetabolites).

PI: controversial use; despite theoretical benefits of normalizing iris configuration and minimizing pigment release, there are no trial data to support its use.

Table 10.5 Glaucoma conditions that may present acutely (symptomatic increased IOP)

Glaucoma type	Critical features	Additional features
Closed angle		
Primary angle closure	Closed angle, shallow AC; fixed mid-dilated pupil; iris bombé	Corneal edema; contralateral angle narrow; may have plateau iris
Angle pulled shut (anterior pathology)		
Neovascular	Rubeosis ± angle zipped shut	Signs of underlying pathology, e.g., diabetes, CRVO
Inflammatory closed angle	Angle zipped shut by PAS	Signs of uveitis
Angle pushed shut (posterior pathology)		
Phacomorphic	Ipsilateral intumescent lens	Appositional closure; contralateral open angle
Lens dislocation	Poor lenticular support permits anterior dislocation	Abnormalities of zonules or lens size
Aqueous misdirection	Shallow AC despite patent PI; no iris bombé	Usually post-surgery in hyperopic eyes
Choroidal pathology	Choroidal detachment, hemorrhage, or effusion	Recent history of surgery or extensive laser
Open angle		
Inflammatory open angle	Elevated IOP with significant flare/cells; open angle	Other signs of cause e.g., uveitis, trauma, surgery
Steroid-induced	Increased IOP associated with steroid use (but may be lag of weeks or months)	Signs of underlying pathology, e.g., uveitis
Posner–Schlossman syndrome	Recurrent unilateral IOP spikes in fairly quiet, white eye	Corneal edema
Pigment dispersion	Mid-peripheral spoke-like TI defects; trabecular pigmentation	Pigment in AC, on cornea, lens, iris; male myopes; 20–45 years; post-exercise
Red cell	Hyphema	Corneal staining
Ghost cell	Vitreous hemorrhage; bleached erythrocytes in AC	
Phacolytic	Lens protein in AC with (hyper)mature cataract	AC cells + flare, open angle ± clumps of macrophages
Lens particle	Retained lens fragment in AC post-surgery/trauma	
Intraocular tumor	Posterior segment tumor	± Cataract; mass seen on US

Neovascular glaucoma (NVG)

Vasoproliferative factors, typically a product of posterior segment ischemia (diabetes or CRVO), promote neovascularization of the angle leading to the formation of a fibrovascular membrane over the trabecular meshwork. Initially, the neovascular vessels cover the trabecular meshwork so that the angle appears open, but with time, peripheral anterior synechiae form and the membrane contracts to zip the angle shut.

Ischemic CRVO and diabetes each account for around a third of the cases of neovascular glaucoma.

Causes include
- Ischemic CRVO (common); risk of progression to NVG is 50%.
- Diabetic retinopathy (common); risk of NVG is highest in PDR.
- Other vascular disorders: ocular ischemic syndrome, central retinal artery (CRAO) and branch retinal vein (BRVO) occlusion.
- Other retinal disease: chronic retinal detachment, sickle cell retinopathy.
- Chronic inflammation.
- Retinal or choroidal tumors.

Clinical features
- Pain is often a feature and may be severe; the predisposing condition may be known or may be suggested by the history (e.g., sudden loss of vision a couple of months previously in cases of CRVO).
- Iris rubeosis: abnormal or nonradial vessels at pupil; increased IOP; AC flare/cells, hyphema; ectropion uvea; conjunctival injection and corneal edema if acute IOP rise or decompensation if chronic; disc changes and field loss as for POAG (p. 269).
- Gonioscopy: abnormal vessels in the angle; fibrovascular membrane overlying the TM (open angle type) or membrane + peripheral anterior synechiae (PAS) zipping angle shut (angle closure type).

Investigation (to determine cause)
- Dilated funduscopy in all cases.
- Carotid Doppler: if no retinal pathology or asymmetric diabetic retinopathy.
- B-scan ultrasound: if poor fundus view (cataract may be associated with chronic retinal pathology such as tumors, detachment, inflammation).

Treatment
- *Underlying pathology:* panretinal photocoagulation (PRP) for retinal ischemia; retinal reattachment for RD; carotid endarterectomy (CEA) for suitable carotid artery stenosis
- *Glaucoma:* mydriatic (e.g., atropine 1% 2×/day) + topical steroid (e.g., prednisolone 1% q1–4h) + ocular hypotensive agents as for POAG. If medical treatment fails, consider trabeculectomy (high rate of failure), tube-shunt procedures, or cyclodestruction (e.g., cyclodiode and cyclocryotherapy) depending on *visual prognosis.*

- *Pain:* if the eye is blind and painful, consider retrobulbar alcohol or evisceration/enucleaton.
- Off-label intravitreal or intracameral injections of recombinant anti–vascular endothelial growth factor (anti-VEGF), bevacizumab (Avastin), or ranibizumab (Lucentis) result in rapid regression of rubeosis and are often used in combination with PRP. Anti-VEGF agents do not reverse ischemia or decrease the production of VEGF, so therapy targeting the underlying process is vital.
- If IOPs permit, many surgeons opt to wait 2 or more days after an anti-VEGF injection, prior to surgery, to reduce the amount of neovascularization, which may decrease the incidence of intraoperative or post-operative hyphema.
- Anti-VEGF agents may also play a role in decreasing tube-shunt or trabeculectomy bleb failure from aggressive fibrous encapsulation.

Inflammatory glaucoma: general

Raised IOP in the context of intraocular inflammation is a common clinical problem. The challenge is to elucidate the time course (acute vs. chronically elevated IOP), the state of the angle (open vs. appositional closure vs. synechial closure), and the underlying mechanism.

Therapy may be made difficult because of marked fluctuations in IOP (ciliary body shutdown → ↓IOP; trabeculitis → ↑IOP, and concerns over whether anti-inflammatory treatment could be making things worse, steroid-induced glaucoma]).

Open-angle type

Acute

- *Mechanism:* acute trabeculitis (particularly with HSV, VZV), trabecular meshwork blockage.

Clinical features
- Elevated IOP; open angle; signs of uveitis with or without keratitis; IOP returns to normal after acute episode of inflammation.

Treatment
- *Inflammatory process:* treatment of underlying cause may be sufficient (e.g., topical steroids and mydriatic for anterior uveitis; p. 325).
- *Increased IOP:* if there are features of concern (e.g., IOP >30 mmHg; sustained increased IOP; vulnerable optic disc), consider topical (e.g., β-blocker, carbonic anhydrase inhibitor) or systemic (e.g., acetazolamide) medication for as long as required.

Chronic

- *Mechanism:* trabecular scarring; chronic trabeculitis.

Clinical features
- Increased IOP; open angle; no active inflammation but may have signs of previous episodes; ± disc changes or field defects (p. 264).

Treatment
- Medical: as for POAG; prostaglandin agonists are occasionally useful but may exacerbate inflammation.
- If medical treatment fails, consider trabeculectomy (which has poorer results than for POAG, but improves if augmented) or tube procedure.
- If surgical treatment fails, consider cyclodestruction (e.g., cyclodiode), but there is a significant risk of phthisis.

Steroid-induced glaucoma

Although related to the treatment rather than the underlying disease process, this is an important differential diagnosis of inflammatory glaucoma. Raised IOP due to steroids requires a reduction in the potency and frequency of topical corticosteroids, whereas if it is due to uncontrolled inflammation, the steroid dose may need to be increased.

If patients require large or frequent doses of steroids or develop an adverse response to steroids, it is often advisable to initiate systemic immunomodulatory therapy (methotrexate, cyclosporine, etc.).

Angle closure type

With seclusio pupillae

- *Mechanism:* 360° posterior synechiae (seclusio pupillae) block anterior flow of aqueous humor, causing iris bombé and appositional angle closure.

Clinical features

- Increased IOP; seclusio pupillae; iris bombé; shallow AC; angle closure (appositional); signs of previous inflammatory episodes.

Treatment

- *Inflammatory process:* minimize posterior synechiae formation by rapid and effective treatment of anterior uveitis (consider subconjunctival steroid injection).
- *Increased IOP:* Nd-YAG PI needs to be larger than is necessary for acute-angle closure glaucoma (AC will be shallow, so watch out for the corneal endothelium), and surgical PI may be necessary if Nd-YAG PI closes, although there is a high chance that PI will close if the inflammatory response is not well controlled. Consider topical (e.g., β-blocker, carbonic anhydrase inhibitor) or systemic (e.g., acetazolamide) medication as a temporary measure or for as long as required.

With synechial closure

- *Mechanism:* peripheral anterior synechiae may zipper the angle closed; the risk of synechial closure is increased in presence of granulomatous inflammation and possibly pre-existing narrow angles.

Clinical features

- Increased IOP, shallow AC, PAS with angle closure, signs of previous inflammatory episodes.

Treatment

- Medical: as for POAG, but some practitioners would advise caution with prostaglandin agonists.
- If medical treatment fails, consider trabeculectomy (augmented) or tube shunt.
- If surgical treatment fails, consider cyclodestruction (e.g., cyclodiode), but there is a significant risk of phthisis.
- If >25% of angle remains open, consider Nd-YAG PI to deal with any pupillary block component.
- Goniosynechiolysis has been shown to be effective if synechiae have been present for <6 months.

Inflammatory glaucoma: syndromes

Posner–Schlossman syndrome (glaucomatocyclitic crisis)

This syndrome of recurrent unilateral episodes of very high IOP typically affects young males. The cause is not known; acute trabeculitis has been postulated, possibly secondary to HSV or cytomegalovirus (CMV).

Clinical features

- Blurring of vision, halos, painless.
- Increased IOP (40–80 mmHg), white eye, minimal flare, occasional cells/fine keratic precipitates, no synechiae (PS or PAS), open angle.

Treatment

- *Inflammatory process:* topical steroid (e.g., dexamethasone 0.1% 4x/day).
- *Increased IOP:* consider topical (e.g., β-blocker, α_2-agonist, carbonic anhydrase inhibitor) or systemic (e.g., acetazolamide) agents according to IOP level.
- Consider oral acyclovir for HSV or valganciclovir for CMV.

Fuchs' heterochromic iridocyclitis

This syndrome of mild chronic anterior uveitis, iris heterochromia, and cataract may be complicated by glaucoma in 10–30% cases. It typically affects young adults and there is no sex bias. It is unilateral in >90% cases.

Clinical features

- Decreased vision due to cataract; floaters; often asymptomatic.
- White eye, white, stellate keratic precipitates (KPs) over whole corneal endothelium, mild flare, few cells, iris atrophy (washed out, moth-eaten), transillumination defects, abnormal iris vessels, iris heterochromia (a dark iris becomes lighter; whereas a light iris may become darker), iris nodules, cataract (posterior cortical/subcapsular), vitritis, increased IOP.
- Gonioscopy: open angle; ± twig-like neovascularization of the angle associated with hyphema during cataract surgery.

Treatment

- *Inflammatory process:* treatment is not usually necessary.
- *Increased IOP:* treat as for POAG (p. 269).

Lens-related glaucoma

Lens-related glaucoma may result from abnormalities of lens size, lens position, release of lens protein (mature cataract, trauma, surgery), and/or the consequent inflammatory response.

Phacomorphic glaucoma

The enlarging lens causes pupillary block and anterior bowing of the iris with secondary angle closure. In an eye of normal axial length, this occurs secondary to an intumescent cataractous lens; in a short eye, this may result simply from the normal increase in lens size with age.

Clinical features
- Increased IOP, shallow AC, fixed semidilated pupil, swollen cataractous lens.
- Ipsilateral closed angle (appositional; sigma sign may be seen on indentation gonioscopy).
- Contralateral angle is open with deep AC (in contrast to PACG).

Treatment
- Medical (topical and systemic): as for PACG.
- Nd-YAG PI to reverse pupillary block component.
- Early cataract extraction is the definitive treatment.

Phacolytic glaucoma

The hypermature cataract loses soluble lens proteins through the anterior capsule, causing trabecular obstruction and subsequent secondary open-angle glaucoma.

Clinical features
- Increased IOP, lens protein in a deep AC (may form a pseudohypopyon), hypermature or mature cataract, open angle (with lens protein); AC tap reveals lens protein and foamy macrophages.

Treatment
- Medical: topical (e.g., β-blocker, $α_2$-agonist, carbonic anhydrase inhibitor) or systemic (e.g., acetazolamide) agents as required.
- Early cataract extraction.

Phacoanaphylactic uveitis

This is an inflammatory reaction to lens protein, usually following traumatic capsular rupture or postoperative retention of lens material (when it must be distinguished from endophthalmitis). This insult may also cause sensitization such that lens protein exposure in the contralateral eye (surgery, hypermature or mature cataract) may be associated with an aggressive inflammatory response.

Clinical features
- Recent trauma or surgery, exposed lens protein, AC flare + cells with or without hypopyon, KPs, synechiae (posterior synechiae + PAS), angle usually open (but may have PAS); IOP may be high, normal, or low.

Treatment
- *Inflammatory process:* topical steroid (e.g., dexamethasone 0.1% hourly) and surgical removal of any retained lens fragments.
- *Increased IOP:* medical: topical (e.g., β-blocker, α_2-agonist, carbonic anhydrase inhibitor) or systemic (e.g., acetazolamide) agents as required.
- Treat for contralateral cataract.

Glaucoma secondary to lens subluxation/dislocation

There is pupillary block by anterior lens subluxation or complete dislocation into the AC; there may also be a coincident angle abnormality (e.g., Marfan syndrome).

Clinical features
- Increased IOP, subluxed/dislocated lens, ± corneal edema (if acute or lenticulocorneal touch).

Treatment
- Positional: dilate and have patient lie supine (to encourage gravity-driven posterior movement of lens), and constrict (to keep lens safely behind pupil); long-term miotic therapy may be needed unless the lens dislocates safely into the vitreous.
- Occasionally, in cases of anterior lens dislocation associated with loose zonules, such as in microspherophakia, miotics are contraindicated, as they decrease tension on zonules and exacerbate anterior dislocation. In these situations, cycloplegics are indicated to maintain tension on zonules and posterior position of the lens diaphragm.
- Consider lens extraction if positional measures fail, if there is complete dislocation into the AC, or if there is a cataract or recurrent problem.

Other secondary open-angle glaucomas

Steroid-induced

Exogenous and occasionally endogenous steroids may decrease outflow facility, leading to increased IOP after days, weeks, or months. In the normal population, 5% will have an IOP increase of >15 mmHg and 30% will have an increase of 6–15 mmHg if given topical steroids for up to 6 weeks. POAG patients are often particularly sensitive to this steroid effect.

Possible mechanisms include prostaglandin inhibition (e.g., PGF2α) and structural changes in the extracellular matrix (glycosaminoglycans) and trabecular meshwork (cross-linking of actins).

A history of steroid administration should be specifically asked for, since patients may not volunteer use of steroid-containing anabolics, skin creams, or episodic courses of steroids (e.g., for exacerbations of asthma or COPD). While steroids by any route may cause increased IOP, pressure elevation is more common with increased frequency and potency of steroid exposure (e.g., more common after intravitreal triamcinolone).

Treatment

Ideally, decrease frequency and potency or stop steroid and/or use other immunomodulators. If it is not possible to reduce steroids, then treat as POAG (p. 269).

Red cell glaucoma

Hyphema (usually traumatic) leads to blockage of the trabecular meshwork by red blood cells. In 10% cases a rebleed may occur, usually at around day 5.

Patients with sickle cell disease/trait do worse and are harder to treat as sickled cells more easily obstruct the TM, and sickled cells within the optic nerve vasculature lead to earlier optic nerve damage. Sickling may be worsened by the acidosis induced by carbonic anhydrase inhibitors.

Treatment

- *Hyphema:* strict bed rest, topical steroid (e.g., dexamethasone 0.1% 4×/day), mydriatic (e.g., atropine 1% 2×/day) (p. 100), avoid anticoagulants (aspirin, NSAIDS), use eye shield.
- *Increased IOP:* topical (e.g., β-blocker, α_2-agonist, carbonic anhydrase inhibitor) or systemic (e.g., acetazolamide) agents as required; surgical: AC paracentesis ± AC washout.

Ghost cell glaucoma

Vitreous hemorrhage leads to blockage of the trabecular meshwork by degenerated red blood cells, usually 2–4 weeks after the hemorrhage. These cells, which may be seen in the AC and the angle, are tan-colored having lost hemoglobin.

Treatment

Medical treatment (as for POAG, p. 269) is usually sufficient. If this fails, consider AC washout + vitrectomy to remove persistent vitreous hemorrhage.

Angle recession glaucoma

Blunt trauma may cause angle recession and associated trabecular damage. Traumatic angle recession carries a 10% risk of glaucoma at 10 years, the risk increasing with extent of recession. Look for asymmetry of AC depth, pupil, and angle.

- *Screening*: periodic IOP check (e.g., 3 months, 6 months, yearly) if known angle recession.
- *Treatment*: as for POAG (p. 269).

Raised episcleral venous pressure

Aqueous drainage is reduced as episcleral venous pressure increases (p. 262). This may occur as a result of vascular abnormalities in the orbit (Sturge–Weber syndrome, orbital varices), cavernous sinus (arterio-venous fistulae), or superior vena cava (SVC obstruction).

Episcleral venous pressure manifests as unilateral or bilateral engorged episcleral veins, chemosis, and proptosis, with blood in Schlemm's canal on gonioscopy.

Treatment

Treatment is primarily directed at the underlying pathology, although medical and occasionally surgical lowering of IOP may be necessary.

Tumors

Tumors may cause increased IOP via open-angle mechanisms (clogging or infiltration of trabecular meshwork with tumor cells) or rubeosis (secondary to ischemia or radiation), or larger posterior segment tumors may cause it via secondary angle closure (anterior displacement of lens–iris diaphragm).

Suspect tumor in atypical unilateral glaucoma; if there is a poor view of posterior segment (usually due to cataract), a B-scan ultrasound is essential. Approximately 20% of malignant melanomas are associated with increased IOP.

Treatment

Treatment is directed by the underlying tumor, although increased IOP itself suggests a poor prognosis.

Other secondary closed-angle glaucomas

Iridoschisis

Bilateral splitting and atrophy of anterior iris leaf is associated with increased IOP usually secondary to angle closure (due to pupillary block), but sometimes due to debris blocking the trabecular meshwork (open angle). It is uncommon and usually occurs in the elderly.

Treatment
Closed-angle closure type is with Nd-YAG PI; open-angle type is the same as for POAG (p. 269).

Iridocorneal endothelial syndrome (ICE)

ICE is a unilateral condition in which abnormal corneal endothelium migrates across the angle, the trabecular meshwork, and the anterior iris, causing significant anterior segment distortion. ICE syndrome is rare, usually occurs in 20- to 40-year-old females, and carries a 50% risk of glaucoma. HSV has been implicated.

Three overlapping syndromes are described: Chandler's syndrome (predominantly corneal), essential iris atrophy (predominantly iris changes, most highly associated with glaucoma), and iris nevus (Cogan–Reese) syndrome (appearance of a diffuse nevus or pigmented nodules that probably represent protrusions of iris stroma).

Clinical features
- Unilateral pain, blurred vision.
- Unilateral fine corneal guttata ("beaten-metal"), corneal edema (increased IOP), iris atrophy corectopia (displaced pupil), pseudopolycoria (accessory pupil).
- Gonioscopy: broad-based PAS, which may insert anterior to Schwalbe's line.

Treatment
- Medical (e.g., β-blocker, α_2-agonist, carbonic anhydrase inhibitor, prostaglandin agonist), surgery (antimetabolite-augmented trabeculectomy or tube procedures), or cyclodestruction as required.

Posterior polymorphous dystrophy (PPMD)

PMMD is a bilateral condition in which abnormal corneal endothelium may form extensive iridocorneal adhesions with angle closure. Clinically, it may appear similar to ICE syndrome but is dominantly inherited, bilateral, and usually detectable in childhood (although it may only be symptomatic later). PPMD carries a 15% risk of glaucoma.

Treat glaucoma as for POAG (p. 269).

Epithelial down-growth

This is a deranged healing response in which trauma or surgery (poorly constructed wound, vitreous incarceration) allows epithelium to proliferate down through the wound and onto the endothelial surface. Once free of its normal environment, the epithelial cells may proliferate unchecked across the corneal endothelium and angle, thus causing glaucoma in a similar manner to ICE syndrome.

Light argon laser application to suspected intraocular epithelial tissue can aid in identifying epithelial down-growth.

Intracameral 5-fluorouracil has been demonstrated to effectively eliminate intraocular epithelial cells, but glaucoma treatment is often very difficult. Lower IOP as for POAG or NVG, depending on presentation.

Iatrogenic glaucoma

Malignant glaucoma

This is also known as aqueous misdirection syndrome, ciliary block, and ciliolenticular block.

It is thought that that posteriorly directed aqueous is trapped in the vitreous, causing anterior displacement of vitreous and lens–iris diaphragm with secondary angle closure.

Risk factors
- Short axial length, chronic angle closure, previous acute angle closure.
- Post-procedure: surgery (trabeculectomy, tube procedures, cataract extraction, peripheral iridectomy); laser (Nd-YAG PI).
- Miotic therapy (rare).

Clinical features
- Asymptomatic unless acute or very high IOP.
- Increased IOP (may be normal initially), shallow or flat AC, no pupillary block (so no iris bombé and occurs despite a patent PI), no choroidal or suprachoroidal cause (detachment/hemorrhage).

Treatment
- Ensure that a patent PI is present (repeat Nd-YAG PI if necessary).
- Dilate (atropine 1% 3×/day + phenylephrine 2.5% 4×/day).
- Systemic IOP lowering: acetazolamide 500 mg IV stat (then 250 mg PO 4×/day) ± mannitol/glycerol.
- Topical aqueous suppressant to lower IOP: β-blocker (e.g., timolol 0.5% stat then 2×/day) + sympathomimetic (e.g., apraclonidine 1% stat then 3×/day).
- If medical treatment fails, consider laser or surgical treatment.

Laser
- Nd:YAG disruption of anterior vitreous face (if aphakia/pseudophakia, perform posterior capsulotomy/hyaloidotomy; if phakic, a hyaloidotomy can be attempted through the patent PI).
- Argon laser to the ciliary processes (through the patent PI; relieves block by causing shrinkage of processes or disruption of hyaloid face).

Surgery
- If phakic: cataract extraction (phacoemulsification or ECCE), posterior capsulotomy, and anterior vitrectomy.
- If aphakic/pseudophakic: pars plana vitrectomy and posterior capsulotomy.

Post-cataract surgery

Acute postoperative increased IOP may be due to retained viscoelastic, crystalline lens particles, inflammatory debris, TM inflammation, vitreous in the AC, or a suprachoroidal hemorrhage. Iris bombé may develop after an ACIOL if a PI is not created.

A single dose of acetazolamide SR 250 mg may be used prophylacticly against the risk of an early postoperative pressure spike. Delayed onset of OHT may arise due to neovascular glaucoma, suprachoroidal hemorrhage, phacoanaphylaxis (p. 284), epithelial down-growth syndrome (p. 289), aqueous misdirection (see above), or uveitis glaucoma hyphema (UGH) syndrome.

Post-vitreoretinal surgery

With intraocular gases, acute postoperative increased IOP is usually due to expansion or overfill of SF6, C3F8 or silicone oil. Determine treatment according to IOP and half-life of the gas, but usually short-term medical treatment is sufficient (e.g., acetazolamide SR 250 mg 2×/day). Otherwise, remove some of the gas.

With scleral buckles, secondary angle closure may occur from ciliary body swelling and choroidal detachment (possibly due to pressure on the vortex veins). This usually resolves spontaneously; treat medically in the interim.

With silicone oil, oil in the AC blocking the trabecular meshwork and overfill of oil causing secondary angle closure or iris bombé (and possibly other mechanisms) can present from days to months after surgery. Sometimes this resolves spontaneously; treat medically in the interim. Consider oil removal, tube-shunt placement, or cyclodestruction if OHT persists. Early removal of oil (<6 months) may decrease IOP. After this period, removal of oil makes little difference because of incorporation of oil into the TM by macrophages.

Vitrectomy may facilitate ghost cell glaucoma (p. 286) and increase the risk of rubeosis in proliferative diabetic retinopathy.

Pharmacology of IOP-lowering agents

Prostaglandin analogues

These analogues of $PGF_{2\alpha}$ increase uveoscleral outflow (see Table 10.6).

- *Ocular side effects:* common: hyperemia, increased pigmentation of iris (and rarely lid skin), thickening and lengthening of lashes; rare: uveitis, CME.
- *Contraindications* may be associated with CME after complicated cataract surgery or if used during active uveitis.

β-Blockers

These agents reduce aqueous production probably by acting on β-receptors on the nonpigmented ciliary epithelium and vasoconstriction of the arterioles supplying ciliary processes.

- *Ocular side effects:* uncommon: allergic blepharoconjunctivitis, punctate keratitis.
- *Contraindications:* asthma/COPD (bronchospasm may occur even with selective β_1-agents), heart block, bradycardia or cardiac failure. Try to avoid β-blocker in nursing mothers as it is secreted in breast milk.
- *Drug interactions:* concurrent use of cardiac-directed Ca^{2+} antagonists such as verapamil may compound bradycardia, heart block, and hypotension.

Carbonic anhydrase inhibitors

These agents reduce aqueous production by inhibiting carbonic anhydrase isoenzyme II (and hence bicarbonate production) in the non-pigmented ciliary epithelium.

- *Ocular side effects:* common: burning, tearing, allergic blepharoconjunctivitis (up to 10%).
- *Contraindications:* sulfonamide sensitivity; renal failure, liver failure (systemic acetazolamide).
- *Drug interactions:* K^+-losing diuretics (e.g., thiazide) may cause profound hypokalemia if used concurrently with acetazolamide. K^+ supplementation is not usually required for acetazolamide used alone.

Sympathomimetics

The highly α_2-selective brimonidine is well tolerated for chronic use, and apraclonidine ($\alpha_1 + \alpha_2$) is useful for short-term use (e.g., after laser iridotomy). Nonselective sympathomimetics such as adrenaline (epinephrine), dipivefrin, and the adrenergic neuron blocker guanethidine are now seldom used because of their frequent side effects.

- *Ocular side effects:* common: allergic blepharoconjunctivitis (up to 15% for brimonidine, 30% for apraclonidine); older agents: scarring, mydriasis, adrenochrome deposits; uncommon: CME in aphakia (possibly pseudophakia).
- *Contraindications:* heart block, bradycardia.
- *Drug interactions:* monoamine oxidase inhibitors.

Table 10.6 Pharmacological groups

Group	Mechanism	Advantages	Systemic effects	Examples
Topical				
Prostaglandin analogues	Increase uveoscleral outflow	IOP by ±30% Well tolerated	Bronchospasm (rare)	Latanaprost 0.005% Travaprost 0.004% Bimatoprost 0.03%
β-Blocker	Decrease aqueous production	20-year follow-up ↓IOP by ±25% Well-tolerated (in most cases)	Bronchospasm Bradycardia Heart block Hypotension Glucose intolerance Lethargy Impotence	*Nonselective* Timolol 0.25/0.5% Carteolol 1% Levobunolol 0.5% β_1-*selective* Betaxolol 0.25/0.5%
Carbonic anhydrase inhibitors	Decrease aqueous production	↓IOP by ±20%	Metallic taste See list below (for systemic)	Brinzolamide 1% Dorzolamide 2%
α_2-Agonists	Decrease aqueous production Increase uveoscleral outflow	IOP by ±20%	Bradycardia Hypotension Insomnia Irritability GI disturbance	Brimonidine 0.2% Apraclonidine 0.5/1%
Miotics	Increase trabecular outflow		Sweating Drooling Nausea Headache Bradycardia	Pilocarpine 0.5–4% Carbachol 0.75–3%
Systemic				
Carbonic anhydrase inhibitor	Decrease aqueous production Acidosis may cause hypotension	↓IOP by ≤65%	Lethargy Depression Anorexia Hypokalemia Renal calculi Blood dyscrasia	Acetazolamide
Hyperosmotic agents	Creates an osmotic gradient	Rapidly IOP (onset 30 min)	Hypertension Vomiting Cardiac failure MI Hyperglycemia (mannitol) Urinary retention	Mannitol Glycerol

Miotics (parasympathomimetics)

Muscarinic receptor agonist leads to ciliary muscle contraction, which pulls on the scleral spur to open the trabecular meshwork. Pilocarpine is sometimes used as a first-line agent in narrow-angle glaucoma; it is sometimes still used in POAG.

- *Ocular side effects:* fluctuating myopia, miosis (constricted visual field, worse night vision).
- *Contraindications:* inflammatory or malignant glaucoma.

Combination agents

In the United States, two combination agents are available and have been demonstrated to have more effective IOP lowering than either of the individual components alone (but not more effective than each of the separate components alone).

Combination agents have benefits of increased convenience for patients as well as improved patient adherence and compliance (since compliance decreases with each additional drop a patient must use).

Mechanism of action, contraindications, and side-effect profiles are the same as for each individual agent.

- Dorzolamide/timolol: first fixed combination agent now available in a generic form.
- Brimonidine/timolol: most recently approved fixed combination agent.

Laser procedures for glaucoma

Nd-YAG peripheral iridotomy (PI)

Indications
- *Treatment:* angle closure with pupillary block—may be acute or subacute; chronic; primary or secondary.
- *Prophylaxis:* occludable narrow angles (including fellow eye in angle closure).

Method
- Consent: explain what the procedure does, why you are treating both eyes, and possible complications, including failure of treatment or need for retreatment, bleeding, inflammation, corneal burns, and visual effects (e.g., photopsias, monocular diplopia).
- Instill pilocarpine 2% (unfolds the iris) + apraclonidine 1% (prevents IOP spike and may reduce bleeding) + topical anesthetic (e.g., proparicaine).
- Set laser (varies according to model): commonly, bursts of one to two pulses of 3–6 mJ (an iris that is thick, velvety, and heavily pigmented may be more easily penetrated with pretreatment by argon laser: ~40 shots/50 μm/0.05 ms/500–700 mW). The beam should be angled (i.e., not perpendicular).
- Position contact lens (usually the Abraham lens; require coupling agent).
- Identify suitable iridotomy sites: superior (hidden by the normal lid position), peripheral, and ideally in an iris crypt (less energy required).
- Focus and fire laser: success is indicated by a forward gush of pigment-loaded aqueous. This usually takes 2–6 shots.

Post-procedure
- Topical steroid (e.g., dexamethasone 0.1% stat, then 4x/day for 1 week).
- Check IOP after 30–60 minutes.
- *Complications:* bleeding (stops with maintained pressure on lens that increases IOP), anterior inflammation (increase topical steroids), corneal burns (caution with a flatter AC), glare (avoid interpalpebral iris).

Laser trabeculoplasty

While argon laser trabeculoplasty (ALT, ~500 nm) has the longest track record and most data, newer laser energy modalities have been developed and offer theoretical advantages.

Selective laser trabeculoplasty (SLT), a 532 nm Q-switched, frequency-doubled Nd:YAG laser, uses less energy than ALT, with microscopic analysis demonstrating less tissue disruption. SLT has also been demonstrated to be repeatable.

Titanium:saphire laser trabeculoplasty (TLT) uses a longer wavelength (790 nm) and is believed to penetrate more deeply into the trabecular meshwork.

Micropulse laser trabeculoplasty (MLT, 810 nm) uses bursts of short diode laser pulses, which theoretically prevent thermal injury. In addition, the same system that powers MLT can be used for photocoagulation, increasing the utility of the machine.

Indications

- Open-angle glaucoma—commonly POAG, PXF glaucoma, or PDS glaucoma.
- Medical and surgical options are undesirable or ineffective.

Method

- Consent: explain what the procedure does and possible complications, including failure (short and long term), bleeding, inflammation, or PAS.
- Instill apraclonidine 1% (to prevent IOP spike; alternatively give 250 mg acetazolamide 30 min beforehand) + topical anesthetic (e.g., proparacaine).
- Argon: #80–100 spots (360°), 50 μm spot size, 0.1 sec duration, 500–1000 mW power (start low, increase as required to obtain light blanching of pigmented TM).
- Diode: 100 μm spot size, 0.1–0.2 sec duration, 800–1200 mW power.
- SLT: #80–100 spots (360°), 400 μm spot size, 0.8–1.1 mJ titrate to obtain fine "champagne bubbles."
- TLT: #100, 30–120 mJ, 200 μm spot size.
- MLT: #65–130 spots, 2 mW, 300 μm spot size, 2 ms micropulse (0.3 ms on, 1.7 ms off).
- Position goniolens (antireflective laser lens).
- Identify trabeculoplasty site: aim for the anterior border of the pigmented trabecular meshwork.
- Focus and fire laser: the ideal reaction is a mild blanching or small bubble; the more pigmented the angle, the less power is usually required. In these cases, consider placing only 50 equally spaced shots over 180°.
- If patient is currently using maximum tolerated medical therapy, consider dividing treatment into two 180° sessions to prevent IOP spike.

Post-procedure

- Topical steroid (e.g., prednisolone qid) and all usual glaucoma medication.
- Check IOP 1 hour later and observe until IOP plateaus.
- Review in 1–2 weeks: if there is an inadequate IOP response, consider laser trabeculoplasty on the remaining 180°.
- *Complications:* bleeding (stops with maintained pressure on lens), anterior inflammation (usually mild), peripheral anterior synechiae, pressure spike.

Laser iridoplasty

Most commonly used for plateau iris syndrome, the laser shrinks the periph-eral iris to widen the angular approach. Iridoplasty may also be used to pull the iris tissue away from a drainage implant tube lumen or trabeculectomy fistula. A contact lens (e.g., Abraham or Goldmann [central part rather than mirrors]) is used to direct the argon laser to the most peripheral iris.

Typical applications are 20–50 burns over 360° (with ≥2 spot sizes between burns) of 200–500 μm spot size, 0.2–0.5 sec duration, and 200–400 mW power.

Post-laser inflammation may promote formation of PAS.

Transscleral cyclophotocoagulation (cyclodiode)

Indications

These include intractable increased IOP, e.g., in rubeotic or synechial angle closure where other treatment modalities have failed, low visual potential, or a poor surgical candidate.

Method

- Consent: explain what the procedure does and the possible complications, including failure of treatment or need for retreatment, hypotony, inflammation, bleeding, vision loss, and sympathetic ophthalmia.
- Set laser (varies according to model)—commonly 2500 mW power, 2000 ms duration.
- Identify ciliary body 0.5–2 mm from limbus. Transillumination helps to identify the dark ciliary body. Place the contact G-probe (of the diode laser) in an anteroposterior manner against the globe, with the heel to the limbus.
- Fire laser: aim to treat up to three quadrants or 360°, using 6–7 shots per quadrant. If laser burn is audible ("pop"), decrease power.

Post-procedure

- Topical steroid (e.g., dexamethasone 0.1% 4×/day until inflammation abates) and all usual glaucoma medication except prostaglandin. Review in 1–2 weeks.
- *Complications:* vision loss, anterior inflammation (may get hypopyon or hyphema), hypotony, scleral thinning, cataract, phthisis, sympathetic ophthalmia.

Alternative

Endoscopic cyclophotocoagulation (requiring surgical incision) is a viable alternative to the external, nonincisional cyclodiode treatment.

Surgery for glaucoma

Glaucoma surgery includes iris procedures (surgical iridectomy), angle procedures (goniotomy, trabeculotomy), filtration procedures (trabeculectomy, deep sclerectomy), artificial drainage tubes, and cyclodestruction (e.g., cyclodiode) (Table 10.7).

In adult glaucoma, the most common operation is trabeculectomy with or without antimetabolites. Antimetabolites are indicated according to risk of fibrosis and previous failure, though they are commonly used for primary trabeculectomies. Artificial drainage tubes have historically been reserved for resistant cases but are being used more commonly as first-line surgical therapy.

Surgical iridectomy and surgical cyclodialysis have become less common since the advent of laser peripheral iridotomy and cyclodiode. Goniotomy and trabeculotomy are generally restricted for congenital glaucoma (p. 630).

Table 10.7 Common surgical procedures in glaucoma

Procedure	Mechanism	Indication
Iris procedures		
Peripheral iridectomy	Relieves pupillary block	Laser PI not possible (patient cooperation, thick iris, poor view, e.g., persistent corneal edema)
Angle procedures		
Goniotomy	Opens the abnormal angle (probably)	Primary congenital glaucoma (primary trabecular meshwork dysgenesis)
Trabeculotomy	Opens Schlemm's canal directly to anterior chamber	Congenital glaucoma, including primary congenital glaucoma and anterior segment dysgenesis
Filtration procedures		
Trabeculectomy	Forms new drainage channel from AC to subconjunctival space	Has a place in most chronic glaucomas (adult and pediatric)
Augmented trabeculectomy	Trabeculectomy with antimetabolite to reduce scarring	Standard trabeculectomy has failed or would be likely to fail
Artificial drainage tube implants	Silicone tube flows from AC via valve to episcleral explant	Augmented trabeculectomy has failed or would be likely to fail

Filtration surgery: trabeculectomy

The Collaborative Initial Glaucoma Treatment Study (CIGTS) compared the safety and efficacy of medical therapy and trabeculectomy and generally found similar outcomes, although patients who presented with more advanced glaucoma maintained more vision with earlier surgery.

Indication

- *When to operate:* this surgery may be first line if there is a high risk of progression or the patient aims to be drop-free; more commonly it is reserved for when medical and/or laser therapy is proven to be inadequate.
- *Which operation:* assess risks of operation failure (e.g., from scarring) against the increased risk of complications from antimetabolite augmentation or tube procedures (see Table 10.8).

Method

The standard trabeculectomy with fornix-based flap is described here.

- Consent: explain what the operation does and possible complications, including scarring with return to high IOP, hypotony, hemorrhage, worsened vision, and risk of acute postoperative infection as well as late-onset endophthalmitis.
- Preoperative: consider stopping aqueous suppressants a couple of days before surgery.
- Prep with 5% povidone iodine and drape.
- Place corneal traction suture.
- Form fornix based: incise at limbus (5 to 8 mm length) (Table 10.9).
- Form scleral flap (rectangular/square/triangular): incise outline of the flap to a depth of 1/2 to ¾ scleral thickness, before anterior lamellar dissection anteriorly into the clear cornea, and free the posterior and lateral aspects of the flap.
- Place a paracentesis obliquely in the temporal cornea.
- Form sclerectomy under scleral flap: make a perpendicular incision at the sclerolimbal junction to form the anterior margin of the sclerectomy. Complete sclerectomy posteriorly by removing a block of sclerolimbal tissue with the punch (e.g., Kelly) or blade or scissors (e.g., Vannas).
- Perform peripheral iridectomy: this should be broad-based but short and peripheral. This stage is primarily to prevent iris blockage of the trabeculectomy, although it will also relieve any coincident pupillary block.
- Suture scleral flap: sutures can either be fixed, releasable (leave access via a corneal groove), or adjustable (can be loosened by massaging posterior aspect of scleral flap). Assess flap by injecting balanced salt solution via the paracentesis.
- Close conjunctiva securely to prevent retraction and consequent leak. This can be achieved with two lateral interrupted and a central mattress suture or a continuous running suture.
- Postoperative: subconjunctival steroid (e.g., dexamethasone), antibiotic (e.g., cefazolin).

Post-procedure

Use topical antibiotic (e.g., gatifloxacin 4×/day) and steroid (e.g., prednisolone acetate 1% every 2 hours initially, tapering down over 2 months).

Review at 1 day and 1 week, then according to result.

Table 10.8 Choice of filtration procedure

Procedure	Indication
Trabeculectomy	
Standard	Low risk of scarring
	Low risk of failure from other causes
Augmented trabeculectomy	
5-fluorouracil (50 mg/mL) or mitomycin C (0.2 mg/mL)	Moderate risk of scarring
	Planned combined trabeculectomy and cataract surgery
	Previous surgery involving the conjunctiva (not trabeculectomy)
Mitomycin C (0.4 mg/mL)	High risk of scarring
	Previous failed trabeculectomy
	Chronic inflammation (conjunctival or intraocular)
	High-risk glaucoma (including aphakic, active neovascular)
Tube procedures	
Molteno, Ahmed, Baerveldt, and alternatives	Previous failed augmented trabeculectomy
	Multiple further operations likely to be necessary
	Inadequate healthy conjunctiva for trabeculectomy
	High-risk glaucoma (including aphakic, active neovascular, aniridia, cellular overgrowth, e.g., ICE, epithelial downgrowth syndrome)

Table 10.9 Comparison of fornix- vs. limbal-based flaps for trabeculectomy

	Fornix-based	Limbal-based
Operative	Easier	Access can be difficult
	Faster	Slower
	Good sclerostomy exposure	Adequate sclerostomy exposure
Use of antimetabolites	Take care to avoid wound margin	Relatively safe
Postoperative manipulation	Easier	More difficult
Postoperative	More conjunctival wound leaks	Fewer conjunctival wound leaks
	Less posterior scarring	More posterior scarring

Fixed, releasable, and adjustable sutures

Optimal bleb drainage is not always achieved. Postoperatively, bleb drainage may be increased by removing or loosening selected scleral sutures. The technique depends on the suture type used:

- *Fixed sutures:* if the suture can be visualized through Tenon's layer, it may be cut by argon laser lysis.
- *Releasable sutures* are tied with a slipknot and loop into a corneal groove to permit access. They can be released at the slit lamp without disturbing the conjunctival flap.
- *Adjustable sutures* can be loosened by massaging the posterior aspect of the scleral flap at the slit lamp.

Filtration surgery: antimetabolites

The control of wound healing is critical to the success of glaucoma filtration surgery. Antimetabolites such as 5-fluorouracil (5-FU) and mitomycin-C (MMC) permit the surgeon to inhibit the fibrosis and scarring that may close off an otherwise satisfactory trabeculectomy.

Since this fibrotic response will vary between patients, the use of antimetabolites can be titrated according to the predicted risk of scarring (see Table 10.8). They should not be used indiscriminately, as they may cause significant side effects (Box 10.4).

Agents
- 5-FU inhibits DNA synthesis and RNA function; usual intraoperative dose is 50 mg/mL.
- MMC alkylates DNA and inhibits DNA and RNA synthesis; usual dose is 0.2–0.4 mg/mL.

Indications
- Moderate risk of scarring: 5-FU (50 mg/mL) or MMC (0.2 mg/mL)
- High risk of scarring: MMC (0.4 mg/mL).

If there is a very high risk or failed augmented trabeculectomy, consider a tube implant procedure (Table 10.8).

Risk factors for scarring
- Age: <40.
- Race: African Caribbean, Indian subcontinent.
- Previous surgery involving conjunctiva: includes trabeculectomy, cataract surgery with scleral tunnel, vitreoretinal surgery.
- Glaucoma type: neovascular, aphakic, inflammatory.
- Chronic inflammation: chronic conjunctivitis, uveitis.
- Topical treatment: β-blockers (low risk), pilocarpine, dipivefin (moderate risk).

Intraoperative use (as part of trabeculectomy, p. 299)
- Select agent and concentration (50 mg/mL 5-FU; 0.2–0.4 mg/mL MMC) according to patient's risk of fibrosis.
- Prepare sponges: sponges need to be cut to size and then soaked in the antimetabolite of choice. Polyvinyl alcohol sponges may be preferred, as they disintegrate less than those made of methylcellulose.
- During trabeculectomy, place sponge under the conjunctival flap (and under scleral flap in resistant cases) for appropriate duration (5 min for 5-FU; 2–4 min for MMC); avoid contact with cornea and conjunctival wound edge. Ensure that there is no intraocular administration.
- Remove sponges; all cytotoxics and used sponges require safe disposal separate to clinical waste.
- Irrigate eye well.

Postoperative use
- Select agent (usually 5-FU).
- Using a small-caliber needle (30g) on a 1 mL syringe (e.g., insulin syringe), administer antimetabolite adjacent to *but not into* the bleb.

The usual dose is 5 mg 5-FU (usually 0.1 mL of 50 mg/mL 5-FU); MMC may also be used (at a dose of 0.02 mg).

Box 10.4 Potential complications of antimetabolites

- Epithelial erosions
- Wound leak
- Bleb leak
- Hypotony
- Blebitis
- Endophthalmitis
- Scleritis

Filtration surgery: complications (1)

Intraoperative complications

- Conjunctival flap damage: may get persistent leak especially if exposed to antimetabolites, button holes especially if previous surgery.
- Scleral flap damage: may not close in controlled manner.
- Bleeding: may be conjunctival, scleral, from the iris, or, most seriously, suprachoroidal.
- Vitreous loss: increased risk with posterior sclerostomy.
- Wound leak from damaged conjunctiva or inadequate closure.

Early postoperative complications

Shallow AC

Grade according to corneal contact: with peripheral iris only (I), with whole iris (II), or with lens (III). Examination by ultrasound should identify the reason for a shallow AC (Table 10.10). If the AC is very shallow, it may not be possible to see if the PI is patent or not.

Specific treatment will depend on the underlying cause, but in general when there is a risk of corneal decompensation from lenticulocorneal touch, urgent measures are required to reform the AC (e.g., balanced salt solution, viscoelastic, or gas). Otherwise there is a risk of early cataract formation.

Low IOP/hypotony

IOP <6 mmHg is associated with flat AC, choroidal detachment, and suprachoroidal hemorrhage. IOP <4 mmHg is also associated with hypotony maculopathy and corneal edema.

General treatment is with topical steroids + mydriatic; stop IOP-lowering agents. Consider surgery (reform AC and/or drain choroidal effusions) if there is corneal decompensation from lens touch (absolute indication), "kissing" choroidal detachments (absolute indication), or marked AC inflammation (relative indication).

Table 10.10 Differential diagnosis of shallow AC after trabeculectomy

	IOP	Seidel	PI	Bleb
Wound leak	Low	+	Patent	Poor/flat
Ciliary body shutdown	Low	–	Patent	Poor/flat
Overfiltration	Low	–	Patent	Good
Pupillary block	High	–	Non-patent	Flat
Malignant glaucoma	High	–	Patent	Flat
Suprachoroidal hemorrhage	Variable	–	Patent	Variable

Wound leak

In milder cases where antimetabolites have not been used, resolution is likely within 48 hours. In the interim, a bandage contact lens may be applied. However, other cases (particularly with antimetabolites) usually require surgical intervention (i.e., suture wound).

Overfiltration

In milder cases, observation, a scleral shell, or autologous blood injection may be sufficient. However, more severe cases (e.g., hypotony maculopathy) may need surgical intervention (partial/temporary closure of overdraining bleb).

High IOP

Pupillary block: PI is either incomplete or blocked by inflammatory debris.
- Perform a new Nd-YAG PI (or complete old iridectomy); then give topical mydriatic + steroids.

Malignant glaucoma: aqueous misdirection may occur especially in short eyes (p. 290).

Filtration failure: obstruction of the sclerostomy and scleral flap may be internal (incarceration of iris, ciliary processes, or vitreous), scleral (fibrin, blood), or external (overly tight scleral flap sutures).
- Consider bleb massage, removal of releasable suture(s), loosening of adjustable suture(s), and argon laser lysis of fixed suture(s).

Infection

Blebitis: presents as a painful red eye, possibly with mucus discharge and photophobia (see Fig. 10.1). The bleb is milky with loculations of pus, conjunctival injection (especially around the bleb), and increasing IOP. Occasionally there is AC activity (cells/flare ± hypopyon).
- Identify organism with culture/swab of bleb.
- Treat with intensive topical antibiotics (e.g., moxifloxacin qh) and systemic antibiotic (e.g., moxifloxacin 400 mg PO qd); adjust according to response and organism identified (commonly staphylococci if early and streptococci and *Haemophilus* if late). Consider addition of topical steroids after 24 hours and add mydriatic if AC activity is present.

Endophthalmitis: clinical features are the same as for blebitis but are more severe, with decreased VA and vitritis.
- Investigate and treat as for other postoperative endophthalmitis. However, endophthalmitis occurring after trabeculectomy tends to run a more aggressive course with a worse prognosis than after cataract surgery.

Visual loss

Wipe-out of the remaining field may occur in the presence of a vulnerable optic nerve (associated with increased IOP or hypotony) or hypotonous changes may lead to reduced acuity (e.g., from maculopathy).

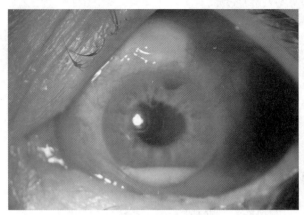

Figure 10.1 Infectious blebitis with associated endophthalmitis and a layered hypopyon in the anterior chamber. See insert for color version.

Filtration surgery: complications (2)

Late postoperative complications

- *Filtration failure:* subconjunctival fibrosis ("ring of steel"), especially with limbal-based flaps, may lead to a poorly filtering encapsulated bleb (tense localized dome). Treat with needling (+ subconjunctival 5-fluorouracil) and post-procedure topical steroids/antibiotics.
- *Leaking bleb:* sweaty or leaking blebs are more common in antimetabolite-associated or nonguarded filtration surgery. If there is a small leak and low risk of infection and the eye is not hypotonous, then the leaking bleb may be monitored initially; it often resolves (though often recurs). Otherwise, consider bandage contact lens, autologous blood injection, compression sutures, or refashioning of bleb.
- *Infection:*(blebitis/endophthalmitis)—see above and p. 254.
- *Visual loss:* postoperative lens opacities probably account for most of the postoperative drop in acuity. Unfortunately, cataract surgery carries a 10% risk of bleb failure. There can also be induced astigmatism, maculopathy, and glaucomatous progression.
- *Ptosis* often resolves spontaneously; it is more common with superior rectus traction sutures (rather than corneal) and in revised trabeculectomies where conjunctiva has been mobilized from the superior fornix.

Glaucoma drainage device (GDD) surgery

The tube versus trabeculectomy (TVT) study compared Baerveldt drainage implants with trabeculectomy with MMC in patients with previous ocular surgery (either a failed trabeculectomy or prior cataract surgery), and at 1 year demonstrated that trabeculectomy patients obtain lower IOPs with fewer medications, but had higher incidences of hypotony and require more reoperations.

The study determined that Baerveldt implants maintain IOP control comparable to that with antimetabolite-augmented trabeculectomy.

Indication

When to operate

Historically, GDD surgery was reserved for patients who were at high risk for failure due to fibrosis of the sclerectomy or conjunctiva. More commonly, GDDs are used for the same indications as for trabeculectomy: inadequate IOP, progression of glaucomatous damage, or intolerance of medical therapy.

GDDs may be more appropriate in children and in patients with lid disease or lifestyles that predispose to trabeculectomy bleb infections (gardening, swimming, etc)

Which tube

Nonvalved implants (Baerveldt/Molteno) require ligation sutures, as resistance is provided by the encapsulated plate. Filtration prior to encapsulation can lead to profound hypotony. Valved implants (Ahmed) have a leaflet-type valve set to around 10 mmHg and require no ligation suture.

Many surgeons use only one type of tube, on the basis of their training and comfort level. Some surgeons vary the type of tube used according to the clinical scenario: a patient with very high IOP (neovascular glacuoma) who needs immediate IOP lowering may receive an Ahmed valve implant; a patient who is intolerant of medications, has moderately elevated IOPs, and can tolerate 4–6 weeks of higher IOPs may receive a Baerveldt implant.

Modifications of the Baerveldt to allow drainage prior to release of the ligation suture involve the placement of small, full-thickness slits in the tube between the anterior chamber and the ligature, allowing some restricted flow out of the tube.

Method

Standard GDD placement with fornix-based limbal incision is described here.

- Consent: explain what the operation does and the possible complications, including encapsulation with return to high IOP, hypotony, hemorrhage, worsened vision, and risk of acute postoperative infection as well as corneal scarring, cataract formation, exposure of the implant, and double vision.
- Preoperative: consider stopping aqueous suppressants a couple of days before surgery.
- Prep with 5% povidone iodine and drape.
- Place corneal traction suture superotemporally.

- 10 mm limbal peritomy with 2 mm radial relaxing incisions at ends of limbal incision.
- Dissect a subtenon's pocket between the superior and lateral rectus.
- Ahmed implant.
  - Prime the Ahmed valve with balanced salt solution (BSS) on a 30g cannula.
  - Measure 8 mm posterior to the limbus and suture the Ahmed plate to globe with partial-thickness scleral passes of 8-0 nylon, rotate knots.
- Baerveldt implant.
  - Ligate tube about 1 mm from plate with 7-0 Vicryl suture (will dissolve and open the tube in about 4–6 weeks).
  - Use BSS on a cannula to verify watertight ligation of tube.
  - Capture superior and lateral rectus muscles with muscle hooks and pass plate wings under muscles.
  - With plate anteriorly against muscle insertions, suture plate to globe with partial-thickness scleral passes of 8-0 nylon, rotate knots.
  - Four or more venting tube slits can be created with a paracentesis blade or the needle of the 7-0 Vicryl suture placed between the anterior chamber and the ligature.
- Create a paracentesis and consider addition of viscoelastic solution.
- Trim the tube to length with a bevel up, aiming for about 2 mm in the eye.
- Use a 23g needle to enter the anterior chamber from about 1.5 mm posterior to the limbus, aiming to have the needle (and ultimately the tube) parallel with the iris, without contacting intraocular structures.
- Verify the tube position; if not ideal, then remove the tube, close the sclerostomy with 10-0 nylonsuture (instead of 8-0 vicryl), and repass the 23g needle in another position.
- Suture the tube to the sclera with 8-0 Vicryl or 10-0 nylon
- Secure scleral reinforcement graft (tutoplast sclera or pericardium) over the tube with 8-0 Vicryl.
- Close conjuctiva with wing or running suture.
- Use topical antibiotic (e.g., gatifloxacin 4×/day) and steroid (e.g., prednisolone acetate 1% four times a day initially, tapering down over 2 months).
- Review at 1 day and 1 week, then according to result.

Glaucoma drainage device: complications

Intraoperative complications

- Conjunctival flap damage: button holes, especially if previous surgery.
- Bleeding may be conjunctival, scleral, from the iris, or, most seriously, suprachoroidal.
- Scleral perforation with retinal damage.
- Damage to crystalline lens from improper needle pass or tube position.
- Wound leak from damaged conjunctiva or inadequate closure.

Early postoperative complications

Shallow AC

Grade as for trabeculectomy. Pay extra attention to the potential for damage caused by tube against corneal endothelium or crystalline lens.

Specific treatment will depend on the underlying cause, but in general, if there is a risk of corneal decompensation from lenticulocorneal and/or tube-corneal touch, urgent measures are required to reform the AC or to restrict flow into the tube (e.g., balanced salts, viscoelastic, or gas).

Low IOP/hypotony

Manage as for trabeculectomy; it may be a result of a non-tight sclerostomy, faulty valve (Ahmed), incomplete ligature (Baerveldt, Molteno), or aqueous hyposecretion.

High IOP

Early

This may result from failure to prime the valved tube, inadequate or absent venting slits on a ligated nonvalved tube, or tube occlusion with fibrin, blood, viscoelastic, vitreous, etc. Many times, IOP will improve with time and can be managed temporarily with topical IOP-lowering agents. Occasionally, AC tap, anterior chamber tissue plasminogen activator (tPA), or tube irrigation or revision is necessary.

If intraocular structures such as the iris are occluding the tube, a 27g needle, argon laser iridoplasty, or Nd:YAG iridotomy can be used to clear the obstruction. Occasionally, surgical revision is necessary.

Late

Valve failure or occlusion (fibrin, vitreous, etc) or encapsulation of plate and mechanical restriction of aqueous diffusion may result in high IOP. Needle bleb (± 5-FU injection), and IOP should decrease. If IOP is still high, then the tube or valve is occluded.

Diplopia

This may improve over time. If persistent in primary gaze, consider tube revision or removal. If present only in extreme gaze and IOPs are well controlled, balance the risk of glaucomatous damage with revision or removal of the implant with disability from diplopia.

Exposure of implant
Excise down-growth of epithelium that prevents proper wound closure. Reinforce exposed portion of implant with donor tissue (sclera, pericardium, cornea, etc). Advance conjunctiva, if possible, or place conjunctival graft. If exposure persists, consider removing implant.

Uveitis

Relevant pages:

Anatomy and physiology

Uveitis describes intraocular inflammation of both the uveal tract itself and neighboring structures (e.g., retina, vitreous, optic nerve). Uveitis is relatively common with an incidence of around 15 new cases per 100,000 population per year. Acute presentations (often recurrences) make a significant contribution to emergency ophthalmic presentations.

Anatomy

The uveal tract comprises the iris, ciliary body, and choroid.

Iris

The *iris* is the most anterior part of the uveal tract. It extends from a relatively thin root in the anterior chamber angle to the pupil. It is divided by a collarette into the central pupillary zone and the peripheral ciliary zone.

The anterior surface is made of connective tissue with an incomplete border layer overlying the stroma that contains the vessels, nerves, and sphincter pupillae. The *sphincter pupillae* is a ring of true smooth muscle supplied by the short ciliary nerves (CN III) under parasympathetic control. The posterior surface comprises an epithelial bilayer.

The anterior layer is lightly pigmented and contains the radial myoepithelial processes of the dilator pupillae that extend from the iris root. These are supplied by two long ciliary nerves (CN V_1) under sympathetic control.

The anterior layer is continuous with the pigmented outer layer of the ciliary body. The posterior epithelial layer is cuboidal, densely pigmented, and continuous with the nonpigmented inner layer of the ciliary body.

Ciliary body

The *ciliary body* comprises the ciliary muscle and ciliary epithelium, arranged anatomically as the pars plana and pars plicata (containing approximately 70–80 ciliary processes). The *ciliary epithelium* is a cuboidal bilayer arranged apex to apex with numerous gap-junctions.

The inner layer is nonpigmented, with high metabolic activity, and posteriorly is continuous with the neural retina. The outer layer is pigmented and posteriorly continuous with the retinal pigmented epithelium (RPE).

Choroid

The *choroid* is a vascular layer extending from the ora serrata (where it is 0.1 mm thick) to the optic disc (0.3 mm thick). From the inside out, it comprises Bruch's membrane (RPE basement membrane, collagen, elastin, collagen, choriocapillaris basement membrane), the choriocapillaris (capillary layer), the stroma (medium-sized vessels in Sattler's layer, large vessels in Haller's layer), and the suprachoroid (a potential space).

Physiology

Iris

Pupillary functions include light regulation, depth of focus, and minimization of optical aberrations. The iris also maintains the blood–aqueous barrier (tight junctions between iris capillary endothelial cells) and contributes to aqueous circulation and outflow (uveoscleral route). In inflammation, there is breakdown of the blood–aqueous barrier, leading to flare and cells in the anterior chamber (AC).

Ciliary body

The nonpigmented layer contributes to the blood–aqueous barrier (tight junctions between nonpigmented epithelial cells). The nonpigmented and pigmented layers together are responsible for aqueous humor production. Contraction of the ciliary muscle permits accommodation and increases trabecular outflow. The ciliary body also contributes to the uveoscleral outflow route.

Choroid

With 85% of the ocular blood flow (cf. <5% for the retina), the choroid provides effective supply of oxygen and nutrients, removal of waste products, and heat dissipation. It may also have a significant role in ocular immunity.

Classification of uveitis (1)

The classification of uveitis may be anatomical, clinical, pathological, or etiological, and all of these may be useful in defining a uveitis entity. Anatomical classification has been formalized by the International Uveitis Study Group (ISUG) and amended by the Standardization of Uveitis Nomenclature (SUN) group (2005) (Table 11.1).

Anterior uveitis accounts for the majority of uveitis cases in Western populations. A much smaller proportion is made up of posterior, intermediate, and panuveitis.

Anatomical classification

Table 11.1 Anatomical classification of uveitis (SUN 2005)

Type	Primary site of inflammation	Includes
Anterior uveitis	Anterior chamber	Iritis Iridocyclitis Anterior cyclitis
Intermediate uveitis	Vitreous	Pars planitis Posterior cyclitis Hyalitis
Posterior uveitis	Retina or choroid	Focal, multifocal, or diffuse choroiditis Chorioretinitis Retinochoroiditis Retinitis Neuroretinitis
Panuveitis	Anterior chamber, vitreous and retina, or choroid	All intraocular structures

Reprinted with permission from Jabs DA, Nussenblatt RB, Rosenbaum JT (2005). Standardization of Uveitis Nomenclature (SUN) Working Group. *Am J Ophthalmol* 140:509–516.

Clinical classification

The most recent clinical classification of uveitis is outlined in Table 11.2. Clinical behavior may be further described in terms of onset, duration, and course of uveitis (Table 11.3).

Pathological classification

Pathological classification separates granulomatous and nongranulomatous uveitis. The term *granulomatous* is sometimes used in the clinical context to describe uveitis with large, greasy, mutton-fat keratic precipitates (macrophages) and iris nodules (which may include Koeppe and Busacca nodules).

Table 11.2 Proposed clinical classification of uveitis (IUSG, 2005)

Group	Subgroup
Infectious	Bacterial
	Viral
	Fungal
	Parasitic
	Others
Noninfectious	Known systemic association
	No known systemic association
Masquerade	Neoplastic
	Non-neoplastic

Table 11.3 Descriptors of uveitis (SUN 2005)

Type	Descriptor	Definition
Onset	Sudden	
	Insidious	
Duration	Limited	≤3 months
	Persistent	>3 months
Course	Acute	Sudden onset + limited duration
	Recurrent	Repeated episodes; inactive periods ≥3 months off treatment
	Chronic	Persistent; relapse in <3 months off treatment

Reprinted with permission from Jabs DA, Nussenblatt RB, Rosenbaum JT (2005). Standardization of Uveitis Nomenclature (SUN) Working Group. *Am J Ophthalmol* 140:509–516.

However, this is strictly a histological term and is not accurate as a clinical descriptor. Indeed, this clinical picture may be seen in diseases with nongranulomatous histopathology, and true granulomatous diseases may present with nongranulomatous uveitis.

Etiological classification

An etiological classification helps define the cause, context, and treatment options for the disease, but in many patients a true etiology is never found.

Classification of uveitis (2)

Differential diagnosis of uveitis by anatomical type

Table 11.4 Differential diagnosis of uveitis by anatomical location

Anterior			JIA
			FHI
			Sarcoidosis
			Syphilis
			Posner–Schlossman
			Behçet's disease
			HSV, VZV
Intermediate			Idiopathic (pars planitis)
			MS
			Sarcoidosis
			IBD
			Lyme disease
Posterior	Retinitis	Focal	Onchocerciasis
			Cysticercosis
			Masquerade
		Multifocal	HSV
			VZV
			CMV
			Sarcoidosis
			Masquerade
			Candidiasis
	Choroiditis	Focal	Idiopathic
			Toxocariasis
			TB
			Masquerade
		Multifocal	Sympathetic ophthalmia
			VKH
			Sarcoidosis
			Serpiginous
			Birdshot
			Masquerade
			MEWDS
Panuveitis			Idiopathic
			Sarcoidosis
			Behçet's disease
			VKH
			Infective endophthalmitis
			Syphilis

CMV, cytomegalovirus; FHI, Fuchs heterochromic iridocyclitis; HSV, herpes simplex virus; IBD, inflammatory bowel disease; JIA, juvenile idiopathic arthritis; MEWDS, multiple evanescent white dot syndrome; MS, multiple sclerosis; POHS, presumed ocular histoplasmosis syndrome; TB, tuberculosis; VKH, Vogt–Koyanagi–Harada syndrome; VZV, varicella zoster virus.

Uveitis: assessment

All patients require a detailed history (ophthalmic and general) and a thorough ophthalmic examination, including dilated funduscopy of both eyes. In some cases a systemic examination may also be necessary (see Table 11.5).

For example, an apparently classic acute anterior uveitis may have posterior segment involvement (notably CME), may be secondary to more posterior disease (e.g., toxoplasmosis retinochoroiditis), or may be part of a panuveitis (e.g., sarcoid) and have systemic involvement.

Table 11.5 An approach to assessing uveitis

Symptoms	Anterior: photophobia, redness, watering, pain, ↓VA; may be asymptomatic
	Intermediate: floaters, photopsia, ↓VA
	Posterior: ↓VA, photopsia, floaters, scotoma
POH	Previous episodes and investigations; surgery/trauma
PMH	Arthropathies (e.g., ankylosing spondylitis), chronic infections (e.g., HSV, TB), systemic inflammation (e.g., sarcoid, Behcet's disease)
Region of systems	Detailed review of all systems
FH	Family members with uveitis or related diseases
SH	Travel or residence abroad, pets, IV drugs, sexual history
Drug history	Including any systemic immunosuppression
Allergies	Allergies or relevant drug contraindications
Visual acuity	Best-corrected/pinhole; near
Visual function	Check for RAPD, color vision
Conjunctiva	Circumcorneal injection
Cornea	Band keratopathy, keratic precipitates (distribution, size, pigment)
AC	Flare/cells, fibrin, hypopyon
Gonioscopy	PAS (consider if ↑IOP)
Iris	Transillumination defects/sectoral atrophy, miosis, posterior synechiae, heterochromia, Koeppe or Busacca nodules
Lens	Cataract, aphakia/pseudophakia
Tonometry	IOP
Dilated funduscopy	Noncontact handheld lens ± indirect/indenting
Vitreous	Haze, cells, snowballs, opacities, subhyaloid precipitates (KP-like but on posterior vitreous face)

Table 11.5 (Contd.)

Optic disc	Disc swelling, glaucomatous changes, atrophy
Vessels	Inflammation (sheathing, leakage), ischemia (B/CRAO, B/CRVO, retinal edema), occlusion
Retina	CME, uni- or multifocal retinitis (blurred white lesions may progress to necrosis, atrophy, or pigmentation)
Choroid	Uni- or multifocal choroiditis (deeper yellow-white lesions), associated exudative retinal detachment

Grading of activity

Grading of AC flare and cells is not difficult and a useful indicator of disease activity (Tables 11.6 and 11.7). Activity within the vitreous is harder to assess: quantification of vitreous cells is of limited use due to their persistence; degree of vitreous haze is a more useful indicator.

Table 11.6 Grading of AC flare

Grade	Description
0	None
1+	Faint
2+	Moderate (iris + lens clear)
3+	Marked (iris + lens hazy)
4+	Intense (fibrin or plastic aqueous)

Reprinted with permission from Jabs DA, Nussenblatt RB, Rosenbaum JT (2005). Standardization of Uveitis Nomenclature (SUN) Working Group. *Am J Ophthalmol* 140:509–516.

Table 11.7 Grading of AC cells (counted with 1 x 1 mm slit)

Activity	Cells
0	<1
0.5+	1–5
1+	6–15
2+	16–25
3+	26–50
4+	>50

Reprinted with permission from Jabs DA, Nussenblatt RB, Rosenbaum JT (2005). Standardization of Uveitis Nomenclature (SUN) Working Group. *Am J Ophthalmol* 140:509–516.

Symptoms of systemic disease in uveitis

Table 11.8 Systemic review that may provide clues to underlying disease

System	Symptom	Associated disease
CVS	Chest pain—pericarditis	TB, RA, SLE
	Chest pain—myocarditis	Syphilis
	Palpitations	Sarcoidosis, ankylosing spondylitis, syphilis, RA, SLE, HIV
	Edema—cardiac failure	TB, sarcoidosis, syphilis, RA, SLE, HIV
	Edema—IVC obstruction	Behçet's disease
RS	Cough	TB, sarcoidosis, Wegener's granulomatosis, HIV, toxocariasis
	Hemoptysis	TB, Wegener's granulomatosis, HIV, RA, SLE, sarcoidosis
	Stridor	Relapsing polychondritis
	Chest pain—pleuritic	Sarcoidosis, TB, Wegener's granulomatosis, SLE, RA, lymphoma, HIV
	Shortness of breath	Sarcoidosis, TB, Wegener's granulomatosis, SLE, RA, HIV
GI	Diarrhea	IBD, Behçet's, HIV
	Blood and/or mucus in stools	IBD, Behçet's, HIV
	Jaundice	IBD (with cholangitis or hepatitis) toxoplasmosis, HIV
GU	Dysuria/discharge	Reiter's, syphilis, TB
	Hematuria	Wegener's granulomatosis, IgA nephropathy, TINU, SLE, TB
	Genital ulcers	Behçet's, syphilis, HLA-B27-related disease
	Testicular pain	Behçet's, HLA-B27-related disease, polyarteritis nodosum
ENT	Deafness or tinnitus	VKH, sympathetic ophthalmia, Wegener's granulomatosis, Cogan's syndrome
	Earlobe pain and/or swelling	Relapsing polychondritis
	Oral ulcers	Behçet's, HSV, HLA-B27-related disease, SLE
	Sinus problems	Wegener's granulomatosis
	Recurrent epistaxis	Wegener's granulomatosis

Table 11.8 (Contd.)

System	Symptom	Associated disease
Musculo-skeletal	Joint pain, swelling, or stiffness	HLA-B27-related arthropathies, JIA, sarcoidosis, RA, SLE, Behçet's, relapsing polychondritis, Wegener's, Lyme
	Lower back pain	HLA-B27-related arthropathies, TB
Skin	Rash—erythema nodosum	Sarcoidosis, Behçet's, TB, IBD
	Rash—vesicular	HSV, VZV
	Rash—other	Psoriasis, syphilis, Lyme, SLE, Behçet's, Reiter's, JIA, TB
	Photosensitivity	SLE
	Vitiligo	SLE, VKH, sympathetic ophthalmia, leprosy
	Alopecia	SLE, VKH
	Raynaud's phenomenon	SLE, RA
CNS	Headaches	Sarcoidosis, VKH, Behçet's, TB, SLE, lymphoma
	Seizures	Sarcoidosis, VKH, Behçet's, SLE, HIV, toxoplasmosis, lymphoma
	Weakness	MS, sarcoidosis, Behçet's, HIV, leprosy, syphilis, toxoplasmosis, lymphoma
	Numbness and/or tingling	MS, sarcoidosis, Behçet's, HIV, leprosy, lymphoma
	Loss of balance	MS, sarcoidosis, Behçet's, VKH, HIV, syphilis, lymphoma
	Speech problems	MS, sarcoidosis, Behçet's, HIV, lymphoma
	Behavior change	VKH, sarcoidosis, Behçet's, SLE, Wegener's granulomatosis, HIV, TB, syphilis, lymphoma
General	Fever/night sweats	JIA, lymphoma, VKH, SLE, RA, IBD, sarcoidosis, Kawasaki disease
	Swollen glands	Sarcoidosis, lymphoma, HIV, JIA, TB, RA, syphilis, toxoplasmosis

HIV, human immunodeficiency virus; HSV, herpes simplex virus; IBD, inflammatory bowel disease; JIA, juvenile idiopathic arthritis; MS, multiple sclerosis; RA, rheumatoid arthritis; SLE, systemic lupus erythematosus; TB, tuberculosis; TINU, tubulointerstitial nephritis with uveitis; VKH, Vogt–Koyanagi–Harada syndrome; VZV, varicella zoster virus.

Investigations in uveitis

When to investigate

Ideally, one would perform the minimum number of investigations to obtain the maximum amount of information. The usefulness of each test will depend on the pretest probability of the diagnosis and the specificity and sensitivity of the test. Consider also the potential morbidity of certain tests (e.g., FA or vitreous biopsy). In general, investigations may be performed for the following:

- *Diagnosis:* by identifying causative or associated systemic disease; by identifying a definite etiology (e.g., an organism).
- *Management:* monitoring disease activity or complications (e.g., OCT for macular edema); monitoring potential side effects of treatment (e.g., blood tests for some immunosuppressants).

Role in diagnosis

The etiology of most cases of uveitis is not known, although an autoimmune or autoinflammatory cause is often theorized. In most cases, a careful history and examination provides most if not all of the information need for diagnosis (see Table 11.9).

Some uveitis syndromes like FHI, Behçet's, and toxoplasmosis are diagnosed purely on clinical grounds. Investigations are helpful in identifying uveitis of infective origin (e.g., TB, HSV) or systemic disease (e.g., lymphoma, sarcoidosis, demyelination). The role of some investigations is controversial (e.g., when to test HLA-B27 status).

Role in management

Monitoring disease

This is done almost entirely by clinical examination; however, in certain situations investigations may be helpful. For example:

- Optical coherence tomography (OCT) is extremely useful in establishing macular causes of worsening vision, particularly where clinical diagnosis is difficult because of poor visualization or pre-existing macular disease (e.g., epiretinal membrane, CME, macular hole); this has largely replaced FA for this purpose.
- Fluorescein angiography (FA) is particularly helpful in assessing retinal vascular involvement and neovascularization.
- Electroretinogram (ERG) is required for monitoring birdshot retinochoroidopathy.
- Visual fields: for monitoring optic nerve damage due to either disease or associated ↑IOP or AZOOR complex disorders.

Monitoring therapies

Regular BP, weight, BM, and urinalysis are recommended for patients on systemic corticosteroids. Blood tests (e.g., CBC, urinalysis, LFT) are necessary for some of the other immunosuppresive agents (p. 709).

Table 11.9 Suggested investigations in diagnosis of uveitis types

	Investigation	Consider
Baseline	CBC	
	ESR	
	Syphilis serology	Syphilis
	ANA (in children)	
	Urinalysis	TINU (protein), diabetes (glucose)
	Chest X-ray	TB, sarcoidosis
Selective	ACE	Sarcoidosis
	ANCA	Wegener's (PR3)
	Toxoplasma serology	Toxoplasmosis
	Toxocara ELISA	Toxocariasis
	Borrelia serology	Lyme disease
	HLA-B27	B27-associated disease
	HLA-A29	Birdshot retinochoroidopathy
	Mantoux test	TB, sarcoidosis
	FA	
	Electrophysiology	
	Ultrasound B-scan	
	High-resolution CT thorax	Sarcoidosis
	CT orbits	
	MRI head scan	Demyelination, sarcoidosis, lymphoma
		Sarcoidosis
	Gallium scan	Demyelination, lymphoma
	Lumbar puncture	Sarcoidosis
	Conjunctival biopsy	
	PCR of intraocular fluid	Infection
	Vitreous biopsy	Infection, lymphoma
	Choroidal biopsy	Lymphoma

Acute anterior uveitis (AAU)

Anterior uveitis accounts for ~75–90% of all cases of uveitis. Representing a wide spectrum of disease, it may be isolated, part of a panuveitis, or part of a systemic disease.

Idiopathic acute anterior uveitis

Approximately 50% of patients with AAU have the disease in isolation (i.e., HLA-B27 negative with no underlying systemic disease). The condition affects any age (biphasic peaking at 30 and 60 years) and both sexes equally. It is almost always unilateral but may affect both eyes sequentially. Recurrences are common.

Clinical features

- Pain, photophobia, redness, blurred vision.
- Limbal injection, keratic precipitates (especially inferior), AC flare/cells, posterior synechiae (PS), vitreous cells.

Treatment

Treat with frequent potent topical steroid (e.g., dexamethasone 0.1% or prednisolone acetate 1% up to every 30 min initially, titrating according to disease) and dilate (e.g., cyclopentolate 1% 3×/day; atropine 1% 3×/day in severe cases)—this may be the only chance to break the synechiae. If there is poor dilation, consider subconjunctival injection of lidocaine/phenylephrine; subconjunctival dexamethasone may also be necessary.

If there is no response after 48 hours of half-hourly drops, the patient may require expert consultation (e.g., consideration of oral steroids). In recalcitrant cases, subtenons triamcinolone injections or immunosuppression may be needed to control the uveitis. More recently, biological agents such as infliximab have also been beneficial for treatment.

HLA-B27-associated AAU

Up to 50% of patients with AAU are HLA-B27 positive (cf. 8% in the general population) (see Table 11.10). HLA-B27-related disease peaks at 30 years of age, is more common in males, and is associated with a positive family history. The diagnosis may be associated with ankylosing spondylitis, Reiter's disease, and, less commonly, psoriasis or inflammatory bowel disease (IBD).

It is almost always unilateral but may affect both eyes sequentially (alternating); rarely, it may become persistent. Inflammation is often more severe and recurrences are more frequent than in idiopathic AAU.

Clinical features

- Pain, photophobia, redness, blurred vision.
- Anterior segment inflammation may be severe: circumlimbal injection, keratic precipitates (especially inferior), AC flare/cells/fibrin ± hypopyon, posterior synechiae, vitreous spillover cells.

Treatment

The treatment is the same as for idiopathic AAU.

Other causes

Although the vast majority of acute anterior uveitis is idiopathic or HLA-B27 related, it is important to be keep an open mind. Atypical features may suggest an alternative diagnosis requiring different treatment. Important differential diagnoses include the following.

Herpes viral group (HSV, VZV, CMV) anterior uveitis

Consider this if there is unilateral persistent anterior uveitis with patchy iris atrophy, transillumination defects, and semidilated pupil, corneal hypoesthesia, and ↑IOP ± evidence of active or previous keratitis (p. 345).

Posner–Schlossman syndrome

Consider PSS with ↑IOP (40–80 mmHg), white eye, few keratic precipitates, minimal flare, occasional AC cells, no synechiae (PS or PAS), and open angle (p. 327). Gonioscopy may demonstrate evidence of keratic precipitates in the angle, suggesting a viral trabeculitis etiology (HSV, VZV, CMV).

Systemic disease

AAU is associated with a number of systemic diseases, some of which may be undiagnosed at the time of presentation. For example, a fibrinous uveitis in a middle-aged adult may be the first presentation of diabetes mellitus.

Systemic diseases to consider include diabetes, sarcoidosis, vascular disease (e.g., carotid artery stenosis), and renal disease (e.g., TINU, IgA nephropathy).

Table 11.10 Comparison of HLA-B27 positive vs. negative AAU

	HLA-B27 positive	HLA-B27 negative
Peak age of onset	30s	40s
Sex ratio (M:F)	2.5:1	1:1
Fibrin in AC	56%	10%
3+ cells in AC	60%	18%
Persistent PS	36%	15%
Low back pain	56%	14%

This table was published in Rothova A, et al. (1987). Clinical features of acute anterior uveitis. *Am J Ophthalmol* 103:137–145. Copyright Elsevier 1987.

Anterior uveitis syndromes

Fuchs heterochromic iridocyclitis (FHI)

This is an uncommon, chronic, nongranulomatous anterior uveitis of unknown etiology. It typically affects young adults and there is no gender bias. It is unilateral in about 90%.

Clinical features
- Floaters, glare; ↓VA due to cataract ± vitreous opacities; often asymptomatic.
- White eye, white stellate keratic precipitates (KPs) over whole corneal endothelium, mild flare, few cells, iris atrophy (washed out, moth-eaten), transillumination defects, abnormal iris vessels, iris heterochromia (becomes bluer), iris nodules; no posterior synechiae; cataract (posterior subcapsular), vitritis, ↑IOP (10–15%).
- Gonioscopy: open angle; ± twig-like neovascularization of the angle; these may lead to hyphema in response to paracentesis or during cataract surgery (Amsler hemorrhages).

Treatment
- *Inflammatory process:* not usually necessary.
- *Cataract:* conventional phacoemulsification but with careful post-operative control of inflammation (p. 249).
- *↑IOP:* treat as for POAG (p. 269), but it may require augmented trabeculectomy or drainage-tube surgery.

Posner–Schlossman syndrome (PSS)

This is an inflammatory glaucoma syndrome characterized by recurrent unilateral episodes of very high IOP. It typically affects young males. The suggested etiology is acute trabeculitis, perhaps secondary to HSV.

Clinical features
- Blurring of vision, halos, painless.
- ↑IOP (40–80 mmHg), white eye, few KPs, minimal flare, occasional AC cells, no synechiae (PS or PAS), open angle.

Treatment
- *Inflammatory process:* topical steroid (e.g., dexamethasone 0.1% or prednisolone acetate 1% 4×/day initially, titrating according to disease).
- *↑IOP:* consider topical (e.g., β-blocker, α-agonist, carbonic anhydrase inhibitor) or systemic (e.g., acetazolamide) according to IOP level.
- Oral antiviral medication (acyclovir) for recurrent disease.

TINU

This is the rare association of tubulointerstitial nephritis (often presenting as acute renal failure) and uveitis. It typically affects young females (median age 15; F:M 3:1) but can occur at almost any age. It is commonly idiopathic but may be associated with drugs (NSAIDs, penicillin, furosemide) or infection (streptococci, staphylococci, etc).

The uveitis is usually anterior (80%) and bilateral (77%) and usually presents after the systemic disease (65%). The uveitis may recur or follow a persistent course in over 50%. Ocular complications include posterior synechiae, ↑IOP, and cataract.

In most cases the renal disease recovers, but chronic renal impairment occurs in 11%, with dialysis being required in 4%. The renal disease is commonly treated with systemic steroids; the uveitis may be treated as for idiopathic AAU.

IgA nephropathy

This is a relatively common renal disease of children in young adults in which recurrent micro- or macroscopic hematuria may be related to respiratory tract infections. In some patients, episodes are associated with an anterior uveitis, which may be treated similarly to idiopathic AAU.

Schwartz syndrome

This is the uncommon association of anterior segment pseudo-inflammation (mild) and ↑IOP (with an open angle) arising from a rhegmatogenous retinal detachment. Detachments most commonly associated with this syndrome are large in area (and macula-off), flat in height, and long in duration.

The postulated mechanism involves mechanical blockage of the angle by photoreceptor outer segments. Refer to a vitreoretinal surgeon for assessment and repair (p. 383). The ↑IOP and anterior uveitis may be treated medically in the interim and tend to resolve rapidly after surgical repair.

Kawasaki disease

This is an uncommon acute vasculitis of children, defined as fever (≥5 days) with four of the following five criteria: conjunctival injection, rash, desquamation of extremities, cervical lymphadenopathy, and mucosal changes (pharyngeal injection, cracked red lips, strawberry tongue).

An anterior uveitis is common in the first week of illness; rarely, disc edema and dilated retinal vessels are seen. Most seriously, cardiac abnormalities (notably coronary artery aneurysms) occur in 20% of patients.

Anterior segment ischemia

This is an uncommon but important cause of anterior uveitis, particularly in the elderly.

Clinical features
- Dull ache, usually unilateral.
- AC with significant flare/moderate cells, sluggish pupil; if part of ocular ischemic syndrome, there may also be dilated irregular retinal veins (not tortuous), attenuated retinal arterioles, midperipheral retinal hemorrhages, rubeosis, and posterior segment neovascularization.
- *Investigate* for carotid artery stenosis with carotid Doppler ultrasound and refer to a vascular surgeon if indicated.

Uveitis with HLA-B27-related arthropathies

HLA-B27 is a type I major histocompatibility complex (MHC; Ch6) molecule: a cell surface polypeptide involved in presenting antigen to the immune system. There are 24 subtypes of HLA-B27, encoded by 26 different alleles. Subtypes vary by ethnic origin, and some are more highly associated with inflammatory disease, notably HLA-B*2705 (the ancestral type), B*2702 (more common in whites), and B*2704 (more common in Asians).

HLA-B27 is present in 8% of the general population but is seen in up to 50% of patients with acute anterior uveitis and is strongly linked to the seronegative spondyloarthropathies. This is a group of overlapping inflammatory conditions that, as the name suggests, are negative for rheumatoid factor (RF) and generally include an axial (spinal) arthritis. They may all be associated with uveitis.

Ankylosing spondylitis (AS)

AS is a chronic spondyloarthropathy, predominantly affecting the spine and sacroiliac joints. AS is more common in males and usually presents in early adulthood. Of those with AS, 95% are HLA-B27 positive; 25% will develop anterior uveitis. Of these, 80% will have involvement of both eyes, but nearly always sequentially.

Clinical features
- *Ophthalmic:* acute anterior uveitis; unilateral but may affect both eyes sequentially (alternating); rarely may become persistent.
- *Systemic:* axial arthritis, sacroiliitis, kyphosis, stiffness, enthesitis, aortic regurgitation.

Treatment
- *Ophthalmic:* as in idiopathic acute anterior uveitis (p. 325).
- *Systemic:* investigation and treatment by rheumatologist. This may include lumbar-spinal X-ray (bamboo spine; sacroiliitis) and HLA-B27 status. Treatment may include oral NSAIDs and physical therapy.
- In advance diseases, immunosuppressive agents (methotrexate, azathioprine) and biological agents (etanercept, infliximab) may be beneficial for both systemic and ocular inflammation.

Reiter syndrome (reactive arthritis)

Reiter syndrome describes a reactive arthritis, urethritis (or cervicitis), and conjunctivitis occurring after a sexually transmitted or dysenteric infection. Candidates include *Chlamydia, Yersinia, Salmonella,* and *Shigella*. In patients with Reiter syndrome, 70% are HLA-B27 positive; 50% will develop conjunctivitis, and 12% will have anterior uveitis.

Clinical features
- *Ophthalmic:* bilateral mucopurulent conjunctivitis; acute anterior uveitis; keratitis (punctate epitheliopathy, supepithelial infiltrates).

- *Systemic:* oligoarthritis (typically knees, ankles, sacroiliac joints), enthesitis (including plantar fasciitis), aphthous oral ulcers, circinate balanitis, keratoderma blenorrhagica (scaling skin rash on the soles)

Treatment
- *Ophthalmic:* conjunctivitis—self-limiting; AAU—as above.
- *Systemic:* investigation and treatment by rheumatologist.

Inflammatory bowel disease
Of patients with ulcerative colitis (UC) and Crohn's disease, around 5% will develop anterior uveitis.

Clinical features
- *Ophthalmic:* acute anterior uveitis; rarely epi/scleritis or retinal vasculitis.
- *Systemic:* gastrointestinal inflammation (patchy, transmural, anywhere from mouth to anus in Crohn's; continuous, superficial, colorectal in UC), cholangitis, chronic active hepatitis, arthritis (oligo- or AS-like), rash (erythema nodosum, pyoderma gangrenosum).

Treatment
- *Ophthalmic:* as in idiopathic acute anterior uveitis (p. 325).
- *Systemic:* investigation and treatment by gastroenterologist.

More recently, intramuscular etanercept has been demonstrated to have excellent activity against the gastrointestinal (GI) diseases, but with limited activity for ocular inflammation. Intravenous infliximab has demonstrated more clinical benefit for both GI and ocular inflammation.

Psoriatic arthritis
Of those with psoriasis, 10% will develop psoriatic arthritis, and of these, 10% will develop anterior uveitis.

Clinical features
- *Ophthalmic:* conjunctivitis; acute anterior uveitis; rarely keratitis (peripheral corneal infiltrates).
- *Systemic:* salmon-pink lesions with silvery scaling that may be in isolated plaques (more common on extensor rather than flexor surfaces) or occur as a pustular rash (soles and palms or, more seriously, generalized); nail changes (pitting, onychlysis, oil drop). Arthritis may be axial (AS-like), oligoarthritis (Reiter's-like), distal interphalangeal joints (osteoarthritis-like) with nail changes, symmetrical peripheral arthropathy (RA-like), or arthritis mutilans.

Treatment
- *Ophthalmic:* the conjunctivitis is self-limiting; treat anterior uveitis as in idiopathic AAU (p. 325).
- *Systemic:* investigation and treatment by dermatologist and rheumatologist.

Uveitis with other arthropathies

Juvenile idiopathic arthritis (JIA)

This condition describes an idiopathic arthritis of >6 weeks duration with onset before the age of 16 years. JIA may be subclassified into systemic, oligoarthritis (≤4 joints), polyarthritis (>4 joints) RF negative, polyarthritis RF positive, psoriatic, enthesitis related, and other/overlap (classification of the International League of Associations of Rheumatologists).

The term *JIA* is meant to replace juvenile chronic arthritis (JCA) and juvenile rheumatoid arthritis (JRA).

Of those with JIA, 20% will develop anterior uveitis, of which 70% will be bilateral and 25% will be severe sight-threatening disease. JIA is more common in females.

Clinical features
Ophthalmic

- Asymptomatic; rarely floaters; ↓VA from cataract.
- White eye, small KPs, AC cells/flare, posterior synechiae, vitritis, CME (rare). Complications include band keratopathy, cataract, inflammatory glaucoma, or phthisis bulbi.
- Arthritis: pattern may be oligoarthritis (<4 joints), polyarthritis (>4 joints), psoriatic type, or enthesitis related.
- Systemic: fever, rash, lymphadenopathy, hepatosplenomegaly, serositis.

In long-standing uveitis, chronic breakdown of the blood–aqueous barrier leads to persistent flare. AC cells are thus a better guide than flare to gauge the level of disease activity.

Screening

Patients diagnosed with JIA should be seen as soon as possible by an ophthalmologist. If ophthalmic examination is normal, regular follow-up is indicated according to risk (see Table 11.11).

Table 11.11 Recommendation for JIA-associated uveitis screening (American Uveitis Society)

Risk	Factors	Screening
High	Onset <6 years age Pauciarticular and ANA+	Every 3 months for 1 year Every 6 months for next 5 years Every 12 months thereafter
Medium	Polyarticular and ANA+ Pauciarticular and ANA–	Every 6 months for 5 years Every 12 months thereafter
Low	Onset >11 years age Systemic onset HLA-B27+	Every 12 months

Treatment
- *Uveitis:* topical steroids and mydriatic; if systemic therapy is required, this should be directed by a pediatrician and pediatric rheumatologist. NSAID and steroid-sparing agents such as methotrexate are commonly used to minimize long-term steroid side effects. Biological agents such as etanercept and infliximab have demonstrated excellent activity against joint disease, with infliximab demonstrating better ocular control.
- ↑*IOP:* initially topical therapy. But up to two-thirds of patients may require surgery (commonly an antimetabolite-augmented trabeculectomy or a drainage-tube procedure).
- *Cataract:* aim to defer surgery until the eye has been quiet for a minimum of 3 months, although weigh this against the risk of amblyopia in younger children. There is considerable debate over the specifics of surgery, including whether to implant a lens or leave the patient aphakic.
- *Band keratopathy:* chelation with EDTA or excimer phototherapeutic keratectomy.

Relapsing polychondritis

This is a rare condition of recurrent inflammation of cartilage affecting the ear, nose, and, most seriously, the trachea and larynx (risk of respiratory obstruction). The ophthalmic features include anterior uveitis, epi/scleritis, and, rarely, corneal involvement (keratoconjunctivitis sicca or peripheral ulcerative keratitis). Anterior uveitis may be treated similarly to that in idiopathic AAU.

Intermediate uveitis

The term *intermediate uveitis* refers to uveitis in which the vitreous is the major site of inflammation. The term *pars planitis* may be used when there is snowbank or snowball formation occurring in the absence of an associated infection or systemic disease (i.e., idiopathic).

Intermediate uveitis accounts for around 10% of all cases of uveitis. It is bimodal, being most common in young adults, but with a second peak in the elderly. Males and females are equally affected. It is bilateral in 80% but is often asymmetric.

Clinical features

- Floaters, ↓VA (may indicate macular edema); may be asymptomatic.
- Vitritis (cells, "snowballs"), exudation at the ora serrata ("snowbanking", commonly inferior but can be 360°), peripheral periphlebitis, rarely vitreous hemorrhage. Some anterior chamber activity is common.
- *Complications:* cystoid macular edema (CME), optic nerve edema, cataract, tractional retinal detachment, peripheral retinal neovascularization, cyclitic membrane, vitreous hemorrhage.

Investigation

Consider CBC, urinalysis, ESR, VDRL, TPHA, urinalysis, CXR for all patients. Further investigation should be directed by clinical indication (see Table 11.12). OCT or FA may be helpful to confirm CME.

Treatment

- *Observation:* if no CME and stable VA >6 months, then monitor only
- *Topical:* if significant AC activity, control with topical corticosteroids and mydriatics (e.g., cyclopentolate 1% 1–2×/day).
- *Periocular/systemic:* if CME or visually disabling floaters, consider periocular corticosteroid (e.g., orbital floor/subtenons methylprednisolone/triamcinolone 40 mg); intravitreal fluocinolone acetonide implant (Retisert) for unilateral disease; or oral corticosteroids (e.g., prednisone initially 1 mg/kg/day and titrating down) ± other immunosuppresives (e.g., methotrexate, azathioprine, cyclosporine) for bilateral or resistant disease.
- *Surgical:* options include cryotherapy (double freeze–thaw technique; there is some benefit for peripheral snowbanking with associated neovascularization) and vitrectomy/lensectomy (may benefit those with resistant disease and disabling media opacity).

Table 11.12 Associations of intermediate uveitis

Group	Cause	Consider
Primary ocular	Idiopathic/pars planitis	After exclusion of other associations
Secondary systemic	MS	MRI brain, lumbar puncture
	Sarcoid	ACE, Ca, CXR, CT thorax
	Inflammatory bowel disease	Bowel studies, biopsy
	CNS/intraocular lymphoma	MRI brain, lumbar puncture
Secondary infective	Toxocara	Serology
	Lyme disease	Serology
	HTLV-1	Serology

Retinal vasculitis

Retinal vasculitis comprises inflammation of the retinal vasculature. It may be a primary ocular disease or secondary to either infection or systemic disease.

Clinical features

- ↓VA, floaters, positive scotomas; may be asymptomatic if peripheral.
- Perivascular sheathing of arteries, veins, or capillaries; retinal hemorrhages; vitritis; disc swelling, CME.
- *Complications:* BRVO or CRVO, neovascularization, vitreous hemorrhage, ischemic maculopathy, tractional retinal detachment (TRD).

Investigations

Use FA for vessel wall staining, vascular leakage, skip lesions, widespread capillary leakage, new vessel leakage, disc leakage, petalloid macular leakage, enlarged foveal avascular zone (FAZ) (ischemia), vascular occlusion, and capillary dropout.

Consider CBC, urinalysis, ESR, VDRL, TPHA, ANA, ANCA, and CXR for all patients. Further investigation should be directed by clinical indication (see Tables 11.13 and 11.14).

Treatment

Where possible, the underlying disease is treated (e.g., with antibiotics for infective cases). However, in most instances, immunosuppression is required.

Corticosteroids are first line and may be periocular, oral (e.g., prednisone 1–2 mg/kg), or IV (e.g., pulsed methylprednisolone 500–1000 mg three doses on alternate days).

Cyclosporine and azathioprine tend to be used second line, although methotrexate, mycophenolate, tacrolimus, infliximab (mainly in Behcet's disease), and cyclophosphamide (mainly in Wegener's granulomatosus) also have their place.

Table 11.13 Causes of retinal vasculitis

Group	Cause	Consider
Primary ocular	Intermediate uveitis	Urine, blood glucose
	Birdshot retinochoroidopathy	HLA-A29
	Eales' disease	PPD skin test, CXR
	VKH	
	Sympathetic ophthalmia	
Secondary infective	CMV	PCR
	HSV	PCR
	VZV	PCR
	HTLV-1	Serology
	HIV	Serology, CD4 count
	Toxoplasmosis	Serology, PCR
	Tuberculosis	PPD skin test, CXR
	Lyme disease	Serology
	Cat scratch disease	Serology, PCR
	Syphilis	Serology (VDRL, TPHA)
	Whipple's disease	PCR
Secondary systemic	Leukemia	CBC ± LP, bone marrow
	Lymphoma	MRI brain ± LP
	SLE	ANA, dsDNA
	Behcet's disease	Pathergy
	Sarcoidosis	ACE, Ca, CXR, HRCT thorax
	Wegener's granulomatosis	c-ANCA (PR3)
	Polyarteritis nodosa (PAN)	p-ANCA, tissue biopsy
	Antiphospholipid syndrome	Anticardiolipin antibodies

ACE, angiotensin-converting enzyme; ANA, antinuclear antibody; ANCA, antineutrophil cytoplasmic antibody; Ca, calcium; CBC, complete blood count; CMV, cytomegalovirus; CXR, chest-X-ray; dsDNA, double-stranded DNA; HIV, human immunodeficiency virus; HRCT, high-resolution computed tomography; HSV, herpes simplex virus; HTLV-1, human T-cell lymphotropic virus type 1; LP, lumbar puncture; PCR, polymerase chain reaction; PPD, posterior polymorphous dystrophy; TPHA, treponema pallidum hemagglutination assay; VDRL, venereal disease research lab test; VKH, Vogt–Koyanagi–Harada syndrome; VZV, varicella zoster virus.

Table 11.14 Diagnostic pointers in retinal vasculitis

Clinical feature	Possible cause of vasculitis
Arteritis	ARN (HSV, VZV)
BRVO	Behcet's disease
RPE changes	TB
	Sarcoidosis
	Lymphoma
Capillary closure	TB
	MS
	Sarcoidosis

Sarcoidosis

This relatively common granulomatous multisystem disorder may be life threatening. The eye is affected in up to 25% of patients. Of these, anterior uveitis occurs in 60%, and posterior segment disease occurs in 25% of patients. Sarcoid affects up to 0.1% of the population, being higher in females and with peaks in the third and sixth decades. It is more common in African Caribbeans, Irish, and Scandinavians.

The cause of sarcoidosis is unknown; there is PCR evidence for several agents (including atypical mycobacteria) that may trigger the disease in susceptible individuals. The T_H1 response predominates in typical sarcoid granuloma, although it appears that a transition to the T_H2 response underlies progressive pulmonary fibrosis.

The presentation may be acute or insidious. An acute presentation, typically with erythema nodosum and bihilar lymphadenopathy (BHL), has a better prognosis. The course tends to be self-limiting, although steroids may hasten recovery. An insidious presentation is more commonly followed by a relentless progression to pulmonary fibrosis.

Clinical features

Ophthalmic

- *Anterior uveitis* (2/3 are persistent, 1/3 acute; unilateral or bilateral; 'granulomatous'): limbal injection, mutton-fat keratic precipitates, AC flare/cells, posterior synechiae, vitreous cells; iris granulomas and nodules.
- *Intermediate uveitis:* vitreous cells, snowballs, snowbanking.
- *Posterior uveitis:* CME (most common cause of ↓VA), periphlebitis (± patchy sheathing ± "candle wax dripping"), occluded vessels (especially BRVO), retinal neovascularization, choroidal neovascularization, retinal, or preretinal nodules (probably granuloma), pigment epithelial changes, disc swelling (from inflammatory papillitis, optic nerve granuloma, or papilledema secondary to CNS disease). Peripheral multifocal chorioretinitis (small punched-out atrophic spots) is highly suggestive of sarcoidosis.
- *Complications:* cataract, glaucoma (↑risk with duration of active disease).

Systemic

- *Respiratory system:* often asymptomatic despite CXR changes, dry cough, dyspnea; BHL, parenchymal disease.
- *Cardiovascular system:* pericarditis, cardiomyopathy, conduction defects, cardiac failure, cor pulmonale.
- *Skin:* erythema nodosum (red, tender, elevated lesions typically on the shins; commonest in younger females); cutaneous granuloma (nontender; nodules, papules, macules; almost anywhere including the lids); lupus pernio (uncommon, bluish plaque, typically on the face or ears).
- *Joints:* arthritis (common in acute sarcoid); bone cysts (usually in the digits).

- *Glands:* swelling of any of lacrimal, salivary, parotid, and submaxillary glands, lymphadenopathy, hepatosplenomegaly.
- *Central nervous system* (neurosarcoidosis, more common in patients with posterior uveitis): cranial nerve palsies (most commonly CN VII; can be bilateral), peripheral neuropathy, myopathy, aseptic meningoencephalitis (typically basal leptomeninges); CNS granuloma may mimic a tumor; optic nerve involvement may present as atypical optic neuritis.

Investigations

The diagnosis is essentially clinical but may be supported by investigations such as serum angiotensin-converting enzyme (ACE) (see also Box 11.1), imaging, and ideally typical histology. In some cases, it may be difficult to distinguish neurosarcoidosis from MS.

- *Serum ACE* (commonly elevated in active sarcoid because of synthesis by activated macrophages), serum Ca^{2+} (less commonly elevated).
- *CXR:* abnormal in >90% with ocular sarcoid: stage 0 (normal); stage 1 (BHL only); stage 2 (BHL + parenchymal disease); stage 3 (parenchymal disease only).
- *High-resolution CT* of the thorax has high sensitivity and specificity; it is particularly useful in those with normal CXR.
- *MRI* of the brain or optic nerves (ideally fat suppressed, gadolinium enhanced, T1) and LP in suspected neurosarcoid.
- *Gallium 67 scan:* typical uptake pattern is lacrimal and parotid glands (panda appearance) or mediastinum (lambda sign).
- *Biopsy:* transbronchial, endobronchial, or conjunctival biopsy may reveal the typical noncaseating granulomata of whorls of eipthelioid cells surrounding multinucleate giant cells. Bronchoalveolar lavage (BAL) may show lymphocytosis with high CD4+/CD8+ ratio, but low specificity.
- *FA:* include ischemia (hypofluorescence), leakage from periphlebitis, new vessels, CME (hyperfluorescence), peripheral patchy hyper- and hypofluorescence.
- *ICG:* choroidal stromal vasculitis, early lobular hypofluorescence, late hyperfluorescence (focal or diffuse).

Treatment

- *Ophthalmic:* anterior segment inflammation—as for idiopathic AAU; posterior segment inflammation—periocular steroid injection or systemic therapy (see below); cataracts—conventional surgery but with tight control of inflammation; glaucoma—medical ± surgical (antimetabolite-augmented trabeculectomy, glaucoma tube shunt).
- *Systemic:* investigation and treatment by a physician (usually respiratory); oral corticosteroids (proven short-term benefits) ± steroid-sparing agents such as methotrexate, azathioprine, and cyclosporine. In patients with recalcitrant diseases or who are intolerant of immunosuppression, biological therapy such as intravenous infliximab is an alternative option.

Sarcoidosis syndromes

- Heerfordt's syndrome (uveoparotid fever): parotid/submandibular gland enlargement, CN VII palsy, uveitis.
- Lofgren's syndrome: fever, erythema nodosum, BHL.
- Mickulicz's syndrome: diffuse swelling of lacrimal/salivary glands (most commonly due to sarcoidosis).

Box 11.1 Differential diagnosis of elevated serum ACE

- Child (peaks at 13 years of age, adult level by 18 years)
- Sarcoidosis.
- Mycobacterial infection (including leprosy and tuberculosis).
- Certain chronic lung diseases (including berylliosis, silicosis, farmer's lung, histoplasmosis, lymphangiomyomatosis).
- Gaucher disease.

Behçet's disease

Possibly first recognized by Hippocrates, the modern description of this disease dates from the Greek Adamantiades and the Turk Behçet. It is an idiopathic, chronic multisystem autoimmune disease and vasculitis characterized by recurrent episodes of acute inflammation. The common ophthalmic presentation is of a sight-threatening panuveitis and retinal vasculitis (see Table 11.15 for diagnostic criteria).

Prevalence is highest along the traditional Silk Route, peaking in Turkey, where up to 0.4% of the population may be affected. It typically affects young adults. There is some geographical variation of risk factors, including gender, family history (more significant in Middle Eastern countries), and the HLA-B51 allele (more significant in Japan with a relative risk of 6.7).

Clinical features

Ophthalmic

- *Anterior uveitis:* acute anterior nongranulomatous uveitis, typically with hypopyon.
- *Posterior uveitis:* vitiritis; macular edema; retinal infiltrates, hemorrhage, edema; occlusive periphlebitis ± BRVO or CRVO, neovascularization ± vitreous hemorrhage or tractional retinal detachment, diffuse capillary leakage.
- *Complications:* cataract, glaucoma, end-stage disease (optic atrophy, retinal atrophy with attenuated vessels; high risk of blindness).

Systemic

- Oral ulceration (aphthous or scarring).
- Genitourinary (GU) (genital ulceration).
- *Skin lesions:* erythema nodosum, pseudofolliculitis, papulopustules, acneiform rash.
- *Joints:* arthritis (mono/poly).
- *Vascular:* thromboses (venous > arterial), including superficial thrombophlebitis, superior (SVC) or inferior (IVC) vena cava obstruction.
- *GI:* nausea, vomiting, abdominal pain, bloody diarrhea.
- *CNS:* meningoencephalitis, sinus thrombosis ± intracranial hypertension, cranial or peripheral neuropathies, focal CNS signs.

Investigations

- Positive pathergy test: sterile pustule appearing 24–48 hours after oblique insertion of 20-gauge needle.
- MRI, MRA, MRV of the brain if there are neurological features.

Treatment

Coordinate care with PCP and rheumatologist; give systemic corticosteroids (e.g., initially 1–2 mg/kg/day prednisone PO). Consider adding steroid-sparing agents, including cyclosporine, azathioprine, and chlorambucil. New therapy with IV infliximab has demonstrated excellent success in treating systemic and ocular inflammation related to Behçet's disease.

Table 11.15 Criteria for diagnosis of Behçet's disease (International Study Group for Behçet's Disease, 1990)

	Diagnostic (classification) criteria
Must have:	• Recurrent oral ulceration (minor, major, or herpetiform) ≥3× in 12 months
Plus two of:	• Recurrent genital ulceration (aphthous or scarring) • Eye lesions: uveitis (anterior, posterior, or cells in the vitreous) or retinal vasculitis • Skin lesions: erythema nodosum, pseudofolliculitis, or papulopustular lesions; or acneiform rash (in postadolescent patient not on corticosteroids) • Positive pathergy test

Vogt–Koyanagi–Harada disease

Vogt–Koyanagi–Harada disease (VKH) is a multisystem inflammatory disease affecting the eyes (bilateral granulomatous panuveitis), ears, brain, skin, and hair (see Table 11.16). It is thought to be a T-cell-mediated autoimmune disease directed against melanocyte antigen(s).

Prevalence is higher in darker-skinned races, including Asians, Native Americans, Hispanics, and those from the Middle and Far East. It is more common in women in their third and fourth decade, but may occur in either sex at any age.

It is associated with HLA-DR4, notably HLA-DRB1*0405, which recognizes various melanocyte proteins. VKH may arise after cutaneous injury, presumably via liberation of melanocyte antigens.

Clinical features

There is often a prodrome of fever, meningismus, and auditory symptoms for a few days before blurring or profound visual loss from the uveitis develops.

Ophthalmic

- *Anterior uveitis:* bilateral granulomatous anterior uveitis, posterior synechiae, iris nodules, AC shallowing.
- *Posterior uveitis:* multifocal chordoditis, multifocal detachments of sensory retina, exudative retinal detachments, choroidal depigmentation ("sunset glow fundus"), Dalen–Fuchs nodules (peripheral yellow-white choroidal granulomas), subretinal fibrosis.
- *Complications:* cataract, glaucoma, choroidal neovascular (CNV) membrane.

Systemic

- *Cutaneous:* late features—vitiligo, alopecia, poliosis.
- *Auditory:* tinnitus, deafness, vertigo.
- *Neurological:* sterile meningitis (headache, neck stiffness), encephalitis, (convulsions, altered consciousness), cranial neuropathies (including ocular motility disturbance).

Investigations

- *FA:* focal areas of delay in choroidal perfusion, multifocal areas of pinpoint leakage, large placoid areas of hyperfluorescence, pooling within subretinal fluid, and optic nerve staining.
- *Ultrasound:* low to medium reflective diffuse choroidal thickening.
- *Lumbar puncture* (not always required): lymphocytic pleocytosis.

Treatment

Coordinate care with PCP; start high-dose systemic corticosteroids (e.g., 1–2 mg/kg/day prednisone PO or methylprednisolone 1 g/day IV for 3 days). For resistant or recurrent disease consider adding steroid-sparing agents such as methotrexate, azathioprine, and cyclosporine.

Table 11.16 Diagnostic criteria for Vogt–Koyanagi–Harada disease

1		No history of penetrating ocular trauma or surgery preceding initial onset of uveitis
2		No clinical or laboratory evidence suggestive of other ocular disease entities
3		Bilateral ocular involvement
	a	*Early*
		1) Diffuse choroiditis (focal subretinal fluid or bullous serous retinal detachments)
		2) If fundus findings equivocal, then there must be characteristic FA findings (see Investigations) AND diffuse choroidal thickening (in the absence of posterior scleritis on US)
	b	*Late*
		1) History suggestive of prior presence of early features AND two or more of the following:
		2) Ocular depigmentation (sunset glow fundus or Sugiura sign)
		3a) Nummular chorioretinal depigmented scars
		3b) Retinal pigment epithelium clumping/migration
		3c) Recurrent or chronic anterior uveitis
4		Neurological and auditory findings
	a	Meningismus (malaise, fever, headache, nausea, abdominal pain, neck and back stiffness)
	b	Tinnitus
	c	CSF pleocytosis
5		Integumentary findings (not preceding ocular or CNS disease)
	a	Alopecia
	b	Poliosis
	c	Vitiligo

Complete VKH requires all criteria (1 to 5).

Incomplete VKH requires criteria 1 to 3 AND either 4 or 5.

Probable VKH (isolated ocular disease) requires criteria 1 to 3.

Reprinted with permission from Read RW, et al. (2001). Revised diagnostic criteria for Vogt–Koyanagi–Harada disease. *Am J Ophthalmol* 131:647–652.

Sympathetic ophthalmia

Sympathetic ophthalmia is a rare bilateral granulomatous panuveitis that bears remarkable parallels to VKH but differs in being causally related to antecedent ocular trauma or surgery. Although this response to injury can occur within a few days or over 60 years later, it usually arises between 1 and 12 months after injury.

It appears to be a T-cell-mediated response to an ocular antigen, presumably liberated during the initial insult. It occurs in 0.1% cases of penetrating ocular trauma and in 0.01% cases of routine vitrectomy. In one prospective study, the most common cause of sympathetic ophthalmia was ocular (particularly vitreoretinal) surgery.

Clinical features

Ophthalmic

- *Anterior:* bilateral granulomatous anterior uveitis with mutton-fat keratic precipitates, posterior synechiae.
- *Posterior:* vitritis, choroidal infiltration, Dalen–Fuchs nodules, macular edema, exudative retinal detachment; the inciting eye may be phthisical.
- *Complications:* cataract, secondary glaucoma, end-stage disease (optic atrophy, chorioretinal scarring).

Systemic

Features are the same as for VKH, but systemic involvement is less common.

Prevention

After trauma, there is a short window of opportunity (~10 days) in which enucleation would could prevent sympathetic ophthalmia. This may be the best option for blind, painful eyes with no hope of useful vision. However, for the many traumatized eyes with visual potential, there is now a strong trend to preserve the eye whenever possible.

Treatment

Once inflammation has developed, the role of enucleation of the exciting eye is controversial; some suggest that it may favorably modify the disease if performed within 2 weeks of initial symptoms.

Immunosuppression is started with high-dose systemic corticosteroids (e.g., 1–2 mg/kg/day prednisone PO or methylprednisolone 1 g/day IV for 3days). For resistant or recurrent disease or unacceptable steroid side effects, consider adding steroid-sparing agents, such as methotrexate, azathioprine and cyclosporine.

With aggressive treatment, 60% of patients may achieve ≥20/60 in the sympathizing eye.

Viral uveitis (1)

Herpes simplex virus

HSV1 (very rarely HSV2) may cause an anterior uveitis that is usually associated with keratitis but may be isolated.

Clinical

- *Anterior:* unilateral persistent anterior uveitis with KPs, posterior synechiae, and patchy iris atrophy (with transillumination defects); semidilated pupil ± corneal scarring, keratitis, ↑IOP, or ↓corneal sensation (p. 174). The uveitis may be granulomatous.
- Glaucoma is common (secondary to trabeculitis or blockage by inflammatory debris).
- *Posterior* (rare): healthy individuals may get acute retinal necrosis (ARN) (see below); those with disseminated HSV or HSV encephalitis may get an occlusive vasculitis (usually bilateral) with relatively few hemorrhages but commonly complicated by retinal detachment.

Treatment

- If there is keratitis, then antiviral coverage is generally required (p. 174).
- For isolated anterior uveitis, titrate topical steroids according to inflammation and taper very slowly (frequency/potency), as HSV uveitisis highly steroid sensitive and relapses are common; add a cycloplegia.
- Treat associated ↑IOP with topical glaucoma drops.
- For frequent recurrences, consider long-term oral antiviral prophylaxis.

Varicella zoster virus

Primary VZV infection (chickenpox) commonly causes a widespread vesicular rash that may be associated with keratitis (superficial, disciform, or stromal), mild anterior uveitis, and very occasionally necrotizing retinitis. Reactivation (shingles) usually occurs in the elderly or immunosuppressed and frequently affects CN V_1 (ophthalmic branch), known as herpes zoster ophthalmicus (HZO).

Of this group, up to 40% have anterior uveitis, with an increased risk if the nasociliary branch is involved (Hutchinson sign: vesicles at side of the nose). Typical ocular inflammation (e.g., disciform keratitis with anterior uveitis) may also occur without the rash (HZO sine herpete).

Clinical

- *Anterior:* unilateral anterior uveitis with KPs, posterior synechiae, and segmental iris atrophy (with transillumination defects) ± conjunctivitis, keratitis, epi/scleritis; the uveitis may be granulomatous.
- Glaucoma is common (up to 40%).
- *Posterior:* ARN or PORN may develop (see below).

Treatment

- For isolated anterior uveitis, titrate topical steroids according to inflammation and taper very slowly (frequency/potency), as VZV uveitis is highly steroid sensitive and relapses are common with steroid withdrawal; add cycloplegia.
- For HZO, see p. 177.

Other viruses

Other common viruses that may cause an anterior or posterior uveitis include measles (with SSPE) mumps, rubella, EBV, CMV, and HTLV-1.

Subacute sclerosing panencephalitis (SSPE)

This rare neurodegenerative syndrome following measles infection exhibits a retinitis with focal pigmentary changes in the fovea ± papilledema or optic atrophy.

Human T-lymphotropic virus type-1 (HTLV-1)

This RNA retrovirus is common in Japan and parts of Africa and causes leukemia and tropical spastic paraparesis. It may cause uveitis in isolation (usually intermediate) or be secondary to leukemia (usually posterior with retinal vasculitis ± secondary infection, e.g., CMV).

Cytomegalovirus (CMV)

CMV retinitis is the leading cause of visual loss in AIDS, but may also occur in patients who are immunosuppressed from therapy (e.g., associated with organ transplants) or other disease (e.g., lymphoma). HIV- and non-HIV-associated infections behave fairly similarly, both being dependent on the degree of immune system suppression/recovery.

Traditionally, HIV-associated CMV retinitis required lifelong maintenance therapy (cf. non-HIV disease). However, with antiretroviral therapy (ART)-induced immune recovery, this is no longer always necessary.

Viral uveitis (2)

Acute retinal necrosis (ARN)

This is a rare syndrome of necrotizing retinitis caused by VZV, HSV1, and occasionally HSV2 infection (children). It may infect healthy individuals of any age. See Table 11.7 for diagnostic criteria.

Clinical findings

- Usually unilateral ↓VA, floaters, discomfort
- It begins predominantly as a peripheral disease comprising occlusive arteritis, full-thickness peripheral necrotizing retinitis (well demarcated, spread circumferentially), and marked vitritis ± AC activity.
- *Complications:* retinal detachment (in up to 75%; rhegmatogenous or tractional), ischemic optic neuropathy.
- *Prognosis:* second eye involvement occurs in around 30% (may occur simultaneously to several years later).

Investigations

- AC tap ± vitreous biopsy with PCR to identify viral DNA.

Treatment

- *For all patients:* antiviral (e.g., acyclovir IV dose 10 mg/kg 3×/day 2 weeks, then PO dose 3 months). Consider systemic steroids (treat inflammation), aspirin (treat arterial occlusion), and barrier laser photocoagulation (treat retinal breaks), but there is no clinical evidence of benefit for these additional therapies. Retinal detachment repair is challenging because of the necrotic retina and number of breaks; vitrectomy with silicone oil injection is most commonly used.
- *If immunosuppressed:* consider lifelong antiviral treatment.

Progressive outer retinal necrosis (PORN)

This very rare devastating necrotizing retinitis is caused by VZV infection in the context of immunosuppression (usually HIV with CD4+ T cell counts <50/mm^3). See Table 11.17 for diagnostic criteria.

Clinical findings

- Uni/bilateral painless rapid ↓VA.
- Rapidly coalescing white areas of outer retinal necrosis (often central as well as peripheral) but with minimal or no vasculitis, retinitis, or vitritis (cf. ARN).

Treatment

This should be coordinated between an ophthalmologist with experience in HIV ocular disease and an infectious disease specialist. Options include intravenous ganciclovir or foscarnet with additional intravitreal ganciclovir, foscarnet, or fomivirsen. The prognosis is very poor, partly due to the extremely high rate of retinal detachment.

Table 11.17 Diagnostic criteria for ARN and PORN

	ARN	PORN
Appearance	One or more foci of full-thickness retinal necrosis with discrete borders	Multiple foci of deep retinal opacification that may be confluent
Location	Peripheral retina (usually adjacent or outside temporal arcades)	Peripheral retina ± macular involvement
Progression	Rapid (but usually responds to treatment)	Extremely rapid
Direction	Circumferential	No consistent direction
Vessels	Occlusive vasculopathy (arterial)	No vascular inflammation
Inflammation	Prominent AC and vitreous inflammation	Minimal or none
Suggestive features	Optic neuropathy/atrophy Scleritis Pain	Perivenular clearing of retinal opacification

This table was published in Engstrom RE Jr, et al. (1994). The progressive outer retinal necrosis syndrome. *Ophthalmology* 101:1488–502. Copyright Elsevier 1994.

HIV-associated disease: anterior segment

The human immunodeficiency virus (HIV-1 and 2) is an RNA retrovirus that infects CD4+ T cells, causing the acquired immunodeficiency syndrome, AIDS. Worldwide, around 33 million people are infected with HIV, with around 4 million new infections and 3 million deaths per year. More than 25 million people have died of HIV since 1981 (United Nations AIDS report). Most of the infected people live in developing countries (notably Sub-Saharan Africa) and under socioeconomic deprivation.

Transmission may be via infected blood or other bodily fluids. Major risk factors include unprotected sexual intercourse, intravenous drug abuse, blood transfusion, and maternal infection (vertical transmission).

The main markers of disease are CD4 level and viral load. The CD4 level is a good indicator of HIV-induced immunocompromise and correlates with susceptibility to infections (Table 11.18). The viral load (i.e., RNA copies/mL) correlates with risk of progression.

Prognosis is greatly improved with antiretroviral therapy (ART). This regimen involves using at least three antiretroviral drugs, usually two nucleoside reverse transcriptase inhibitors and either a protease inhibitor or a non-nucleoside reverse transcriptase inhibitor.

Management of eye disease should be coordinated between an ophthalmologist with experience in HIV and an infectious disease specialist.

Conjunctival microvasculopathy

Microvascular abnormalities of the conjunctiva are common (see Table 11.19). The mechanism may be related to vascular damage due to high viral load. Irregular-caliber vessels are seen, which may be in a corkscrew pattern. Conjunctival microvasculopathy may be associated with abnormalities of the retinal microvasculature (p. 353).

Keratouveitis

VZV keratouveitis is common in HIV, with or without the typical dermatomal rash of HZO. The features include a moderate anterior uveitis, ↑IOP, and iris atrophy. Treatment is with systemic antiviral (e.g., acyclovir or famciclovir) (p. 177).

HSV keratouveitis is less common, with probably equal prevalence to that of the general population. In HIV patients, however, it tends to be limbal and more severe and have more recurrences, and dendrites may be larger and less defined. Treatment is with topical ± systemic antiviral (e.g., acyclovir) (p. 174).

Microsporidial keratouveitis presents with bilateral irritation and photophobia and punctate keratopathy, often with a follicular conjunctivitis and/or an anterior uveitis.

HIV status is a relative contraindication for refractive surgery. There is an increased risk of dry eyes, postsurgical corneal infection, and reactivation of keratouveitis.

Table 11.18 CD4 level and typical diseases relevant to the eye

CD4 count Cells/mm³	Ocular disease
250–500	Herpes zoster ophthalmicus Tuberculosis
150–250	Lymphoma Kaposi's sarcoma
50–150	Pneumocystosis Toxoplasmosis Microsporidiosis VZV retinitis
<50	CMV retinitis

Table 11.19 Ophthalmic complications of HIV infection

	Infective	Tumor	Other
Adnexae	HZO Molluscum contagiosum Preseptal cellulitis	Kaposi sarcoma Squamous cell carcinoma	Conjunctival microvasculopathy
Orbit	Orbital cellulitis	Non-Hodgkin lymphoma	
Anterior segment	Viral keratitis (VZV, HSV) Bacterial keratitis (S. aureus, S. epidermidis, P. aeruginosa) Protozoan keratitis (microsporidia)		Conjunctival microvasculopathy Vortex keratopathy (antivirals, atovaquone) Dry eye Anterior uveitis
Posterior segment	CMV retinitis VZV retinitis (including PORN, ARN) HSV retinitis (incl. ARN) Toxoplasma retinochoroiditis Syphilis retinitis Pneumocystis choroiditis Cryptococcus choroiditis Tuberculous choroiditis	Ocular-CNS non-Hodgkin lymphoma	Retinal micro-vasculopathy Ischemic maculopathy Immune recovery uveitis
Neuro-ophthalmic	Cerebral toxoplasmosis Cryptococcal meningitis Neurosyphilis Progressive multifocal leukoencephalopathy	Ocular-CNS non-Hodgkin lymphoma	Optic neuritis Optic atrophy Ocular motility disorders

Anterior uveitis

Anterior uveitis is seen in over half of all patients with HIV. VZV and HSV tend to cause relatively mild inflammation (often with ↑IOP and iris atrophy). However, posterior uveitis associated with toxoplasma or syphilis may also cause significant anterior chamber inflammation.

Uveitis may also be caused by concurrent therapy, notably rifabutin (anti-atypical mycobacteria) and cidofivir (anti-CMV).

Mycobacterium tuberculosis

Mycobacterium tuberculosis is a rare cause of intraocular inflammation in HIV patients. This is an acid-fast obligate aerobe transmitted by aerosolized droplet. Tuberculosis should be ruled out in any HIV patient with a past history of TB exposure or symptoms of pulmonary TB with granulomatous anterior uveitis, choioretinitis, retinal vasculitis, and choroidal lesions.

Clinical findings

- Chronic granulomatous anterior uveitis.
- Papillitis.
- Intermediate uveitis.
- Choroidal tubercles and granulomas.
- Multifocal choroiditis or serpiginous like choroiditis.
- Retinal vasculitis.

Diagnostic testing

- Purified protein derivative (PPD) test.

Interpretation of the PPD test: In patients with HIV/AIDS, 5 mm induration is considered a positive reaction. Medical personnel or individuals in close contact with TB patients need reactions of only ≥10 mm induration to be counted as positive. Individuals with no risk factors or exposure to TB patients need >15 mm induration.

- Sputum culture.
- Bronchoscopy.
- Chest X-ray or CT scan.
- PCR with analysis of anterior chamber or vitreous sample.
- FA can be useful in evaluation of choroidal lesions and in confirming the presence of macular edema. Choroidal tubercles initially show hypofluorescene or very minimal hyperflourescence that increases in the late phases of disease.
- Quantiferon gold.

Treatment

Treat with rifampin, isoniazid, pyrazinamide, and ethambutol for 9–12 months. Unfortunately in HIV/AIDS, the choroiditis can progress despite this treatment.

HIV-associated disease: posterior segment

CMV retinitis

This may affect up to 40% of patients with AIDS, but usually only when CD4 <50/mm^3. Since the advent of ART, there has been a dramatic reduction in the incidences of CMV retinitis.

Clinical features

- Floaters, ↓VA, and/or field loss.
- *Anterior:* AC inflammation (± distinctive stellate KPs) is usually mild or absent (depending on degree of immunosuppression).
- *Posterior:* vitritis (usually mild or absent) with retinitis that may be
  - Hemorrhagic retinitis: hemorrhage and necrosis with loss of fundus details (pizza pie appearance).
  - Granular retinitis: relatively indolent, with minimal hemorrhage and no vascular sheathing.
  - Perivascular retinitis: "frosted branch angiitis," which spreads along the course of the retinal vessels.

Complications include retinal detachment (up to 30%), retinal atrophy, and optic nerve disease (5%).

Treatment

ART

Sustaining a CD4 count >50/mm^3 is effective prophylaxis against CMV retinitis. Late introduction of ART to patients with CMV retinitis is still likely to induce an immune recovery; in such patients, anti-CMV treatments are required at least until immune recovery occurs.

Specific anti-CMV treatment

This involves induction and maintenance therapy. Commonly used agents include systemic antivirals (e.g., valganciclovir, ganciclovir, foscarnet, or cidofovir), intravitreal implants (ganciclovir), or injections (ganciclovir, fomivirsen, foscarnet) or a combination. Lifelong maintenance treatment is recommended for all patients without immune recovery.

Toxoplasma retinochoroiditis

This is decreasing in frequency given the toxoplasmacidal effect of prophylactic agents actually intended to eliminate *Pneumocystis*-related lung disease. Ocular toxoplasmosis in HIV is more severe, often multifocal (even bilateral), associated with moderate to severe anterior uveitis and vitritis, and is commonly associated with neurotoxoplasmosis. In contrast to the immunocompetent situation, it always requires treatment (and should not be given with corticosteroids (p. 358).

Pneumocystis carinii choroiditis

This is relatively uncommon, particularly among those on systemic prophylaxis for *Pneumocystis carinii* pneumonia (co-trimoxazole) instead of inhalational form (pentamidine). The choroiditis is often bilateral and comprises yellow choroidal patches of 1/4 to 2 DD in size around the posterior pole with minimal vitritis. It is often asymptomatic. Treatment is with systemic co-trimoxazole or pentamidine.

Cryptococcus choroiditis

This rare condition is usually associated with cryptococcal meningitis and may be associated with an optic neuropathy or papilledema. It is characterized by multifocal off-white choroidal lesions, occasionally with a retinitis or endophthalmitis. Treatment is with a systemic antifungal (e.g., amphotericin-B or fluconazole).

Immune recovery uveitis

Eyes with inactive CMV retinitis may show a paradoxical worsening of inflammation as T-cell recovery takes place. The noninfectious inflammation is due to the reconstituted immune system responding to viral antigens present in the eye. Presentation includes moderate to severe vitritis, tractional retinal detachment, CME, and neovascularization.

Syphilis choroiditis/chorioretinitis

Coinfection with syphilis may occur via sexual transmission. Syphilis may cause protean ocular and systemic manifestations (p. 357).

HIV microvasculopathy

Around 75% of HIV-infected individuals develop microvascular abnormalities of the retina and/or conjunctiva (p. 349). It is not clear if this is due to HIV-induced thrombotic tendency or an immune phenomenon or is a direct result of HIV infection of the vessels.

Retinal microvasculopathy

In the retina there may be tortuosity of the vessels with cotton-wool spots, telangiectasia, intraretinal hemorrhages, and venous or arterial occlusions. These clinical findings are noninfectious in nature and are related to HIV viremia-associated damage of the retinal vasculature.

Mycobacterial disease

Tuberculosis

Worldwide, more than 1 billion people are infected by *Mycobacterium tuberculosis*, a facultative intracellular bacterium. Tuberculosis (primary or post-primary) develops in around 10%, and of these individuals ocular disease develops in around 1%.

Widespread chronic inflammation develops with characteristic caseating granuloma. This immune reaction or occasionally direct ocular penetration may lead to uveitis.

Ocular TB may be difficult to diagnose because of its protean manifestations and the frequent absence of any clinical or radiological evidence of respiratory disease.

Clinical features

Ophthalmic
- *External:* lid abscess, conjunctival infiltration/nodules, phlyctenulosis, scleritis (usually anterior necrotizing), interstitial keratitis
- *Anterior:* typically granulomatous anterior uveitis with mutton-fat KPs, iris granuloma, posterior synechiae, but can be nongranulomatous
- *Posterior:* vitritis, vasculitis (periphlebitis ± BRVO or CRVO ± ischemia), macular edema, choroidal granuloma (usually multifocal around the posterior pole ± inflammatory retinal detachment); optic neuropathy; Eales' disease (retinal vasculitis with neovascularization and high risk of vitreous hemorrhage, typically in young males)

Systemic
- *Respiratory system:* pneumonia, pleural effusion, fibrosis.
- *GI:* ileocaecal (may obstruct), peritoneum (ascites).
- *GU:* sterile pyuria, epididymitis, salpingitis + infertility (in females).
- *CNS:* meningitis, CNS tuberculoma (may mimic tumor).
- *Skeletal:* arthritis, osteomyelitis.
- *Skin:* lupus vulgaris.
- *Cardiovascular system:* constrictive pericarditis, pericardial effusion.
- *Adrenal:* hypoadrenalism (Addison's disease).
- *Lymph nodes:* lymphadenopathy, scrofula.

Investigation
- *Microbiology:* sputum, early-morning urine (acid-fast bacillus, stains with Ziehl–Neelsen stain).
- *Chest X-ray:* classically apical infiltrates or cavitation; also consolidation, pleural effusion, hilar lymphadenopathy; normal in 50% of cases of ocular TB.
- *Tuberculin testing:* standard testing involves intradermal injection of 0.1 mL of 1:1000 strength tuberculin PPD (i.e., 10 tuberculin units) and measuring the induration 72 hours later. Interpret with caution (see Box 11.2), as the response can be highly variable with up to 17% false negatives and BCG vaccination inducing false positives (but usually only if within 5 years). A 1:10,000 strength tuberculin PPD may be used if active TB is suspected, since an intense reaction may become necrotic.

- QuantiFERON-TB Gold is a newly developed blood test that can differentiate previous TB exposure from BCG vaccination and other atypical myobacteria exposure.

Box 11.2 Interpretation of Mantoux testing (CDC recommendations, 2005)

- For high-risk individuals (immunosuppressed, contacts of active TB, typical CXR changes), the test is considered positive if induration ≥5 mm.
- For moderate risk (e.g., health workers, those with chronic disease, children, immigrants from endemic areas), induration must be ≥10 mm.
- For low risk, the test is only considered positive if induration ≥15 mm.

Treatment

Standard unsupervised treatment

If patient adherence or compliance is likely to be good, treatment is unsupervised with a daily regimen, usually using combination tablets. The initial 2 months of therapy consists of rifampin, isoniazid, pyrazinamide, and ethambutol. Continuation treatment for 4 additional months is with rifampin and isoniazid only.

Supervised and extended treatment

Otherwise, directly observed therapy (DOT) is instituted, with higher doses of the same drugs given three times per week. Treatment may be prolonged for 9 months if the patient is immunosuppressed or has disseminated disease.

Additional treatment

For ocular complications such as CME, retinal vasculitis, and persistent inflammation, consider oral corticosteroids but only if the patient is on effective anti-TB treatment.

Monitoring

Urinalysis and liver function tests (LFTs) should be checked before starting treatment with rifampin, isoniazid, and pyrazinamide. VA should be checked before starting treatment with ethambutol and the patient advised to report any visual disturbance (↓VA, ↓color vision, ↓visual field).

Leprosy (Hansen disease)

Worldwide, around 15 million people have leprosy, of whom about two-thirds are in Asia. The spectrum of leprosy is cased by the interaction of the obligate intracellular bacterium *Mycobacterium leprae* with the host's immune system.

A poor cell-mediated immune response leads to the lepromatous form, which is generalized and commonly affects the eyes. A strong response leads to tuberculoid leprosy, which is more localized and rarely affects the eye.

Clinical features

Ophthalmic

- *External:* madarosis, trichiasis, lagophthalmos (CN VII palsy), conjunctivitis, epi/scleritis, keratitis (neurotrophic, exposure, or secondary infection).
- *Anterior:* anterior uveitis is usually persistent; less commonly, acute anterior uveitis; "iris pearls" at the pupillary margin may enlarge and drop into the AC; iris atrophy; miosis.

Systemic

- *Tuberculoid:* thickened and tender nerves associated with hypopigmented anesthetic patches and muscle atrophy.
- *Lepromatous:* nerve changes are less marked but with widespread infiltration, including skin, ears, nose (saddle-nose), face (leonine appearance), and larynx (hoarse voice).

Investigation and treatment

This should include skin and nasal mucosa smears for noncultivable acid-fast bacilli. Systemic treatment should be coordinated by a referral center with multidisciplinary support. Treatment of eye disease is usually with topical steroids.

Spirochetal and other bacterial uveitis

Syphilis

The spirochete *Treponema pallidum* is usually transmitted by sexual contact or transplacentally. Acquired syphilis is divided into primary, secondary, and tertiary stages. Congenital syphilis may be divided into early (equivalent to acquired secondary stage) and late (equivalent to acquired third stage) (see Table 11.20).

Clinical features (Table 11.21)

Anterior uveitis

This is the most common ocular feature of both secondary and tertiary syphilis.

- Granulomatous or nongranulomatous; variable severity; ± roseolae (vascular fronds on the iris); ± iris atrophy; nodules on the iris or iridocorneal angle occur in tertiary disease only.

Posterior uveitis

This may be uni- or bilateral, uni- or multifocal, and choroiditis or chorioretinitis.

- Yellow plaque-like lesions with overlying vitritis ± serous retinal detachment. Resolution of the lesions results in a pigmentary retinopathy.

Investigation

- *Nontreponemal serology* (Table 11.22): venereal disease research laboratory (VDRL) tests disease activity; it may become negative in later-stage syphilis. Rapid plasma reagin (RPR) is a simple test used in screening; it has a high false-positive rate and also turns negative in many patients with tertiary and neurosyphilis.
- *Treponemal serology* (Table 11.22): fluorescent treponemal antibody absorption (FTA-ABS) and hemagglutination tests (TPHA) test previous or current infection. They do not distinguish from other treponematoses (e.g., yaws).
- Dark-ground microscopy of chancre or mucocutaneous lesion
- *Lumbar puncture:* consider if there is active ocular disease, suspected neurosyphilis, or HIV. Cerebrospinal fluid (CSF) typically shows raised protein, pleocytosis, and positive VDRL.
- HIV test; coinfection is increasingly observed.

Treatment

Management of syphilitic eye disease should be in conjunction with an infectious disease physician. Treatment requires high-dose intravenous procaine penicillin G with an extended regimen for late latent and tertiary syphilis. Spirochete death may transiently worsen inflammation (Jarish–Herxheimer reaction).

Consider topical steroids for interstitial keratitis and anterior uveitis. Systemic steroids must be used with caution but have a role in sight-threatening posterior uveitis or scleritis.

Table 11.20 Stages of syphilis

Stage	Main features
Congenital	
Early <2 years of age	Mucocutaneous rash; periostitis and osteochondritis; Chorioretinitis and retinal vasculitis producing characteristic salt-and-pepper fundus
Late >2 years of age	Saddle nose, frontal bossing, saber shins, Hutchinson's teeth; interstitial keratitis
Acquired	
Primary (from 2 weeks post-infection)	Painless ulcer (chancre) with regional lymphadenopathy appears 2–6 weeks post-infection and resolves within a further 6 weeks
Secondary (from 8 weeks post-infection)	Diffuse maculopapular rash (including palms/soles) often with generalized lymphadenopathy, malaise, and fever Anterior or posterior uveitis
Tertiary (from 5 years post-infection)	Around one-third progress to this stage. Aortitis may cause aortic regurgitation and dissection. Neurosyphilis may cause meningitis, CNS vasculitis, and parenchymatous degeneration, resulting in the syndromes of tabes dorsalis and generalized paresis of the insane (GPI). Anterior or posterior uveitis; interstitial keratitis

Table 11.21 Ophthalmic complications of syphilis

Adnexae	Gummata	Madarosis
Anterior segment	Conjunctival chancre Papillary conjunctivitis Epi/scleritis	Interstitial keratitis Anterior uveitis
Posterior segment	Multi- or unifocal choroiditis, chorioretinitis	Neuroretinitis Retinal vasculitis
Neuro-ophthalmic	Argyll Robertson pupils Papilledema Retrobulbar neuritis	Optic neuritis Ocular motility disorders Visual field defects

Table 11.22 Serological tests for syphilis

	Primary		Secondary	Tertiary	Treated
	Early	Late			
VDRL	–/+	+	+	+	– or low +
Titer	Rising titer		Titer α activity	Titer may wane	Falling titer
FTA-ABS	+	+	+	+	+
TPHA	–/+	+	+	+	+

False-positive VDRL may occur in other conditions including EBV, mycoplasma, autoimmune disease, chronic liver disease, and malignancy.

Other bacteria

Other bacteria that may cause uveitis include the spirochetes *Borrelia burdorferi* (Lyme disease) and *Leptospira interrogans* (leptospirosis, including Weil's disease), the gram-positive bacillus *Tropheryma whippelii* (Whipple's disease), and the gram-negative bacilli *Bartonella henselae* (cat-scratch disease) and *Brucella* (brucellosis).

Lyme disease

Lyme disease is caused by the infectious organism *Borrelia burgdorferi* through a tick-borne transmission. The organism is found in rodents, deer, birds, cats, and dogs and is transmitted to humans by the ticks *Ixodes dammini* (east) or *Ixodes pacificus* (west). The first reported case of the disease was discovered in 1975 in Lyme, Connecticut.

While most patients do not recall exposure to ticks or tick bite, 80% of affected patients develop a classic skin lesion of erythema chronicum migrans. After several weeks, the organism may spread systemically and is associated with annular skin lesions, meningitis, cranial or peripheral neuritis, migratory musculoskeletal pain, and carditis. Months to years later, chronic arthritis or neurological symptoms may develop.

Clinical features: systemic

Stage I
- Classic triad of nonspecific follicular conjunctivitis (10%), skin rash, and flu-like symptoms.
- Erythema chronicum migrans is a spreading target lesion skin rash often forgotten by the patient (60–80% of patients).
- Headache, stiff neck, malaise, myalgias, arthralgias, and fever.

Stage II
- 1–4 months after infection, further invasion brings neurological, musculoskeletal, and cardiac findings.
- Neurological (30–40%): Bell's palsy, encephalitis, meningitis.
- Cardiac (8%): myocarditis, heart block.
- Musculoskeletal: arthritis, tendonitis, joint effusions.

Stage III
- After 5 months of infection.
- Chronic atrophic skin changes, keratitis, chronic arthritis, ataxia, chronic encephalomyelitis, acute respiratory distress syndrome (ARDS).

Clinical features: ophthalmic
- Follicular conjunctivitis early (11% of patients).
- Chronic iridocyclitis.
- Vitritis.
- Peripheral retinal vasculitis.
- Diffuse choroiditis.
- Panuveitis.
- Intermediate uveitis.
- Optic neuritis.
- Neuroretinitis.
- Orbital myositis.
- Cranial nerve palsies.

Diagnostic
- Lyme immunofluorescent antibody titer (IFA).
- ELISA for IgM and IgG should be in early stage I, ELISA is only 50% sensitive early on, and 80% later.
- High rate of false positives due to cross-reactivity with *T. pallidum*.
  - Western blot for confirmation of positive ELISA and IFA.

Treatment
- Oral tetracycline or doxycycline, erythromycin, amoxicillin for early disease course.
- Neurological or neuro-ophthalmologic manifestation needs IV ceftriaxone or penicillin.

Protozoan uveitis

Toxoplasmosis

The protozoan *Toxoplasma gondii* is an obligate intracellular parasite that is estimated to infect up to 50% of the world's population. Lifetime risk of ocular toxoplasmosis is around 18/100,000 but up to 20 times this level in West Africa and South America.

The definitive host is the cat; livestock and humans are only intermediate hosts. Oocysts are excreted in cat feces, which are ingested by humans and livestock in which they may become encysted (bradyzoite) or actively proliferate (tachyzoite). Human infection arises from contact with cat feces or contaminated soil, ingestion of undercooked meat (bradyzoites), contaminated water, or transplacentally.

In the past, most toxoplasmosis was thought to be congenital, but acquired disease is increasingly recognized. Vertical transmission rate (transplacental) increases from 15% in the first trimester to 60% in the third trimester; disease severity is much greater if acquired in early pregnancy.

Clinical features
Ophthalmic
Affects both eyes in 40%, but if simultaneously active, suspect immunocompromise.

- Asymptomatic finding, floaters, ↓VA.
- Vitritis (may have "vitreous precipitates" akin to KPs on posterior surface of PVD), retinitis (white, fluffy area when active; becomes circumscribed and pigmented as it heals; atrophic scar with pigmented border when inactive; satellite lesions with old scars commonly seen); retinal vasculitis (periphlebitis); may have an anterior uveitis often with ↑IOP.
- Other presentations include scleritis, punctate outer retinitis (with quiet vitreous), large lesions (especially in the elderly), endophthalmitis-like, neuroretinitis, serous retinal detachments, and pigmentary retinopathy.
- Complications include cataract, glaucoma, and CNV membrane.

Systemic
- *Congenital:* the impact of transplacental infection is greatest early in pregnancy; complications include hydrocephalus, cerebral calcification, hepatosplenomegaly, and retinochoroiditis (more commonly bilateral and affecting the macula).
- *Acquired:* if the patient is immunocompetent, the disease is usually asymptomatic, but the patient may have fever and lymphadenopathy. If immunocompromised, they may have life-threatening disease, including encephalitis, intracerebral cysts, hepatitis, and myocarditis.

Investigation
This is essentially a clinical diagnosis. Interpret positive serological tests with caution. Many of the adult population are positive for anti-toxoplasma IgG; however IgM antibodies do suggest acquired infection, and negative serology in undiluted serum makes the diagnosis unlikely. Matched early and convalescent samples are not required. PCR of intraocular samples may also be used.

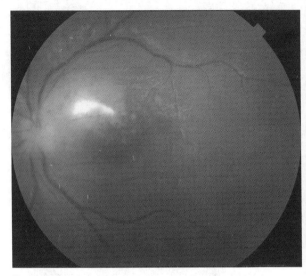

Figure 11.1 Active macular toxoplasmosis retinochoroiditis with overlying vitreous cells and associated optic disc edema. See insert for color version.

Treatment

Box 11.3 **Indications for treatment**

- Lesions involving optic disc, macula or papillomacular bundle
- Lesions threatening a major vessel
- Marked vitritis
- Any lesion in an immunocompromised patient

Systemic treatment is with ≥4 weeks of prednisone AND cotrimoxazole OR clindamycin/sulfadiazine OR pyrimethamine/sulfadiazine/folinic acid (weekly CBC required) OR atovaquone. Steroids must not be used without effective antitoxoplasmosis therapy and should not be given if the patient is immunosuppressed.

For maternal infection acquired during pregnancy, use spiramycin (named-patient basis) to reduce transplacental spread. Atovaquone may theoretically reduce recurrences, as it is active against bradyzoites as well as tachyzoites.

Prognosis

In immunocompetent patients, the disease is self-limiting and hence does not require treatment unless sight threatening. Recurrence is common; mean number of recurrences is two, but a wide variation is seen.

Pregnancy

Education is key (Table 11.23). Some countries perform serial antenatal serological screening to detect active toxoplasmosis to enable early initiation of treatment. Treat maternal infection that is acquired during pregnancy with spiramycin.

Microsporidiosis

Microsporidia are protozoan obligate intracellular parasites, of which four genera may cause the human disease, microsporidiosis. This is usually seen in the immunosuppressed (notably in AIDS), where it may present as chronic diarrhea, respiratory infection, or keratoconjunctivitis. Microsporidial keratoconjunctivitis presents with bilateral irritation and photophobia, and punctate keratopathy, often with a follicular conjunctivitis and/or an anterior uveitis.

Table 11.23 Toxoplasmosis and pregnancy

Advice	Wash all fruit and vegetables
	Avoid unpasteurized goat's milk
	Cook all meat thoroughly
	Avoid handling cat litter (or use rubber gloves)
Risk of transmission	15–60% risk if acquired during pregnancy
	No risk otherwise (even if recurrence of active disease during pregnancy)

Nematodal uveitis

Toxocariasis

The ascarid *Toxocara canis* is one of the most common of all nematode infections and is a significant cause of visual loss worldwide. The definitive hosts are puppies (or kittens for the less common *T. catis*).

Ova excreted in feces are inadvertently ingested by humans, where they develop into larvae. The larvae invade the gut wall and spread hematogenously throughout the body, notably to the liver, lung, brain, heart (visceral larva migrans), or eye (ocular toxocariasis). Larval death causes an intense inflammatory reaction.

Infection by *Toxocara* usually occurs <3 years of age, although some ocular disease may not present until adulthood.

Clinical features
Ophthalmic
Ocular toxocariasis is unilateral. Presentation may vary with age.
• Diffuse chronic endophthalmitis (age 2–9 years): ↓VA + floaters;
  white eye with chronic anterior uveitis, posterior synechiae, vitritis,
  snowbanking, macular edema, exudative retinal detachment;
  complications include tractional retinal detachment, cyclitic membrane,
  cataract, hypotony.
• Posterior pole granuloma (age 6–14 years): ↓VA; yellow-white
  granuloma 1–2 DD at the macula/papillomacular bundle with retinal
  traction and vitreous bands.
• Peripheral granuloma (age 6 years–adult): usually asymptomatic until
  significant traction; yellow-white granuloma anterior to the equator
  with vitreous bands. Traction may cause macula heterotopia or retinal
  detachment (tractional or rhegmatogenous).
• Less common presentations include isolated anterior uveitis,
  intermediate uveitis, optic papillitis, and vitreous abscess.

Systemic (visceral larva migrans)
Systemic features usually occur in patients <4 years of age.
• Fever, pneumonitis + bronchospasm, hepatosplenomegaly, fits,
  myocarditis, death (rare); eosinophilia.

Investigation
This is essentially a clinical diagnosis, although ELISA for serum antibodies may be supportive and B-scan ultrasound may help differentiate it from other diagnoses.

Treatment
For ocular toxocariasis use systemic or periocular steroids titrated according to disease severity; antihelminthics (e.g., thiabendazole) are of limited use. Consider vitrectomy to clear debris, relieve traction, and repair retinal detachments.

Diffuse unilateral subacute neuroretinitis (DUSN)

DUSN is an increasingly recognized cause of posterior uveitis in young people in which a solitary nematode persists in the subretinal space for years, causing progressive damage. Two unknown nematodes may cause the syndrome. They have different sizes (0.5 mm and 1–2 mm) and occur in different geographical distributions.

Signs include a unilateral vitritis, optic disc swelling (later atrophy), deep retinal gray-white lesions, and sometimes the worm itself. Treatment is difficult. If directly visualized, the worm may be killed by argon laser; if not, use antihelminthics (e.g., thiobendazole). Steroids suppress inflammation but do not alter outcome.

Onchocerciasis

Worldwide onchcocerciasis (river blindness) affects around 20 million people, causing visual impairment in 10%.

The filarial nematode *Onchocerca volvulus* is spread between humans (definitive host) by bites of the Simulium blackfly (vector). Having entered the subcutaneous tissue, the larvae mature into adult worms (up to 80 cm long) and mate to produce microfilariae within large subcutaneous nodules. The microfilariae then spread to nearby tissues, which may include the eye.

The Simulium breeds in areas of fast flowing water that also tend to be those regions that are most fertile and heavily farmed.

Ocular disease from the microfilariae includes sclerosing keratitis (with an opaque apron over the inferior cornea), chorioretinitis, sclerosis of the retinal vessels, optic neuritis, and optic atrophy. Microfilariae may best be seen in the AC after face-down posturing. Histology may be obtained from skin nodules.

Treatment was traditionally with diethylcarbamazine (which induces the severely itchy Mazzotti reaction), but has now been replaced with ivermectin.

Fungal uveitis

Candidiasis

Candida albicans is a higher-order fungus of the class Blastomycetes. It is yeast-like (i.e., reproduces by budding) and imperfect (i.e., no sexual stage has yet been identified). It is often a commensal of skin, mouth, and vagina, but opportunistic systemic infection may arise from hematogenous spread, notably in intravenous drug abuse, indwelling venous catheters, and immunosuppression.

Uveitis in an intravenous drug abuser should be considered fungal until proven otherwise.

Clinical features
- *Risk group:* intravenous drug abuse, indwelling catheters (hemodialysis, parenteral nutrition), immunosuppression (AIDS, steroids, cytotoxics, long-term antibiotics), systemic debilitation (malignancy).
- ↓VA, floaters, pain; often bilateral.
- Multifocal retinitis (yellow-white fluffy lesions ≥1 DD in size) ± vitritis (colonies appear as "cotton balls" that may be joined together, forming a "string of pearls") ± anterior uveitis.
- *Complications:* retinal necrosis, tractional retinal detachment.

Investigation and treatment
- Vitrectomy (send whole vitrectomy cassette) for microscopy/culture to confirm diagnosis.
- Intravitreal antifungals (e.g., 5 µg amphotericin B).
- Systemic antifungals: coordinate care with infectious disease specialist; oral fluconazole (usually 400 mg initially then 200 mg 2×/day) ± flucytosine is generally effective. Consider intravenous amphotericin B (dose according to preparation) for known systemic involvement or resistant cases; duration of treatment is usually ≥4 weeks.
- Review frequently; hospital admission may be helpful especially if poor adherence or compliance to medical regimen is likely or intravenous treatment is necessary.

Aspergillosis

Aspergillus may occasionally cause an endogenous endophthalmitis similar to *Candida*. It generally occurs in those with chronic pulmonary disease who are severely immunosuppressed. It is more aggressive than candidal infection, with pain and rapid visual loss being marked.

A confluent yellowish infiltrate is seen in the subretinal space that progresses to a subretinal hypopyon. Other features include intraretinal hemorrhages, dense vitritis, and AC hypopyon. Treatment is similar to *Candida* but usually requires IV amphotericin B.

Histoplasmosis and POHS

Histoplasma capsulatum is a higher dimorphic fungus that grows as a yeast at 37°C and as a mycelium in soil. It is endemic in southern Europe, southern United States, Central America, and Asia.

Ocular disease from direct infection of the globe is rare, usually occurs in the very young or the immunosuppressed, and may involve posterior or panuveitis or endophthalmitis. Treatment is with ketoconazole or amphotericin B.

More commonly, *H. capsulatum* is invoked as the possible agent underlying the presumed ocular histoplasmosis syndrome (POHS), albeit via an abnormal immune response. The evidence for *H. capsulatum* being the causative agent is, however, inconclusive.

Epidemiology indicates that while there is correlation between regions of high prevalence of *H. capsulatum* and POHS, an apparently identical syndrome is seen in nonendemic areas (such as the UK, northern Europe, and northern US).

The ocular disease is most common in the fourth decade. It is usually bilateral but sequential, with a mean interval of 4 years between onset of symptoms in each eye.

Clinical features

- Well-demarcated atrophic choroidal scars (≤1 DD) around posterior pole/mid-periphery ("histo" spots); peripapillary atrophy; peripheral linear atrophic streaks; no significant vitritis.
- *Complications:* choroidal neovascularization (type 2); this is often the presenting feature of otherwise asymptomatic disease.

Investigation and treatment

Diagnosis is clinical but FA is required if CNV is suspected. Antifungals have no benefit. Active lesions at the macula are often treated with immunosuppression (commonly corticosteroids).

For extrafoveal and juxtafoveal CNV, conventional laser photocoagulation is of benefit (Macular Photocoagulation Study: severe vision loss at 5 years is 42% for untreated vs. 12% for argon-treated extrafoveal).

For subfoveal membranes, photodynamic therapy (PDT), submacular surgery, and anti-VEGF therapy (membrane excision) should be considered.

White dot syndromes (1)

Acute posterior multifocal placoid pigment epitheliopathy (APMPPE)

This is an uncommon condition of young adults that is usually bilateral and may be preceded by a flu-like illness. There appears to be an association with HLA-B7 and HLA-DR2.

Clinical features
- Acute ↓VA sequentially in both eyes (usually after a few days interval).
- Postequatorial lesions of the RPE (initially gray-white but fade over weeks with irregular depigmentation and pigmentation), mild vitritis.

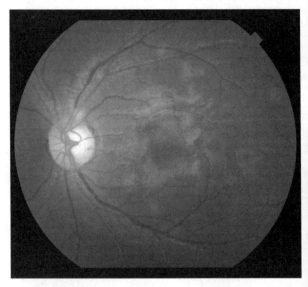

Figure 11.2 APMPPE lesions of the left eye. Multiple subretinal yellow lesions are in the posterior pole with involvement of the macula. See insert for color version.

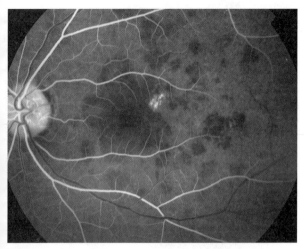

Figure 11.3 Early fluorescein angiogram demonstrated corresponding area of choroidal hypofluorescence in the location of APMPPE lesions. See insert for color version.

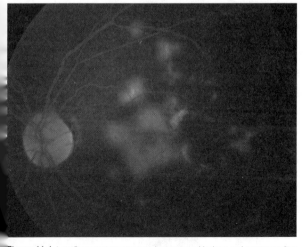

Figure 11.4 Late fluorescein angiogram demonstrated leakage and corresponding area of hyperfluorescence in the location of APMPPE lesions. See insert for color version.

Investigations and treatment

FA shows early dense hypofluorescence and late staining of lesions. There is spontaneous recovery within 2–3 months, so treatment is not usually indicated.

Serpiginous choroidopathy

This is a rare bilateral condition of the middle-aged patient that may superficially resemble APMPPE but has a much worse prognosis.

Clinical features

- ↓VA but often asymptomatic until macular involvement.
- Peripapillary lesions at the level of the RPE/inner choroid (gray-white, spread centrifugally from the disc but may skip, becomes atrophic over months with irregular depigmentation and pigmentation), mild vitritis.
- *Complications*: extensive subretinal scarring, CNV membrane (≤30%).

Investigations and treatment

FA shows early dense hypofluorescence and late staining of lesions. Corticosteroids and other immunosuppressives are commonly used in the acute phase, although there is no clear evidence of benefit.

CNV membranes may be treated by laser, PDT, anti-VEGF therapy, or submacular surgery.

Birdshot retinochoroidopathy (BSRC)

This is an uncommon bilateral condition of middle-aged Caucasian adults, with a slight female preponderance. Around 95% are HLA-A29 positive.

Clinical features

- ↓VA, ↓color vision, floaters, nyctalopia.
- Lesions at the level of the RPE (oval, cream-colored, radiate from the optic disc to the equator, associated with large choroidal vessels; become atrophic but not pigmented), moderate vitritis, vasculitis, CME.
- *Complications*: CNV membrane, optic atrophy.

Investigations and treatment

This is one condition in which treatment should be directed by FA and electrodiagnostic results rather than the clinical picture alone.

- ERG: ↓b-wave amplitude and latency; EOG: ↓Arden ratio.
- HLA testing: HLA-A29 positive in 95%. If HLA-A29 negative, consider sarcoid in the differential diagnosis as this can give a similar picture.

Corticosteroids, intravitreal flucinolone implant and other immunosuppressives are used to treat any CME, retinal vasculitis, retinal degeneration, with guarded final outcome.

CNV membranes may be treated by laser, PDT, anti-VEGF therapy, or submacular surgery.

More recently, intravenous daclizumab has demonstrated excellent success in controlling disease activity in BSRC.

WHITE DOT SYNDROMES (2)   **371**

White dot syndromes (2)

Multifocal choroiditis with panuveitis (MCP) and punctate inner choroidopathy (PIC)

These are uncommon bilateral conditions that may simulate POHS (sometimes called pseudo-POHS). Both are more common in women, but PIC tends to affect a younger age group. A viral etiology has been suggested.

Clinical features
- ↓VA, scotomas, photopsia.
- *MCP:* choroidal lesions (gray, peripheral + posterior polar), vitritis, anterior uveitis, CME, subretinal fibrosis, CNV membrane.
- *PIC:* quiet eye (no vitritis) with lesions at the level of the inner choroid or retina (initially yellow-white but become atrophic pigmented scars similar to POHS; posterior polar), serous retinal detachment, CNV membrane.

Investigations and treatment
- FA: early hypofluorescence and late staining of lesions.
- Corticosteroids are commonly used for acute lesions or CME.
- CNV membrane: medical treatment, laser, PDT, anti-VEGF therapy or submacular surgery.

Multiple evanescent white-dot syndrome (MEWDS)

This is a rare unilateral condition, typically in young women, which may be preceded by a flu-like illness.

Clinical features
- Acute ↓VA, scotomas ± photopsia.
- Small white dots at level of outer retina/RPE, tiny orange-white dots at the fovea, mild vitritis.

Investigations and treatment
- FA: early punctate hyperfluorescence and late staining of lesions.
- ERG: ↓a-wave.

Spontaneous recovery occurs within 2–3 months, so treatment is not usually indicated.

Acute zonal occult outer retinopathy (AZOOR)

This may form part of a spectrum of disease comprising MEWDS, MCP, PIC, and the acute idiopathic blind-spot enlargement syndrome (AIBES). AZOOR is an uncommon condition affecting one or both eyes, typically in myopic young to middle-aged women after a flu-like illness.

Clinical features
- Acute sctomas, worse in bright light; photopsia.
- Acutely may have vitritis; later may have zonal atrophy or irregular pigmentation (RP-like).

Investigations and treatment
- ERG: variably abnormal in a patchy distribution and often asymmetric.
- Immunosuppression is common during the acute phase but is of limited proven benefit.

Table 11.24 Summary of white dot syndromes

Syndrome	Age	Sex	Laterality	Vitritis	Lesion size	Prognosis
PIC	20–40	F > M	Bilateral	–	1/10 DD	Guarded
POHS	20–50	M = F	Bilateral	–	1/3 DD	Guarded
MEWDS	20–40	F > M	Unilateral	+	1/5 DD	Good
APMPPE	20–40	M = F	Bilateral	+	1 DD	Good
Serpiginous choroidopathy	30–60	M = F	Bilateral	+		Poor
Birdshot retino-choroidopathy	23–79	F > M	Bilateral	++	1/4–1/2 DD	Guarded
Multifocal choroiditis with panuveitis	30–60	F > M	Bilateral	++	1/10 DD	Guarded

Vitreoretinal

Anatomy and physiology

Anatomy

Vitreous

The *vitreous* makes up 80% of ocular volume or around 4.0 mL. It is a transparent gel consisting of hyaluronic acid and collagen (types II, IX, and a V/XI hybrid). Collagen fibrils connect the vitreous to the retinal internal limiting membrane. The vitreous base is a band of adherent vitreous 3–4 mm wide overlying the ora serrata and peripheral retina.

Retina and choroid (p. 406)

The *retina* is a transparent light-transforming, laminated structure comprising photoreceptors, interneurons, and ganglion cells overlying the retinal pigment epithelium (RPE). Superficial retinal vessels form four major arcades over the surface of the retina.

Within the suprachoroidal space are the long posterior ciliary nerves and arteries, which can be seen peripherally at 3 and 9 o'clock. Similarly, the vortex ampullae (which drain into the vortex veins) may be seen at all four diagonal quadrants just posterior to the equator.

Vitreoretinal adhesions

Normal attachments are strongest at the optic disc, the fovea, and especially the ora serrata/vitreous base, which remains adherent even when posterior vitreous detachment is otherwise complete.

Abnormal attachments include areas of lattice degeneration (posterior border), white without pressure, congenital cystic tufts, pigment clumps, and condensations around retinal vessels.

Physiology

Forces of attachment

The retinal position is maintained by hydrostatic forces and, to a lesser extent, by adhesion of the interphotoreceptor matrix. The hydrostatic forces are both active (the RPE pump) and passive (the osmotic gradient).

Forces of detachment

Vitreoretinal traction may be dynamic (from eye movement) or static (purely from vitreoretinal interaction, e.g., diabetic fibrovascular proliferation). The direction of static forces may be tangential, bridging, or anteroposterior. Gravitational forces are probably a significant factor in superior breaks.

Vitreous liquefaction

The aging vitreous becomes progressively liquefied (syneresis), resulting in optically empty lacunae and a reduction in its shock-absorbing capacity. Liquefaction occurs earlier in myopia, trauma, inflammation, and many disorders of collagen and connective tissue. A break in the cortical vitreous permits vitreal fluid to flow through, causing separation and collapse of the remaining vitreous (posterior vitreous detachment).

Retinal detachment: assessment

Retinal detachment (RD) is a relatively common sight-threatening condition with an incidence of around 1/10,000/year (for assessment see Table 12.1; for differentiating features see Tables 12.2 and 12.3).

Rhegmatogenous retinal detachment (RRD) is usually an ophthalmic emergency (p. 383). It is the most common form of retinal detachment and arises from a full-thickness break in the retina. Untreated, it almost always leads to a blind eye, but with appropriate early treatment it may have an excellent outcome.

In *tractional* and *exudative retinal detachment* (TRD, ERD) there are usually no breaks in the retina; it is either pulled (tractional) or pushed (exudative) from position. Tractional detachments (p. 385) tend to be slowly progressive but may be static for long periods. Exudative detachments (p. 386) may fluctuate according to the underlying disease process.

Table 12.1 An approach to assessing retinal detachments

Visual symptoms	Asymptomatic; flashes, floaters, distortion, "curtain" field defect, ↓VA
POH	Refractive error, surgery (e.g., complicated cataract extraction), laser treatment, trauma
PMH	Connective tissue syndromes (e.g., Stickler), diabetes, anesthetic history
FH	Retinal problems or detachments, connective tissue syndromes
SH	Driver; occupation
Allergy history	Allergies or relevant drug contraindications
Visual acuity	Best-corrected/pinhole
Pupils	RAPD (if extensive RD)
Cornea	Clarity (for surgery)
AC	Cells/flare (mild activity is common)
Lens	Cataract
Tonometry	IOP may be low, normal, or high
Vitreous	Hemorrhage, pigment ("tobacco dust")
Fundus	Retinal detachment: location, extent, age (atrophy, intraretinal cysts, pigment demarcation lines), proliferative vitreoretinopathy (vitreous haze, retinal stiffness, retinal folds), retinal break(s): location, associated degeneration
Macula	On, threatened or off
Other eye	Degenerations, breaks, other disease

Indirect funduscopy with indentation of both eyes

Table 12.2 Differentiating features of retinal detachments

	RRD	**ERD**	**TRD**
Vitreous	Pigment ± blood	No pigment ± inflammatory cells	No pigment
Fluid	Fairly static	Dependent shifting fluid	Little fluid, nonshifting
Shape	Convex corrugated	Convex smooth	Concave
Retinal features	Break(s) ± degeneration	Normal or features of underlying disease	Preretinal fibrosis

Table 12.3 Differentiating features of RRD vs. retinoschisis

	RRD	**Retinoschisis**
Dome	Convex corrugated	Convex smooth
Laterality	Unilateral	Usually bilateral
Field defect	Relative	Absolute
Chronic changes	Demarcation line	No demarcation line
Breaks	Present	Absent or small inner leaf holes
Response to laser	No uptake	Good uptake

Peripheral retinal degenerations

Almost all eyes have some abnormality of the peripheral retina. Only about 1 in 40 of the population develops any form of retinal break. Identification of different types of peripheral retinal degeneration facilitates risk stratification and selective treatment of those lesions that are likely to progress (see Table 12.4).

Lattice degeneration

Lattice is present in about 6% of the normal population but in 30% of all rhegmatogenous retinal detachments. It is more common in myopes and connective tissue syndromes (e.g., Stickler).

- Areas of retinal thinning with criss-cross white lines ± small round holes within the lesion; typically circumferential but may be radial (more common in Stickler syndrome).
- Retinal tears may occur at posterior margin (due to strong vitreous adhesion) and lead to retinal detachment.

Snail track degeneration

Snail track is relatively common in myopes.

- Long circumferential areas of retinal thinning with a glistening appearance ± large round holes.
- Large round holes within the lesion may lead to retinal detachment.

Peripheral cystoid degeneration

Peripheral cystoid degeneration increases with age to become almost universal.

- Close-packed, tiny cystic spaces at the outer plexiform/inner nuclear level ± retinoschisis.

Retinoschisis (degenerative type)

Retinoschisis is present in about 5% of the normal population but is more common in hypermetropes. It is usually bilateral. It is asymptomatic unless anterior extension causes a significant field defect.

- Splitting of retina usually at outer plexiform/inner nuclear level leads to inner leaf ballooning into the vitreous cavity; usually inferotemporal and arising in areas of peripheral cystoid degeneration.
- Rarely, a combination of small inner leaf holes and the less common larger outer leaf breaks may lead to retinal detachment.

White without pressure

White without pressure is fairly common in young and heavily pigmented patients. It represents the vitreoretinal interface and is probably of no significance.

- Whitened ring of retina just anterior to the retina and underlying the vitreous base.

Snowflake degeneration

Snowflake degeneration may represent vitreous attachments to retinal Müller cells. It is probably of no significance; rare familial cases probably reflect a different process.

- Diffuse frosted appearance with white dots.

Pavingstone degeneration

Pavingstone degeneration is common with increasing age and myopia.
• Irregular patches of atrophy with absent RPE and choriocapillaris forming windows to the large choroidal vessels and sclera ± mild retinal thinning.

Cobblestone degeneration

Cobblestone degeneration is more common with increasing age and is of no significance.
• Small drusen-like bodies with pigment ring at level of Bruch's membrane.

Reticular pigmentary degeneration (honeycomb pigmentation)

Reticular pigmentary degeneration is more common with increasing age and is of no significance.
• Honeycomb pattern of peripheral pigmentation.

Meridional folds

Meridional folds do not increase risk of retinal detachment, but in cases of detachment the hole(s) may be closely related to these folds.
• Small radial fold of retina in axis of dentate process ± small hole at base.

Retinal tufts

Retinal tufts are common lesions and often associated with holes. However, they are usually within the vitreous base and thus of no significance.
• White inward projections of retina due to abnormal traction ± small holes.

Table 12.4 Peripheral retinal degenerations

Moderate risk	Low risk
Lattice	Peripheral cystoid degeneration
Snail track	Retinoschisis
	White without pressure
	Snowflake degeneration
	Pavingstone degeneration
	Cobblestone degeneration
	Reticular pigmentary degeneration
	Meridional folds
	Retinal tufts

Retinal breaks

Around 2.5% of the population has an identifiable full-thickness retinal defect (break). Since progression to retinal detachment is rare and retinopexy (laser or cryotherapy) is not without risk, attempts have been made to identify and treat only the high-risk group.

High risk may be a function of the type of break (e.g., fresh horseshoe tear associated with acute PVD), the eye (e.g., high myopia), events in the contralateral eye (e.g., giant retinal tear), or the patient as a whole (e.g., Stickler syndrome).

Hole

This is a full-thickness retinal defect due to atrophy without vitreoretinal traction. It may be associated with peripheral retinal degeneration (e.g., lattice or snail track). An operculated hole is used to denote a hole caused by PVD where the operculum has avulsed and is now free floating in the vitreous.

Tear

This is a full-thickness horseshoe-shaped defect due to PVD. It is associated with abnormal vitreous adhesions, (e.g., lattice degeneration). Ongoing vitreoretinal traction at the flap apex causes progression to RRD in at least a third of cases (see Tables 12.5 and 12.6).

Giant retinal tear

A giant retinal tear is a tear of more than 3 clock-hours in extent. They are normally located in the peripheral retina just posterior to the ora. They are associated with systemic disease (e.g., Marfan and Stickler syndromes), trauma, and high myopia.

Dialysis

This is a full-thickness circumferential break at the ora serrata. It may arise spontaneously or after trauma. It is not related to PVD. It is usually inferotemporal, but post-trauma cases may be superonasal.

Treatment of retinal breaks

Treatment is controversial. Common practice is that all horseshoe tears (especially if acute) should be treated, usually with laser photocoagulation or, less commonly, cryotherapy.

Asymptomatic small, round holes are commonly not treated. Dialyses are treated with scleral buckling if there is associated RD or with laser/cryotherapy if there is no or limited RD.

Fellow eye treatment is also controversial. In giant retinal tears the fellow eye is often treated (e.g., with 360° cryotherapy or laser retinopexy). In a case of simple RRD, lattice in the fellow eye is often not treated unless there is an additional risk factor (e.g., high myopia, aphakia, etc.).

A retinal detachment warning should be given in all cases (i.e., advise patient to seek urgent ophthalmic review if further episodes of new floaters, flashes, a "curtain" field defect, or drop in vision occur).

Table 12.5 Risk factors for RRD according to type of break

High risk	Low risk
Horseshoe tear, large hole, or dialysis	Asymptomatic small, round holes
Giant retinal tear in the other eye	Breaks within the vitreous base

Table 12.6 Risk factors for RRD according to other ocular and systemic features

Ocular	General	Trauma (blunt or penetrating) Surgery
	Refractive	Myopia
	Lenticular	Aphakia Pseudophakia (especially complicated surgery) Posterior capsulotomy
	Retinal	Lattice degeneration Retinoschisis Retinal necrosis (CMV, ARN/PORN)
	Other eye	Previous contralateral retinal detachment (especially giant retinal tear)
Systemic		Stickler syndrome Marfan syndrome Ehlers-Danlos syndrome

Posterior vitreous detachment

With age, the vitreous becomes progressively liquefied (syneresis). This results in optically empty spaces and a reduction in its shock-absorbing capability. The liquefaction process occurs earlier in myopia, trauma, inflammation, and many disorders of collagen and connective tissue.

When a break in the cortical vitreous occurs, vitreal fluid can flow through to cause separation of the vitreous and retina, with collapse of the remaining vitreous—posterior vitreous detachment (PVD). This is of significance because 1) it is very common, 2) it may be associated with a retinal tear, and 3) the symptoms are similar to retinal detachment.

Clinical features

- Flashes, floaters (usually a ring or cobwebs; the less common shower of black specks suggests hemorrhage and is often associated with a retinal tear).
- Vitreous: Weiss ring (indicates detachment at the optic disc), visible posterior hyaloid face; occasionally vitreous and optic nerve hemorrhage.
- *Complications:* retinal break(s), vitreous hemorrhage, retinal detachment.

It is critical to achieve a complete fundal examination to rule out any associated retinal breaks.

Treatment

- *Uncomplicated PVD:* reassure patient but give retinal detachment warning (i.e., advise patient to seek urgent ophthalmic evaluation if further episodes of new floaters, flashes, a "curtain" field defect, or drop in vision occur).
- *PVD complicated by vitreous hemorrhage:* clear visualization of whole retina to ora serrata is necessary to rule out breaks and early RRD. If this is not possible, then use B-scan ultrasound (Table 12.7); follow up frequently as an outpatient until hemorrhage has cleared.
- *PVD complicated by retinal tear:* treat (e.g., by laser photocoagulation; [focal argon retinopexy]).

Table 12.7 Ultrasonic features of vitreoretinal pathology

Posterior vitreous detachment	Faintly reflective posterior hyaloid face may appear incomplete except on eye movement
	Eye movement induces staccato movement with 1 sec after-movement
	Low reflectivity on A-scan
	No blood demonstrated on color flow mapping
Rhegmatogenous retinal detachment	Highly reflective irregular convex membrane
	Eye movement induces undulating after-movement (unless PVR)
	High reflectivity on A-scan.
	Blood demonstrated on color flow mapping
Tractional retinal detachment	Highly reflective membrane tented into vitreous
	Eye movement induces no after-movement of membrane
	Blood demonstrated on color flow mapping
Choroidal detachment	Highly reflective regular dome-shaped membrane
	Attached to the vortex ampulla/vein
	Blood demonstrated on color flow mapping both in retina (6–8 cm/sec) and choroid (8–10 cm/sec)
Vitreous hemorrhage	Reflective particulate matter within the vitreous space (indistinguishable from vitritis)

Rhegmatogenous retinal detachment

Rhegmatogenous retinal detachment (RRD) is usually an ophthalmic emergency. Untreated, it usually progresses to blindness and even phthisis. However, with appropriate early treatment, it may have an excellent outcome. It is the most common form of retinal detachment, with an incidence of 1/10,000/year.

RRD occurs when vitreous liquefaction and a break in the retina allows fluid to enter the subretinal space and lift the neural retina from the RPE.

Clinical features

- Flashes (usually temporal, more noticeable in dim conditions), floaters (distinct, e.g., Weiss ring, or particulate, e.g., blood), curtain-type field defect, ↓VA (suggests macula involvement).
- Vitreous: PVD + vitreal pigment ("tobacco dust") ± blood.
- Retinal break(s): usually horeshoe tear (occasionally giant, i.e., >3 clock-hours); sometimes large round holes or dialysis. The upper temporal quadrant is the most common location (60%). Identification of the primary break may be assisted by considering the effect of gravity on the subretinal fluid (Box 12.1, modified from Lincoff's rules, p. 384). However, multiple breaks are common, and a meticulous view of the whole peripheral retina is essential.
- Retinal detachment: unilateral corrugated convex dome of retina and loss of RPE/choroidal clarity; usually peripheral (subretinal fluid extends to ora serrata) but occasionally posterior polar if secondary to a macular or other posterior hole.
- Chronic changes (Table 12.8): retinal thinning, demarcation lines from 3 months, intraretinal cysts from 1 year; some develop proliferative vitreoretinopathy (Table 12.9). May have RAPD (if extensive), relative field defect, ↓IOP (but may be normal or high), and mild AC activity.

Investigation

- Consider ultrasound if unable to adequately visualize (e.g., dense cataract or hemorrhage).
- B-scan ultrasound: highly reflective irregular convex membrane; eye movement induces undulating after-movement (unless PVR).

Treatment

Urgent vitreoretinal referral

Posture patient so that dependent fluid moves away from macula: it is mainly useful for upper bullous attachments and giant retinal tears (position so tear is unfolded). Traditional posturing for superior detachments usually involves being flat on one's back with ipsilateral cheek on pillow for temporal detachments (i.e., right cheek for right eye) and contralateral cheek on pillow for nasal detachments (i.e., left cheek for right eye).

Surgery: scleral buckling and vitrectomy have advantages in different contexts. Vitrectomy is now the more commonly used procedure (around 80% cases), but there is still considerable intersurgeon variation.

Scleral buckling is suitable for most simple RRD cases; determine segmental (single breaks or multiple breaks within 1 clock-hour) vs. encircling (more extensive breaks).

Vitrectomy is indicated for retinal detachments with posterior retinal breaks, giant retinal tears, proliferative, and vitreoretinopathy but is also increasingly used for bullous retinal detachments of all types, including those with high-risk features (e.g., aphakia/pseudophakia).

Table 12.8 Features of a chronic retinal detachment

- Retinal thinning
- Demarcation lines (high water marks)
- Intraretinal cysts
- Proliferative vitreoretinopathy

Table 12.9 Proliferative vitreoretinopathy

Type	A	Vitreous haze/pigment
		± pigment on inner retina
	B	Retinal wrinkling + stiffness
	C	Rigid retinal folds ("starfolds")
Subtypes of C		
Location	Pre- vs.	Anterior
	post- equatorial	Posterior
Extent	1–12	Number of clock-hours
Contraction	Type 1	Focal
	Type 2	Diffuse
	Type 3	Subretinal
	Type 4	Circumferential
	Type 5	Anterior

Box 12.1 Locating the primary retinal break

In superior retinal detachments
- For superonasal or superotemporal detachments, the break is usually near the superior border of the detachment.
- For symmetric superior detachments crossing the vertical meridian (i.e., superonasal and superotemporal), the break is usually near 12 o'clock.

In inferior retinal detachments
- For inferior detachments, the break is usually on the side with the most fluid (i.e., the higher fluid level) BUT
    1) it may be quite inferior (i.e., not related to the superior border) and
    2) slower fluid accumulation means that non-midline breaks may still result in symmetrical inferior detachments.
- For bullous inferior detachments, break is usually above the midline.
- A peripheral track of detached retina extending superiorly from a retinal detachment will contain the primary break near its apex.

Source: Lincoff H, Gieser R (1971). *Arch Ophthalmol* 85:565–569.

Tractional retinal detachment

Tractional retinal detachment is uncommon. It arises from a combination of contracting retinal membranes, abnormal vitreoretinal adhesions, and vitreous changes. It is usually seen in the context of diseases that induce a fibrovascular response (e.g., diabetes) (see Table 12.10).

Clinical features

- Often asymptomatic; distortion (if macular involvement).
- Retinal detachment: concave tenting of retina that is immobile and usually shallow ± macular ectopia (drag); slowly progressive.
- May also have relative field defect, metamorphopsia on Amsler grid, ↓VA, and evidence of underlying disease process (e.g., diabetic retinopathy).
- *Complications:* may develop a break to become a rapidly progressive combined tractional-rhegmatogenous retinal detachment.

Treatment

Surgery is difficult and is often deferred until the macula is threatened or detached. It usually requires removal of tractional forces by vitrectomy and membrane peel, or delamination followed by tamponade with either a long-acting gas or silicone oil if needed (retinal break).

Table 12.10 Causes of tractional retinal detachments (selected)

- Proliferative diabetic retinopathy
- Retinopathy of prematurity (ROP)
- Sickle-cell retinopathy
- Vitreomacular traction syndrome
- Incontinentia pigmenti
- Retinal dysplasia
- Familial exudative vitreoretinopathy

Exudative retinal detachment

Exudative (serous) retinal detachment (ERD) is relatively rare. It arises from damage to the outer blood-retinal barrier, allowing fluid to access the subretinal space and separate retina from the RPE (see Table 12.11).

Clinical features

- Distortion and ↓VA (if macula involved), which may fluctuate; relative field defect; floaters (if uveitic).
- Retinal detachment: smooth, convex dome that may be shallow or bullous; in bullous ERDs the fluid moves rapidly to the most dependent position ("shifting fluid"); the fluid may be clear or cloudy (lipid-rich); no retinal breaks or evidence of traction.
- May also have irregular pigmentation of previously detached areas and evidence of underlying disease (e.g., abnormal Coats' vessels).

Investigation and treatment

This is directed toward the underlying disease process. All patients require a full ophthalmic and systemic examination, blood pressure, and urinalysis. Consider B-scan ultrasound, especially if posterior scleritis is suspected.

Table 12.11 Common causes of exudative retinal detachments

Congenital		Uveal effusion syndrome
		Familial exudative vitreoretinopathy
Acquired	Vascular	Exudative ARMD
		Coats' disease
		Central serous chorioretinopathy
		Vasculitis
		Malignant hypertension
		Pre-eclampsia
	Tumors	Choroidal tumors
	Inflammatory	Posterior uveitis (notably Vogt–Koyanagi–Harada syndrome (sympathetic ophthalmia)
		Posterior scleritis
		Postoperative inflammation
		Extensive panretinal photocoagulation
		Orbital cellulitis
		Idiopathic orbital inflammatory disease

Retinoschisis

Retinoschisis is by definition a splitting of the retina layers, usually occurring at the outer plexiform/inner nuclear level. Degenerative retinoschisis is common, being present in about 5% of the normal adult population.

Degenerative retinoschisis

Degenerative retinoschisis is more common in hypermetropes and is usually bilateral. In typical senile retinoschisis, the break is at the outer plexiform/inner nuclear level. In the less common reticular type, the split is at the nerve fiber layer (i.e., as in X-linked juvenile retinoschisis, p. 389).

Clinical features

- Asymptomatic (unless very posterior extension); absolute field defect.
- Retinoschisis: split retina with inner leaf ballooning into the vitreous cavity; usually inferotemporal; arises in areas of peripheral cystoid degeneration.

Complications

- Inner leaf breaks (small/round) and/or outer leaf breaks (less common; large with rolled edges).
- Retinal detachment: either low-risk limited type (outer leaf break only with fluid from the schisis cavity causing local retinal elevation) or high-risk rhegmatogenous type (inner and outer leaf breaks with retinal elevation).

Investigations

This is mainly a clinical diagnosis, but laser uptake by the posterior leaf or OCT findings can differentiate from retinal detachment (Table 12.12).

Treatment

No treatment is necessary unless retinoschisis is complicated by retinal detachment.

X-linked juvenile retinoschisis (p. 389)

This rare condition is seen in males and may present in childhood with maculopathy. It results in retinal splitting at the nerve fiber layer (cf. typical degenerative retinoschisis). Visual prognosis is poor.

Table 12.12 Differentiating retinoschisis from chronic RRD

	Retinoschisis	RRD
Vitreous	Clear	Pigment ± blood
Dome	Convex smooth	Convex corrugated
Laterality	Usually bilateral	Unilateral
Field defect	Absolute	Relative
Signs of chronicity	No demarcation line	Demarcation line
Breaks	Absent or small inner leaf holes	Present
Response to laser	Good uptake	No uptake

Hereditary vitreoretinal degenerations

These are rare, inherited conditions characterized by premature degeneration of vitreous and retina. Interestingly, the primary abnormality may be vitreal with secondary retinal changes (e.g., Stickler syndrome) or retinal with secondary vitreous abnormalities (e.g., X-linked juvenile retinoschisis).

Stickler syndrome

This condition arises from abnormalities in type II collagen (COL2A1, Ch12q) and is autosomal dominant with complete penetrance but variable expressivity. Also known as hereditary arthro-ophthalmopathy, it is the most common syndrome of this group of conditions.

Clinical features

- High myopia, optically empty vitreous, perivascular pigmentary changes (lattice-like).
- *Complications:* retinal tears, giant retinal tears, retinal detachments, cataract (comma-shaped cortical opacities), ectopia lentis, glaucoma (open-angle).
- *Systemic:* epiphyseal dysplasia → degeneration of large joints, cleft palate, bifid uvula, midfacial flattening, Pierre–Robin sequence, sensorineural deafness, mitral valve prolapse.

Investigations and treatment

Essentially this is a clinical diagnosis, although genetic testing is available. Multidisciplinary care may include genetic counseling. Treat myopia early to prevent amblyopia. Consider annual dilated funduscopy. Retinal detachments are common (up to 50%) and carry a poor prognosis.

X-linked juvenile retinoschisis

This rare condition appears to arise from abnormalities in an intercellular adhesion molecule (located on Xp22), which results in retinal splitting at the nerve fiber layer. It is seen in males and may present in early childhood with maculopathy. Visual prognosis is poor.

Clinical features

- Foveal schisis with spoke-like folds separating cystoid spaces (superficially resembles CME but no leakage on FA); later nonspecific atrophy; peripheral retinoschisis ± inner leaf breaks (may coalesce to leave free-floating retinal vessels).
- Complications: vitreous hemorrhage, retinal detachment.

Investigations

This is essentially a clinical diagnosis. Scotopic ERG shows selective loss of B-wave and oscillatory potentials. There is absolute visual field loss in schisis areas.

Treatment

There is no indication for prophylactic treatment of schisis, but combined schisis-detachment requires vitrectomy/gas (or silicone oil)/panretinal photocoagulation (PRP) and scleral buckling.

Goldmann–Favre syndrome

This very rare condition is similar to juvenile retinoschisis but is autosomal recessive with more marked peripheral abnormalities (RP-like changes with whitened retinal vessels).

Familial exudative vitreoretinopathy

This rare condition usually shows autosomal-dominant inheritance (Ch11q).

Clinical features

- Abrupt cessation of peripheral retinal vessels at the equator (more marked temporally), vitreous bands in the periphery.
- *Complications:* neovascularization, subretinal exudation (akin to Coats' disease), macular ectopia (akin to ROP), retinal detachment.

Other hereditary vitreoretinal degenerations

These include Wagner syndrome, erosive vitreoretinopathy, Knobloch syndrome, Goldmann–Favre syndrome, autosomal-dominant neovascular inflammatory vitreoretinopathy, and autosomal-dominant vitreoretinochoroidopthy.

Choroidal detachments and uveal effusion syndrome

Choroidal detachments

Choroidal detachments are usually seen in the context of acute hypotony, for example, after glaucoma filtration surgery or cyclodestructive procedures (Table 12.13). They are usually easily distinguished from retinal detachments (Table 12.14).

Clinical features

There is a smooth convex dome(s) of normal or slightly dark retinal color; it arises from extreme periphery (may include ciliary body, and ora serrata becomes easily visible), but posterior extension is limited by vortex vein adhesions to the scleral canals. Choroidal detachments may touch ("kissing choroidals").

Treatment

Management is either by observation (e.g., if this reflects an appropriate post-trabeculectomy fall in IOP) or by treating the underlying disease process. Choroidal hemorrhage may require surgical drainage.

Uveal effusion syndrome

This is a rare syndrome arising from impaired posterior segment drainage associated with scleral thickening.

Clinical features

There are combined choroidal detachments and exudative retinal detachments.

Treatment

Surgery: scleral windows may decompress the vortex veins.

Table 12.13 Common causes of choroidal detachment

Effusion	Hypotony
	Extensive PRP
	Extensive cryotherapy
	Posterior uveitis
	Uveal effusion syndrome
	Nanophthalmos
Hemorrhage	Intraoperative
	Trauma
	Spontaneous

Table 12.14 RRD vs. choroidal detachment

	RRD	**Choroidal detachment**
Color	Pale	Darker/normal color
Dome	Convex corrugated	Convex smooth
Breaks	Present	Absent
Ora serrata	Visible with indentation	Easily visible
Maximal extent	Anterior: ora serrata Posterior: unlimited	Anterior: ciliary body Posterior: vortex veins

Epiretinal membranes

Common synonyms for the disease reflect its appearance (macular pucker, cellophane maculopathy) and uncertain pathogenesis (premacular fibrosis, idiopathic premacular gliosis). The condition is more common with increasing age (present in 6% of those over 50 years), in females, and after retinal insults (Box 12.2).

The membranes are fibrocellular and avascular and are thought to arise from the proliferation of retinal glial cells that have migrated through defects in the internal limiting membrane (ILM); such defects probably arise most commonly during posterior vitreous detachment.

Clinical features

- Asymptomatic, metamorphopsia, ↓VA.
- Membrane may be transparent (look for glistening light reflex), translucent or white; retinal striae; vessels may be tortuous, straightened, or obscured; pseudohole. The features are well demonstrated on red-free light.
- *Complications:* fovea ectopia; tractional macular detachment; CME; intra- or preretinal hemorrhages.

Investigations

- OCT is not usually required, but may differentiate pseudo- vs. true hole and the thickness of membrane.
- FA is not essential but nicely demonstrates vascular abnormalities and any associated CME. Some surgeons compare pre- and postoperative FA.

Treatment

- *Indications:* severely symptomatic membranes; ensure that macular function is not limited by an additional underlying pathology (e.g., ischemia due to a vein occlusion).
- *Surgery:* vitrectomy/membrane peel; some surgeons assist visualization by staining with triamcinolone acetonide or indocyanine green.
- *Complications:* cataract (up to 70% rate of significant nuclear sclerosis within 2 years), retinal tears/detachment, worsened acuity (up to 15%), and symptomatic recurrence (5%).

Prognosis

The disease is fairly stable, with over 75% patients showing no further reduction in VA after diagnosis. With surgery, 60–85% patients show visual improvement (≥2 Snellen lines).

Poor prognostic features are duration of symptoms before surgery, underlying macular pathology, and lower preoperative acuity (but may still show significant improvement).

Box 12.2 Causes of epiretinal membranes

- Idiopathic
- Retinal detachment surgery
- Cryotherapy
- Photocoagulation
- Trauma (blunt or penetrating)
- Posterior uveitis
- Persistent vitreous hemorrhage
- Retinal vascular disease (e.g., BRVO)

Macular hole

The incidence of macular hole is around 1/10,000/year; it is more common in women (2:1 F:M) and has a mean age of onset of 65 years. In some cases, a predisposing pathological condition is identified (Box 12.3).

In the remaining idiopathic cases, abnormal vitreomacular traction may be observed clinically and with OCT. Release of this traction appears to underlie the success of vitrectomy in treating this condition.

Staging

The developing macular hole may initially be asymptomatic but can cause a progressive drop in acuity to around 20/200. Worsening acuity approximately correlates with the pathological stages described by Gass.

Clinical features

- Stage 1: no sensory retinal defect.
  - a: small yellow foveolar spot ± loss of foveal contour.
  - b: yellow foveolar ring.
- Stage 2: small (100–200 μm) full-thickness sensory retinal defect.
- Stage 3: larger (>400 μm) full-thickness sensory retinal defect with cuff of subretinal fluid ± yellow deposits in base of hole.
- Stage 4: as for stage 3 but with complete vitreous separation.
- Watzke–Allen test (thin beam of light projected across the hole is seen to be broken) may help differentiate between pseudo- and lamellar holes.

Investigations

OCT may assist diagnosis and staging where required.
FA is not usually indicated, but usually shows a window defect.

Treatment

- Refer to vitreoretinal surgeon; delay affects surgical outcome (worse results if present >6 months).
- *Surgery:* vitrectomy, ILM peel, and gas (will require face-down posturing). Adjunctive agents such as autologous serum/platelets may be used.
- *Complications:* cataracts (50% rate of significant nuclear sclerosis within 2 years), retinal tears or detachment (around 1%), failure (anatomical up to 10%; visual up to 20%), late reopening of hole (5%) and endophthalmitis.

Prognosis

Stage 1 holes spontaneously resolve in 50% of cases. Without surgery, stage 2 holes almost always progress, resulting in final VA of around 20/200. With surgery, early stage 2 holes show anatomical closure in >90% and visual success (≥2 Snellen lines) in 80%. Around 10–20% develop a macular hole in the other eye.

Box 12.3 Causes of macular holes

- Idiopathic
- Trauma
- CME
- Epiretinal membrane/vitreomacular traction syndrome
- Retinal detachment (rhegmatogenous)
- Laser injury
- Pathological myopia (with posterior staphyloma)
- Hypertension
- Diabetic retinopathy

Laser retinopexy and cryopexy for retinal tears

Laser retinopexy (slit lamp or indirect delivery systems)

Mechanism

Laser light is absorbed by target tissue, generating heat and causing local protein denaturation (photocoagulation) adhering the neural retina to the RPE. Green light is mainly absorbed by melanin and hemoglobin.

Indication

- Retinal break with risk of progression to rhegmatogenous retinal detachment (usually horseshoe tears) and without excessive subretinal fluid.
- Equatorial and postequatorial lesions can be reached with a slit-lamp delivery system; more anterior lesions require indirect laser with indentation or cryotherapy.

Method

- *Consent*: explain what the procedure does, the likely success rate (around 80%), and possible complications, including the need for retreatment (around 20%), and possible detachment despite treatment (9%, half of which are from a different break).
- *Ensure maximal dilation* (e.g., tropicamide 1% + phenylephrine 2.5%) and topical anesthesia (e.g., proparacaine 1%).

Slit lamp

- *Set laser* (varies according to model): commonly spot size of 500 μm, duration 0.1 sec, and low initial power, e.g., 100 mW.
- *Position contact lens* (usually a wide field lens e.g., transequator or the 3-mirror; require coupling agent).
- *Focus and fire laser* to generate 2–3 rings of confluent gray-white burns (adjust power appropriately).

Indirect ophthalmoscope

- *Set laser* (varies according to model): commonly duration 0.1 sec and low power, e.g., 100 mW.
- *Insert speculum* and coat cornea with hydroxypropylmethylcellulose or ensure regular irrigation to maintain clarity.
- While *viewing* with indirect ophthalmoscope, gently indent to clearly visualize lesion.
- *Focus and fire laser* to generate 2–3 rings of confluent gray-white burns (adjust power appropriately).
- *Complications*: failure resulting in retinal detachment, retinal/vitreous hemorrhage, epiretinal membrane formation, CME.

Cryopexy

Mechanism

Freezing causes local protein denaturation adhering the neural retina to the RPE.

Indication
- Retinal break with risk of progression to rhegmatogenous retinal detachment (usually horseshoe tears) and without excessive subretinal fluid.
- Cryotherapy is most suitable for pre-equatorial lesions. It has advantages over laser retinopexy when there is a small pupil or media opacity.

Method
- *Consent*: explain what the procedure does, the likely success rate, and possible complications, including treatment failure or need for retreatment, discomfort, inflammation, and retinal/choroidal detachment.
- *Ensure maximal dilation* (e.g., tropicamide 1% + phenylephrine 2.5%).
- *Give local anesthesia* (e.g., by subconjunctival or retrobulbar injection as this preserves mobility).
- *Insert speculum* and coat cornea with hydroxypropylmethylcellulose or ensure regular irrigation to maintain clarity.
- While *viewing* with indirect ophthalmoscope, gently indent with the cryoprobe to clearly visualize lesion.
- *Surround* the break with a single continuous ring of applications. The duration of each application should be just long enough for the retina to whiten, but the probe should not be removed until thawing has occurred.
- *Post-procedure*: consider mild topical steroid/antibiotic combination.
- *Complications*: inflammation, failure resulting in retinal detachment, retinal/vitreous hemorrhage, epiretinal membrane formation.

Scleral buckling procedures

Scleral buckling

Mechanism

It is suggested that the buckle closes the break by multiple mechanisms, including moving the RPE closer to the retina and moving the retina closer to the posterior vitreous cortex. It is postulated that these may reduce flow through the break (including the amount of fluid pumped through during eye movements) and relieve vitreous traction on flap tears.

Indications

- *Most simple RRD and dialysis:* procedure of choice in situations where there is no pre-existing PVD, since a vitrectomy would require the induction of a PVD during surgery (highly difficult maneuver).
- *Segmental buckles:* for single breaks or multiple breaks within 1 clock-hour.
- *Encircling bands:* traditionally for extensive or multiple breaks or breaks in the presence of high-risk features (e.g., aphakia/pseudophakia, etc); however the majority of these would now have a vitrectomy.

Method

- *Consent:* explain what the operation does and the possible complications, including failure, diplopia, refractive change, inflammation, infection, hemorrhage, explant extrusion, and worsened vision.

Perform appropriate conjunctival peritomy

- *Inspect sclera* for thinning and anomalous vortex veins; place traction sutures around selected rectus muscles to assist positioning.
- *Identify break* by indirect ophthalmoscope and indentation using the cryoprobe (or one of a number of instruments specifically designed for this purpose).
- *Perform cryopexy* by surrounding break(s) with a continuous ring of applications. Each application should last just long enough for the retina to whiten; the probe should not be removed until thawing has occurred. Mark the external position of the break on the sclera using indentation and a marker pen.
- *Select buckle size:* this should cover double the width of the retinal tear; position so that it extends from ora serrata to cover the posterior lip of the break.
- *Place partial-thickness 5–0 nonabsorbable sutures* using a spatulated needle. These are usually mattress-type sutures and are placed at least 1 mm away from the buckle on either side. Wider separation of sutures may result in a higher buckle. The number of sutures depends on the size of explant.
- *Tighten sutures.* Tighter sutures results in a higher buckle.
- *Confirm buckle position* is correct and that arterial perfusion of the optic nerve is unaffected.
- *Close conjunctiva* (e.g., with 7–0 absorbable suture).

Complications
- *Intraoperative:* scleral perforation, subretinal fluid (SRF) drainage problems (retinal incarceration, choroidal/subretinal hemorrhage).
- *Postoperative:* infection, glaucoma, extrusion, choroidal effusion/detachment, epiretinal membrane, CME, diplopia, refractive change, diplopia.

Prognosis
Anatomical success >90%, but only around 50% achieve a VA of 20/50 (macula-on detachments).

Options
Choice of buckle

Table 12.15 Buckle options

Material	Solid silicone rubber vs. Silicone sponge
Orientation	Segmental vs. encircling
Size	Wide range available (and can be cut to size)

Drainage procedures
Trans-scleral drainage of subretinal fluid with a 27–30 gauge needle is possible but is generally not necessary. This is sometimes combined with the injection of intravitreal air in the DACE (drain-air-cryotherapy-explant) procedure.

Vitrectomy: outline

Vitrectomy

Mechanism

Vitrectomy removes dynamic tractional forces exerted on the retina; static tractional forces arising from membranes/fibrovascular proliferation can be removed at the same time. Vitrectomy also allows access to the retina to permit drainage of subretinal fluid and insertion of tamponade agents.

Indications

Retinal detachments

- RRD: traditionally reserved for those with posterior retinal breaks, giant retinal tears, proliferative vitreoretinopathy, or media opacity; now usage is widened to include most bullous detachments, and detachments associated with aphakia/pseuodophakia (or other higher-risk features).
- TRD.

Other

- Diagnostic: e.g., biopsy for endophthalmitis, lymphoma.
- Pharmacological: e.g., administration of antibiotics, steroids.
- Macular pathology: macular holes, epiretinal membranes.
- Trauma: e.g., removal of foreign body.
- Persistent media opacity: vitreous hemorrhage, inflammatory debris, floaters (severe).
- Complications of cataract surgery: dropped nucleus, dislocated IOL.

Method

- *Consent:* explain what the operation does, the presence of a postoperative gas bubble, the importance of posturing, and possible complications, including failure, inflammation, infection, hemorrhage, and worsened vision.
- *Make 3 sclerostomies* 4 mm (phakic) or 3.5 mm (aphakic/pseudophakic) behind the limbus, placed inferotemporally, superotemporaly, and superonasally.
- *Secure the infusion cannula* to the inferotemporal port. The infusion is used to both maintain the globe (thus permitting aspiration) and increase pressure if intraocular bleeding occurs.
- *Insert the light-pipe and then the vitrector* through the two superior ports under visualization (contact lens or indirect microscope system with inverter).
- *Vitrectomy:* of the posterior vitreous face and extending out to the periphery.
- *Replace the infusion fluid with a tamponade agent* (usually gas, sometimes silicone oil for complicated cases).
- *Close the sclerostomies.*
- *Postoperative care:* advise patient regarding posturing and warn against air travel until gas is resorbed.

Complications
- *Intraoperative:* retinal breaks (posterior, peripheral), choroidal hemorrhage.
- *Postoperative:* retinal breaks/RRD, cataract, glaucoma, inflammation, endophthalmitis (1/2000), hypotony, corneal decompensation, sympathetic ophthalmia (0.01% of routine vitrectomy).
- *Tamponade gas-associated:* ↑IOP, posterior subcapsular "feathering" of the lens, anterior IOL movement (if pseudophakic).
- *Silicone oil-associated:* ↑IOP, emulsified silicone oil ("inverse hypopyon"), adherence to silicone IOL, silicone oil keratopathy (if oil in AC), peri-oil fibrosis.

Prognosis
Anatomical success for simple RRD is >90%.

Vitrectomy: heavy liquids and tamponade agents

Perfluorocarbon ("heavy") liquids

- *Indications:* these may be useful in repositioning of giant retinal tears, in flattening PVR-associated retina, in floating up dislocated lens fragments or IOLs, and in assisting hemostasis.

Agents
Perfluoro-*n*-octane is the most commonly used agent.

Tamponade

Indications

- *Simple retinal detachment:* consider air or SF6/air mix.
- *Complicated retinal detachment* (e.g., PVR, giant retinal tear, multiple recurrences): consider C3F8/air mix or silicone oil. Overall, these are similarly effective in PVR, although silicone oil is associated with better final VA in anterior disease, requires no postoperative posturing, and allows easier intraoperative and immediate postoperative visualization.

When vitrectomy has been performed for indications other than RD, there may be no need for tamponade.

Agents

Table 12.16 Common tamponade agents

Agent	Symbol	Expansion if 100%	Nonexpansile concentration (mixed with air)	Duration
Air	Air	None	100%	≤1 week
Sulfur hexafluoride	SF6	×2	20%	1–2 weeks
Perfluoropropane	C3F8	×4	12%	8–10 weeks
Silicone oil	Si oil	None	100%	Until removal

Complications

↑IOP (may be related to overfill), posterior subcapsular "feathering" of the lens, anterior IOL movement (if pseudophakic).

Posturing

The aim of postoperative posturing by the patient is to achieve effective tamponade of the break by the gas bubble and keep the gas bubble away from the crystalline lens. Posturing should start as soon as possible (same day of surgery), for as much of each day as possible (commonly 50 min in every hour, and adopt appropriate sleeping posture), and continues for ~2 weeks (with some variation according to tamponade agent).

The posture required will depend on the location of the retinal break but aims to move the break as superiorly as possible. Advise patient not to fly until the gas bubble has resolved.

Medical retina

Anatomy and physiology

The retina is a remarkable modification of the embryonic forebrain that gathers light, codes the information as an electrical signal (transduces), and transmits it via the optic nerve to the processing areas of the brain.

Embryologically, it is derived from the optic vesicle (neuroectoderm), with an outer wall that becomes the retinal pigment epithelium, a potential space (the subretinal space), and an inner wall that becomes the neural retina.

Anatomy

Retinal pigment epithelium (RPE)

The RPE is a monolayer of hexagonal cells. The apices form microvilli that envelop the photoreceptor outer segments. Near the apices, adjacent RPE cells are joined by numerous tight junctions to form the outer blood–retinal barrier.

The base of the RPE is crenellated (to increase surface area) and mitochondrion rich. The basement membrane of the RPE forms the inner layer of Bruch's membrane. Anteriorly, the RPE is continuous with the pigmented layer of the ciliary body.

Neural retina

This is a 150–400 μm thick layer of transparent neural tissue, comprising photoreceptors (rods, cones), integrators (bipolar, horizontal, amacrine ganglion cells), the output pathway (nerve fiber layer), and the support cells (Müller cells). Anteriorly, the neural retina is continuous with the nonpigmented layer of the ciliary body.

The macula is defined histologically by a multilayered ganglion cell layer (i.e., more than one cell thick) and approximates to a 5500 μm oval centered on the fovea and bordered by the temporal arcades. It is yellowish from the presence of xanthophyll. The macula is further divided into perifovea (1500 μm wide band defined by 6 layers of bipolar cells), parafovea (500 μm wide band defined by 7–11 layers of bipolar cells), and fovea (1500 μm diameter circular depression). The fovea comprises a rim, a 22 slope, and a central floor, the foveola (350 μm diameter, 150 μm thin). The umbo is the center of the foveola (150 μm diameter); maximal cone density equates to highest acuity.

Blood supply

Branches of the ophthalmic artery include the central retinal artery, which supplies retinal circulation, and the three posterior ciliary arteries, which provide choroidal circulation. Anatomically, the retinal circulation supports the inner two-thirds of the retina, whereas the choroidal circulation supports the outer third; the watershed is at the outer plexiform layer. Physiologically, this equates to two-thirds of the retina's oxygen and nutrient requirements being supplied by the choroidal circulation.

The retinal circulation comprises a small part of ocular blood flow (5%) but with a high level of oxygen extraction (40% arteriovenous difference), contrasting with figures of 85% and 5% for the choroidal circulation. In the retinal circulation, the arterial branches lie in the nerve fiber layer but give rise to both an inner capillary network (ganglion cell layer) and an outer capillary network (inner nuclear layer). However, there are no capillaries in the central 500 μm, the foveal avascular zone (FAZ).

The outer blood–retinal barrier is formed by the tight junctions of the RPE cells, whereas the inner is formed by the nonfenestrated endothelium of the retinal capillaries.

Physiology

RPE

The RPE is vital to the normal function of the neural retina. Functions include maintenance of the outer blood–retinal barrier, maintenance of retinal adhesion, nutrient supply to the photoreceptors, absorption of scattered excess light (by melanosomes), production and recycling of photopigments, and phagocytosis of damaged photoreceptor discs (each sheds >100 discs per day).

Neural retina

Each human eye contains around 120 million rods and 6.5 million cones. The rods subserve peripheral and low-light (scotopic) vision, whereas the cones permit normal (photopic), central, and color vision. The rods reach their highest density at 20° from the fovea, in contrast to blue cones, which are densest in the perifovea, and red and green cones, which are densest (up to $385,000/mm^2$) at the umbo.

The outer segments of photoreceptors contain transmembrane photopigment molecules (rhodopsin in rods, iodopsins in cones) that undergo *cis-trans* isomerization on absorption of a photon of light (440–450 nm for blue, 535–555 nm for green, and 570–590 nm for red cones).

Activation of a single photopigment molecule starts a cascade of activation (transducin activates phosphodiesterase which in turn hydrolyses cGMP) with 100-fold amplification at every stage. Falling cGMP levels cause closure of Na channels, with photoreceptor hyperpolarization. The resting potential is then restored by the action of recoverin, which activates guanylate cyclase to cGMP and reopen Na channels.

Rods synapse with "on" bipolar cells, which in turn synapse with amacrine and ganglion cells. Cones synapse with "on" and "off" bipolar cells, which in turn synapse with "on" and "off" ganglion cells. Negative feedback is provided by the laterally interacting horizontal cells (between photoreceptors) and amacrine cells (between bipolar cells and ganglion cells). This contributes to the center-surround phenomenon exhibited by ganglion cells in which they are activated by stimulation in the center of their receptive field but inhibited by stimulation of the surround. Ganglion cell representation is maximal at the fovea, where the cone: ganglion cell ratio approaches 1:1.

Ganglion cells are divided into two main populations. The parvocellular system subserves fine visual acuity and color. These cells are mainly foveal, have small receptive fields, and show spectral sensitivity. The magnocellular system subserves motion detection and coarser form vision. These ganglion cells are mainly peripheral, have larger receptive fields and high luminance and contrast (but no spectral) sensitivity, and are sensitive to motion. This division is preserved in the lateral geniculate nucleus (layers 1–2 magnocellular, 3–6 parvocellular) and visual cortex.

Age-related macular degeneration (1)

Age-related macular degeneration (AMD) is the leading cause of blindness for those over age 50 in the Western world. Its prevalence increases with age. Estimates vary according to the exact definition of AMD. One study found visually significant disease (VA ≤20/30) in around 1% for age 55–65 years, 6% for 65–75 years, and 20% for >75 years.

Drusen (not necessarily with ↓VA) are increasingly common with age. Other risk factors include gender (female > male), ethnic origin (white >> black), diet, cardiovascular risk, smoking, pigmentary changes in the macula, family history of macular degeneration, and hypermetropia.

Non-neovascular (dry) AMD

Accounting for 90% of AMD, this tends to lead to gradual but potentially significant reduction in central vision. It is characterized by drusen (hard or soft) and RPE changes (focal hyperpigmentation or atrophy).

Histology

There is a gradual loss of the RPE/photoreceptor layers, thinning of the outer plexiform layer, thickening of Bruch's membrane, and atrophy of choriocapillaris, exposing the larger choroidal vessels on examination.

Drusen are PAS-positive amorphous deposits lying between the RPE membrane and the inner collagenous layer of Bruch's membrane; they may become calcified. Additional abnormal basement membrane deposit lies between the RPE membrane and RPE cells; it is not visible clinically.

Clinical features

- ↓VA, metamorphopsia, scotomas; usually gradual in onset.
- Hard drusen (small, well-defined, of limited significance), soft drusen (larger, poorly defined, increased risk of CNV), RPE focal hyperpigmentation, RPE atrophy ("geographic" if well-demarcated) (see Fig. 13.1).

Investigation

FA is not usually necessary. Fundus autofluorescence is useful for delineating the area of disease and following disease progression.

Treatment

- *Supportive:* low vision aid counseling, and linking to support group and social services.
- *Refraction:* with increased near-add; low-vision aid assessment and provision are often best arranged in a dedicated low-vision clinic.
- *Intraocular telescope:* implantable telescope after cataract extraction can provide patients with moderate disease an enlarge image for reading daily activities within a 3 meters range; patient selection is highly important for this procedure.
- *Amsler grid:* regular use of an Amsler grid allows the patient to detect new or progressive metamorphopsia, prompting him/her to seek ophthalmologic examination.
- *Lifestyle changes:* vitamin supplementation (AREDS formula) and smoking cessation may slow progression.

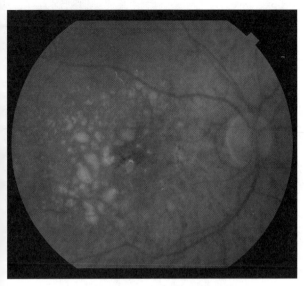

Figure 13.1 Severe dry AMD with extensive area of large confluent drusen, pigmentary changes, and early RPE atrophy. See insert for color version.

Age-related macular degeneration (2)

Neovascular (wet) AMD

Although much less common, neovascular AMD leads to rapid and severe loss of vision. It accounts for up to 90% of legal blindness due to AMD.

Histology

New fragile capillaries grow from the choriocapillaris through the damaged Bruch's membrane and proliferate in the sub-RPE (type I membranes) and/or subretinal space (type 2 membranes). There may be associated hemorrhage, exudation, retina or RPE detachment, or scar formation.

Type I membranes are more common in AMD with diffuse RPE and Bruch's membrane disease; type 2 are more common in younger patients with focal disease of the RPE and Bruch's membrane (e.g., with POHS).

Clinical features

- ↓VA, metamorphopsia, scotoma; may be sudden in onset.
- A gray membrane is sometimes visible; more commonly, it is deduced from associated signs, including subretinal (red) or sub-RPE (gray) hemorrhage (Fig. 13.2), subretinal/sub-RPE exudation, retinal or pigment epithelial detachment, CME, or subretinal fibrosis (disciform scar).

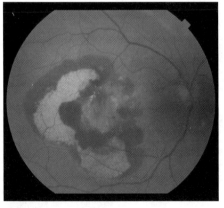

Figure 13.2 Neovascular AMD with a large choroidal neovascular complex and extensive subretinal and sub-RPE hemorrhage. See insert for color version.

Investigation

Urgent FA is vital for accurate diagnosis and plan for treatment.

- Classic choroidal neovascular membrane (CNV): early well-demarcated lacy hyperfluorescence with progressive leakage (Fig. 13.3).
- Occult CNV type I: fibrovascular pigment epithelial detachment seen as irregular elevation (on stereoscopic view) with stippled pinpoint hyperfluorescence beginning at 1–2 min post-injection (Fig. 13.4).
- Occult CNV type II: late leakage of undetermined source, poorly demarcated hyperfluorescence 5–10 min post-injection.

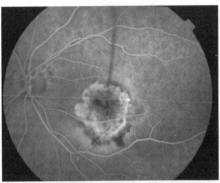

Early phase: well-demarcted lacy hyperfluorescence

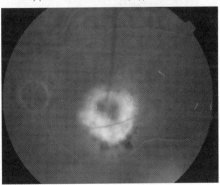

Late phase: progressive lakage

Figure 13.3 FA of classic choroidal neovascular membrane.

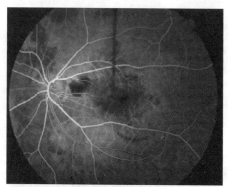

Early phase: stippled hyperfluorescence usually maximal at 1–2 min
masking by blood adjacent to disc

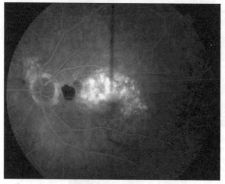

Late phase: progressive leakage

Figure 13.4 FA of occult choroidal neovascular membrane.

Treatment

Supportive

Offer counseling, refraction, Amsler grid, and low-vision aids and encourage lifestyle changes as for non-neovascular AMD.

Laser photocoagulation (usually argon green)

- Extrafoveal CNV—if well demarcated, treat with confluent burns over the whole lesion and up to 100 µm beyond its circumference.
- Juxtafoveal CNV—if well demarcated, treat the parts away from the fovea as for extrafoveal CNV (i.e., up to 100 µm beyond the lesion), but on the foveal side only treat up to the perimeter of the lesion. Consider anti-VEGF and PDT if this cannot be performed without significant risk to the fovea.

Photodynamic therapy (PDT)

For subfoveal CNV, if it is 100% classic or predominantly classic, then treat with photodynamic therapy. Also consider PDT for 100% occult lesions if CNV ≤4 DD in size and/or with a recent decrease in VA.

Anti-VEGF therapy

The two most commonly injected anti-VEGF drugs are ranibizumab (Lucentis) and bevacizumab (Avastin). Ranibizumab (Lucentis) is an FDA-approved murine antigen-binding (Fab) antibody fragment with high affinity for all isoforms of VEGF molecule. Bevacizumab is the full-length antibody for the VEGF molecule.

Ranibizumab is a humanized agent and further affinity maturated, giving ranibizumab a 20-fold higher binding affinity than that of bevacizumab. In the ANCHOR and MARINA clinical trials, intravitreal injections of ranibizumab helped 34–40% of patients with neovascular AMD regain vision. This benefit was sustained over the course of the 2-year study. This data was significantly better than the results achieved with PDT and intravitreal pegaptanib (Macugen).

Age-related macular degeneration (3)

Differential diagnosis of CNV

Table 13.1 Common causes of CNV

Degenerative	AMD
	Pathological myopia (lacquer crack)
	Angioid streaks
Trauma	Choroidal rupture
	Laser
Inflammation	POHS
	Multifocal choroiditis
	Serpiginous choroidopathy
	Bird-shot retinochoroidopathy
	Punctate inner choroidopathy
	VKH
Dystrophies	Best's disease
Other	Chorioretinal scar (any cause)
	Tumor
Idiopathic	

Anti-VEGF therapy

Pegaptanib (Macugen) was the first FDA-approved anti-VEGF agent for the treatment of neovascular AMD. The drug is a 28-base ribonucleixribo-nucleotide aptamer, with high affinity for VEGF165 isoform. Two concurrent clinical trials (VISION trials) demonstrated that 70% of pegaptanib vs. 55% of sham injections lose <15 letters of visual acuity at 1 year. On average, the patient during the first 2 years of treatment continues to lose vision, although at a significantly slower rate.

Two additional anti-VEGF drugs are used for treatment of neovascular AMD, the FDA-approved ranibizumab and the off-label parent antibody molecule bevacizumab. Ranibizumab may offer several theoretical advantages over bevacizumab, such as deeper penetration of the retina (smaller molecule), higher binding affinity, and being less immunogenic. These theoretical advantages have yet to be proven in clinical application.

Any differences between the two anti-VEGF agents are likely to be small and may be demonstrated by the results of the ongoing CATT (Comparison of AMD Treatment Trial) study. Several phase III clinical trials (ANCHOR, MARINA, PIER) have demonstrated excellent success using ranibizumab to treat all angiographic forms of AMD. Exciting results included average increase of 6.5 ETDRS letters of improvement in 2 years of follow-up; 1 of 3 patients experienced improvement of 3 or more lines of vision at 2 years.

Risk of intravitreal anti-VEGF injections

- Vitreous hemorrhage.
- Intraocular inflammation (pseudo-endophthalmitis).
- Infectious endophthalmitis.
- Increase IOP.
- Retinal detachment.
- Traumatic cataract.
- Theoretical risk of systemic vascular thrombosis.

Intravitreal injection of bevacizumab and ran-bizumab

- Discus with the patient the risks and benefits of the procedure and obtain informed consent.

Procedure

- Prepare the injection in a sterile environment.
- Provide anesthesia (topical anesthesia, subconjunctival anesthesia).
- Prepare the surgical area, including the eyelid, with 50% betadine.
- Instill 50% betadine into the fornix.
- Measure with caliper the location of the injection (3 mm in pseu-dophakic, 4 mm in phakic patients).
- Firmly grasp the conjunctiva and inject 0.05cc of bevacizumab or ranbizumab.
- Confirm arterial perfusion by vision evaluation or IOP check.
- Give postoperative antibiotics per physician preference.

Photodynamic therapy (PDT)

Photodynamic therapy describes the laser stimulation of a photoactivated dye that results in the production of free radicals and the occlusion of choroidal neovascular membranes (CNV). The aim of this technique is to selectively destroy the membrane while minimizing damage to the retina above or to the RPE and to choroid below.

The most common indication is AMD, but it may be used for other choroidal neovascular membranes (e.g., in myopia, inflammatory membranes).

Mechanism

Verteporfin is a photoactivated dye that binds to lipoproteins and becomes concentrated in the proliferating vascular bed of the CNV. Laser light of 689 nm wavelength is directed onto the CNV, thereby activating the dye.

The energy level used (600 mW/cm^2 x 83 sec = 50 J/cm^2) is too low to cause thermal damage but is sufficient to activate the dye, which catalyses the formation of the free-radical "singlet oxygen." This causes local endothelial cell death and occlusion of the blood supply to the CNV.

PDT in practice

In advance

Discuss with the patient the procedure and obtain informed consent. Explain its purpose (to slow progression of disease) and risks and the practicalities, such as what protective clothing to wear (Box 13.1).

On day of procedure

- Calculate spot size (greatest linear diameter + 1000 μm).
- Confirm informed consent—purpose, risks (Box 13.1).
- Ensure safety precautions (hat, long sleeves, resuscitation equipment is available).
- Insert IV cannula in a large vein (e.g., antecubital fossa).
- Reconstitute 15 mg powder with 7 mL water for injections to produce a 2 mg/mL solution, then dilute requisite dose (6 mg/m^2 body surface area) with glucose 5% to a final volume of 30 mL and give over 10 min.
- At 15 min since start of infusion, start 83 sec of laser (689 nm, variable spot size, 600 mW/cm^2).

Follow-up

Review with FA at 12 weeks. If recurrent leakage occurs, PDT may be performed up to 4 times/year. If severe ↓VA of ≥4 lines occurs within 1 week of treatment do not retreat unless VA returns to a pretreatment level.

Evidence for PDT in subfoveal CNV due to AMD

Predominantly classic CNV (include classic with no occult)

Treatment benefit demonstrated in the TAP (Treatment of AMD with Photodynamic therapy) study is as follows:
- TAP1: fewer than 15 letters lost in 67% vs. 39% at 1 year ($p < 0.001$)
- TAP2: fewer than 15 letters lost in 59% vs. 31% at 2 years ($p < 0.001$)

Minimally classic CNV

There is emerging evidence for treatment benefit in those cases where there is documented progression of lesion (↑lesion size on FA or ↓VA).

100% occult CNV

Treatment benefit demonstrated (mainly for small lesions or worse VA) in the VIP (Verteporfin in Photodynamic therapy) study was overall. The TAP study showed a trend toward benefit.

- VIP2: fewer than 15 letters lost in 45% vs. 32% at 1 year ($p = 0.03$); subgroup analysis suggests that the main benefit is for smaller lesions (<4 disc areas) or worse VA (<20/50).
- TAP2: fewer than 15 letters lost in 56% vs. 30% at 2 years ($p = 0.06$)

Evidence for PDT in subfoveal CNV due to myopia

Treatment benefit was overall; most lesions were predominantly classic. It is unclear whether there is benefit for minimally classic or occult lesions.

- VIP1: fewer than 8 letters lost in 72% vs. 44% at 1 year ($p < 0.01$)

Box 13.1 Patient advice regarding PDT

Side effects

- Injection-site reactions: inflammation, leakage, hypersensitivity
- Back pain: 2%
- Transient visual disturbances
- Significant visual loss: up to 4%

Contraindications

- Liver failure
- Porphyria
- Allergy to any of the components

Advice to patient

For 48 hours post-PDT, avoid direct sunlight and bright lights (including solaria, halogen, or strip-lights and undraped windows). If it is necessary to go outside during daylight hours (e.g., returning from PDT clinic), wear a wide-brimmed hat, sunglasses, long-sleeved shirt, trousers, and socks.

Diabetic eye disease: general

Diabetes mellitus is estimated to affect 200 million people worldwide. It is the most common cause of blindness in the working population, being associated with a 20-fold increase in blindness.

The World Health Organization (WHO) divides diabetes into type I (insulin dependent) and type II (non–insulin dependent). Type I is typically of juvenile onset and is characterized by insulin deficiency. Type II is typically of adult or elderly onset and is characterized by insulin resistance.

Clinical features

Systemic disease

Presentation

- Type I: acutely with diabetic ketoacidosis (DKA) or subacutely with weight loss, polyuria, polydipsia, fatigue.
- Type II: incidental finding (may have long asymptomatic period); or symptoms of weight loss, polyuria, polydipsia, fatigue; or complications.

Systemic complications

- Macrovascular: myocardial infarction (3–5× risk), peripheral vascular disease, stroke (>2× risk).
- Microvascular: nephropathy, neuropathy.

Ophthalmic

- *Retinopathy and sequelae:* risk varies according to type of disease (I vs. II), duration of disease, glycemic control, hypertension, hypercholesterolemia, nephropathy, pregnancy, and possibly intraocular surgery. In type I diabetes, retinopathy is rare at diagnosis but present in over 90% after 15 years. In type II disease, retinopathy is present in 20% at diagnosis but only rises to 60% after 15 years.
- Cataract occurs at a younger age and can progress quickly.
- *Other:* numerous ocular conditions occur more frequently in diabetes, including dry eye, corneal abrasions, anterior uveitis, rubeosis, neovascular glaucoma, ocular ischemic syndrome, papillitis, AION, orbital infection, and cranial nerve palsies (pp. 547–553).

Diagnosis

- Random plasma glucose level >200 mg/dL.
- Fasting plasma glucose >126 mg/dL.
- Oral glucose tolerance test (usually performed by physician) with a 2-hour value of >200 mg/dL.
- Hemoglobin A1c > 6.5%.

DCCT and UKPDS

These large multicenter randomized, controlled trials have provided a wealth of information about the natural history and the risk factors in type I and type II diabetes.

For type I disease, the Diabetes Control and Complication Trial (DCCT) demonstrated that tight control (HbA1c 7.2% vs. 9%) was associated with 76% reduction in retinopathy, 60% reduction in neuropathy, and 54% reduction in nephropathy.

For type II disease, the United Kingdom Prospective Diabetic Study (UKPDS) demonstrated that tight control (HbA1c 7% vs. 7.9%) was associated with 25% reduction in microvascular disease. Additionally tight BP control (144/82 vs. 155/87) was associated with a 37% reduction in microvascular disease and 32% reduction in diabetes-related deaths.

Diabetic eye disease: assessment

When assessing the diabetic patient (Tables 13.2), the ophthalmologist aims to 1) assess risk factors for eye disease (and, to a lesser extent, other systemic complications), 2) ensure that modifiable risk factors are treated, 3) detect and grade eye disease (e.g., Fig. 13.5; see Table 13.3), and 4) institute ophthalmic treatment where necessary.

Table 13.2 An approach to assessing diabetic eye disease

Visual symptoms	Asymptomatic; ↓VA, distortion, floaters
POH	Previous diabetic eye complications; laser treatment; surgery; concurrent eye disease
PMH	Diabetes: age of diagnosis, type and duration; hypertension, hypercholesterolemia, smoking; pregnancy; ischemic heart disease, cerebrovascular disease, peripheral vascular disease, nephropathy, neuropathy
SH	Driver; occupation
Drug history	Treatment for diabetes (diet, oral hypoglycemics, insulin types and frequency), hypertension, hypercholesterolemia; aspirin or antiplatelet agents
All	Allergies or relevant drug contraindications
Visual acuity	Best-corrected/pinhole/near
Cornea	Tear film
Iris	Rubeosis
Lens	Cataract
Tonometry	IOP
Vitreous	Hemorrhage, asteroid hyalosis, vitreous macular traction
Fundus	Retinopathy (microaneurysms, hemorrhages, exudates, intraretinal microvascular abnormalities, venous beading, venous loops, neovascularization), maculopathy (fluid, exudates, retinal thickening), tractional or rhegmatogenous retinal detachment, arterial or venous occlusion, ocular ischemia
Disc	New vessels, papillitis, AION

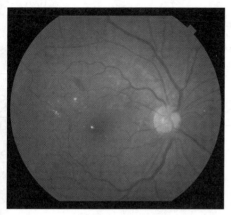

Figure 13.5 Nonproliferative diabetic retinopathy (NPDR) with exudates and associated clinically significant macular edema. See insert for color version.

Table 13.3 Definitions in diabetic eye disease

Disease severity level	Clinical finding on dilated ophthalmoscopy
Diabetic retinopathy disease severity scale	
No apparent retinopathy	No abnormalities
Mild NPDR	Microaneurysms only
Moderate NPDR	More than just microaneurysms but less than severe NPDR
Severe NPDR	Any of the following (4–2-1 rule) and no signs of PDR: • >20 intraretinal hemorrhage in each of the four quadrants • Definite venous beading in two or more quadrants • Prominent IRMA in one or more quadrants
PDR	One or both of the following: Neovascularization Vitreous/preretinal hemorrhage
Diabetic macular edema (DME) disease definition in the ETDRS	
DME absent	No apparent retinal thickening or hard exudates in posterior pole
DME apparently present	Thickening of retina and/or hard exudates within one disc diameter of center of the macula
CSME	Retinal thickening at or within 500 μm of center of the macula Hard exudates with associated retinal thickening at or within 500 μm of center of the macula Retinal thickening one disc area in size within one disc diameter of center of the macula

CSME, clinically significant macular edema; ETDRS, Early Treatment of Diabetic Retinopathy Study; IRMA, intraretinal microvascular abnormality; NPDR, nonproliferative diabetic retinopathy; PDR, proliferative diabetic retinopathy.

Diabetic eye disease: management

Optimal diabetic care (Table 13.4) can best be achieved by a multidisciplinary approach. This includes doctors (PCP, endocrinologist, and appropriate specialists according to need), specialist nurses, podiatrists, ophthalmologists, and others. Education to encourage the patient in self-management is critical.

Treatment—ophthalmic

Table 13.4 An approach to diabetic eye disease

Retinopathy	
None	Routine screening annually
Preproliferative	Observe 4 monthly
Proliferative (active)	Panretinal photocoagulation (1–2 sessions x ≥1000 x 200–500 µm x 0.1 sec); review every 3 weeks
Proliferative (regressed)	Observe every 4–6 months
Maculopathy	
Focal leakage	Focal laser photocoagulation (*n* x 50–100 µm x 0.08–0.1 sec); review at 3–4 months
Diffuse leakage	Grid laser photocoagulation (*n* x 100–200µm x 0.1sec); review at 3–4 months
Ischemic	FA to confirm diagnosis
Persistent maculopathy	Intravitreal triamcinolone (4 mg under sterile conditions) and bevacizumab
Resolved maculopathy	Observe every 4–6 months
Rubeosis	
Rubeosis + clear media	Urgent panretinal photocoagulation ± IV bevacizumab
Rubeosis + vitreous hemorrhage	Vitrectomy + endolaser ± IV bevacizumab
Rubeotic glaucoma	Urgent panretinal photocoagulation
	↓IOP with topical medication/cyclodiode/augmented trabeculectomy/tubes
Vitreous hemorrhage	
No view of fundus	Ultrasound to ensure retina is flat + review every 2–4 weeks until adequate view, ± IV bevacizumab
Adequate view	Ensure retina is flat + panretinal photocoagulation
Persistent	Vitrectomy + endolaser ± IV bevacizumab

Treatment—general

Glycemic control
- Aim for an HbA1c 6.5–7%.
- For type I disease, insulin regimens include 1) twice-daily premixed insulins, 2) ultrafast or soluble insulins with each meal and long-acting insulin at night (see Table 13.5).
- For type II disease, start with diet, followed by metformin and then a sulfonylurea (e.g., glipizide or glyburide); a glitazone (e.g., rosiglitazone) may be used as an alternative to either of these; insulin may be required.

Blood pressure control
- Aim for BP <130/80 or <125/75 if there is proteinuria.
- Effective antihypertensives include angiotensin-converting enzyme (ACE) inhibitors, angiotensin II receptor (AIIR) antagonists, β-blockers, and thiazide diuretics.

Cholesterol control
- Aim for lipid lowering if there is >30% 10-year risk of coronary heart disease (current recommendations, although ideally, treat all with risk >15%). This can be calculated from the Framingham equation.
- A statin is the drug of choice; fibrates may be helpful if ↑TG and ↓HDL.

Support renal function
- Microalbuminuria is indicative of early nephropathy and is associated with increased risk of macrovascular complications.
- ACE inhibitors or AIIR antagonists are preferred.

Lifestyle
- Smoking cessation: smoking greatly increases macrovascular disease, and strategies to help the patient stop smoking should be explored.
- Weight control is advised mainly in type II disease, particularly with body mass index (BMI) >25.
- Exercise >30 min/day ↓weight, ↓BP, ↑insulin sensitivity, and improves lipid profile.

Table 13.5 Insulin types (and examples)

Short-acting	Insulin Aspart (NovoLog)
	Insulin Lispro (Humalog)
	Insulin glulisine (Apidra)
Intermediate	Insulin NPH (Novolin N, Humulin N)
Long-acting	Insulin Zn suspension (Levemir)
	Insulin glargine (Lantus)

Diabetic eye disease: screening

What is screening?
Screening is the systematic testing of a population (or subgroup) for signs of asymptomatic or ignored disease.

Screening for diabetic eye disease
The classification systems for diabetic retinopathy range from the very detailed Arlie House system (generally for use in trials) to the dichotomous nonproliferative vs. proliferative division. In terms of clinical management, the commonly used preproliferative (mild, moderate, severe) and proliferative grading is familiar and has been adopted by practicing ophthalmologists and retina specialists.

Although screening may be performed by dilated funduscopy, quality assurance can be more readily achieved when there is a photographic record. Hence, a regional program of diabetic retinopathy telemedicine screening is recommended. Digital photography could be performed in mobile clinics, in selected primary or secondary care clinics, or by community optometrists and ophthalmologists. Grading of the photographs could be performed by the same clinics or the photographs could be sent to an approved reading center.

Patients with evidence of disease are referred to a local vitreoretinal specialist for treatment and/or further evaluation (Table 13.6).

Table 13.6 Management recommendations for patients with diabetes

Severity of retinopathy	Follow-up (months)	Panretinal photocoagulation	Focal or grid laser
Normal NPDR	12	No	No
Mild NPDR	9–12	No	No
Moderate NPDR	6–9	No	No
Severe NPDR	2–4	Sometimes	No
Non-high-risk PDR	2–4	Sometimes	No
High-risk PDR	2–4	Yes	No
CSME	2–4	No	Yes
Inactive PDR	6	No	No

Central serous chorioretinopathy (CSCR or CSR)

The etiology of central serous chorioretinopathy (also called central serous retinopathy, CSR) is unknown, but ICG studies suggest that local congestion of the choroidal circulation causes ischemia, hyperpermeability, fluid accumulation, RPE detachment, disruption of outer blood–retinal barrier (RPE tight junctions), and subsequent detachment of the sensory retina.

Risk factors

The disease typically affects adult males (20–50 years) and is reportedly associated with type A personalities, stress, pregnancy, Cushing's disease (5% prevalence), and numerous drugs (notably corticosteroids).

Clinical features

- Unilateral sudden ↓VA, positive scotoma (usually central), metamorphopsia, increased hypermetropia.
- Shallow detachment of the sensory retina at the posterior pole ± deeper small yellow elevations (RPE detachments) (Fig. 13.6); pigmentary changes suggest chronicity; occasionally fluid tracks inferiorly from the posterior pole to cause a bullous, nonrhegmatogenous detachment of the inferior peripheral retina.

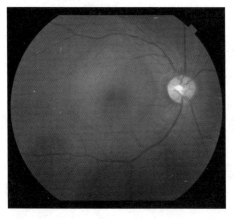

Figure 13.6 Central serous chorioretinopathy with a large, serous elevation of the macula. See insert for color version.

Investigations

- *FA:* one or more points of progressive leakage and pooling (Fig. 13.7) classically in a smokestack or ink-blot pattern (10%) (Fig. 13.8).
- *ICG:* when performed, shows bilateral multifocal hyperfluorescence of greater extent than that seen clinically or on FA.

Treatment

Argon laser treatment

- *Indications:* persistence >6 months, contralateral persistent visual defect from CSCR, multiple recurrences, occupational needs.
- *Technique:* mild burns to the leakage site (usually <10 burns, 50–200 µm, 0.1 sec, power adjusted to produce very gentle blanching only).

PDT

Recent case series suggest that PDT may be beneficial for those with severe/chronic disease who are not amenable to conventional laser treatment.

Prognosis

In 80% of patients, there is spontaneous recovery to near-normal VA (≥6 months) within 1–6 months. Subtle metamorphopsia may persist. Chronic (5%) or recurrent episodes (in up to 45%) may be associated with more significant visual loss.

Differential diagnosis

Other causes of serous retinal detachments include optic disc pits, CNV, IPCV, optic neuritis, papilledema, VKH, sympathetic ophthalmia, uveal effusion syndrome, choroidal tumors, macular holes, vitreous traction, and hypertension.

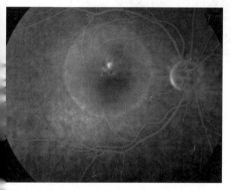

Figure 13.7 Late fluorescein angiogram demonstrated pinpoint area of leakage with pooling of the fluorescein in the subretinal space. See insert for color version.

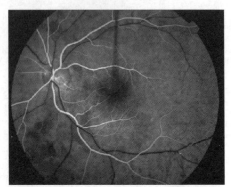

Early phase

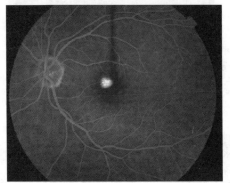

Late phase: point of progressive leakage in an ink-blot type pattern

Figure 13.8 FA of central serous chorioretinopathy.

Cystoid macular edema (CME)

This important macular disorder is a common pathological response to a wide variety of ocular insults (Table 13.7). It is thought that prostaglandin secretion and vascular endothelial damage cause fluid accumulation in the outer plexiform layer.

The relatively loose intercellular adhesions of this layer then permit the formation of cystoid spaces, especially in the macular region of layer of Henle. It most commonly arises after cataract surgery (Irvine–Gass syndrome; p. 257) or in association with diabetic maculopathy, retinal vein occlusions, and posterior uveitis.

Clinical features

- Asymptomatic, ↓VA (may be severe), metamorphopsia, scotomas.
- Loss of foveal contour, retinal thickening, cystoid spaces; central yellow spot, small intraretinal hemorrhages, and telangiectasia (occasional).
- Associated features depend on the underlying cause (e.g., diabetic retinopathy, B/CRVO, uveitis).
- *Complications*: lamellar hole (irreversible ↓VA).

Investigations

- *FA*: typically dye leakage from the parafovea into the cystoid spaces (petalloid pattern) and from the optic disc.
- *OCT*: detection rate is equal to FA and OCT can measure degree of retinal thickening.

Treatment

Although there may be some variation according to the underlying cause, a stepwise approach is recommended. Review the diagnosis if condition is atypical or slow to respond. One approach is as follows:

1. Topical: steroid (e.g., dexamethasone 0.1% or prednisolone acetate 1% 4x/day) + NSAID (e.g., ketoro-lac 0.3% 3x/day).

Review in 4–6 weeks; if no response or persisting, then:

2. Periocular steroid (e.g., transeptal/subtenons; methylprednisolone/ triamcinolone) and continue topical agent. Follow up in 3–4 weeks for IOP check.

Review in 4–6 weeks; if persistent, then:

3. Consider repeating periocular or giving intravitreal steroid (triamcinolone 4 mg); vitrectomy with epiretinal or internal limiting membrane peeling; systemic steroids (e.g., prednisone 40 mg 1x/day, titrating over 3 weeks; or IV methylprednisolone 500 mg single dose); oral acetazolamide (500 mg/day; limited evidence).

Prognosis

Prognosis varies according to the underlying pathology. Most patients with CME arising after cataract surgery will attain VA ≥20/30 within 3–12 months of their operation.

Table 13.7 Causes of CME

- Postoperative (cataract, corneal, or vitreoretinal surgery)
- Post-cryotherapy
- Post-laser (peripheral iridotomy, panretinal photocoagulation)
- Uveitis (posterior > intermediate > anterior)
- Scleritis
- Retinal vein obstruction
- Diabetic maculopathy
- Ocular ischemia
- Choroidal neovascular membrane
- Retinal telangiectasia
- Hypertensive retinopathy
- Radiation retinopathy
- Epiretinal membrane
- Retinitis pigmentosa
- Autosomal dominant CME
- Tumors of the choroid or retina
- Medication

Degenerative myopia

Myopia is common and is regarded as physiological if less than −6D. Of those with high myopia (> −6D), there is a subset in whom the axial length may never stabilize (progressive myopia) and who are at risk of degenerative changes.

The prevalence of progressive myopia varies from 1 to 10%, with geographic variation (highest in Spain and Japan). It is a significant cause of blindness in the developed world and affects the working population.

Risk factors include genetic influences (autosomal dominant/recessive, sporadic; see also Table 13.8) and environmental factors (excessive near work).

Clinical features

- Increasing myopia, ↓VA, metamorphopsia, photopsia (occasional).
- *Fundus:* pale, tessellated with areas of chorioretinal atrophy both centrally and peripherally; breaks in Bruch's membrane ("lacquer cracks") may permit CNV formation, macular hemorrhage, and subsequent pigmented scar (Förster–Fuchs spot); posterior staphyloma (Fig. 13.9); lattice degeneration.
- *Optic disc:* tilted, atrophy temporal to the disc ("temporal crescent").
- *Vitreous syneresis:* posterior vitreous detachment (at younger age).
- *Other associations:* long axial length, deep AC, zonular dehiscence, pigment dispersion syndrome.
- *Complications:* CNV, macular hole, macular schisis, peripheral retinal tears, rhegmatogenous retinal detachment.

Investigations

- *Ultrasound* can confirm a staphyloma and can monitor axial length.
- *FA:* if CNV is suspected.
- *OCT* is used to determine presence of vitreomacular traction and macular schisis.

Treatment

Choroidal neovascular membranes

- *Extrafoveal:* consider argon laser photocoagulation. With time, there is often significant expansion of the resultant atrophic zone.
- *Subfoveal:* PDT is associated with a reduction in visual loss (cf. placebo).
- Anti-VEGF therapy with pegaptanib (macugen), bevacizumab (avastin) or ranibizumab (lucentis) intravitreal injections.

Prognosis

High myopia is the most common cause of CNV in young patients, accounting for >60% of CNV in those under 50 years of age. Risk factors for CNV development are lacquer cracks (29% develop CNV) and patchy atrophy (20% develop CNV). At 5 years following onset of myopic CNV (untreated), around 90% of patients have a VA ≤20/200.

Table 13.8 Associations of myopia

- Stickler syndrome
- Marfan syndrome
- Ehlers–Danlos syndrome
- Down syndrome
- Gyrate atrophy
- Congenital rubella
- Albinism

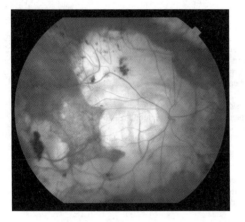

Figure 13.9 Myopic degeneration with a large macular staphyloma. See insert for color version.

Angioid streaks

Angioid streaks are breaks in an abnormally thickened and calcified Bruch's membrane. This type of brittle Bruch's membrane may result from a number of endocrine, metabolic, and connective tissue abnormalities (Table 13.9), but in about half of cases no underlying cause is found.

Clinical features

- Asymptomatic; ↓VA, metamorphopsia.
- *Angioid streaks:* narrow, irregular streaks radiating from a peripapillary ring; the color of the streaks varies from red to dark brown depending on background pigmentation.
- *Associated features:* peripapillary chorioretinal atrophy; local/diffuse RPE mottling ("peau d'orange"; common in PXE); disc drusen.
- *Complications:* CNV, choroidal rupture (after minor trauma) with subfoveal hemorrhage.

Investigations

Use FA if CNV is suspected; angioid streaks show hyperfluorescence due to window defect.

Treatment

- *Conservative:* advise patient to avoid contact sports and risk of trauma.
- *Extrafoveal/juxtafoveal CNV:* consider argon laser photocoagulation.
- *Subfoveal CNV:* preliminary results suggest that PDT may be of benefit.

Table 13.9 Causes of angioid streaks

- Pseudoxanthoma elasticum
- Ehlers–Danlos syndrome
- Paget's disease
- Acromegaly
- Hemaglobinopathies
- Hereditary spherocytosis
- Neurofibromatosis
- Sturge–Weber
- Tuberous sclerosis
- Idiopathic (50%)

Choroidal folds

These are corrugations in the choroid and Bruch's membrane that are seen as a series of light and dark lines. They are usually horizontal and lie over the posterior pole, although they can be vertical, oblique, or jigsaw-like. They are distinguished from retinal striae by being deeper and broader.

FA shows alternating lines of hyperfluorescence (peaks) and hypofluorescence (troughs). Although they may in themselves cause visual dysfunction, their main significance is to prompt a thorough investigation for an underlying disease (see Table 13.10).

Table 13.10 Causes of choroidal folds

- Idiopathic
- Hypermetropia
- Retrobulbar mass
- Posterior scleritis
- Uveitis
- Idiopathic orbital inflammatory disease
- Thyroid eye disease
- Choroidal mass
- Hypotony
- Papilledema

Toxic retinopathies (1)

A number of prescribed and nonprescribed drugs may cause retinal injury, usually via damage to the RPE layer. A high level of clinical suspicion may be required as these conditions are seen infrequently and use of the drug is often not volunteered.

Be alert to the possibility of toxicity when there is unusual pigmentary disturbance or crystal deposition. Withdrawal of the drug (coordinate with the prescribing physician; see Table 13.11) may lead to halting and even regression of the retinopathy; in some cases, however, it may continue to progress.

Chloroquine and hydroxychloroquine

These aminoquinolones are widely used as antimalarials and immunomodulators (e.g., in RA and SLE). Doses of >3.5 mg/kg/day for chloroquine and >6.5 mg/kg/day for hydroxychloroquine may result in retinopathy and maculopathy; risk increases with increasing dose, increasing duration, and reduced renal function.

Clinical features
- Asymptomatic, central/paracentral scotomas, ↓VA.
- Altered foveal reflex → irregular central macular pigmentation → depigmentation of surrounding zone (bull's eye maculopathy), → end-stage disease (generalized atrophy, RP-like peripheral pigmentation, arteriolar attenuation, optic atrophy).
- Associated features: vortex keratopathy.

Prevention and screening
Current prescribing practice (<3.5 mg/kg/day for chloroquine and <6.5 mg/kg/day for hydroxychloroquine) very rarely causes retinopathy.

Table 13.11 Summary of recommendations to prescribing physician

Pretreatment	Ask about visual impairment or eye disease. Arrange for a pretreatment evaluation with documentation of visual acuity, color vision, and visual field with red target.
Treatment	Do not exceed recommended dose (6.5 mg/kg/day hydroxychloroquine). Annual evaluation with documentation of visual acuity, color vision, and visual field. Multi-focal ERG may be more sensitive for detection of early disease.

Vigabatrin

This anticonvulsant is used in the treatment of complex partial seizures and certain other types of epilepsy. In around a third of cases, visual field defects may be noted.

Clinical features

- Usually asymptomatic with good central VA.
- May develop optic atrophy.
- Bilateral visual field defects: generalized constriction or binasal; generally static once established, with no improvement on withdrawal of treatment.
- Normal retinal appearance.

Prevention and screening

Table 13.12 Summary of recommendations

Pretreatment	Perform baseline visual field examination (Humphrey 120 to 45* or Goldmann).
Treatment	Reassess every 6 months for 3 years. Reassess annually thereafter.

Toxic retinopathies (2)

Thioridazine

This phenothiazine is used second line in the treatment of schizophrenia. Doses of >1 g/day for just a few weeks may result in retinopathy.

Clinical features

- Asymptomatic, scotomas (paracentral or ring), ↓VA, nyctalopia, brownish visual discoloration.
- Pigmentary disturbance at the posterior pole; geographic areas of chorioretinal atrophy.

Prevention

Current prescribing practice (maintenance <300 mg/day) should not lead to retinopathy.

Chlorpromazine

This phenothiazine is used in schizophrenia and other psychoses. Doses of >2 g/day for a year may result in retinopathy.

Clinical features

- Usually asymptomatic.
- Pigmentary disturbance.
- Associated features include corneal endothelial deposits and anterior lens granules.

Prevention

Current prescribing practice (<300 mg/day) should not lead to retinopathy.

Tamoxifen

This estrogen antagonist is used in the treatment of breast cancer. Doses of >180 mg/day for a year may result in retinopathy.

Clinical features

- Asymptomatic or mild ↓VA.
- Crystalline maculopathy with fine white refractile deposits in the inner retina centered around the fovea.
- Associated features include vortex keratopathy and optic neuritis.

Prevention

Current prescribing practice (<40 mg/day) rarely leads to retinopathy.

Deferoxamine

This chelating agent is commonly used to treat overload of iron (e.g., after multiple transfusions in chronic anemias such as thalassemia) and aluminium (e.g., dialysis patients). There appears to be no "safe" dose; retinopathy occurred in one instance after a single administration.

Clinical features
- ↓VA, nyctalopia, abnormal color vision, scotomas (usually central/ centrocecal).
- Central and peripheral pigmentary disturbance.

Didanosine

This nucleoside analog antiretroviral is used in the treatment of HIV infection. It is a reverse transcriptase inhibitor commonly used as a part of the ART regimen. In children it has occasionally been observed to cause a retinopathy.

Clinical features
- Asymptomatic or mild peripheral field loss.
- Peripheral well-defined areas of retinal/RPE atrophy.

Clofazimine

This antimycobacterial is used in the treatment of leprosy and AIDS-related *Mycobacterium avium* infection.

Clinical features
- Unusually extensive bull's-eye maculopathy with irregular pigment and atrophy extending beyond the arcades.

Retinal vein occlusion (1)

Retinal vein occlusions are common, can occur at almost any age, and range in severity from asymptomatic to the painful, blind eye. They are divided into branch, hemi- or central retinal vein occlusions (equating to occlusion anterior or posterior to the cribriform plate), and ischemic or nonischemic types.

Most occlusions occur in those over age 65, but up to 15% may affect patients under 45. BRVO is three times more common than CRVO.

Central retinal vein occlusion (CRVO)

Although the division of nonischemic from ischemic CRVO is an arbitrary cutoff based on disc area of nonperfusion determined by FA findings, it is a useful predictor of visual outcome and risk of neovascularization. The clinical picture also differs.

Clinical features

Nonischemic

- Painless ↓VA (mild to moderate), metamorphopsia.
- Dilated, tortuous retinal veins with retinal hemorrhages in all four quadrants; occasional cotton-wool spots (CWS); mild optic disc edema.
- *Complications:* CME.

Ischemic

- ↓VA (severe); painless (unless neovascular glaucoma has developed).
- As for nonischemic but RAPD, deep hemorrhages (Fig. 13.10), widespread CWS (5–10 is borderline; >10 is significant); rarely vitreous hemorrhage, exudative retinal detachment.
- *Chronic:* venous sheathing, resorption of hemorrhages, macular pigment disturbance, collateral vessels at the arcade and optociliary shunt vessels on the optic nerve.
- *Complications*: CME, neovascularization (of the iris [NVI] > of the optic disc [NVD] > elsewhere [NVE]), neovascular (90-day) glaucoma.

Investigations

For all patients

- BP, CBC, ESR, glucose, lipids, protein electrophoresis, TFT, and ECG. Further investigation is directed by clinical indication and may include CRP, serum ACE, anticardiolipin, lupus anticoagulant, autoantibodies (RF, ANA, anti-DNA, ANCA), fasting homocysteine, CXR, and thrombophilia screen (e.g., proteins C and S, antithrombin, factor V Leiden).

FA

- *Nonischemic:* vein wall staining, microaneurysms, dilated optic disc capillaries.
- *Ischemic:* as for nonischemic but capillary closure (5–10 disc areas is borderline; >10 is significantly ischemic), hypofluorescence (blockage due to extensive hemorrhage), leakage (CME, NV).

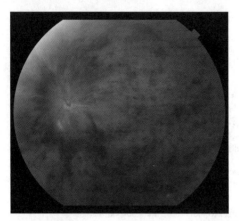

Fig. 13.10 Central retinal vein occlusion with extensive nerve fiber layer and intraretinal hemorrhage with associated diffuse retinal and optic nerve edema. See insert for color version.

Treatment

There is no proven treatment. The following are common practice (see also Table 13.13):

- ↓IOP: if elevated (in either eye).
- Panretinal photocoagulation for neovascularization or high risk.
- Intravitreal triamcinolone acetonide or intravitreal dexamethasone implant for treatment of CME.
- Intravitreal bevacizumab and ranibizumab for treatment of CME and neovascularization.
- Pars plana vitrectomy and endolaser for vitreous hemorrhage secondary to neovascularization.
- Treat underlying medical conditions (Table 13.14): coordinate care with a PCP.

Prognosis

- *Nonischemic:* recovery to normal VA is <10%.
- *Nonischemic:* progression to ischemic is 15% by 4 months, 34% by 3 years.
- *Ischemic:* progression to rubeosis is 37% by 4 months. Highest risk is with VA <20/200 or ≥30 disc areas of nonperfusion on FA.
- Risk of CRVO in contralateral eye is 7% by 2 years.

Table 13.13 Summary of recommendations for management of CRVO

Ischemic with no NV	Examination (including gonioscopy) monthly for first 6 months then every 3 months for 1 year; can be discharged if stable by 24 months
Ischemic with NVI (angle or iris)	PRP (1500–2000 × 500 µm × 0.05–0.1 sec) Follow-up as above
Neovascular glaucoma with visual potential	↓IOP with topical agents or cycloablation
Neovascular glaucoma in blind eye	Keep comfortable with topical steroids and atropine
Nonischemic	Every 3 months for first 6 months; can usually be discharged if stable by 24 months

Table 13.14 Associations of CRVO

Atherosclerotic	• Hypertension • Hypercholesterolemia (including secondary to hypothyroidism) • Diabetes • Smoking
Hematological	• Protein S, protein C, or antithrombin deficiency • Activated protein C resistance • Factor V Leiden • Multiple myeloma • Waldenstrom macroglobulinemia • Antiphospholipd syndrome
Inflammatory	• Behçet's disease • Polyarteritis nodosa • Sarcoidosis • Wegener's granulomatosis • SLE • Goodpasture syndrome
Ophthalmic	• Glaucoma (open or closed angle) • Trauma • Orbital pathology

Retinal vein occlusion (2)

Branch retinal vein occlusion (BRVO)

Clinical features
- May be asymptomatic; ↓VA, metamorphopsia, visual field defect (usually altitudinal).
- *Acute:* retinal hemorrhages (dot, blot, flame), CWS, edema in the distribution of a dilated, tortuous vein; superotemporal arcade most commonly affected; usually arise from an arteriovenous (AV) crossing.
- *Chronic:* venous sheathing, exudates, pigment disturbance, collateral vessels.
- *Complications:* CME, neovascularization (NVE > NVD > NVI), recurrent vitreous hemorrhage.

Investigations
Hypertension is the most common association with BRVO. BRVO may be investigated similarly to CRVO (see Treatment, p. 440).
   Use FA if diagnosis is uncertain or when VA <20/40 at 3 months.

Treatment (see Table 13.15)
- Macular grid laser (after FA): if macular edema, VA ≤20/40 and no spontaneous improvement by 3–6 months.
- Sectoral PRP: if neovascularization.
- Fill-in PRP: if neovascularization progresses or vitreous hemorrhage.

Prognosis
- Recovery to ≥20/40: 50%.
- Risk of macular edema: 57% (for temporal BRVO).
- Risk of retinal neovascularization: 20%, usually within the first 6–12 months.

Hemispheric BVO

In around 20% eyes, the central retinal vein forms posterior to the lamina cribrosa from superior and inferior divisions. These are generally regarded as a variant of CRVO. Ischemic hemispheric vein occlusions have an intermediate risk of rubeosis (compared to ischemic BRVO and CRVO) but a greater risk of NVD than either ischemic BRVO or CRVO. Treatment (in particular the role of laser) is as for BRVO.

Table 13.15 Summary of recommendations for management of BRVO

Ischemia >1 quadrant with no NV	Review at 3 months, then every 3–4 months; if stable can usually be discharged by 24 months
Ischemia with NVD or NVE	Sectoral PRP (400–500 × 500 μm × 0.05–0.1 sec) Follow-up as above
Macular edema	If VA <20/40, then perform FA at >3 months and grid laser (20–100 × 100–200 μm × 'gentle') at 3–6 months
Nonischemic	Review at 3 months, then every 3–6 months; if stable can usually be discharged by 24 months

Retinal artery occlusion (1)

Retinal artery occlusion is an ocular emergency in which rapid treatment *may* prevent irreversible loss of vision. CRAO has an estimated incidence 0.85/100,000/year and causes almost complete hypoxia of the inner retina. Experimental evidence shows that this causes lethal damage to the primate retina after 100 min. Acute coagulative necrosis is followed by complete loss of the nerve fiber layer, ganglion cell layer, and inner plexiform layer.

Central retinal artery occlusion (CRAO)

Clinical features

- Sudden painless, unilateral ↓VA (usually CF or worse).
- White swollen retina with a cherry-red spot at the macula (Fig. 13.11); arteriolar attenuation + box-carring; RAPD; visible emboli in up to 25%.
- *Variants:* a cilioretinal artery (present in 30%) may protect part of the papillomacular bundle, allowing relatively good vision; ophthalmic artery occlusion causes choroidal ischemia with retinochoroidal whitening (no cherry-red spot) and complete loss of vision (usually NLP).
- *Complications:* neovascularization (NVI in 18%; NVD in 2%); rubeotic glaucoma; optic atrophy; ocular ischemic syndrome (if ophthalmic artery occlusion).

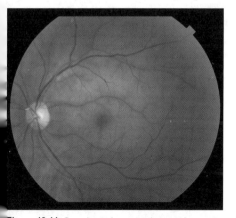

Figure 13.11 Central retinal artery occlusion with extensive retinal edema, whitening, and a cherry-red spot in the fovea. See insert for color version.

Investigations

In the acute setting, the diagnosis is not usually in doubt, so the urgent priority is to rule out underlying disease (such as giant cell arteritis [GCA]) that may threaten the contralateral eye. When presentation is delayed, the clinical picture is less specific and may require ancillary tests.

Identify cause

Most importantly, consider GCA (if age >50 years then get ESR, CRP, CBC, followed by temporal artery biopsy; p. 524). More common causes are atherosclerosis (check BP, blood glucose) and particularly carotid artery disease (may have carotid bruit).

Further investigation is directed by clinical indication and may include PTT, APTT, thrombophilia screen (e.g., proteins C and S, antithrombin, factor V Leiden), antiphospholipid screen, vasculitis autoantibodies (ANA, ANCA), syphilis serology (VDRL, TPHA), blood cultures, ECG, echocardiography, and carotid Doppler scans (Table 13.16).

Table 13.16 Associations of CRAO

Atherosclerotic	• Hypertension (60%) • Diabetes (25%) • Hypercholesterolemia • Smoking
Embolic sources	• Carotid artery disease • Aortic disease (including dissection) • Cardiac valve vegetations (e.g., infective endocarditis) • Cardiac tumors (e.g., atrial myxoma) • Arrhythmias • Cardiac septal defects • Post-intervention (e.g., angiography, angioplasty)
Hematological	• Protein S, protein C, or antithrombin deficiency • Activated protein C resistance • Antiphospholipd syndrome • Leukemia or lymphoma
Inflammatory	• Giant cell arteritis • Polyarteritis nodosa • Wegener's granulomatosis • SLE • Kawasaki disease • Pancreatitis
Infective	• Toxoplasmosis • Mucormycosis • Syphilis
Pharmacological	• Oral contraceptive pill • Cocaine
Ophthalmic	• Trauma • Optic nerve drusen • Migraine

Treatment

Treat affected eye (if within 24 hours of presentation).

- ↓IOP with 500 mg IV acetazolamide, ocular massage ± AC paracentesis (all common practice, but no proven benefit); ocular massage. Selective ophthalmic artery catheterization with thrombolysis is performed in some centers.

Protect other eye, e.g., treat underlying GCA with systemic steroids immediately (p. 524).

Prognosis

Visual outcome: 94% of cases are CF or worse at presentation; about 1/3 show some improvement (with or without treatment).

Retinal artery occlusion (2)

Branch retinal arteriolar occlusion (BRAO)

Most BRAOs are due to emboli that are often visible clinically. The most common emboli are as follows:

- Cholesterol (Hollenhorst plaque): small, yellow, refractile (Fig. 13.12).
- Fibrinoplatelet: elongated, white, dull.
- Calcific: white, nonrefractile, proximal to optic disc.

Antiphospholipid syndrome is associated with multiple BRAO.

Clinical features

- Sudden painless unilateral altitudinal field defect.
- White swollen retina along a branch retinal arteriole; branch arteriolar attenuation + box-carring; visible emboli common in over 60%.

Investigations and treatment

Identify underlying cause (as for CRAO). GCA is extremely rare as a cause of BRAO and does not need investigation in the absence of other supporting evidence.

There is no proven treatment for BRAO.

Cilioretinal artery occlusion

Present in up to 30% of the population, this branch from the posterior ciliary circulation perfuses the posterior pole. Occlusion may be

- Isolated: usually in the young, associated with systemic vasculitis, relatively good prognosis.
- Combined with CRVO: usually in the young, possibly a form of papillophlebitis, relatively good prognosis (as for nonischemic CRVO).
- Combined with AION: usually in the elderly, associated with GCA, very poor prognosis.

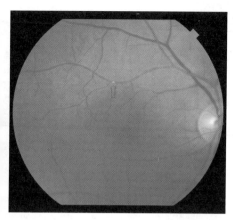

Figure 13.12 Hollenhorst plaque (arrow) lodged in a peripheral retinal artery. See insert for color version.

Hypertensive retinopathy

Systemic hypertension is one of the most common diseases of the Western world, where it may affect up to 60% of those over 60 years of age. Risk factors include age, gender (males > females), ethnic origin (blacks > whites), and society (industrialized > agricultural). Exercise is protective.

Most cases of hypertension are chronic and of unknown cause ("essential"). It causes sclerosis and narrowing of the arterioles in both the retinal and, more severely, the choroidal circulation.

In about 1% of cases, hypertension is acute and severe (accelerated or "malignant" hypertension). This causes fibrinoid necrosis of arterioles and accelerated end-organ damage.

This medical emergency requires urgent assessment, treatment, and identification of an underlying cause. Untreated, accelerated hypertension carries a 90% mortality rate at 1 year.

Chronic hypertension

There is no absolutely safe BP and therefore no absolute definition of hypertension. However, intervention is currently recommended for BP >140 mmHg systolic or >90 mmHg diastolic occurring on two separate occasions (Table 13.17).

Clinical features

Systemic
- Usually asymptomatic.
- May have evidence of end-organ damage (cardiovascular, cerebrovascular, peripheral vascular, renal disease).

Ophthalmic
- Narrowing/irregularity of arterioles (copper and silver-wiring), arteriovenous nicking, CWS, blot or flame hemorrhages.
- *Complications*: macroaneurysms, nonarteritic AION, CRVO, BRVO, CRAO, BRAO.

Investigation and treatment

Alert the primary care physician who will monitor, assess vascular risk, and treat as required (see Tables 13.17 and 13.18). The target is 140/85 for most patients, 130/80 for those with diabetes mellitus, and 125/75 for diabetics with proteinuria.

Malignant hypertension

This is characterized by severe ↑BP (e.g., >220 mmHg systolic or >120 mmHg diastolic) with papilledema or fundal hemorrhages and exudates.

Clinical features

Systemic
- Headache.
- Accelerated end-organ damage (e.g., myocardial infarct, cardiac failure, stroke, encephalopathy, renal failure).

Ophthalmic
- Scotoma, diplopia, photopsia, ↓VA.
- Retinopathy: focal arteriolar narrowing, CWS, flame hemorrhages.
- Choroidopathy: infarcts that may be focal (Elschnig's spots) or linear along choroidal arteries (Siegrist's streaks), serous retinal detachments.
- Optic neuropathy: disc swelling ± macular star.

Investigation and treatment
Refer to a medical team for admission and cautious lowering of blood pressure; too rapid a reduction may be deleterious (e.g., stroke).

Table 13.17 Adult hypertension clinical guidelines

Classification	SBP	DBP	Lifestyle modification	Drugs
Normal	<120	<80	Encourage	No
Prehypertension	120–139	80–89	Yes	No
Stage 1 hypertension	140–159	90–99	Yes	Yes 1 drug
Stage 2 hypertension	>160	>100	Yes	Yes 2 drugs

Treatment determined by the highest BP category

Table 13.18 Common antihypertensives

Group	Example	Contraindication	Side effects
Thiazide diuretic	Hydrochlorothiazide	Renal/hepatic failure, persistent ↓K⁺, ↓Na⁺	↓K⁺, ↓Na⁺, postural hypotension, impotence
B-blocker	Atenolol	Asthma; caution in cardiac failure	Bronchospasm, cardiac failure, lethargy, impotence
ACE inhibitor	Lisinopril	Renal artery stenosis, aortic stenosis,	Cough, ↑K⁺, renal failure, angioedema
AIIR antagonist	Losartan	Caution in renal artery stenosis, aortic stenosis	Mild hypotension, ↑K⁺
Ca²⁺-channel antagonist	Nifedipine	Cardiogenic shock, within 1 month of MI	Dependent edema, flushing, fatigue
A-blocker	Doxazosin	Aortic stenosis	Dependent edema, fatigue, postural hypotension

Hematological disease

Hemoglobinopathies

Normal adult hemoglobin (HbA) comprises two α- and two β-globin chains associated with a heme ring. In sickle hemoglobinopathies, there is a mutant hemoglobin, such as HbS (β-chain residue 6 Glu → Val), which behaves abnormally in response to hypoxia or acidosis. This causes "sickling" and hemolysis of red blood cells.

Many other mutant hemoglobins have been described, the most common one being HbC. In thalassemias the problem is one of inadequate production of one or more of the α- or β-chains.

Although systemic disease is most severe in sickle-cell disease (HbSS), ocular disease is most severe in HbSC and HbS-Thal disease. Sickle hemoglobinopathies are seen in Africans and their descendents (Table 13.19); thalassemias are mainly seen in Africans and in Mediterranean countries.

Clinical features
- Proliferative retinopathy (see Table 13.20).
- *Nonproliferative retinopathy:* arteriosclerosis, venous tortuosity, equatorial "salmon patches" (preretinal/superficial intraretinal hemorrhages), and "black sunbursts" (intraretinal hemorrhage disturbing RPE with pigment migration), macular ischemia, and atrophy ('macular depression sign'); occasional CWS, microaneurysms.
- *Other:* conjunctival comma-shaped capillaries, sectoral iris atrophy.

Table 13.19 Sickle hemoglobinopathies

Disease	Hb	Prevalence in African-American population
Sickle trait	HbAS	5–10%
Sickle-cell disease	HbSS	0.4%
Hemoglobin SC disease	HbSC	0.2%
Sickle-cell thalassemia	HbS-Thal	0.5–1.0%; 0.03% severe

Table 13.20 Goldberg staging of proliferative Sickle cell retinopathy

Stage 1	Peripheral arteriolar occlusions
Stage 2	Arteriovenous anastamosis
Stage 3	Neovascular proliferation ("sea-fans")
Stage 4	Vitreous hemorrhage
Stage 5	Retinal detachment

Investigation
- Hb electrophoresis, CBC.

Some patients with HbSC or HbS-Thal may be unaware of their disease.

Treatment
- Observation.
- Consider laser photocoagulation in proliferative sickle retinopathy. Its use is controversial, as most sea-fans spontaneously regress. The rationale is to remove the drive to neovascularization by ablating the ischemic retina.
- Consider vitreoretinal surgery for persistent vitreous hemorrhage (e.g., >6 months) and tractional retinal detachment, although the results are generally disappointing, and specialist perioperative care is required.

Anemia

Retinal findings increase with severity of anemia, particularly in the presence of thrombocytopenia. The retinopathy is usually an incidental finding, thus investigation and treatment should already be under way with the hematologist.

Clinical features
- *Retinopathy:* usually asymptomatic; hemorrhages, cotton wool spots, venous tortuosity.
- *Other:* subconjunctival hemorrhages, optic neuropathy (if ↓B12).

Leukemia

Retinal findings are more common with acute rather than chronic leukemias. Leukemic complications may be due to direct infiltration or secondary anemia and hyperviscosity.

Clinical features
- *Retinopathy:* usually asymptomatic; hemorrhages, CWS, venous tortuosity, pigment epitheliopathy ("leopard spot" from choroidal infiltration), neovascularization (rare).
- *Other:* spontaneous hemorrhage (subconjunctival or hyphema), infiltration (iris → anterior uveitis ± hypopyon; orbit proptosis; optic nerve → optic neuropathy ± disc swelling).

Hyperviscosity

Hyperviscosity arises from abnormally high levels of blood constituents, either cells (e.g., primary or secondary polycythemia, leukemias) or protein levels (e.g., multiple myeloma, Waldenstrom's macroglobulinemia).

Clinical features
- *Retinopathy:* usually asymptomatic; hemorrhages, CWS, venous tortuosity, and dilation.
- *Other:* optic disc swelling in polycythemia and multiple myeloma, conjunctival/corneal crystals, iris/ciliary body cysts in multiple myeloma.

Vascular anomalies

Retinal telangiectasias

Retinal telangiectasia describes abnormalities of the retinal vasculature, usually with irregular dilation of the capillary bed, and segmental dilation of neighboring venules and arterioles. Most commonly, they are acquired secondary to another retinal disorder (e.g., CRVO).

Congenital forms represent a spectrum of disease from the severe and early onset of Coats' disease to the more limited and later onset of idiopathic juxtafoveal telangiectasia (see Table 13.21).

Coats' disease

This uncommon condition is the most severe of the telangiectasias. It affects mainly males (M:F 3:1) and the young, although up to a third may be asymptomatic until their 30s. Although often considered a unilateral disease, around 10% cases are bilateral.

Clinical features
- May be asymptomatic; ↓VA, strabismus, leukocoria.
- Telangiectatic vessels, "light bulb" aneurysms, capillary dropout, exudation (may be massive), scarring.
- *Complications*: exudative retinal detachment, neovascularization, vitreous hemorrhage, rubeosis, glaucoma, cataract.

Investigations
FA highlights abnormal vessels, leakage, and areas of capillary dropout.

Treatment
Consider laser photocoagulation (or cryotherapy) of leaking vessels; treat directly rather than with a scatter approach. Anti-VEGF therapy may decrease vascular leakage and reduce the degree of exudation and subretinal fluid. Scleral buckling with drainage of subretinal fluid may be performed for significant exudative detachment but carries a guarded prognosis.

Table 13.21 Causes of retinal telangiectasias

Congenital	Coats' disease
	Leber's miliary aneurysms
	Idiopathic juxtafoveal telangiectasia
Acquired	Retinopathy of prematurity (ROP)
	Retinitis pigmentosa
	Diabetic retinopathy
	Sickle retinopathy
	Radiation retinopathy
	Hypogammaglobulinemia
	Eales' disease
	CRVO, BRVO

Leber's miliary aneurysms

This is essentially a localized, less severe form of Coats' disease presenting in adults with unilateral ↓VA, fusiform and saccular aneurysmic dilation of venules and arterioles, and local exudation. Direct photocoagulation of abnormal vessels may be beneficial.

In the area of extensive subretinal fluid, anti-VEGF therapy may aid the reduction resolution of subretinal fluid before laser photocoagulation, or cryotherapy may be used.

Idiopathic juxtafoveal retinal telangiectasia

This rare condition presents in adulthood with mild ↓VA due to telangi-ectatic juxtafoveal retinal capillaries with local exudation. Described by Gass in 1982, it may be subdivided as follows:

- *Group 1A*: unilateral parafoveal telangiectasia of the temporal macula; early middle-aged males; VA around 20/40, focal laser treatment may be effective. Additional options include intravitreal triamcinolone acetonide or anti-VEGF drugs.
- *Group 1B*: unilateral parafoveal telangiectasia of ≤1 clock-hour at the edge of the FAZ; middle-aged males, laser treatment is not indicated.
- *Group 2*: bilateral symmetrical parafoveal telangiectasia; late middle-age; gradual ↓VA occurs due to foveal atrophy or CNV.
- *Group 3*: bilateral perifoveal telangiectasia; adulthood; gradual ↓VA occurs due to capillary occlusion.

Macroaneurysm

This is a focal dilatation of a retinal arteriole occurring within the first three orders of the retinal arterial tree. They tend to be 100–250 μm in size with a fusiform or saccular shape.

Typically they occur in hypertensive females over the age of 50.

Clinical features

- ↓VA (if macular exudate or vitreous hemorrhage); often asymptomatic.
- Saccular or fusiform dilatation of retinal artery often near AV crossing; hemorrhage (sub-, intra-, or preretinal and vitreal) (Fig. 13.13); exudation (often on the temporal arcades with circinates).

Investigations

- FA shows immediate complete filling (partial filling suggests thrombosis) with late leakage (see Fig. 13.14).

Treatment

There is a high rate of spontaneous resolution, particularly of the hemor-rhagic (rather than exudative) lesions. Consider photocoagulation (either direct or to the surrounding capillary bed) if symptomatic due to exud-ation at the macula. Vitrectomy may be required for nonclearing vitreous hemorrhage.

Idiopathic polypoidal choroidal vasculopathy (IPCV, PCV)

This is a recently recognized abnormality of the choroidal vasculature. Risk factors include female sex and hypertension; although originally described in African Caribbeans, it may occur in any race.

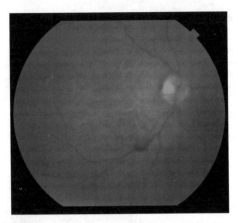

Figure 13.13 Retinal macroaneurysm surrounded by an area of retinal hemorrhage. See insert for color version.

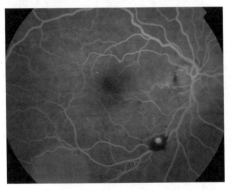

Figure 13.14 Fluorescein angiogram demonstrates a small area hyperfluorescence in the location of the dilated retinal macroaneurysm. The surrounding area is hypofluorescent due to blockage by the retinal hemorrhage. See insert for color versio

The underlying abnormality is of polypoidal aneurysmal dilation abnormal choroidal vasculature usually around the posterior pole. The result in the clinical picture of recurrent multiple serous or hemorrhag detachments of retina/RPE in the absence of features suggestive of AM (e.g., drusen) or intraocular inflammation.

The choroidal aneurysms can be confirmed on ICG, assisting different tion from AMD or other neovascular processes. Prognosis is variable.

Radiation retinopathy

Irradiation of the globe, orbit, sinuses, or nasopharynx may lead to retinal damage. This usually occurs after a delay of 6 months to 3 years, which is thought to be the turnover time for endothelial cells of the retinal vasculature.

Risk of retinopathy increases with radiation dose: 90% of brachytherapy patients receiving a macular dose of ≥7500 rad developed maculopathy; over 50% of patients receiving orbital/nasopharyngeal irradiation may develop retinopathy. Retinopathy is unlikely following doses of ≤2500 rad given in fractions of ≤200 rad.

Clinical features

- Focal dropout and irregular dilatation of the capillary bed at the posterior pole; microaneurysms, telangiectasia, exudation, fine intraretinal hemorrhages.
- *Acute response to high-dose radiation:* ischemic retinal necrosis with widespread vascular occlusion, CWS, widespread superficial and deep hemorrhages; intraretinal microvascular abnormalities; neovascularization ± tractional retinal detachment/vitreous hemorrhage.
- *Papillopathy* (usually accompanied by retinopathy): acute disc hyperemia, edema, peripapillary hemorrhage, and CWS; chronic severe optic atrophy.

Treatment

Consider focal photocoagulation for macular exudation and panretinal photocoagulation for proliferative radiation retinopathy, although less intensive treatment is usually required than in diabetic retinopathy.

Retinitis pigmentosa

Retinitis pigmentosa (RP) is the most common of the retinal dystrophies, affecting around 1 in 4000 of the population. It comprises a spectrum of conditions in which abnormalities of over 100 different genes may cause loss of predominantly rods (rod-cone dystrophy) or cones (cone-rod dystrophy).

It may be sporadic or inherited (autosomal dominant or recessive, or X-linked). Autosomal disease is the most common form (but the least severe), whereas X-linked disease is the least common (but the most severe). A number of specific syndromes are also described (Table 13.22). For selected gene involvement see Table 13.23.

Clinical features

- Nyctalopia, tunnel vision, ↓VA.
- Mid-peripheral "bone-spicule" retinal pigmentation, waxy pallor of the optic disc, arteriolar attenuation; cataract.
- *Complications:* CME.

Investigations

- ERG: scotopic affected before photopic; b-waves affected before a-waves. This test can be used to monitor disease.
- EOG is abnormal.
- Visual fields initially may have ring scotomas before developing frank tunnel vision.
- OCT demonstrates cystoid macular edema.
- Fundus autofluorescence demonstrates peripheral area of RPE lost and hyperfluoresence.

Treatment

- Supportive measures including counseling, low-vision aids, and social services must not be neglected.
- *Medical:* vitamin A palmitate (15,000IU/day) appears to slow disease progression slightly; acetazolamide (250–500mg/day) and topical carbonic anhydrase inbitors may be effective in RP-related CME.
- *Cataract surgery:* reduce operating light levels, prophylactic postoperative acetazolamide.

Variants

RP variants include unusual distributions (sectoral or central RP) and odd patterns, such as retinitis punctata albescens (scattered white dots predating more typical RP changes).

Table 13.22 Associations of retinitis pigmentosa (selected)

Isolated	• Sporadic
	• Familial (AD, AR, X-linked)
Systemic	• Usher syndrome
	• Bardet–Biedl syndrome
	• Laurence–Moon syndrome
	• Kearns–Sayre syndrome
	• Batten disease
	• Mucopolysaccharidoses I–III
	• Abetalipoproteinemia
	• Refsum disease
	• Osteopetrosis

Table 13.23 Genes involved in retinitis pigmentosa (selected)

AD RP	• Rhodopsin
	• Peripherin-RDS
	• NRL
	• RP1
	• FSCN2
	• PRPC8
AR RP	• PDEB
	• PDEA
	• CNCG
	• Rhodopsin
	• RLB1
	• TULP1
	• ABCR
	• RPE65
	• RP12
X-linked RP	• RPGR

Congenital stationary night blindness

This group of disorders shares the feature of early, but nonprogressive, nyctalopia (night blindness). They may be divided into those with normal fundus (with autosomal dominant [AD], autosomal recessive [AR], and X-linked subtypes) and those with fundal abnormalities (Oguchi's disease, fundus albipunctatus). Autosomal dominant CSNB has been traced back in family pedigrees as far as the 17th century (Nougaret pedigree).

CSNB with normal fundi

There are a number of different subclassifications based on inheritance, ERG findings, or presence of myopia. Mutations in rhodopsin, rod cGMP-PDE, and rod transducin have all been identified in AD CSNB.

Clinical features

In general, AD CSNB shows nonprogressive nyctalopia alone, whereas AR and X-linked disease show additional features, such as ↓VA, nystagmus, and myopia.

Investigations and treatment

On ERG, AD CSNB shows the Riggs ERG abnormality, whereas AR and X-linked CSNB show the Schubert–Bornschein ERG abnormality.

Treatment is supportive and dependent on the type of disease.

CSNB with abnormal fundi

Oguchi's disease

This rare autosomal recessive disease may arise from mutations in arrestin (Ch2) and rhodopsin kinase. In addition to nonprogressive nyctalopia, there is an abnormal golden-yellow fundal reflex that normalizes with dark adaptation (Mizuo phenomenon). There is also a delay in dark adaptation (with normalization of the ERG after several hours).

Fundus albipunctatus

This rare autosomal recessive disease is due to mutations in the gene for 11-*cis* retinol dehydrogenase. In addition to nonprogressive nyctalopia with delayed dark adaptation, there are numerous tiny white dots covering most of the fundus except the macula and far-periphery.

Macular dystrophies (1)

A number of retinal dystrophies show a predilection for the macula, usually causing loss of photoreceptors and the accumulation of a yellow material around the level of the RPE. This causes varying degrees of central vision loss.

There is no effective treatment for any of these conditions. Therefore, the priority of the clinician should be to provide effective diagnosis, counseling, and supportive care as required.

Stargardt's disease and fundus flavimaculatus

These are two clinical presentations of the same disease and are the most common of the macular dystrophies at around 7% of all retinal dystrophies. Most patients are autosomal recessive from a mutation in the ATP-binding cassette (ABCA4, Ch1p). Rare dominant disease links to the *ELOVL4* gene, Ch6q.

Histologically, there is accumulation of a lipofuscin-like material throughout the RPE. In the *ABCA4* knockout mouse model this has been found to be a toxic bis-retinoid.

Clinical features

- *Stargardt's disease:* rapid ↓VA (20/60–20/200) usually in childhood, initially with minimal visible signs; then posterior polar changes, including pigmentary disturbance, "beaten-bronze" atrophy of the macula, yellowish flecks in the peripheral retina.
- *Fundus flavimaculatus:* widespread pisciform flecks throughout the fundus, usually occurring in adulthood with relative preservation of vision.

Investigations

ERG and EOG are normal in early disease, mild reduction shows later.

FA shows classically dark choroid (due to blockage by the abnormal deposit) early in the disease process. In chronic disease, there are extensive window defects due to loss of RPE.

Best's disease

This is a rare condition with very variable expression such that some family members may have the genotype but be completely unaffected. It is autosomal dominant, arising from a mutation in the RPE transmembrane protein bestrophin (*VMD2*, Ch11q). Onset is usually in childhood.

Clinical features

- It is usually asymptomatic in early stages; ↓VA may be as low as 20/200 but most individuals retain reading and even driving vision in one eye.
- It is most easily recognized when there is a yolk-like lesion at the posterior pole; this may later be replaced by nonspecific scarring, atrophy, or even CNV formation (see Table 13.24).

Investigations

- EOG: reduced Arden ratio (<150%); ERG: near-normal.

Table 13.24 Staging of Best's disease

1.	Pre-vitelliform	EOG findings only
2.	Vitelliform	Yolk-like macular lesion
3.	Pseudohypopyon	Partial absorption leaving level
4.	Vitelliruptive	"Scrambled" appearance
5.	End stage	Scarring or atrophy

Adult vitelliform degeneration

Adult vitelliform degeneration (includes adult-onset foveomacular vitelliform dystrophy of Gass) describes a vitelliform appearance occurring in minimally symptomatic adults with a near-normal EOG. There is no clear inheritance pattern, although some cases with mutations of *VMD2* and peripherin/RDS have been described.

Familial drusen

This is a rare autosomal dominant condition with variable expression. The different patterns seen have traditionally been described separately as Doynes honeycomb dystrophy and malattia leventinese. However, it is thought that these reflect the varied phenotype of the same condition, all arising from mutations in *EFEMP1*. It appears that these mutations result in abnormal basement membrane formation at the level of the RPE.

Clinical features

Usually only mild symptoms occur; yellow-white drusen are at the posterior pole, are often confluent, and may be small or large

Investigations

ERG: normal; EOG: mild abnormality.

Pattern dystrophy

This rare group of conditions shows abnormal pigment patterns at the level of the RPE. Different phenotypes may be seen in the same family, hence they are probably best grouped collectively rather than separately under the traditional descriptive names—butterfly dystrophy, etc.

Inheritance is usually autosomal (recessive > dominant) and is in some cases linked to mutations in the peripherin/RDS gene.

Clinical features

Usually only mild symptoms occur; abnormal pigment patterns are at the posterior pole.

Investigations

ERG is normal; EOG shows mild abnormality.

Macular dystrophies (2)

Dominant CME

This very rare autosomal dominant disease (Ch7q) appears to selectively affect Muller's cells, causing multilobulated cystoid spaces arising from the inner nuclear layer. Clinically and on FA the appearances are of typical CME.

Sorsby's macular dystrophy

This very rare autosomal dominant disease arises from mutations in a regulator of extracellular matrix (TIMP3, Ch22). It usually causes significant ↓VA from age 40 years, when exudative maculopathy develops with subsequent scarring, atrophy, and even choroidal neovascularization.

North Carolina macular dystrophy

This rare autosomal dominant disease was initially described in North Carolina but has been identified in a number of families worldwide. It links to *MCDR1*, Ch6q. Onset is from birth. The phenotype varies from normal VA with a few drusen to hand movements (HM) acuity with a macular coloboma or subsequent CNV.

The macular lesions are present at birth and are stable in each individual but can be highly variable within family members.

Progressive bifocal chorioretinal atrophy

This rare autosomal dominant disease has only been described in the UK, and, like North Carolina macular dystrophy, links to Ch6q. This is a bizarre pattern of progressive chorioretinal atrophy that spreads from two foci located just temporal and just nasal to the disc.

Onset is from birth, and the visual loss is severe.

Cone degenerations

This group of disorders causes selective loss of cone photoreceptors with ↓VA, color vision abnormalities, and central scotomata. The macula may show only a mild granularity or marked central atrophy.

Central areolar choroidal dystrophy

This rare autosomal dominant disease links to Ch17p and usually presents in young adults. There is slowly progressive loss of central vision, with central geographic atrophy, including loss of the underlying choriocapillaris.

Choroidal dystrophies

The choroidal dystrophies are inherited, potentially blinding conditions in which the primary clinical abnormality is atrophy of the RPE and choroid. The codependence of retina and choroid is well demonstrated by the discovery that in choroideremia the underlying defect is probably in the rod photoreceptors, where stop mutations in the *CHM* gene prevents its normal production of Rab escort protein (REP-1).

Choroideremia

This rare X-linked recessive condition causes significant disease from childhood in males, but usually only asymptomatic "moth-eaten" peripheral pigmentary disturbance in female carriers.

Clinical features

- Nyctalopia, visual field loss (e.g., ring scotoma), later ↓VA (usually in middle age).
- *RPE/choroidal atrophy:* initially mid-peripheral, patchy, and superficial (choriocapillaris); later central, diffuse, and deeper choroidal atrophy to expose the sclera; retinal vessels and optic disc are relatively preserved.
- *Other:* cataract (posterior subcapsular), early vitreous degeneration.

Investigations and treatment

There is reduction in ERG (rod responses affected before cone responses) with prolongation of b-wave implicit time.

Useful vision is retained until late in the disease course; supportive treatment and genetic counseling may be offered.

Gyrate atrophy

This rare autosomal recessive condition arises from mutations in the *OAT* gene. This encodes for ornithine aminotransferase, which, with cofactor B6, catalyses the conversion of ornithine to glutamic-γ-semialdehyde and then to proline.

Two clinical subtypes are seen according to whether treatment with B6 lowers plasma ornithine levels. Responders appear to have a milder form of disease. Disease is usually symptomatic from late childhood.

Clinical features

- Nyctalopia, peripheral field loss, later ↓VA.
- *RPE/choroidal atrophy:* well-defined circular patches initially mid-peripheral and superficial (choriocapillaris); later confluent, diffuse fundus (relative sparing of macular, retinal vessels, and optic disc) and deeper choroidal atrophy; ERM, CME.
- *Other:* myopia, cataract (posterior subcapsular).

Investigations

- Early reduction in ERG (rod responses affected before cone responses); less marked changes in B6-responsive group.
- Plasma ornithine: 10–15× normal level; also elevated in urine and CSF.

Treatment
- Low-protein diet: with arginine restriction, ornithine levels may be controlled; control of ocular disease was demonstrated at least in the OAT–/– knockout mouse.
- Vitamin B6 reduces ornithine levels in the responsive subgroup, but there is little evidence for improved control of eye disease.

Other choroidal atrophies

These include diffuse choroidal atrophy and central areolar choroidal dystrophy, which are usually autosomal dominant, may be linked to abnormalities of peripherin/RDS, and carry a very poor prognosis.

Albinism

Abnormalities in the synthesis of melanin result in pigment deficiency of the eye alone (ocular albinism) or of the eye, skin, and hair (oculocutaneous albinism). Although there is wide phenotypic variation, the visual acuity is generally reduced because of macular hypoplasia. In most patients there also appears to be increased decussation of the temporal fibers at the chiasm.

Ocular albinism

Classic ocular albinism (Nettleship–Falls albinism) represents 10% of all albinism. It is X-linked, the *OA1* gene being implicated in melanosomes function. Ocular features may be severe despite an otherwise normal appearance. Female carriers may show mild, patchy features of the disease, including a "mud-splattered" fundus.

Clinical features
- ↓VA, photophobia.
- Nystagmus, strabismus, ametropia, iris hypopigmentation/transillumination, macular hypoplasia, fundus hypopigmentation.

Treatment
The main priority is to correct ametropia (± tinted lenses for photophobia) and prevent amblyopia. Consider surgery for strabismus and some cases of nystagmus.

Oculocutaneous albinism

Oculocutaneous disease is autosomal recessive and accounts for most albinism. It arises from abnormalities in several components of melanogenesis: type I = tyrosinase (Ch11q), type II = *p* product (Ch15q, probably a transporter), and type III = tyrosinase-related protein 1 (Ch9p) (Table 13.25).

Clinical features
- *Ophthalmic:* as for ocular albinism.
- *Systemic:* there is variable hypopigmentation of skin and hair (blond).

Treatment
- As for ocular albinism.

Table 13.25 Classification of oculocutaneous albinism

Type I	Tyrosinase	Subtype A	Severe variant
		Subtype B	Yellow variant
		Subtype MP	Minimal pigment
		Subtype TS	Temperature sensitive
Type II	Substance p	Prader–Willi	Learning difficulties, obesity, hypotonia
		Angelmann	Learning difficulties, ataxia, abnormal facies
		Hermansky–Pudlak	Low platelets, pulmonary/renal abnormalities; Puerto-Rican ancestry
		Chediak–Higashi	Immunocompromised secondary to abnormal leukocyte chemotaxis
Type III	TRP1		

Laser procedures in diabetic eye disease

Panretinal photocoagulation

Indication
- Active proliferative retinopathy, some cases of high-risk pre-proliferative retinopathy in patients with poor control of glucose or poor follow-up.

Method
- *Consent*: explain what the procedure does (the aim is to stop disease progression; that further laser treatment may well be required), what it does not do (it does not improve vision; is not an alternative to glycemic control), what to expect, and possible complications, e.g., pain, loss of peripheral field (with driving implications), scotoma, worsened acuity (e.g., macular decompensation), choroidal or retinal detachment.
- *Instill topical anesthetic* and position fundus contact lens (e.g., transequator) with coupling agent.
- *Set argon laser* for 200–500 µm spot size, 0.1 sec, and adjust power to produce a gently blanching burn.

Consider placing a temporal barrier at least 2–3 disc diameters from the fovea to help demarcate a "no-go" zone. Then place ≥1000 burns outside the vascular arcades, leaving burn-width intervals between them. A second session of ≥1000 is usually performed a few weeks later.

The power may need to be adjusted according to variable retinal take-up. Follow up monthly until there is evidence of neovascular regression, ± fill-in PRP until there is a response.

Macular laser (focal or grid)

Indication
- Clinically significant macular edema (Table 13.3).

Method
- *Consent*: explain what the procedure does (reduce sight loss; further laser treatment may be required), what to expect, and possible complications, e.g., pain, scotomata, worsened acuity, retinal detachment.
- *Instill topical anesthetic* and position fundus contact lens (e.g., area centralis) with coupling agent.
- *Set argon laser* for 50–200 µm spot size, 0.08–0.1 sec, and adjust power to produce a very gently blanching burn. Generally, smaller spot sizes and shorter durations are used for more central burns.

- *For focal treatment:* apply burns to leaking microaneurysms 500–3000 μm from the center of the fovea. Lesions as near as 300 μm to the fovea may be treated, provided this would not be within the FAZ.
- *For grid treatment:* place similar burns ≥1 burn-width apart in a grid arrangement around the fovea. They must be at least 500 μm from the center of the fovea and from the disc margin.
- *Review* at 3 months or sooner.

Intravitreal injection in retinal diseases

Indications
These include cystoid macular edema, diabetic macular edema, posterior uveitis, neovascular glaucoma, proliferative diabetic retinopathy, choroidal neovascular membrane, and neovascular age-related macular degeneration.

Method
- Explain to the patient the rationale for the injection and the possible need for future injections.
- Provide local or topical anesthetic. Prepare the injection site with 50% Betadine solution.
- Measure and mark the proper location of the injection with a sterile caliper.
- The injection is placed in the inferior sclera, especially for triamcinolone injections, to prevent short-term loss of vision due to clouding of the vitreous.
- The intraocular pressure is checked to ensure central retinal artery perfusion.

Orbit

Related pages:

Orbital and preseptal cellulitis in children 📖 p. 623

Anatomy and physiology

The bony orbit forms a pyramid comprising a medial wall lying anteroposteriorly, a lateral wall at 45°, a roof, and a floor (Table 14.1). It has a volume of around 30 mL and contains most of the globe and associated structures: extraocular muscles (p. 572), optic nerve (p. 514), cranial nerves (p. 516), vascular supply, and lacrimal system (p. 128) (see also Table 14.2).

Being effectively a rigid box, the only room for expansion is forward. Most orbital pathology, therefore, presents initially with proptosis, followed by disruption of eye movements.

Table 14.1 Orbital bones

Wall	Bones	Rim	Bones
Roof	Frontal Sphenoid (lesser wing)	Superior	Frontal
Lateral	Sphenoid (greater wing) Zygomatic	Lateral	Zygomatic Frontal
Floor	Zygomatic Maxilla Palatine	Inferior	Zygomatic Maxilla
Medial	Maxilla Lacrimal Ethmoid Sphenoid	Medial	Maxilla Lacrimal

Table 14.2 Orbital apertures

Aperture	Location	Contents
Optic canal	Apex (lesser wing sphenoid)	Optic nerve, sympathetic fibers Ophthalmic artery
Superior orbital fissure	Apex (greater/lesser wings sphenoid)	III, IV, V_1, VI, sympathetic fibers Orbital veins
Inferior orbital fissure	Apex	Zygomatic and infraorbital nerve (V_2) Orbital veins
Zygomaticofacial	Lateral wall	Zygomaticofacial nerve (V_2) and vessels
Zygomaticotemporal	Lateral wall	Zygomaticotemporal nerve (V_2) and vessels
Ethmoidal foramen	Medial wall (frontal & ethmoidal bones)	Ethmoidal arteries (anterior, posterior)
Nasolacrimal canal	Medial wall (maxilla/lacrimal)	Nasolacrimal duct

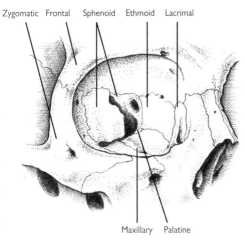

Zygomatic Frontal Sphenoid Ethmoid Lacrimal

Maxillary Palatine

Figure 14.1 The bones of the orbit.

Orbital and preseptal cellulitis

Orbital cellulitis is an ophthalmic emergency that may cause loss of vision and even death. Assessment, imaging, and treatment should be under the combined care of an ophthalmologist and ENT specialist (and pediatrician in children). Part of the ophthalmologist's role is to assist in differentiating orbital cellulitis from the much more limited preseptal cellulitis.

In younger children in whom the orbital septum is not fully developed, there is a high risk of progression, thus it should be treated similarly to orbital cellulitis. For orbital and preseptal cellulitis in children, see p. 623.

Orbital cellulitis

Infective organisms include *Streptococcus pneumoniae*, *Staphylococcus aureus*, *Streptococcus pyogenes*, and *Hemophilus influenza*.

Risk factors
- *Sinus disease:* ethmoidal sinusitis (common), maxillary sinusitis.
- Infection of other adjacent structures: preseptal or facial infection, dacryocystitis, dental abscess.
- *Trauma:* septal perforation.
- *Surgical:* orbital, lacrimal, and vitreoretinal surgery.

Clinical features
- Fever, malaise, painful, swollen orbit.
- Inflamed lids (swollen, red, tender, warm) ± chemosis, proptosis, painful restricted eye movements ± optic nerve dysfunction (↓VA, ↓color vision, RAPD).
- *Complications:* exposure keratopathy, ↑IOP, CRAO, CRVO, inflammation of optic nerve.
- *Systemic:* orbital or periorbital abscess, cavernous sinus thrombosis, meningitis, cerebral abscess.

Investigation
- Temperature.
- CBC, blood culture.
- CT (orbit, sinuses, brain): diffuse orbital infiltrate, proptosis ± sinus opacity.

Treatment
- Admit for intravenous antibiotics (e.g., either floxacillin 500–1000 mg 4×/day or cefuroxime 750–1500 mg 3×/day with metronidazole 500 mg 3×/day).
- ENT to assess for sinus drainage (required in up to 90% of adults).

Preseptal cellulitis

Preseptal cellulitis is not truly an orbital disease. It is much more common than orbital cellulitis, from which it must be differentiated (Table 14.3). The main causative organisms are *Staphylococci* and *Streptococci* spp. It is generally a much less severe disease, at least in adults and older children.

Risk factors
- Infection of adjacent structures (dacryocystitis, hordeolum) or systemic (e.g., upper respiratory tract infection).
- *Trauma*: laceration.

Clinical features
- Fever, malaise, painful, swollen lid/periorbita.
- Inflamed lids but no proptosis, normal eye movements, normal optic nerve function.

Investigation
Investigation is not usually necessary unless there is concern over possible orbital or sinus involvement.

Treatment
- Daily review until resolution (admit young or unwell children).
- Treat with oral antibiotics (e.g., floxacillin 500 mg 4×/day for 1 week and metronidazole 400 mg 3×/day for 1 week).

Table 14.3 Orbital vs. preseptal cellulitis

	Orbital	Preseptal
Proptosis	Present	Absent
Ocular motility	Painful + restricted	Normal
VA	Reduced (in severe cases)	Normal
Color vision	↓ (in severe cases)	Normal
RAPD	Present (in severe cases)	Normal

Mucormycosis (phycomycosis)

This is a rare, very aggressive life-threatening fungal infection caused by *Mucor* species or *Rhizopus*. Mucormycosis is a disease of the immunosuppressed, most commonly seen in patients who are also acidotic, such as in diabetic ketoacidosis or renal failure. However, the disease also occurs in malignancy and therapeutic immunosuppression. It represents fungal septic necrosis and infarction of tissues of nasopharynx and orbit.

Clinical features
• Black crusty material in nasopharynx, acute evolving cranial nerve palsies (II, III, IV, V, VI) ± obvious orbital inflammation.

Investigation
• Biopsy: fungal stains show nonseptate branching hyphae.
• CBC, UA, Glu.

Treatment
• Admit and coordinate care with microbiologist and infectious disease specialist, ENT specialist, ± PCP.
• Correct underlying disease (e.g., diabetic ketoacidosis) where possible.
• Intravenous antifungals (as guided by microbiology; e.g., amphotericin B).
• Early surgical debridement by ENT specialist ± orbital exenteration (for severe or unresponsive disease).

Thyroid eye disease: general

Thyroid eye disease (TED; also called thyroid ophthalmopathy, dysthyroid eye disease, Graves eye disease) is an organ-specific autoimmune disease that may be both sight threatening and disfiguring. Acute progressive disease is an ophthalmic emergency as it may threaten the optic nerve and cornea (see Box 14.1).

While most patients with TED have clinical and/or biochemical evidence of hyperthyroidism or hypothyroidism, some are euthyroid—at least at the time of presentation. Thyroid dysfunction may precede, be coincident with, or follow thyroid eye disease.

Incidence is around 10/100,000/year.

Risk factors

- Female sex (F:M 4:1).
- Middle age.
- HLA-DR3, HLA-B8, and the genes for CTLA4 and the thyroid-stimulating hormone (TSH) receptor.
- Smoking.
- Autoimmune thyroid disease.

Autoimmune thyroid disease

TED is most commonly associated with Graves' disease but may occur in 3% of Hashimoto's thyroiditis.

Graves' disease

This is the most common cause of hyperthyroidism. Anti-TSH receptor antibodies cause overproduction of thyroxine (T4) and/or T3. Classic features include hyperthyroidism, goiter, thyroid eye disease, thyroid acropachy (clubbing), and pretibial myxedema.

Autoimmune thyroiditis (e.g., Hashimoto's thyroiditis)

This is the most common cause of hypothyroidism. It may have a transient hyperthyroid stage, before leaving the patient hypothyroid. The associated goiter is usually firm.

Pathogenesis of TED

The cause is unclear. The target antigen is likely shared between the extraocular muscles and thyroid gland. Activated T cells probably act on cells of the fibroblast-adipocyte lineage within the orbit, thus stimulating adipogenesis, fibroblast proliferation, and glycosaminoglycan synthesis.

Clinical features

Ophthalmic

- Ocular irritation, ache (worse in mornings), red eyes, cosmetic changes, diplopia.
- Proptosis (exophthalmos), lid retraction (upper > lower) (Fig. 14.2), lid lag (on downgaze), conjunctival injection/chemosis, orbital fat prolapse, keratopathy (exposure/superior limbic keratoconjunctivitis or keratoconjunctivitis sicca), restrictive myopathy, optic neuropathy.

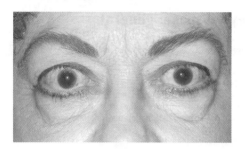

Figure 14.2 Thyroid eye disease with bilateral exophthalmos associated with lid retraction and scleral show. See insert for color version.

Box 14.1 Emergencies in thyroid eye disease

Acute progressive optic neuropathy
Optic neuropathy in TED may arise from compression of the nerve by involved tissues (mainly muscles) or proptosis-induced stretch.
- Assess optic nerve function (VA, color, visual fields, pupillary reactions).

Treatment
- Systemic immunosuppression (coordinate with endocrinologist). This is usually oral corticosteroids (e.g., 1 mg/kg 1×/day PO prednisone) but may be pulsed (e.g., 500 mg IV methylprednisone 1×/day for the first 3 days); other immunosuppresives may be added for additional control and as steroid-sparing agents.
- If this fails, then urgent surgical decompression is required. This varies in extent but must decompress the orbital apex where compression is often maximal. Some medical centers also use orbital radiotherapy in the acute setting.

Exposure keratopathy
Exposure keratopathy in TED may arise from proptosis and lid retraction.
- Assess corneal integrity, tear film, lid closure, and proptosis.
- Treatment: lubricants, acute immunosuppression (e.g., systemic corticosteroids) ± orbital decompression (or lid-lengthening surgery).

Systemic
Systemic signs depend on the thyroid status (over- or underactivity) and underlying disease (goiter in Graves' or Hashimoto's; pretibial myxedema, thyroid acropachy in Graves') (see Table 14.4).

Additionally, there is an increased frequency of other autoimmune diseases in association, e.g., pernicious anemia, vitiligo, diabetes mellitus, and Addison's disease.

Table 14.4 Common systemic features of thyroid dysfunction

	Hyperthyroidism	**Hypothyroidism**
Symptoms	<ul><li>Weight loss</li><li>Heat intolerance</li><li>Restlessness</li><li>Diarrhea</li><li>Poor libido</li><li>Amenorrhea</li><li>Poor concentration</li><li>Irritability</li></ul>	<ul><li>Weight gain</li><li>Cold intolerance</li><li>Fatigue</li><li>Constipation</li><li>Poor libido</li><li>Menorrhagia</li><li>Poor memory</li><li>Depression</li></ul>
Signs	<ul><li>Warm peripheries</li><li>Hair loss</li><li>Tachycardia</li><li>Atrial fibrillation</li><li>Proximal myopathy</li><li>Tremor</li><li>Osteoporosis</li></ul>	<ul><li>Dry coarse skin</li><li>Dry thin hair</li><li>Bradycardia</li><li>Pericardial/pleural effusions</li><li>Muscle cramps</li><li>Slow relaxing reflexes</li><li>Deafness</li></ul>

Thyroid eye disease: assessment

The diagnosis and management of thyroid eye disease depends on accurate clinical assessment. Grading systems aim to formalize this process but generally are not a substitute for careful clinical documentation of disease status (severity and activity). Similarly, while investigations may support a diagnosis of TED, they are not diagnostic in their own right.

Rundle's curve

The natural history of thyroid eye disease can be described in terms of an active phase of increasing severity, a regression phase of declining severity, and an inactive plateau phase (Rundle's curve). While specific to each patient, these time courses can be plotted graphically and broadly categorized according to mild, moderate, marked, or severe disease (Rundle a–d).

Assessment of disease severity

Grading systems used to document severity include the NOSPECS classification (Table 14.5). This is now used sparingly by ophthalmologists, who generally wish to document disease severity and extent in greater detail. It is still widely used by PCPs and endocrinologists.

Assessment of disease activity

The most widely used score of clinical activity is the *Mourits* system, although a standardized protocol based on comparison to clinical photographs has also been devised (Table 14.6).

Table 14.5 NOSPECS disease severity score

0	N	No signs or symptoms
1	O	Only signs, no symptoms
2	S	Soft tissue involvement
3	P	Proptosis
4	E	Extraocular muscle involvement
5	C	Corneal involvement
6	S	Sight loss (↓VA)

On Werner's modified NOSPECS, categories 2–6 can be further graded as o, a, b, or c (e.g., degree of visual loss for category 6).

Investigation

- *Thyroid function tests:* usually TSH and free T4, but check free T3 (the active metabolite) if there is strong clinical suspicion but otherwise normal biochemistry (Table 14.7).
- *Thyroid autoantibodies:* anti-TSH receptor, antithyroid peroxidase, and antithyroglobulin antibodies (Table 14.8).
- *Orbital imaging:* CT head gives better bony resolution and is preferred for planning decompression. MRI (T2-weighted and STIR) gives better soft tissue resolution and identifies active disease; the bellies of the muscles show enlargement and inflammation but the tendons are spared (Fig. 14.3).
- *Orthoptic review* may include field of binocular single vision, field of uniocular fixation, Hess/Lees chart, and visual fields.

Table 14.6 Clinical activity score

Pain	Painful, oppressive feeling on or behind globe	+1
	Pain on eye movement	+1
Redness	Eyelid redness	+1
	Conjunctival redness	+1
Swelling	Swelling of lids	+1
	Chemosis	+1
	Swelling of caruncle	+1
	Increasing proptosis (≥2 mm in 1–3 months)	+1
Impaired function	Decreasing eye movement (≥5° in 1–3 months)	+1
	Decreasing vision (≥1 line pinhole VA on Snellen chart)	+1
Total		/10

Source: Mourits MP, et al. (1989). Clinical criteria for the assessment of disease activity in Graves' ophthalmopathy: a novel approach. *Br J Ophthalmol* 73:639–644.

Table 14.7 Biochemical investigations in thyroid eye disease

Thyroid function tests	Hyperthyroid	Hypothyroid
TSH	↓	↑
Free T4	↑	↓

Table 14.8 Immunological investigations in thyroid eye disease

Autoantibody	Association	
Anti-TSH receptor	>95% Graves' disease	
	40–95% TED	
Anti-thyroid peroxidase	80% Graves' disease	90% Hashimoto's thyroiditis
Anti-thyroglobulin	25% Graves' disease	55% Hashimoto's thyroiditis

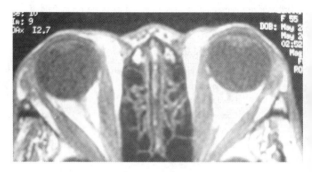

Figure 14.3 Thyroid eye disease MRI with enlargement of all the rectus muscles. See insert for color version.

Thyroid eye disease: management

Treatment of eye disease

General

- Multidisciplinary input from endocrinologist and ophthalmologist.
- Supportive: counseling, ocular lubricants, tinted glasses, bed-head elevation, prisms for diplopia, support group.

Medical

Consider immunosuppression in active disease, particularly if function (motility or vision) is threatened. This is usually by systemic corticosteroids but cyclosporine, methotrexate, and azathioprine have all been used. Radiotherapy is popular in some centers; it may transiently worsen disease.

Surgical

For acute disease

Acute progressive optic neuropathy or corneal exposure may require emergency orbital decompression.

For burnt-out disease

Surgery (usually staged) may improve function and cosmesis. Decompression, motility, or lid surgery are performed as required, and in that order. Decompression can be 1-, 2-, or 3-wall and by a variety of approaches (e.g., coronal, lower lid, etc.) to hide scars.

Prognosis

TED is a self-limiting disease that usually resolves within 1–5 years. Once stable, dramatic improvements in ocular motility and appearance can be achieved with a staged surgical approach. However, good long-term vision depends on successfully guarding against sight-threatening complications in the acute phase (see Box 14.2).

Box 14.2 Poor prognostic factors in TED

- Older age of onset
- Male
- Smoker
- Diabetes
- ↓VA
- Rapid progression at onset
- Longer duration of active disease

Treatment of hyperthyroidism

Carbimazole and propylthiouracil

Carbimazole or propylthiouracil is used to block the production of thyroid hormones. The initial dose (15–40 mg for carbimazole; 200–400 mg for propylthiouracil) is continued until the patient is euthyroid and then gradually reduced while maintaining normal free T4 levels. Therapy is generally required for 12–18 months.

An alternative regimen is blocking-replacement, in which higher doses of carbimazole are given simultaneously with thyroxine replacement.

Patients should be warned of the risk of agranulocytosis and to seek medical review (including CBC) if they develop infections, particularly sore throat.

Radioactive iodine

A single dose of radioactive sodium iodide (I_{131}) is given. The patient must avoid close contact with others, particularly children, for a period after administration. Subsequent hypothyroidism is common and requires thyroxine replacement.

There is some controversy over the possibility that radioactive iodine worsens TED (or whether this is related to a subsequent hypothyroid dip); typically, patients with moderate to severe TED will have progression of disease during radioactive iodine therapy. Patients with mild eye disease typically do not have progression. It is common practice to give prophylactic oral steroids when administering radioactive iodine in this higher-risk group of patients.

Surgical (ablation/thyroidectomy)

This may be used for large goiters or in patients who have moderate to severe eye disease and significant risk progression with radioactive iodine therapy.

In pregnancy and breast-feeding

Carbimazole and propylthiouracil cross the placenta and can cause fetal hypothyroidism. Consequently, the lowest dose possible should be used and the blocking-replacement regimen avoided.

Radioactive iodine is contraindicated in pregnancy.

Treatment of hypothyroidism

Levothyroxine

Thyroxine replacement is started at a dose of 25–100 µg (50 µg if >50 25 µg if cardiac disease) and cautiously increased at intervals of 4week to a maintenance dose of 100–200 µg. Treatment is monitored against thyroid function tests and clinical status.

Rapid increases or excessive doses may result in angina, arrhythmias and features of hyperthyroidism.

Other orbital inflammations

A number of inflammatory diseases may affect the orbit (Table 14.9). These may be purely orbital or related to systemic disease (e.g., thyroid eye disease). The purely orbital diseases may be diffuse (e.g., idiopathic orbital inflammatory disease) or focal (e.g., myositis).

Idiopathic orbital inflammatory disease (pseudotumor)

This is an uncommon chronic inflammatory process of unknown etiology. It may simulate a neoplastic mass (hence the term *pseudotumor*), but histology shows a pure inflammatory response without cellular atypia.

It is a diagnosis of exclusion and may in fact represent a number of poorly understood entities. It may occur at almost any age. It is usually unilateral.

Clinical features

- Acute pain, redness, lid swelling.
- Conjunctival injection, chemosis, lid edema, proptosis, restrictive myopathy, orbital mass.

Investigation

- *Orbital imaging:* B-scan (low to medium reflectivity, acoustic homogeneity); MRI (hypointense, cf. muscle on T1; hyperintense, cf. muscle on T2; moderate enhancement with gadolinium).
- *Biopsy* is required when there is diagnostic doubt.

Treatment

- Immunosuppression: usually with systemic corticosteroids, although cytotoxics (e.g., cyclophosphamide) and radiotherapy are sometimes used.

Idiopathic sclerosing inflammation of the orbit

This is a rare, relentlessly progressive idiopathic fibrosis akin to retroperitoneal fibrosis. There is no known cause and no effective treatment, and visual deterioration is common.

Table 14.9 Inflammatory diseases affecting the orbit (selected)

Isolated	Diffuse	Idiopathic orbital inflammatory disease
		Idiopathic sclerosing inflammation of the orbit
	Focal	Myositis
		Dacryoadenitis
		Tolosa–Hunt syndrome
Systemic		Thyroid eye disease
		Wegener's granulomatosis
		Sarcoidosis

Myositis

In myositis, the inflammatory process is restricted to one or more extraocular muscles, most commonly the superior or lateral rectus. The disease may occur at almost any age and is usually unilateral.

Clinical features

- Acute pain (especially on movement in the direction of the involved muscle), injection over muscle ± mild proptosis.

Investigations

- Orbital imaging: MRI gives better soft tissue resolution; the whole of the muscle and tendon shows enlargement and inflammation (cf. TED).

Treatment

- Immunosuppression: normally very sensitive to systemic corticosteroids.

Tolosa—Hunt syndrome

In this rare condition, there is focal inflammation of the superior orbital fissure ± orbital apex. The disease presents with orbital pain, multiple cranial nerve palsies, and sometimes proptosis.

It must be differentiated from other causes of the superior orbital fissure syndrome: carotid-cavernous fistula, cavernous sinus thrombosis, Wegener's granulomatosis, pituitary apoplexy, sarcoidosis, mucormycosis, and other infections. The condition is very sensitive to steroids.

Dacryoadenitis

Lacrimal gland inflammation may be isolated or occur as part of diffuse idiopathic orbital inflammatory disease. It presents with an acutely painful swollen lacrimal gland that is tender to palpation, has reduced tear production, and results in an S-shaped deformity to the lid.

The condition must be differentiated from infection and tumors of the lacrimal gland. Isolated dacryoadenitis does not usually require treatment.

Wegener's granulomatosis

This is an uncommon necrotizing granulomatous vasculitis that may have ophthalmic involvement in up to 50% of cases and orbital involvement in up to 22%. It is more common in males (M:F 2:1) and in middle age.

Clinical features

Ophthalmic

- *Orbital disease:* pain, proptosis, restrictive myopathy, disc swelling, ↓VA.
- *Other ocular disease:* epi/scleritis, peripheral ulcerative keratitis, uveitis, and retinal vasculitis.

Systemic

- Pneumonitis, glomerulonephritis, sinusitis, nasopharyngeal ulceration.

Investigation

- ANCA: most cases are c-ANCA positive.

Treatment

Treatment (coordinated by rheumatologist and physician) is usually with combined corticosteroids and cyclophosphamide.

Cystic lesions

Dacryops (lacrimal ductal cyst)

These cysts of the lacrimal duct tissue are relatively common and may arise from any lacrimal tissue (including the accessory lacrimal glands of Krause and Wolfring). Dacryops are often bilateral and protrude into the superior fornix. Treatment, if required, is by aspiration.

Dermoid cyst

Dermoids are a type of choristoma (congenital tumors of tissues abnormal to that location). They probably represent surface ectoderm trapped at lines of embryonic closure and suture lines.

They are most commonly located on the superotemporal orbital rim, but may extend deceptively far posteriorly. They comprise stratified squamous epithelium (with epidermal structures such as hair follicles and sebaceous glands) surrounding a cavity that may contain keratin and hair.

Clinical features
Superficial dermoids
- Present in infancy.
- Slowly growing firm smooth, round, nontender mass.

Deep dermoids
- Present from childhood on.
- Gradual proptosis, motility disturbance, ↓VA.
- May extend beyond the orbit into the frontal sinus, temporal fossa, or cranium.

Investigation
Orbital imaging: CT shows well-circumscribed lesion with heterogenous center; B-scan US shows well-defined lesion with high internal reflectivity.

Treatment
They should be excised completely without rupture of the capsule to avoid severe inflammation and recurrence. Intracranial spread of deep dermoid cysts requires coordination with neurosurgeons.

Mucocele

A *mucocele* is a slowly expanding collection of secretions resulting from blockage of the sinus opening. This may be due to a congenital narrowing or arise secondary to infection, inflammation, tumor, or trauma. Over time, erosion of the sinus walls permits the mucocele to encroach into the orbit. Orbit-involving mucoceles usually arise from frontal, ethmoidal, or, occasionally, the maxillary sinus.

Clinical features
These include headache, gradual nonaxial proptosis or horizontal displacement, and a fluctuant tender mass in medial or superomedial orbit.

Investigation
Orbital imaging: CT shows opacification of frontal or ethmoidal sinus (+loss of ethmoidal septae) with a bony defect allowing intraorbital protrusion. B-scan US shows a well-defined lesion with low internal reflectivity.

Treatment
Refer to an ENT specialist to excise the mucocele, restore sinus drainage, or obliterate the sinus cavity (in recurrent cases).

Cephalocele

These are developmental malformations resulting in herniation into the orbit of brain (encephalocele), meninges (meningocele), or both (meningoencephalocele). They may be anterior (frontoethmoidal bony defects) or posterior (sphenoid dysplasia). Encephaloceles may be associated with other craniofacial or ocular abnormalities; posterior encephaloceles may be associated with neurofibromatosis-1 and morning glory syndrome.

Clinical features
Pulsatile proptosis may increase with Valsalva maneuver but have no bruit (cf. arteriovenous fistulae).

Anterior lesions
The encephalocele may be visible, and proptosis is usually anterotemporal.

Posterior lesions
The encephalocele is not visible and the proptosis is usually antero-inferior.

Investigation
Orbital imaging: CT shows a defect in the orbital wall.

Orbital tumors: lacrimal and neural

Lacrimal gland

Pleomorphic adenoma

This is the most common lacrimal neoplasm and accounts for up to 25% of all lacrimal fossa lesions. The tumor derives from epithelial and mesenchymal tissue, hence the term *benign mixed cell tumor*. It may arise from either lobe, most commonly the orbital.

The neoplasm occurs in middle age with a slight male bias (M:F 1.5:1). Malignant transformation occurs at around 10% in 10 years.

Clinical features

- Gradual painless proptosis (inferonasal), ophthalmoparesis, choroidal folds, palpable mass of the superomedial orbit (orbital lobe tumors may not be palpable).

Investigation

- US shows a round lesion with medium to high reflectivity and regular acoustic structure.
- CT/MRI shows a well-defined round lesion ± bone remodeling.

Treatment

This involves surgical removal of the whole tumor with intact capsule without prior biopsy (risk of seeding). This is usually done with an anterior (palpebral lobe tumors) or lateral (orbital lobe tumors) orbitotomy. Prognosis is excellent with complete excision.

Lacrimal carcinomas

The most common malignant tumor of the lacrimal gland is the adenoid cystic carcinoma, followed by the mucoepidermoid carcinoma and the pleomorphic adenocarcinoma. They occur at a similar age to that of adenomas but cause more rapid proptosis and ophthalmoparesis, and orbital pain from perineural spread is common.

Imaging shows an irregular, poorly defined lesion with bony destruction. Treatment is seldom curative but consists of exenteration ± radiotherapy. Prognosis is very poor.

Neural

Optic nerve glioma

This is an uncommon slow-growing tumor of astrocytes that usually occurs in children and has a strong association with neurofibromatosis-1. It usually presents with gradual ↓VA (although this often stabilizes), disc swelling or atrophy, and proptosis. Isolated optic nerve involvement occurs in 2%, but most cases involve the chiasm (72%), often with midbrain and hypothalamic involvement.

Imaging shows fusiform enlargement of the optic nerve ± chiasmal mass. Observation is recommended for patients with isolated optic nerve involvement distant from the chiasm, good vision, and nondisfiguring proptosis. Progress is monitored with serial MRI scans.

Surgical excision is indicated for pain, severe proptosis, or posterior spread threatening the chiasm. Chiasmal or midbrain involvement may be an indication for chemotherapy or radiotherapy.

Prognosis for life is good for optic nerve–restricted tumors but worsens with more posterior involvement.

Optic nerve sheath meningioma

This is a rare benign tumor of meningothelial cells of the meninges that usually occurs in middle age and has a slight female bias (F:M 1.5:1). There is an association with neurofibromatosis-2. It usually presents with gradual ↓VA, disc swelling or atrophy, optociliary shunt vessels (30%), proptosis, and ophthalmoparesis.

Imaging shows tubular enlargement of the nerve with "tram-track" enhancement of the sheath ± calcification. Observation is recommended if VA is good.

Surgical excision is indicated for blind eyes, severe proptosis, or threat to the chiasm. Prognosis for life is good.

Neurofibroma

Neurofibromas are uncommon benign tumors of peripheral nerves.

Plexiform neurofibroma presents in childhood and is strongly associated with neurofibromatosis-1. Anterior involvement results in a "bag-of-worms" mass causing an S-shaped lid deformity. The tumor is poorly defined and not encapsulated. Surgical excision is difficult and may require repeated debulking.

Isolated neurofibroma presents in adulthood with gradual proptosis. The tumor is well circumscribed, and surgical excision is usually straightforward.

Schwannoma

This is an uncommon slow-growing tumor of peripheral or cranial nerves that is usually benign but may be malignant. The tumor usually presents in adulthood. There is an association with neurofibromatosis.

It is usually located in the superior orbit and presents as a gradually enlarging nontender mass (often cystic) with proptosis, ↓VA, and restricted motility.

Treatment is with complete surgical excision, which has a good prognosis.

Orbital tumors: vascular

Cavernous hemangioma

This is the most common benign orbital neoplasm of adults. It is a hamartoma but does not usually present until young adulthood, most notably during pregnancy (accelerated growth). It is usually intraconal.

Clinical features

- Proptosis (usually axial due to intraconal location); later restricted motility, choroidal folds, and ↓VA.

Investigation

- US: well-circumscribed intraconal lesion with high internal reflectivity.
- CT/MRI: well-circumscribed intraconal lesion with mild to moderate enhancement.

Treatment

Most may be observed, but symptomatic lesions should be completely excised, if possible. For apical lesions, decompression may be indicated to preserve vision.

Capillary hemangioma

This is a type of hamartoma (congenital tumors of tissues normal to that location). Very large tumors may be consumptive (Kasabach–Merritt syndrome: ↓platelets, ↓Hb, ↓clotting factors) or cause high-output cardiac failure.

Superficial lesions (strawberry nevus)

These are bright red tumors that usually appear before 2 months of age, reach full size by 1 year, and involute by 6 years. They may be disfiguring and/or may cause amblyopia by obscuration of the visual axis or, more commonly, associated astigmatism. In these cases, treatment (usually with systemic propranolol or corticosteroids) may be indicated.

Deep lesions

These may not be visible but cause variable proptosis (worsens with Valsalva maneuver or crying). With time, partial involution occurs in most of these lesions, but large tumors may be treated (with corticosteroids or radiotherapy).

Lymphangioma

This is a rare hamartoma of lymph vessels that usually presents in childhood. They increase in size with head-down posture, Valsalva maneuver, and viral illness. Superficial lesions are visible as cystic spaces of the lid or conjunctiva that may also contain blood. Deep lesions may cause gradual proptosis or present acutely with orbital pain and ↓VA due to hemorrhage ("chocolate cyst").

Most lesions are observed. If a sight-threatening bleed occurs, the lesion may be drained, but surgery is difficult. Injection of cyanoacrylate glue or fibrin glue may aid in surgical debulking.

Orbital tumors: lymphoproliferative

Benign reactive lymphoid hyperplasia

This is an uncommon polyclonal proliferation of lymphoid tissue that usually occurs in the superoanterior orbit, often involving the lacrimal gland. It may present with gradual proptosis and/or a palpable firm rubbery mass. It usually responds to corticosteroids or radiotherapy, although some cases require cytotoxics. Progression to lymphoma occurs in up to 25% by 5 years.

Atypical lymphoid hyperplasia is intermediate between benign reactive hyperplasia and lymphoma and is characterized by a very homogeneous pattern with larger nuclei.

Malignant orbital lymphoma

This is an uncommon low-grade proliferation of B cells (non-Hodgkin's type) usually arising in the elderly. It usually presents with gradual proptosis and/or a palpable firm rubbery mass. It is usually unilateral, but bilateral involvement occurs in 25%; systemic involvement is present in 40% at diagnosis and in 60% within 5 years.

Treatment (radiotherapy or chemotherapy) depends on the grade and spread of tumor; a systemic workup is necessary in all cases.

Langerhans cell histiocytosis (LCH)

This is a rare proliferative disorder of childhood. It comprises a spectrum of disease from the unifocal, relatively benign eosinophilic granuloma to the disseminated Letterer–Siwe form. In eosinophilic granuloma, orbital involvement is common and presents as rapid proptosis with a superotemporal swelling.

Surgical curretage with injection of intralesional corticosteroids is usually curative. Bilateral proptosis may occur in disseminated LCH.

Orbital tumors: other

Rhabdomyosarcoma

This is the most common primary orbital malignancy in children. It usually arises in the first decade and has a slight male bias (M:F 1.6:1). The tumor arises from pluripotent mesenchymal tissue.

Histologically, it may be differentiated into embryonal (most common), alveolar, and pleomorphic types. It is usually intraconal (50%) or within the superior orbit (25%).

Clinical features

- Acute/subacute proptosis, ptosis and orbital inflammation; it may therefore mimic inflammatory conditions such as orbital cellulitis.

Investigation

- B-scan US: irregular but well-defined edges, low to medium reflectivity.
- CT/MRI: irregular but well-defined mass ± bony erosion.

Treatment

A biopsy (to confirm diagnosis) and systemic workup (to establish spread) are necessary in all cases. Surgical excision is possible for well-circumscribed localized tumors. Combined radiotherapy and chemotherapy is given for more extensive tumors.

Fibrous histiocytoma

This is an uncommon tumor that may affect middle-aged adults or children who have had orbital radiotherapy. It may be benign or malignant. The tumor is usually located superonasally and presents with gradual proptosis, ↓VA, and restricted motility. Treatment is by surgical excision, but recurrences are common.

Metastases

Orbital metastases are uncommon. In around half of all cases, they precede the diagnosis of the underlying tumor (Table 14.10). They usually present aggressively with fairly rapid proptosis, restricted motility, cranial nerve involvement, and orbital inflammation. Scirrhous tumors (e.g., some breast, prostate, and gastric tumors) may cause enophthalmos.

Table 14.10 Primary tumors metastasizing to the orbit

Adults	Children
Breast	Neuroblastoma
Lung	Nephroblastoma
Prostate	Ewing sarcoma
Gastrointestinal	

Vascular lesions

Orbital varices

These are congenital venous enlargements that may present from childhood on. They are usually unilateral and located in the medial orbit.

Clinical features
• Intermittent proptosis and/or visible varix (worse with increased venous pressure, i.e., Valsalva maneuver and in head-down position); occasional thrombosis or hemorrhage.

Treatment
Surgery is difficult but is indicated if the condition is severe or sight threatening. Incomplete excision is common.

Arteriovenous fistula

These are abnormal anastamoses between the arterial and venous circulation. The *carotid–cavernous fistula* is a high-flow system arising from direct communication between the intracavernous internal carotid artery and the cavernous sinus.

The *dural shunt* (also known as indirect carotid–cavernous fistula) is a low-flow system arising from dural arteries (branches of the internal and external carotid arteries) communicating with the cavernous sinus.

Arteriovenous fistulae may be congenital (e.g., Wyburn–Mason syndrome), secondary to trauma (particularly in young adults), or occur spontaneously (most cases in older people).

Clinical features
Carotid–cavernous fistula (direct)
• ↓VA, diplopia, audible bruit.
• Pulsatile proptosis with a bruit, orbital edema, injected chemotic conjunctiva, ↑IOP, variable ophthalmoplegia (usually involving CN III and CN VI), retinal vein engorgement, RAPD, disc swelling.

Dural shunt (indirect carotid–cavernous fistula)
• May be asymptomatic; pain, cosmesis.
• Chemosis, episcleral venous engorgement, ↑IOP.

Investigation
Orbital imaging: B-scan US, CT, and MRI show a dilated superior ophthalmic vein and mild thickening of the extraocular muscles.

Treatment
• High-flow carotid–cavernous fistulae may cause visual loss in up to 50% of cases and require closure by catheter embolization.
• Low-flow dural shunts spontaneously close by thrombosis in up to 40% cases. Intervention is reserved for cases with glaucoma, ↓VA, diplopia, or severe pain.

Intraocular tumors

Iris tumors

Uveal melanoma

Uveal melanoma is the most common primary malignant intraocular tumor of Caucasian adults, with a lifetime incidence of around 0.05%. Risk factors include race (light >> dark pigmentation), age (old > young), and underlying disorders such as ocular melanocytosis and dysplastic nevus syndrome. It is slightly more common in men than women.

Tumors arise from neuroectodermal melanocytes of the choroid, ciliary body, or iris.

Iris melanoma

Compared to the other uveal melanomas, iris tumors are less common (8% of uveal tumors), present at a younger age (40–50 years), and have a better prognosis. Histologically, they usually comprise spindle cells alone or spindle cells with benign nevus cells. See Table 15.1 for differential diagnosis.

Clinical features

- Usually asymptomatic; patient may note a spot or diffuse color change.
- Iris nodule is most commonly light to dark brown, well-circumscribed, usually inferior iris. It may be associated with hyphema, increase of intraocular pressure (IOP) (tumor or pigment cell blockage of trabecular meshwork), or cataract. Transcleral illumination may help demarcate posterior extension.

Risk factors for malignancy

These include size (>3 mm diameter, >1 mm thickness), rapid growth, prominent intrinsic vascularity, pigment dispersion, increased IOP, and iris splinting (uneven dilation).

Investigations

- *B-scan ultrasound:* size, extension, composition.
- *Biopsy:* consider fine needle aspiration (simple, safe, but scanty sample with no architecture) or incisional biopsy (corneal/limbal wound, risk of hyphema, and potential for monocular diplopia).

Treatment

Specialist consultation and advice should be obtained. Options include the following:

- *Observation:* small, asymptomatic tumors with no evidence of growth; intervention may not be necessary.
- *Excision:* consider iridectomy/iridocyclectomy.
- *Radiotherapy:* proton beam radiotherapy or brachytherapy.
- *Enucleation:* rarely indicated (nonresectable, extensive aqueous seeding or painful, blind eye).

Prognosis

Most patients do well and never develop metastatic disease. Poor prognostic features include large tumor size, ciliary body or extrascleral extension, and diffuse or annular growth pattern.

Table 15.1 Differential diagnosis of iris melanoma

Pigmented	• Nevus
	• ICE syndrome
	• Adenoma
	• Ciliary body tumors
Nonpigmented	• Iris cyst
	• Iris granuloma
	• IOFB
	• Juvenile xanthogranuloma
	• Leiomyoma ciliary body tumors
	• Iris metastasis

Box 15.1 Suspicious features in an iris nevus

- Size (>3 mm diameter, >1 mm thickness)
- Rapid growth
- Prominent intrinsic vascularity
- Pigment dispersion
- ↑IOP
- Iris splinting (uneven dilation)
- Pupillary peaking
- Uveal ectropion

Iris nevus

These common lesions require yearly ophthalmic observation unless there are suspicious features (Box 15.1), which require closer observation and photography.

Clinical features

- Usually asymptomatic; patient may note a spot on the iris.
- Small (<3 mm diameter, <0.5 mm thick), defined, pigmented stromal lesion; pupillary peaking or uveal ectropion occasionally occur in nevi.

Iris metastasis

These are typically amelanotic solid tumors, which may cause complications such as secondary open-angle glaucoma (clogging or infiltration of trabecular meshwork with tumor cells), hyphema, and pseudohypopyon. In most cases patients are already known to have a malignancy elsewhere, but in some patients the iris lesion is the presenting feature and requires extensive workup with an oncologist.

Ciliary body tumors

Ciliary body melanoma

These account for around 12% of all uveal melanomas (p. 494). They most commonly present around 50–60 years of age. In contrast to iris melanomas, they usually contain the more anaplastic epithelioid melanoma cells and carry a worse prognosis (see Table 15.2).

Clinical features
• Usually asymptomatic; occasionally visual symptoms.
• Ciliary body mass (may only be visible with full dilation); dilated episcleral sentinel vessels; anterior extension onto the iris or globe; lens subluxation or secondary cataract; anterior uveitis.

Investigation
• *B-scan ultrasound:* size, extension, composition.
• *Biopsy:* consider fine needle aspiration.

Treatment
Specialist consultation and advice should be obtained. Options include the following:
• Excision may be possible for smaller lesions.
• Radiotherapy: brachytherapy or proton beam.
• Enucleation for larger lesions or significant extension.

Medulloepithelioma

This is a rare, slow-growing tumor derived from immature epithelial cells of the embryonic optic cup. It usually arises from the nonpigmented ciliary epithelium, but iris and retinal sites are occasionally seen. Overall, local invasion is common but metastasis is rare.

Age of onset ranges from infant (congenital) to adult but is usually under the age of 10; both sexes are equally affected.

Clinical features
• Red eye, decreased VA, iris color and contour change/mass.
• Injection, ciliary body mass (amelanotic, often cystic), cyclitic membrane.
• Complications: neovascular glaucoma, lens coloboma/subluxation/cataract.

Investigation and treatment
Diagnosis may be assisted by ultrasound. Iridocyclectomy may be curative for small, well-defined, benign tumors; for most others, enucleation is still required.

Table 15.2 Differential diagnosis of ciliary body melanoma

Pigmented	• Metastasis
	• Ciliary body adenoma
Nonpigmented	• Ciliary body cyst
	• Uveal effusion syndrome
	• Medulloepithelioma
	• Leiomyoma
	• Metastasis

Choroidal melanoma

Choroidal melanomas account for 80% of all uveal melanomas. They usually present around 50–60 years of age.

They are classified according to size: small (<10 mm diameter or <3 mm in thickness), medium (10–15 mm diameter or up to 10 mm in thickness), and large (>15 mm diameter or >10 mm in thickness).

Histologically, they may comprise spindle cells (types A and B), epithelioid cells, or a mixture (most common type). Necrosis may prevent cell typing in 5% of cases.

Clinical features

- Often asymptomatic; decreased visual acuity, visual field loss, "ball of light" slowly moving across vision.
- Elevated sub-RPE mass that is commonly brown but may be amelanotic; commonly associated with orange pigment (lipofuscin) and exudative retinal detachment (Fig. 15.1). Some (20%) may rupture through Bruch's membrane and RPE to form a "mushroom." There is occasional vitreous hemorrhage, increased IOP, cataract, and uveitis.

The key diagnostic dilemma is to distinguish a malignant melanoma from a benign nevus (p. 500). Suspicious features are listed in Box 15.2. See also Table 15.3.

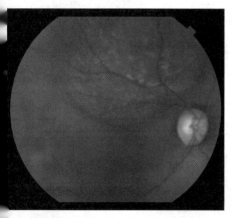

Figure 15.1 Large peripapillary choroidal melanoma with lipofuscin pigment in the tumor with associated serous detachment of the retina. See insert for color version.

Box 15.2 Suspicious features suggestive of choroid melanoma

- Symptomatic
- Juxtapapillary
- Subretinal fluid/retinal detachment
- Lipofuscin on the surface
- Large size (e.g., >2 mm thickness)
- Significant growth
- ↑IOP

Table 15.3 Differential diagnosis of choroidal melanoma

Pigmented	• Nevus
	• CHRPE
	• Melanocytoma
	• Metastasis
	• BDUMP syndrome
Nonpigmented	• Choroid granuloma
	• Posterior scleritis
	• Retinal detachment
	• Choroidal detachment
	• Choroidal neovascular membrane
	• Hematoma (subretinal/subRPE/suprachoroidal)
	• Choroidal osteoma
	• Choroidal hemangioma
	• Metastasis

Investigations

- *Ultrasound:* mass, acoustically hollow, low internal reflectivity, with choroidal excavation. Retinal detachment can be present.
- *CT and MRI* may detect extraocular extension but cannot reliably differentiate between types of tumor.
- *Biopsy:* fine needle aspiration biopsy may be performed in selected cases.
- *Systemic assessment:* CBC, LFT, liver/abdominal US (or CT, MRI).

At the time of presentation, most patients (98%) do not have detectable metastatic disease. The remaining 2% usually have large intraocular tumors with extraocular spread.

Treatment

Specialist consultation and advice should be obtained. Options include the following:

- *Observation* for small choroidal melanocytic lesions without suspicious features.

- *Transpupillary thermotherapy* (TTT): consider for small (<10 mm diameter, <3 mm thick), heavily pigmented lesions, which are outside the macula and not touching the optic disc. However, increased incidence of recurrence has been noted when TTT is the only treatment.
- *Radiotherapy:* plaques (4 mm larger in diameter than the lesion; deliver around 80–100 Gy to the tumor apex) or proton beam irradiation (usually 50–70 Gy in 4–5 fractions). Plaque radiotherapy has fewer local side effects than proton beam and was shown to be as effective as enucleation for medium-sized melanomas (Collaborative Ocular Melanoma Study [COMS]). Side effects include radiation retinopathy, cataracts, and neovascular glaucoma.
- *Local resection* may be suitable for smaller anterior tumors. Unlike enucleation, it preserves vision and cosmesis and avoids long-term complications of irradiation. However, the surgery is difficult with significant risk of complications (vitreous hemorrhage, retinal detachment, cataract).
- *Enucleation* is usually performed for large tumors (>15 mm diameter, 10 mm thick), optic nerve involvement, or painful blind eyes. No benefit has been demonstrated for pre-enucleation radiotherapy (COMS).
- *Orbital exenteration* is controversial; occasionally it is performed for massive orbital extension or recurrence after enucleation.

Prognosis

Poor prognostic features include large tumor size, extrascleral extension, older age, epithelioid cell type, and certain mutations (monosomy 3 and partial duplication of 8q).

Choroidal nevus

Uveal nevi are benign melanocytic tumors. They may occur in up to 6% of adult Caucasians, making them the most common of all intraocular tumors. Rarely, they may become malignant (1 in 5000). Their main significance lies in the need to differentiate them from a malignant melanoma. Choroidal nevi are usually incidental findings on routine eye examinations.

Clinical features

- Asymptomatic, rarely decreased visual acuity.
- Small (<5 mm diameter, <1 mm thick), homogenous gray-brown; may have drusen; absence of lipofuscin or subretinal fluid.

Differentiating a nevus from a malignant melanoma

With time, a malignant melanoma may declare itself by continued, often rapid, growth. However, it may be possible to identify probable melanomas at the time of presentation from the presence of suspicious characteristics. Features suggestive of malignancy include the following:

- **T**hickness (>2 mm).
- **F**luid (subretinal).
- **S**ymptoms.
- **O**range pigment.
- **M**argin touching disc.
- **H**ollowness on ultrasound.

In the absence of any of the first six features, a small melanocytic lesion is very unlikely to be a choroidal melanoma (only 3% show significant growth at 5 years). The presence of one feature increases the risk to 38%, and of two or more, to >50%. The following mnemonic has been suggested: TFSOM: To Find Small Ocular Melanomas.[1]

Investigation and treatment

If no suspicious features are present, these lesions can be followed yearly. The nevus should be photographed for future comparison.

Melanocytoma of the optic disc

These consist of a distinctive cell type—the polyhedral nevus cell. They are heavily pigmented benign tumors involving the optic disc, which may cause axonal compression and consequent visual field defects.

1 Shields C, Shields JA (2002). Clinical features of small choroidal melanoma. *Curr Opin Ophthalmo* 13:135.

Choroidal hemangiomas

Choroidal hemangiomas are benign vascular hamartomas. Although congenital, they are usually asymptomatic until adulthood when secondary degenerative changes of the overlying RPE and retina may cause visual loss.

Two clinical patterns are seen: circumscribed and diffuse. Histologically, they comprise mainly cavernous vascular channels (with normal endothelial cells and supporting fibrous septa) but with some capillary-like vessels (especially in the diffuse form).

Circumscribed choroidal hemangioma

This form is isolated, may be asymptomatic, and has no systemic associations. It is usually static but may grow in pregnancy.

Clinical features

- Poorly demarcated, elevated, orange-red choroidal mass; usually 3–7 mm diameter, 1–3 mm thick; located around the posterior pole (within 3 mm of disc or foveola) (Fig. 15.2).
- *Complications*: fibrous change of RPE, cystic change, or serous detachment of the retina.

Investigations

- *Ultrasound:* high internal reflectivity
- *FA:* early hyperfluorescence of intralesional choroidal vessels, followed by diffuse hyperfluorescence of the whole lesion (Fig. 15.3).
- *ICG:* early cyanescence of intralesional choroidal vessels, followed by intense cyanescence of the whole lesion and subsequent central fading (washout).

Treatment

Specialist consultation and advice should be sought. Options include observation, photodynamic therapy (PDT), transpupillary thermotherapy, thermal laser therapy, or irradiation.

Diffuse choroidal hemangioma

This form is usually associated with other ocular and systemic abnormalities, forming part of the Sturge–Weber syndrome.

Clinical features

- Deep-red (cf. normal other eye) thickened choroid, particularly at the posterior pole; may have tortuous retinal vessels, fibrous change of RPE, cystic change, or serous detachment of the retina and disc cupping.
- *Complications:* fibrous change of RPE, cystic change or serous detachment of the retina, glaucoma.

Investigations

- *Ultrasound:* diffuse choroidal thickening with high internal reflectivity.
- *MRI brain:* if CNS hemangioma suspected as part of Sturge–Weber syndrome (Table 15.4).

Treatment

Specialist consultation and advice should be sought. Options include PDT, TTT, or irradiation. Coordinate care with a neurologist if there is cerebral involvement.

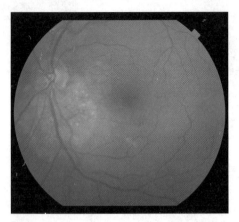

Figure 15.2 Peripapillary choroidal hemangioma with slight elevation of the mass and associated RPE atrophy. See insert for color version.

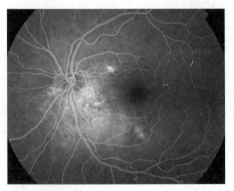

Figure 15.3 Fluorescein angiogram of the choroidal hemangioma demonstrated area of hyperfluroscence due to window defects early in the study and leakage late on the angiogram. See insert for color version.

Table 15.4 Features of Sturge–Weber syndrome

Ocular	Extraocular
Episcleral hemangioma	Nevus flammeus of the face
Culinary body/iris hemangioma	CNS hemangioma
Choroid hemangioma (diffuse)	
Glaucoma	

Other choroidal tumors

Choroidal osteoma

This is a rare, benign tumor of the choroid. Originally thought to be a choristoma, it is now felt to be an acquired neoplasm in which mature bone replaces choroid with damage to overlying RPE and retina.

Typically, it is seen in young adult women (F:M 9:1); it may be bilateral in 20%.

Clinical features

● Gradual decreased visual acuity, metamorphopsia.
● Yellow well-defined geographic lesion, usually abutting or surrounding optic disc; superficial abnormalities include prominent inner choroidal vessels and irregular RPE changes.
● *Complications*: CNV.

Investigations and treatment

● *US:* highly reflective with acoustic shadow.
● *CT:* bone-like signal from posterior globe.
● *FA:* early mottled hyperfluorescence and late diffuse hyperfluorescence. Although treatment of the tumor itself is not indicated, CNV may be treated conventionally.

Choroidal metastasis

These are the most common intraocular malignant neoplasms. Usually patients are already known to have a primary tumor (Box 15.3), but in around 25% of cases the first clinical manifestation may be an ocular problem.

Although the choroid is the primary site, metastasis may occur in the iris, ciliary body, retina, and vitreous, and the optic nerve may be involved. Bilateral involvement is seen in around 20% of patients.

Clinical features

● ↓VA, metamorphopsia; may be asymptomatic.
● Yellow-white (breast, lung, GI tract) ill-defined lesion (Fig. 15.4); it usually fairly flat but may have associated exudative retinal detachment.
● Color variation: consider cutaneous malignant melanoma if lesion is black, renal cell carcinoma or follicular thyroid carcinoma if red-orange, and carcinoid if golden-orange.

Investigations and treatment

Ocular

● *US:* high internal reflectivity.
● *FA:* no or few large vessels within the tumor, early hypofluorescence, and late diffuse hyperfluorescence. ICG may show tumors not detected on FA.
● Fine needle aspiration (FNA): consider FNA if there is diagnostic uncertainty and no extraocular tissue available for biopsy.

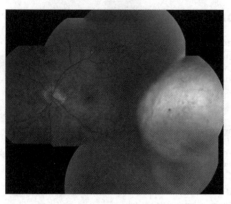

Figure 15.4 Large peripheral subretinal metastatic ovarian carcinoma. See insert for color version.

Systemic
This should be coordinated with a PCP and/or oncologist and include a complete examination (including breasts, prostate, lymph nodes, skin) and selected testing (e.g., CXR, mammography).

Treatment will depend on the lesion, visual status of the eye, and general health of the patient. Options include observation, chemotherapy, radiotherapy (plaque, proton-beam), or occasionally enucleation.

Box 15.3 Most common primary tumors metastasizing to the eye

- Lung
- Breast
- Gastrointestinal
- Kidney
- Thyroid
- Testis
- Skin

Retinoblastoma (Rb)

This is the most common primary malignant intraocular tumor of child-hood. Lifetime incidence is 1 in 15,000. It is rare after the age of 6 years, with median presentation between 1 and 2 years of age (earlier for bilat-eral disease). There is no gender or racial predilection.

The tumor arises from primitive retinoblasts of the developing retina with loss of function of the Rb tumor suppressor gene (*Ch13q14*). Loss or inactivation of both Rb copies is required (Knudson's two-hit hypothesis); in 60% of cases both mutations are acquired, whereas in 40%, one of the abnormal genes is inherited.

Over 90% of cases are sporadic (with no family history). In most of these cases the mutation is somatic (arising sufficiently late not to be heritable) and gives rise to isolated unilateral disease.

In contrast, the familial cases and around one-third of the sporadic cases result from germline mutations, which are heritable and give rise to bilat-eral multifocal disease. Germline mutations carry a 90% penetrance: 90% of these patients will develop retinoblastoma.

Characteristic histological features include abnormal patterns of retinoblasts such as the Flexner–Wintersteiner rosettes, Homer-Wright rosettes, and fleurettes.

Clinical features

- Leukocoria (60%) (see Box 15.4), strabismus (20%), decreased VA, acute red eye, orbital inflammation.
- White, round retinal mass with endophytic (towards vitreous), exophytic (toward RPE/choroid), mixed, or diffuse infiltrating growth pattern.
- Endophytic tumors tend to be friable with prominent superficial vessels and vitreous seedings.
- Exophytic tumors are associated with exudative retinal detachments (which are often large and may even be total).
- Diffuse infiltrating tumors show generalized retinal thickening with vitreous (and even aqueous) seeding but no calcification.
- *Complications*: glaucoma, buphthalmos/corneal edema, iris invasion, pseudohypopyon, rubeosis, hyphema, orbital inflammation, phthisis bulbi, invasion of optic nerve or brain, metastasis.

Investigations

- *US*: intralesional calcification with high internal reflectivity and acoustic shadow.
- *CT/MRI*: CT is better for imaging the retinoblastoma itself (calcification high density), but MRI is preferred for assessing any intracranial involvement (extension or associated tumors).

Treatment

This requires significant multidisciplinary input and should be coordinated by a recognized center. Various options can be considered.

Photocoagulation or transpupillary thermotherapy:

Consider for small posterior tumors without optic nerve involvement or vitreous seeding.

Cryotherapy

Consider for similar small tumors that are equatorial or pre-equatorial.

Radiotherapy

Consider plaque radiotherapy for larger tumors not involving the optic nerve or macula and with only limited vitreous seeding; consider external beam radiotherapy for larger or multiple tumors, optic nerve involvement, or significant vitreous seeding, or when other measures have failed.

Complications include cataract, orbital growth abnormalities, radiation retinopathy, and secondary malignancies (significant risk in patients with germinal mutations).

Chemotherapy

Consider for bilateral disease, large tumors (chemoreduction combined with local treatment), extraocular involvement, metastasis, or recurrence. Common regimens include carboplatin, etopside, and vincristine.

Enucleation

Consider for advanced disease (particularly if unilateral/asymmetric). Aim to remove >10 mm length of optic nerve, which is the main exit route for tumor cells. An implant may be inserted at the initial surgery unless residual tumor is suspected.

Prognosis

Most untreated tumors proceed to local invasion and metastasis to cause death within 2 years; rarely, however, the tumor may spontaneously stop growing to form a retinoma, or necrose to cause phthisis bulbi.

Most small to medium-sized tumors without vitreous seeding can be successfully treated while preserving useful vision. Overall, there is a 95% survival rate (in the developed world).

Poor prognostic factors include size of tumor, optic nerve involvement, extraocular spread, and older age of child. Patients with germinal mutations are at increased risk of pineoblastoma (trilateral retinoblastoma), ectopic intracranial retinoblastoma, and osteogenic or soft tissue sarcomas. Risk is also increased with radiation exposure.

Box 15.4 Differential diagnosis of leukocoria

- Retinoblastoma
- Cataract
- Persistent fetal vasculature syndrome
- Inflammatory cyclitic membrane
- Coats' disease
- ROP
- Toxocara
- Incontinentia pigment
- Familial exudative vitreoretinopathy
- Retinal dysplasia (e.g., Norrie's disease, Patau's syndrome, Edward's syndrome)
- Other posterior-segment tumors (e.g., combined hamartoma of RPE and retina)

Retinal hemangiomas

Capillary hemangioma

This is an uncommon benign hamartoma of the retinal (or optic disc) vasculature consisting of capillary-like vessels. It may present at any age but is most commonly diagnosed in young adults. Isolated capillary hemangiomas are usually not related to systemic disease, but most multiple and bilateral tumors are seen in the context of von Hippel–Lindau syndrome (VHL) (Table 15.5).

Histologically, there are endothelial cells, pericytes, and stromal cells. The VHL mutation may be restricted to the stromal cells, suggesting that despite their innocent appearance, they are the underlying neoplastic cell.

Clinical features

- ↓VA; asymptomatic (may be diagnosed on family screening).
- Red nodular lesion with tortuosity and dilatation (often irregular) of feeding artery and draining vein, exudation, exudative retinal detachment, rubeosis/neovascular glaucoma, epiretinal membranes, tractional retinal detachment, vitreous hemorrhage.
- Optic disc hemangiomas are less well defined and do not have obvious feeder vessels.

Investigation

- FA: rapid sequential filling of artery, hemangioma, and vein; extensive late leakage. Leakage into vitreous may appear hazy on late images.

Treatment

Systemic disease

If VHL is suspected, multidisciplinary care with physician and clinical geneticist is required.

Ocular disease

- Photocoagulation for small (<3 mm diameter) tumors requires confluent burns covering the entire tumor and feeder artery; multiple treatment sessions are usually required.
- Cryotherapy is used for peripheral or larger tumors, usually double freeze-thaw technique. Multiple treatment sessions are often required.
- Radiotherapy.
- Excision.

Table 15.5 Features of von Hippel–Lindau syndrome

Ocular	Extraocular
Retinal capillary hemangioma	Hemangioblastoma of cerebellum, spinal cord, or brainstem
	Renal cell carcinoma
	Pheochromocytoma
	Islet cell carcinoma
	Epididymal cysts/adenomas
	Visceral cysts

Cavernous hemangioma

This is an uncommon benign hamartoma of the retinal (or optic disc) vasculature that consists of large-caliber, thin-walled vessels. It is usually isolated but familial bilateral cases do occur.

Clinical features
- Usually asymptomatic; occasional ↓VA or floaters.
- Cluster of intraretinal blood-filled saccules (a plasma level may separate out due to the slow flow); otherwise normal retinal vasculature; vitreous hemorrhage.

Investigation and treatment
- FA shows slow filling, hyperfluorescence, and no leakage.
- Treatment is not usually necessary.

Racemose hemangioma

These are rare retinal arteriovenous malformations (AVMs) and are there-fore not true tumors. Although congenital, they progress with age and are usually detected in early adulthood.

These may be isolated or associated with ipsilateral AVMs of the CNS (Wyburn–Mason syndrome; Table 15.6).

Clinical features
- Usually asymptomatic; occasional ↓VA.
- Enlarged tortuous vascular abnormality with direct connection between arterial and venous circulations with similar color throughout.

Investigation and treatment

This is usually a clinical diagnosis. There is no effective treatment for ret-inal AVMs, although intracranial AVMs have been successfully treated with surgery, radiotherapy, and embolization.

Table 15.6 Features of Wyburn–Mason syndrome

Ocular	Extraocular
Retinal AVM	Cerebral/brainstem AVM
Orbital/periorbital AVM	

Other retinal tumors

Astrocytoma

This is a rare, benign tumor of the neurosensory retina that is composed of astrocytes. There is debate as to whether it is acquired or actually a hamartoma. Typically, it presents in childhood or adolescence; both sexes are equally affected.

Isolated astrocytomas are usually not associated with systemic disease, but most multiple and bilateral tumors are seen in the context of tuberous sclerosis (Table 15.7). An association with neurofibromatosis (NF) is also suggested.

Clinical features

- ↓VA, but often asymptomatic.
- Superficial white, well-defined lesion (translucent to calcified "mulberry" type; flat or nodular), exudative retinal detachment.

Investigation and treatment

Further evaluation is not usually required other than ruling out possible syndromic associations.

Table 15.7 Features of tuberous sclerosis

Ocular	Extraocular
Retinal astrocytoma	Adenoma sebaceum
	Ash leaf spots
	Shagreen patches
	Subungual fibromas
	Cerebral astrocytomas (with epilepsy and ↓IQ)
	Visceral hamartomas (e.g., renal angiomyolipoma, cardiac rhabdomyoma)
	Visceral cysts
	Pulmonary lymphangioleiomyomatosis

RPE tumors

Congenital hypertrophy of the retinal pigment epithelium (CHRPE)

This is a common benign congenital proliferation of the RPE occurring in around 1% of the population (typical form). The typical form is unilateral and either solitary or, more commonly, grouped ("bear tracks"). They are unrelated to systemic disease. The atypical form is bilateral and multifocal and is associated with familial adenomatous polyposis (FAP) and its variants (Table 15.8).

Histologically, the RPE cells are of increased height with increased numbers of melanin granules.

Clinical features
Typical CHRPE
- *Solitary:* black, well-defined, flat, round lesion, often with depigmented lacunae within it, deep to the neurosensory retina; usually 2–5 mm.
- *Grouped:* similar smaller lesions, grouped to form "bear tracks"; usually <2 mm.

Atypical CHRPE
- Bilateral, multiple, widely separated, black oval lesions with irregular depigmentation; usually <2 mm

Investigation and treatment
Typical CHRPE does not require investigation. Atypical CHRPE should prompt an investigation of family history and consideration of referral to a gastroenterologist. If FAP is diagnosed, prophylactic colectomy is recommended. In untreated FAP, the development of colonic carcinoma is almost universal.

Table 15.8 Features of familial adenomatous polyposis (FAP)

Ocular	Extraocular
Atypical CHRPE	Colonic polyps and carcinoma
	Gardner's variant: bone cysts, hamartomas, soft tissue tumors
	Turcot's variant: CNS neuroepithelial tumors

Combined hamartoma of the RPE and retina

This is a rare, benign hamartoma of the RPE, retinal astrocytes, and retinal vasculature. It is usually not related to systemic disease but may be associated with NF-2 and, rarely, NF-1 (see Tables 15.9 and 15.10).

Clinical features
- Decreased VA, floaters, leukocoria.
- Elevated lesion with whitish sheen superficially (epiretinal membranes and intraretinal gliosis), tortuous vessels, and variable deeper pigmentation; usually juxtapapillary but may be peripheral; usually 4–6 mm in diameter.

Investigation and treatment
Assess for the possibility of underlying neurofibromatosis.

Table 15.9 Features of neurofibromatosis-1 (NF-1)

Ocular	Extraocular
Optic nerve glioma*	Café-au-lait spots (≥6; each >0.5 cm pre-puberty or >1.5 cm post-puberty)*
Lisch nodules (≥2)*	Axillary/inguinal freckling*
Lid neurofibroma	Neurofibromas (≥1 plexiform type or ≥2 any type)*
Choroidal nevi	
Retinal astrocytoma	Characteristic bony lesion (sphenoid dysplasia which may →pulsatile proptosis; long bone cortex thinning/dysplasia)*
	First-degree relative with NF-1*

Table 15.10 Features of neurofibromatosis-2 (NF-2)

Ocular	Extraocular
Early-onset posterior subcapsular or cortical cataracts	Acoustic neuroma
	Meningioma
	Glioma
Combined hamartoma of the RPE and retina	Schwannoma
	First-degree relative with NF-2

Definite NF-2

- Bilateral acoustic neuroma, OR
- First-degree relative with NF-2 AND either unilateral acoustic neuroma (at <30 years) or two of the other diagnostic features

Probable NF-2

- Unilateral acoustic neuroma (at <30 years) AND one of the other diagnostic features; OR
- Multiple meningiomas AND one of the other diagnostic features.

Lymphoma

Although this is an uncommon tumor of the eye, ocular lymphoma is increasing in incidence. It is both sight threatening and life threatening and is easily missed, as it may masquerade as a number of other conditions. Risk factors include immunosuppression (e.g., therapy-associated, AIDS).

Epstein–Barr virus (EBV) is strongly associated with ocular-CNS lymphoma in AIDS patients. The cell type is usually large-cell, non-Hodgkin's B-cell lymphoma, although T-cell NHL is also seen. Two patterns of disease are seen: ocular-CNS and systemic.

Ocular-CNS type

This is the most common type and is a uveitis "masquerade" syndrome.

Clinical features
- *Typical:* "vitritis" (cellular infiltrate), yellowish sub-RPE plaques with overlying pigment clumping; 90% bilateral.
- *Atypical:* may mimic CMV retinitis, ARN, and uveitis associated with sarcoidosis, TB, and syphilis.

Systemic (or visceral) type

This is less common and has a uveal pattern of disease and a better prognosis than that of the ocular-CNS type.

Clinical features
- *Typical:* more diffuse yellowish choroidal thickening (may be multifocal), with minimal if any vitritis.
- *Atypical:* may mimic melanoma (or other choroidal tumors), posterior scleritis, uni- or multifocal choroiditis.

Investigation
Consider diagnostic vitrectomy, FNA or even incisional biopsy (if chorioretinal involvement) to obtain cytology and histology. Multiple vitreous biopsies may be needed to make the diagnosis. The vitreous specimen requires careful handling and should be spun down. An IL10:IL6 ratio of >1.0 performed on the specimen fluid may be suggestive of intraocular lymphoma (but is not 100% sensitive or specific).

Systemic assessment and treatment should be coordinated by an oncologist and usually includes lumbar puncture and MRI brain (for ocular-CNS type) and abdominal-pelvis imaging (for systemic type).

Treatment
Treatment options include radiotherapy (external beam or plaque) and chemotherapy (systemic or intravitreal). CNS involvement may require aggressive treatment with combined intrathecal and intravenous chemotherapy and radiotherapy.

Neuro-ophthalmology

Anatomy and physiology (1)

Within the retina, photoreceptors transduce photons into electrical impulses that are relayed via bipolar cells to the retinal ganglion cell. The ganglion cells can be divided into two populations: the parvocellular system for fine visual acuity and color, and the magnocellular system for motion detection and coarser form vision. This division is preserved in both the lateral geniculate nucleus and the visual cortex.

Optic nerve

The optic nerve is about 50 mm long, carries 1.2 million axons, and runs from the optic disc to the chiasm. It may be divided into the following:

- *Intraocular part* (1 mm long): unmyelinated axons pass through the channels of the lamina cribrosa to become myelinated, thus doubling in diameter (1.5 mm prelaminar to 3.0 mm retrolaminar).
- *Intraorbital part* (25 mm long): this portion has a full meningeal sheath of tough outer dura (continuous with sclera anteriorly and periosteum of sphenoid posteriorly), arachnoid, subarachnoid space, and inner pia mater. It has around 8 mm of slack to allow free ocular motility.
- *Intracanalicular part* (5–9 mm long): the nerve enters the optic foramen to travel through the optic canal within the lesser wing of the sphenoid.
- *Intracranial part* (12–16 mm long; 4.5 mm diameter): the nerve runs up, posteriorly, and medially to form the chiasm. Neighboring structures include the frontal lobes superiorly, the internal carotid artery (ICA) laterally, and the ophthalmic artery inferolaterally.

Blood supply

The ophthalmic artery originates from the ICA. It lies inferolaterally to the intracranial optic nerve and inferiorly to the intracanalicular part and perforates the intraorbital part 8–12 mm behind the globe to become the central retinal artery.

The intracranial, intracanalicular, and intraorbital portions of the optic nerve are supplied by the pial plexus fed by branches of the ophthalmic artery and, most posteriorly, by superior hypophyseal artery. The intraocular part (optic nerve head) is supplied by the circle of Zinn–Haller, an anastomosis fed mainly by the short posterior ciliary arteries.

Optic chiasm

The optic chiasm (8 mm long, 12 mm wide) represents the joining of both optic nerves, hemidecussation of the nasal fibers, and emergence of the optic tracts. The chiasm usually lies directly above the pituitary gland (80%) but may be relatively anterior (prefixed) or posterior (postfixed).

The pituitary itself lies within the sella turcica of the sphenoid, roofed by the diaphragma sellae, a sheet of dura between anterior and posterior clinoids. Neighboring structures include the cavernous sinus and ICA inferolaterally and the third ventricle lying posteriorly.

Within the chiasm, fibers from superonasal retina are found to decussate relatively posteriorly while inferonasal fibers decussate more anteriorly; some of these inferonasal fibers appear to loop so far forward as to join the contralateral optic nerve to form Wilbrand's knee. Macular fibers decussate in the central and posterior chiasm.

Optic tract and lateral geniculate nucleus (LGN)

The optic tract runs from the chiasm to the LGN, during which axons from corresponding locations of each retina start to become associated. Within the tract, parvocellular fibers run centrally with magnocellular fibers on the outside.

The LGN is organized into six layers: contralateral fibers synapse with layers 1 (magnocellular), 4, and 6 (parvocellular); ipsilateral fibers with layers 2 (magnocellular), 3, and 5 (parvocellular). There may be other modifying pathways (akin to K cells in primates) between these layers.

Axons from superior retina synapse medially, from inferior retina laterally. Macular fibers synapse in the central and posterior LGN. The blood supply is from branches of the middle cerebral artery and thalamogeniculate branches of the posterior cerebral artery.

Optic radiation

Axons of the optic radiation project from the LGN to the visual cortex. Fibers from the superior retina project posteriorly through the parietal lobe. Fibers from the inferior retina project through the temporal lobe but deviate laterally around the inferior horn of the lateral ventricle to form Meyer's loop. Macular fibers generally lie between these two sets of projections. The blood supply is from internal carotid, middle, and posterior cerebral arteries.

Visual cortex

The primary visual cortex (V_1, Brodmann area 17, striate cortex) is located on the medial surfaces of both occipital lobes on either side of the calcarine sulcus. V_1 is organized into six layers: optic tracts synapse mainly with layer IV; layers II and III project to secondary visual cortex; layer IV to superior colliculus; and layer VI back to LGN.

Superior retina is represented superiorly, inferior retina inferiorly, macula most posteriorly, and extreme temporal periphery (temporal crescent) anteriorly. The blood supply is mainly from the posterior cerebral artery but with middle cerebral artery contributions at the anterior and lateral margins.

Visual cortex cells are arranged into basic processing units representing discrete areas of the visual field. These hypercolumns comprise right and left ocular dominance columns and orientation columns. The orientation columns are divided into blobs (color) and interblobs (orientation).

Cell types range in complexity. Least discriminatory are the circularly symmetrical cells, which respond to small central stimulus regardless of orientation and movement. Simple cells require a centrally located single contrast stimulus that must be correctly orientated and moving in the correct direction. Complex cells are similar but do not require the stimulus to be centrally located. Hypercomplex cells require that the stimulus is also of a particular length.

Further processing occurs in the visual association areas, which may also integrate information from nuclei involved with head and eye movement. Subspecialization occurs in V_3 (depth perception, dynamic form), V_4 (color), and V_5 (motion, maintenance of fixation).

Anatomy and physiology (2)

Ocular motor nerves

Third nerve

The CN III nucleus lies in the midbrain anterior to the periaqueductal gray matter at the level of the superior colliculus. It consists of a single central nucleus innervating both levator palpebrae superioris (LPS) muscles, and separate subnuclei for each superior rectus (SR) (contralateral innervation), medial rectus, inferior rectus (MR), and inferior oblique (IO) (all ipsilateral innervation).

The CN III fasciculus travels anteriorly through the medial longitudinal fasciculus (MLF), the red nucleus, and the cerebral peduncle. On leaving the midbrain, it emerges within the interpeduncular fossa and passes anteriorly beneath the posterior cerebral artery, above the superior cerebellar artery, and lateral to the posterior communicating artery (Fig. 16.1). It travels within the lateral wall of the cavernous sinus, dividing into superior and inferior branches that enter the orbit via the superior orbital fissure and annulus of Zinn.

The superior branch innervates LPS and SR, whereas the inferior branch innervates MR, IR, IO, and the pupillary sphincter. Parasympathetic fibers from the Edinger–Westphal nucleus travel in the IO branch as far as the ciliary ganglion and then in the short ciliary nerves to the globe, where they innervate the ciliary muscle and pupillary sphincter.

Fourth nerve

The CN IV nucleus lies just below the CN III nucleus in the lower midbrain at the level of inferior colliculus. The fasciculus decussates within the anterior medullary velum and exits the midbrain posteriorly.

It then curves round the midbrain, passes anteriorly between the posterior cerebral and superior cerebellar arteries, and travels within the lateral wall of the cavernous sinus (inferolateral to CN III, superior to CN V$_1$). It then enters the orbit through the superior orbital fissure (but superior to the annulus of Zinn) and terminates in the superior oblique muscle.

Sixth nerve

The CN VI nucleus lies in the lower pons anterior to the fourth ventricle at the level of the facial colliculus. Although most axons innervate the ipsilateral LR, about 40% of axons project via the MLF to the contralateral MR subnucleus. The fasciculus travels anteriorly through the medial leminiscus and corticospinal tract, just medial to the trigeminal nuclear complex and vestibular nuclei.

After emerging at the pontomedullary junction, it ascends in the subarachnoid space between the pons and the clivus, before turning anterior over the petrous apex of the temporal bone and under the petroclinoid ligament to enter the cavernous sinus. Here it runs within the sinus itself just lateral to the ICA and inferomedial to CN III, IV, and V$_1$, which run in the sinus wall. It then enters the orbit via the superior orbital fissure and annulus of Zinn to terminate in the LR muscle.

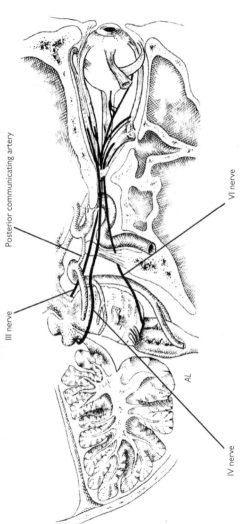

Posterior communicating artery

VI nerve

III nerve

IV nerve

AL

Figure 16.1 Cranial nerves III, IV, and VI.

Anatomy and physiology (3)

Autonomic supply

Sympathetic

The first-order neurons originate in the posterior hypothalamus and descend through the brainstem to synapse in the spinal cord at the ciliospinal center of Budge (C8-T2).

The second-order neurons emerge anteriorly in the ventral root (close to the lung apex) and then ascend in the sympathetic chain to synapse at the superior cervical ganglion.

The third-order neurons ascend along the ICA to the cavernous sinus and then via the nasociliary branch of CN V$_1$ into the orbit and subsequently the long ciliary nerves, terminating in the dilator pupillae.

Parasympathetic

The light and near reflexes are both mediated by the parasympathetic supply from the Edinger–Westphal nucleus. The afferent arm for the light reflex is by 1) retinal ganglion cells that synapse in the ipsilateral pretectal nucleus and then 2) interneurons that innervate bilateral Edinger–Westphal nuclei. The inputs for the near reflex are less well-defined but probably include cortical influences (frontal and occipital lobes) mediated by a midbrain center (anterior to the pretectal nucleus).

The efferent arm for both reflexes comprise 1) preganglionic neurons from the Edinger–Westphal nucleus that travel in CN III and then the inferior division of CN III to the inferior oblique before synapsing at the ciliary ganglion, and 2) postganglionic neurons that run via the short ciliary nerves to terminate in the constrictor pupillae and ciliary muscle.

Cerebrospinal fluid (CSF)

CSF is produced by the choroid plexus in the lateral ventricles and the third ventricle. It flows from the lateral ventricles via the foramen of Munro to the third ventricle and then via the aqueduct of Sylvius to the fourth ventricle. From there, it leaves either via the lateral foramina of Luschka or the medial foramen of Magendie to bathe the spinal cord and cerebral hemispheres in the subarachnoid space.

CSF is then absorbed into the cerebral venous system by the arachnoid granulations. The subarachnoid space is continuous with the optic nerve sheath.

Optic neuropathy: assessment

The optic nerve is vulnerable to injury from numerous local and systemic diseases (see Table 16.1). Clinical features often include ↓VA, relative or complete afferent pupillary defect, ↓light sensitivity, ↓color vision, visual field defects, and optic disc abnormalities, such as pallor.

Table 16.1 An approach to assessing optic nerve disease

Visual symptoms	Blurring, washout of colors, blind spots; may be asymptomatic; check duration, speed of onset and recovery, precipitants, associations (diplopia, proptosis, red eye)
POH	Previous or current eye disease; refractive error
PMH	Vascular risk factors and disease; neurological disease (e.g., MS); connective tissue disease (e.g., SLE, RA); granulomatous disease (e.g., sarcoidosis, TB)
Review of systems	Detailed review of all systems; particularly any headache or abnormalities of sensation, motor system, speech, balance, or hearing
SH	Driver; profession; diet, alcohol intake, toxin exposure (e.g., lead, tin, or carbon monoxide)
FH	Family members with visual problems
Drug history	Previous or current toxic drugs (e.g., anti-TB)
Allergy history	Allergies or relevant drug contraindications
Visual acuity	Best-corrected/pinhole/near
Visual function	Check for RAPD, color vision, red desaturation, visual fields (formal perimetry)
Orbit	Proptosis
AS	Features suggestive of glaucoma, uveitis, CCF
Tonometry	IOP
Optic disc	Size, cup, color, edema; congenital abnormalities; flat, elevated, tilted, crowding; peripapillary edema or hemorrhages; retinociliary collateral vessels
Macula	Abnormalities that may cause central scotoma
Fundus	Abnormalities (e.g., retinoschisis) that may cause peripheral field loss; posterior uveitis; or vasculitis
Vessels	Arteriosclerosis, hypertensive changes, occlusions
CNS/PNS	Cranial nerves (including ocular motility), sensory, motor, cerebellar function, speech, mental state
CVS	Pulse, heart sounds, carotid bruits
Systemic review	Including respiratory, gastrointestinal, genitourinary, ENT systems

Consider also retinoscopy to rule out refractive error.

Diagnosis is more difficult in early symmetric disease where there may be no objective signs. Electrodiagnostic tests are often helpful in such cases. Also, typical optic neuropathy features may be seen in other diseases (e.g., central scotoma, ↓color vision, or secondary optic atrophy in retinal disorders). The challenge is thus first to recognize the optic neuropathy and then elucidate the cause (Tables 16.2 and 16.3).

Unexplained optic neuropathy requires urgent investigation (p. 523) to elucidate the cause and rule out serious disease such as compression secondary to a tumor.

Table 16.2 Clinical features of optic nerve vs. macular disease

	Optic neuropathy	Macular disease
History		
Main complaint	Gray/darkness	Distortion
Scotoma	Negative	Positive
Associated symptoms	May have retrobulbar pain, e.g., on eye movement	May have micropsia, hyperopic shift
Examination		
VA	Variable ↓	↓↓
Color vision	↓ or ↓↓	Normal or mild ↓
RAPD	+	−
Testing		
Perimetry	Central, centrocecal, arcuate, or altitudinal defects	Central scotoma
Amsler grid	Scotoma	Metamorphopsia
VEP latency	↑	Normal or mild ↑

Table 16.3 Differential diagnosis of acute or subacute optic neuropathy

Optic neuritis (typical)	Ages 20–50 years, unilateral, ↓VA over hours/days, recovery starts within 2 weeks, retrobulbar pain
Compressive	Progressive ↓VA, disc pallor ± pain, involvement of other local structures
Sphenoid sinus disease	Persistent severe pain, pyrexia, history of sinusitis; consider fungal disease in the immunosuppressed or in diabetic ketoacidosis
Sarcoidosis	Progressive ↓ VA ± uveitis, symptoms or signs of sarcoidosis, very steroid sensitive
Vasculitis (e.g., SLE)	Progressive ↓ VA ± uveitis, symptoms or signs of vasculitis
Syphilis	Progressive ↓ VA ± uveitis; symptoms or signs of syphilis; may be HIV+
Anterior ischemic optic neuropathy (AION)	Sudden painless ↓ VA, altitudinal field loss, swollen optic disc (may be segmental), usually older age group; features of arteritic or nonarteritic disease
Toxic or nutritional	Slowly progressive symmetrical ↓VA with central scotomas; relevant nutritional, therapeutic, or toxic history
Leber's hereditary optic neuropathy (LHON)	Severe sequential ↓VA over weeks or months, telangiectatic vessels around optic disc (acutely); usually young adult males; family history
Postviral demyelination	Often bilateral ↓VA few weeks postviral or postvaccination, usually in children or young adults; ± acute disseminated encephalomyelitis (ADEM)

Optic neuritis: assessment

Inflammation of the optic nerve may be divided into papillitis (where the disc is swollen), retrobulbar neuritis (where the disc is spared), and neuroretinitis (with retinal involvement, "macular star"). The most common cause of optic neuritis is demyelination, although a number of important differential diagnoses must be considered.

Acute demyelinating optic neuritis

Incidence within the general population is around 5/100, 000/year, but it occurs in up to 70% of patients with known MS. Most of the patients are female (F:M 3:1) and are usually aged 20–50 years. The disease is usually unilateral, although bilateral involvement may be seen in children.

Clinical features
• Rapid ↓VA over hours or days (rarely become NPL); recovery starts within 2 weeks and may continue for a few months; ↓contrast sensitivity, ↓color vision, field loss (variable pattern), retrobulbar pain (present in 90%; often worse on eye movement, usually precedes ↓VA), photopsia.
• RAPD (may be absent if pre-existing contralateral disease), disc swelling (only 1/3 of cases); disc should not be pale in the acute stages of a first episode; may have few hemorrhages, retinal exudates, and mild vitritis.

Investigations
If the episode is entirely typical (Box 16.1), the diagnosis may be made on clinical grounds alone.

> **Box 16.1 Features of typical optic neuritis (from Optic Neuritis Treatment Trial)**
>
> • Ages 20–50 years
> • Unilateral
> • Worsens over hours/days
> • Recovery starts within 2 weeks
> • Retrobulbar pain (may be worse on eye movement)
> • ↓Color vision
> • RAPD

If the episode is atypical, investigate to rule out a progressive optic neuropathy (see below).

Treatment
This is indeed controversial. Intravenous methylprednisolone hastens visual recovery but does not affect long-term outcome (conclusion of Optic Neuritis Treatment Trial). On this basis, IV steroid treatment may be offered to those with poor vision in the other eye or with severe pain.

In those at high risk (>2 plaques on MRI), interferon β1a appears to reduce or at least delay both the clinical diagnosis of MS (i.e., a further significant demyelinating episode) and the accumulation of further silent MRI lesions (CHAMPS: Controlled High-risk Avonex MS Prevention Study; ETOMS: Early Treatment of MS Study).

Prognosis

Visual recovery

All patients will have some improvement, with >90% attaining 20/30 in the affected eye. However, even if RAPD resolves and VA recovers to ≥20/20 abnormalities of color perception, contrast sensitivity, stereopsis, or field may persist. Around one-third of patients have a further episode (either eye) within 5 years. On MRI, poor visual prognosis is associated with length of optic nerve involvement and intracanalicular segment involvement.

Probability of developing MS

Risk factors are female sex, multiple white matter lesions on MRI, and CSF oligoclonal bands. Five-year probability of MS increases from 16% with a normal MRI to 51% if >2 white matter lesions are found.

Devic's disease

Devic's disease (neuromyelitis optica) is characterized by bilateral optic neuritis with transverse myelitis. Patients present with rapid, severe bilateral ↓VA and paraplegia.

Atypical optic neuritis

If an acute optic neuropathy does not fulfill the criteria for typical optical neuritis (e.g., not improving at 2 weeks), it must be investigated further to exclude a compressive lesion or other serious pathology (see Table 16.3, p. 521).

Investigations may include MRI (gadolinium enhanced), CXR, CBC, ESR, CRP, UA, Glu, LFT, ACE, ANA, ANCA, syphilis serology, LHON, and LP (CSF analysis for microscopy, protein, glucose, oligoclonal bands, and cytology).

A diagnosis of demyelinating disease is supported by typical white matter plaques on MRI and oligoclonal bands in CSF (but not in serum).

Anterior ischemic optic neuropathy (1)

AION is a significant cause of acute visual loss in the elderly population, affecting up to 10/100,000/year of those over 50 years of age. In 5–10% of cases, the etiology is arteritic (giant cell arteritis); in 90–95% it is non-arteritic. Giant cell arteritis (GCA) is an ophthalmic emergency requiring immediate assessment and appropriate institution of systemic steroid treatment.

Arteritic AION

In arteritic AION, short posterior ciliary artery vasculitis leads to ischemic necrosis of the optic nerve head.

Clinical features
- Sudden ↓VA (<20/200 in 76%); headache, scalp tenderness, jaw claudication, weight loss, night sweats, myalgia (association with polymyalgia rheumatica); may have a warning episode of transient ↓VA (short obscurations or longer amaurosis fugax–like episodes).
- RAPD, swollen disc (typically pale; rarely segmental), ± peripapillary hemorrhages and cotton wool spots, abnormal temporal arteries (thickened, tender, nonpulsatile).
- *Associations:* CRAO, BRAO, cilioretinal artery occlusion, CN III, IV, VI palsy.

Investigations
- Immediate ESR, CRP, CBC: ↑ESR, ↑CRP, and ↑Plt are all supportive of GCA (Table 16.4). Consider urgent temporal artery biopsy (aim to perform it within a few days, although positive results may be obtained up to 7 days after corticosteroid treatment). ESR should be interpreted in context (Box 16.2). See also diagnostic criteria in Box 16.3.

Treatment
Give immediate adequate steroid treatment (e.g., 1 g methylprednisolone IV 1×/day for 1–3 days) followed by oral prednisolone 1–2 mg/kg 1×/day). Aspirin may have additional benefit. Once disease is controlled, steroids may be titrated according to symptoms and inflammatory markers (CRP responds more quickly than ESR).

Treatment may last several years so osteoporosis prophylaxis is important. The elderly are particularly vulnerable to the side effects of steroids.

Prognosis
The risk of second eye involvement ranges from 10% (if treated) to 95% (untreated). Other complications of GCA include TIA, stroke, neuropathies, thoracic artery aneurysms, and death.

Table 16.4 Investigations in GCA

	Sensitivity	Specificity
Histological		
Temporal artery biopsy	80–90% (unilateral biopsy) 95–97% (bilateral biopsy)	≤100%
Hematological		
Biopsy-proven GCA vs. normal controls (Hayreh et al.)*		
↑ESR	92%	94%
↑CRP	100%	
↑ESR + ↑CRP		97%
Biopsy-positive vs. biopsy-negative patients with clinical suspicion of GCA (Foroozan et al.)**		
↑ESR + ↑Plt	51%	91%

*Hayreh et al. defined ↑ESR as >47mm/h and ↑CRP > 2.45mg/dL. *Am J Ophthalmol* 1997; 123:392–395.

**Foroozan et al. defined ↑ESR as > age/2 for men or > (age +10)/2 for women and ↑Plt as >400 × 10³/μL. *Ophthalmology* 2002; 109:1267–1271.

Box 16.2 Interpretation of ESR results

- The upper limit of normal for ESR has traditionally been approximated to age/2 for men and (age + 10)/2 for women. However, it is increasingly thought that this upper limit may be rather generous: a lower upper limit may need to be considered.
- ESR will be lower in the presence of polycythemia, hemoglobinopathies, hereditary spherocytosis, congestive cardiac failure, and anti-inflammatory medications.
- ESR will be elevated by anemia, malignancy, infection, and inflammation.

Box 16.3 ACR traditional criteria (1990) for diagnosis of GCA

- Age ≥50 years at disease onset
- New onset of localized headache
- Temporal artery tenderness or decreased pulse
- ESR ≥50 mm/h
- Arterial biopsy with necrotizing arteritis with a predominance of mononuclear cell infiltrates or granulomatous process with multinuclear giant cells

The presence of three or more out of five of the above criteria was associated with 93.5% sensitivity and 91.2% specificity.

Anterior ischemic optic neuropathy (2)

Nonarteritic AION

Nonarteritic AION comprises 90–95% of AION cases (see Table 16.5). It is proposed that an insufficient circulation to a crowded optic nerve head may lead to local edema, causing further vascular compromise and subsequent infarction. Identified vascular risk factors should be modified to prevent further ophthalmic and systemic complications.

Risk factors

The main risk factors appear to be diabetes, hypertension, and optic disc morphology ("disc at risk"—crowded disc with a small cup). Other proposed risk factors include smoking, hyperlipidemia, hypotension, anemia, hypermetropia, and obstructive sleep apnea.

Clinical features

- ↓VA (usually sudden but can be progressive; VA >20/200 in 61%; ≥20/40 in 18%); commonly occurs overnight; occasional pain.
- RAPD, field loss (45% inferior altitudinal; 15% superior altitudinal), swollen optic disc (typically hyperemic, ± segmental, telangiectasia).
- *Associations:* "disc at risk" in fellow eye.

Investigations

- First rule out GCA (assessment, p. 524).
- If nonarteritic, then obtain BP, glucose, lipids, CBC. If patient is <50 years of age, then consider also vasculitis screen.

Treatment

There is no proven benefit for any treatment (including steroids, optic nerve sheath fenestration, hyperbaric oxygen, dopamine, and aspirin); however, aspirin (e.g., 81 mg/day) is commonly prescribed.

Refer to the physician for vascular assessment and treatment.

Prognosis

The risk of second eye involvement is around 19% over 5 years, with an increased risk after cataract surgery. Additionally, cardiovascular and cerebrovascular diseases are more common, possibly with increased mortality.

Posterior ischemic optic neuropathy

This rare condition describes ischemia of the more posterior (retrolaminar) optic nerve. It appears to result from watershed infarction, associated with hypotension or low hematocrit (typically after back surgery). Clinically, there is sudden visual loss with an RAPD (if unilateral) but normal optic disc; bilateral involvement is common.

Table 16.5 Arteritic and nonarteritic AION

	Arteritic AION	**Nonarteritic AION**
Incidence	1/100,000/year	10/100,000/year
Cause and possible associations	Giant cell arteritis	*Major:* diabetes mellitus, hypertension, optic disc morphology *Minor:* smoking, hyperlipidemia, hypotension, anemia, hypermetropia, obstructive sleep apnea
Age (mean)	70 years	60 years
VA + field	Sudden ↓ Usually <20/200	Sudden ↓ Usually >20/200 Often altitudinal field loss
Associated symptoms	Scalp tenderness, jaw claudication, headache	Usually none
Disc	Swollen Commonly pale	Swollen (often sectoral) Commonly hyperemic Predisposed (small + crowded)
ESR	↑↑ (mean = 70 mmHg)	Normal
CRP	↑↑	Normal
Plt	↑	Normal
Risk to fellow eye	10% (if treated) to ≤95% (untreated)	19% over 5 years
Prognosis	Up to 15% improve	40% improve (by ≥2 Snellen lines)

Other optic neuropathies and atrophies

Leber's hereditary optic neuropathy (LHON)

This rare condition is maternally inherited, arising from point mutations in mitochondrial DNA. It may present at almost any age but typically in young adult males (M:F 3:1). Family history is present in around 50%. The mutations identified are 11,778 (the most common comprising 95%), 3460, and 14,484, all of which affect complex I of the respiratory chain.

Clinical features

- Sudden painless sequential ↓VA (usually affects second eye within 2 months; typically 20/200–HM).
- Large, dense, centrocecal scotoma, ↓color vision; disc may show peripapillary telangiectasia and peripapillary nerve fiber layer swelling (early) and temporal pallor (late). Pupillary reactions usually normal.

Investigations and treatment

Perform mitochondrial DNA analysis for LHON mutations (peripheral blood); consider also screening for differential diagnosis, including toxins and deficiencies. There is no effective treatment. Most patients have a poor visual prognosis, although some spontaneous recovery is seen with the uncommon 14,484 mutation.

Nutritional and toxic optic neuropathies

These uncommon acquired optic neuropathies all behave in a similar manner, probably because of a common disruption of mitochondrial oxidative phosphorylation. Tobacco-alcohol amblyopia may represent a combination of toxin (cyanide in tobacco smoke) and nutritional deficiency (low B12 associated with alcohol excess). Numerous other agents have been identified (Table 16.6).

Clinical features

- Subacute painless bilateral ↓VA (typically 20/30–20/200).
- Small central/centrocecal scotomas, ↓color vision; ± swelling of disc or peripapillary nerve fiber layer (early) and temporal pallor (late).

Investigations and treatment

A detailed history may reveal the cause. Consider obtaining B1, B2, B12, and folic acid levels (peripheral blood) and heavy metal screening (including 24-hour urine).

Treat deficiency with oral supplementation, except for B12 (IM and must be given with folate). In alcoholics, consider prophylactic vitamin supplementation. Identify and prevent route of toxin exposure (which may affect others, e.g., family members).

Inherited optic atrophy

Autosomal dominant

Kjer syndrome is the most common isolated optic atrophy and is due to a mutation in 3q. Bilateral symmetrical ↓VA (usually 20/30–20/120) occurs insidiously in mid- to late childhood.

Autosomal recessive

- Isolated: this is rare, severe, and presents early (age <4 years).
- Behr syndrome: optic atrophy ± nystagmus, ataxia, spasticity, ↓IQ.
- Wolfram syndrome (DIDMOAD): diabetes insipidus, diabetes mellitus, optic atrophy, deafness.

Table 16.6 Causes of nutritional and toxic optic neuropathies

Nutritional	B1 (thiamine) deficiency
	B2 (riboflavin) deficiency
	B6 deficiency
	B12 deficiency
	Folate deficiency
Toxic	Amiodarone
	Ethambutol
	Methanol
	Carbon monoxide
	Cyanide
	Isoniazid
	Lead
	Triethyl tin

Table 16.7 Causes of optic atrophy

Inherited		Kjer syndrome
		Behr syndrome
		Wolfram syndrome
		LHON
Compression	Extrinsic tumor	Pituitary
		Craniopharyngioma
		Meningioma
		Metastasis
	Intrinsic tumor	ON glioma
		ON sheath meningioma
	Other	Aneurysm
		Mucocele
Vascular		CRAO
		AION or PION
Inflammatory		Acute demyelinating optic neuritis
		Sarcoidosis
		Vasculitis (e.g., SLE, PAN)
Infection		Bacterial (e.g., TB, syphilis)
		Rickettsial (e.g., Lyme disease)
		Viral (e.g., measles, mumps, varicella)
		Fungal (e.g., *Aspergillus*)
Nutritional		See above
Toxic		See above
Other		Trauma
		Disc edema (e.g., papilledema)
		Retinal disease (e.g., RP)

Papilledema

Papilledema describes optic disc swelling (usually bilateral) arising from raised intracranial pressure (ICP); the term should not be used to describe other causes of disc edema (see Table 16.8). Raised ICP is transmitted from the subarachnoid space via the optic nerve sheath to cause axoplasmic hold-up and consequent disc edema.

The urgent priority is to rule out an intracranial mass (e.g., tumor, abscess, hemorrhage); however, the most common cause of papilledema is idiopathic intracranial hypertension (see Table 16.9).

Clinical features

- Visual obscurations (transient ↓VA, few seconds duration, up to 30x/day, uni- or bilateral, may be precipitated by posture, straining, etc.); diplopia; field defects (usually enlarged blind spot). Sustained ↓VA is a serious sign of irreversible damage—it may occur early in aggressive disease or late in chronic papilledema.
- ↑ICP leads to headache (often worse lying down or straining), nausea, vomiting, and pulsatile tinnitus.
- Disc swelling is usually bilateral; however, swelling may not occur in an already abnormal optic disc or nerve sheath (e.g., congenital anomaly, optic atrophy, high myopia).

Staging of papilledema

- *Early:* hyperemic, blurred + elevated margin, subtle peripapillary nerve fiber layer edema, dilated disc capillaries, distended retinal veins, absent spontaneous venous pulsation (SVP).
- *Acute:* as listed above + peripapillary hemorrhages, cotton wool spots, increased nerve fiber layer edema (may obscure retinal vessels).
- *Chronic:* ↓hyperemia, ↓cotton-wool spots or hemorrhages, variable swelling, usually still elevated; ± drusen-like deposits and optociliary shunt vessels at the disc (in which case this is sometimes called vintage papilledema).
- *Atrophic/late:* pale atrophic disc, ↓swelling, attenuated arterioles.

Investigation

Urgent neuroimaging (preferably MRI with gadolinium enhancement) may reveal primary pathology, hydrocephalus, or empty sella; consider the following:

- *MRV:* check cerebral venous sinuses.
- *LP:* check opening pressure (normal <20 cmH$_2$O or <25 cmH$_2$O in the obese), glucose, protein, protein electrophoresis, microscopy, culture.
- *FA* (if diagnostic uncertainty): late leakage from dilated disc capillaries.

Treatment

Intervention depends on the underlying cause and severity and may range from weight loss to extensive neurosurgery. Shared care with another specialty (neurosurgery, neurology, oncology, medicine) is often necessary. However, regular ophthalmic assessment of acuity, color vision, fields, and optic disc status is invaluable to preserving vision.

Table 16.8 Causes of apparent optic disc swelling

True disc swelling	Papilledema	↑ICP	Tumors, etc. (Table 16.9)
	Local disc swelling	Inflammatory	Optic neuritis
			Uveitis
			Scleritis
		Granulomatous	Tuberculosis
			Sarcoid
		Infiltrative	Leukemia
			Lymphoma
		Vascular	AION
			CRVO
			Diabetic papillitis
		Tumors	Of optic nerve (meningioma, glioma)
			Of orbit
		Hereditary	LHON
No true disc swelling	Pseudopapilledema	Structural	Disc drusen
			Tilted discs
			Hypermetropic discs
			Myopic discs
			Myelinated peripapillary nerve fibers

Table 16.9 Causes of raised intracranial pressure

Mass effect	Tumor
	Hemorrhage
	Trauma (hematoma/edema)
Increased CSF production	Choroid plexus tumor
Reduced CSF drainage	Stenosis of formen/aqueduct (congenital or secondary to tumor, cyst, infection, etc.)
	Damage to arachnoid granulations (meningitis, subarachnoid hemorrhage)
	Idiopathic intracranial hypertension
Other	Malignant hypertension

Pseudopapilledema

A number of optic disc anomalies may resemble papilledema.

Disc drusen: may cause the most diagnostic confusion as they may not be clinically obvious (buried) and may cause visual loss. Their prevalence is around 0.5% in Caucasians. They may be inherited (autosomal dominant). They are usually bilateral and become more obvious throughout life.

The disc has a lumpy appearance and absent cup and the vessels emerge centrally and then show abnormal branching (trifurcation); opto-ciliary shunt vessels may be present. VA is usually normal, but field defects occur in 75% of cases (arcuate, blind spot enlargement, generalized constriction). They are associated with CNV. Their presence may be demonstrated by their autofluorescence or on B-scan US or CT.

Hypermetropic discs may appear crowded and elevated.

Myopic discs are often elevated nasally and may show staining on FA.

Tilted discs are usually elevated superotemporally.

Idiopathic intracranial hypertension

Idiopathic intracranial hypertension (formerly known as benign intracranial hypertension and pseudotumor cerebri) is the most common cause of papilledema. It is a diagnosis of exclusion made in the presence of normal neuroimaging and CSF analysis, but with an elevated CSF opening pressure. The prevalence is around 0.9/100,000 in the general population but up to 19/100,000 in obese young women.

Risk factors

It typically affects obese young women, but there is a wide age range of presentation. The strongest risk factors are obesity and recent weight gain, although many other associations have been suggested (Table 16.10).

Clinical features

- Visual obscurations (transient ↓VA, few seconds duration, uni- or bilateral, up to 30×/day, may be precipitated by posture, straining, etc.); diplopia; field defects (usually enlarged blind spot); sustained ↓VA may be early in aggressive disease (usually an indication for shunting).
- Headache (in 94% of cases; often worse lying down or straining), retrobulbar pain, pulsatile tinnitus.
- Disc swelling (usually bilateral; p. 530).

Investigation

- *MRI* with gadolinium enhancement and MRV: aim to rule out all other causes of ↑ICP.
- *LP:* check opening pressure, glucose, protein, protein electrophoresis, microscopy, and culture. Normal opening pressure in adults is usually <20 cm H_2O, or <25 cm H_2O in the obese; in children, lower levels are normal.

Treatment

Titrate treatment against symptoms and risk of visual loss (monitor VA, color vision, fields, discs). The evidence base for treatment is weak. Treatment may include the following:

- Weight loss.
- *Medical:* acetazolamide (up to 500 mg 4×/day), or consider furosemide.
- *Surgical:* optic nerve sheath fenestration is effective for vision preservation but may not address headaches or tinnitus. Unilateral surgery occasionally positively affects the contralateral side.
- *Neurosurgical:* lumboperitoneal or ventriculoperitoneal shunting (but significant complications).
- *If pregnant:* acetazolamide appears to be safe after 20 weeks gestation; weight loss is not advised.

Table 16.10 Associations of idiopathic intracranial hypertension

Drugs	Tetracycline
	Corticosteroids
	OCP
	Vitamin A derivatives
	Nalidixic acid
Endocrine	Hypoparathyroidism
	Adrenal adenomas
Habitus	Obesity
	Obstructive sleep apnea syndrome
Hematological	Cerebral venous thrombosis

Congenital optic disc anomalies

Congenital optic disc anomalies range from common variations with minimal sequele (e.g., tilted discs) to severe abnormalities associated with poor vision and CNS abnormalities (e.g., morning glory anomaly).

Tilted disc

In this common bilateral but often asymmetric condition, the optic nerves insert obliquely into the globe. It is often associated with myopia and oblique astigmatism. The bitemporal field defects are unlike chiasmal lesions: they do not respect the vertical midline, they are static, and in some cases they may be resolved with refractive correction.

Clinical features
- Normal VA; may have superotemporal field defects.
- Disc is usually orientated inferonasally with elevation of the superotemporal rim, thinning of the inferonasal RPE/choroid, and situs inversus of the retinal blood vessels.

Optic disc pit

This rare usually unilateral condition may cause significant visual problems. Its origin is unclear, but it represents a herniation of neurectodermal tissue into a depression within the optic nerve.

Clinical features
- Often asymptomatic; ↓VA if complications; visual field defects (commonly paracentral arcuate scotoma).
- Gray pit usually in the temporal part of the optic disc; disc itself is larger than in the unaffected eye.
- *Complications:* macular retinoschisis and subsequent serous retinal detachment may occur in up to 45% of cases; this can be treated with vitrectomy and gas tamponade.

Optic nerve hypoplasia

This describes a reduced number of axons within the optic nerve. Optic nerve hypoplasia is a significant cause of poor vision in childhood. It may be isolated or be associated with a range of CNS abnormalities (Table 16.11)

Clinical features
- Variable VA (normal to NLP), visual field defects, color vision, pupil reactions.
- Small, gray disc surrounded by an inner yellow ring of chorioretinal atrophy and an outer pigment ring (double-ring sign).
- Other features may include aniridia, microphthalmos, strabismus, and nystagmus.

Table 16.11 Associations of optic disc hypoplasia

Syndromic	De Morsier syndrome (septo-optic dysplasia)
Non-syndromic	Isolated midline CNS abnormalities
	Endocrine abnormalities

Optic disc coloboma

This rare condition arises from incomplete closure of the embryonic fissure (inferonasal), with variable involvement of the adjacent retina and choroid. It may be sporadic or autosomal dominant and may be isolated, part of a syndrome, or occasionally associated with transsphenoidal encephalocele (Table 16.12).

Clinical features
- ↓VA (according to severity of coloboma), superior visual field defect.
- Glistening white bowl-shaped excavation within the disc (inferior part predominantly affected) ± chorioretinal/ciliary body or iris colobomata.

Morning glory anomaly

This very rare condition describes a usually unilateral excavation of the posterior globe that includes the optic disc and may even include the macula ("macula capture").

Clinical features
- Severe ↓VA.
- Enlarged pink disc located within the excavation and surrounded by an elevated and irregularly pigmented annular zone. Vessels are abnormally straight, with arteries and veins being of similar appearance.
- *Complications:* serous retinal detachments may occur in 30%.
- *Associations:* syndrome of transsphenoidal encephalocele with hyertelorism, flat nasal bridge, midline cleft lip/palate, and often panhypo-pituitarism.

Megalopapilla

Megalopapilla describes an unusually large but essentially normal disc. The patients have a high cup–disc ratio that may be confused with glaucomatous change.

Table 16.12 Associations of optic disc hypoplasia

Chromosomal	Patau's syndrome (trisomy 13)
	Edward's syndrome (trisomy 18)
	Cat-eye syndrome (trisomy 22)
Other syndromes	Aicardi syndrome
	CHARGE syndrome
	Walker–Warburg syndrome
	Goltz syndrome
	Goldenhar syndrome
	Meckel–Gruber syndrome

Chiasmal disorders

The chiasm enables the hemidecussation of visual information from the temporal fields so that information from the right visual field of both eyes is processed in the left visual cortex and vice versa. It lies in an anatomically crowded region, so chiasmal syndromes may be accompanied by other neurological or endocrine abnormalities.

The most common and best-described disorder of the chiasm is a pituitary adenoma causing bitemporal hemianopia; however, a wide range of other lesions and clinical presentations may be seen (Table 16.13).

Clinical features

- Often asymptomatic unless central (decrease VA) or advanced peripheral field loss; in advanced cases, a pre-existing phoria may lead to hemifield slide due to loss of overlap between the two eyes (can also cause diplopia). During close work, an object placed just beyond fixation may disappear (postfixation blindness).
- Field loss: classically bitemporal but often asymmetric and dependent on exact site of lesion (Table 16.14).
- Headache (usually frontal).

Associated features

- Involvement of CN III, IV, V_1, V_2, and VI and sympathetic nerve fibers may result in abnormalities of pupils (including Horner's syndrome), ocular motility, and facial sensation. Rarely, seesaw nystagmus may occur.
- ↑ICP may cause nausea, vomiting, pulsatile tinnitus, and papilledema. Hydrocephalus (blockage of foramen of Munro from posterior chiasmal lesions) may cause abnormal gait, urinary incontinence, drowsiness, and Parinaud's syndrome.
- Functioning pituitary tumors may cause acromegaly or gigantism (↑GH; large hands and feet and coarsening of features or abnormal height), Cushing's syndrome (↑ACTH; moon face, truncal obesity, hypertension), and hyperprolactinemia (impotence and galactorrhea).
- Pituitary destruction causes hypopituitarism with loss of LH/FSH (↓libido, amenorrhea; may present as primary infertility), GH (silent unless pubertal), TSH (hypothyroidism), and ACTH (secondary hypoadrenalism with collapse). Hypothalamic involvement may cause diabetes insipidus (↓ADH; polydipsia, polyuria).

Investigations

- Accurate visual field testing and interpretation is vital.
- Urgent neuroimaging: MRI (gadolinium enhanced) is preferred, although CT is better at detecting bony involvement.
- Consider endocrinological consultation and LP for CSF analysis.

Treatment

The ophthalmologist's role is to diagnose, refer for appropriate treatment (e.g., to endocrinology, neurosurgery, or often to a multispecialty pituitary team; see Table 16.15), and monitor the patient's vision long term (VA, color vision, visual fields). Late loss of vision may represent tumor recurrence or be the result of treatment (radiotherapy).

Table 16.13 Causes of chiasmal syndromes

Pituitary	Adenoma (functioning or nonfunctioning)
	Apoplexy (e.g., Sheehan's syndrome)
	Lymphocytic hypophysitis
Suprasellar	Meningioma
	Craniopharyngioma
Chiasm	Optic glioma
	Chiasmatic neuritis
Other	ICA aneurysm
	AVM (e.g., Wyburn–Mason syndrome)
	Cavernous hemangioma
	Germinoma
	Lymphoma
	Sarcoidosis
	Langerhans cell histiocytosis
	Metastasis
	Radionecrosis

Table 16.14 Localization by field defect

Superior bitemporal loss	Inferior lesion (e.g., pituitary adenoma)
Inferior bitemporal loss	Superior lesion (e.g., craniopharyngioma)
Junctional (central scotoma with superotemporal field loss in contralateral eye)	Anterior chiasmal lesion to side of central scotoma (e.g., sphenoid meningioma)
Bitemporal central hemianopic scotomas	Posterior chiasmal lesion (e.g., hydrocephalus)
Nasal loss	Lateral lesion (e.g., ectasia of the ICA)

Table 16.15 Treatment options for chiasmal lesions

Pituitary adenoma	Medical (bromocriptine or cabergoline if prolactin secreting; octreotide if growth hormone secreting)
	Surgical resection (e.g., transsphenoidal route)
	Radiotherapy
Pituitary apoplexy	Hormone replacement (including high-dose corticosteroids)
	Trans-sphenoidal decompression
Meningioma	Surgical resection ± radiotherapy
Craniopharyngioma	Surgical resection ± radiotherapy
Optic glioma	Controversial (conservative vs. surgery vs. radiotherapy)

Retrochiasmal disorders

Most retrochiasmal disorders are associated with significant additional neurological morbidity. Hence such patients tend to have already been assessed, investigated, and started on treatment and rehabilitation before seeing an ophthalmologist. However, lesions that are otherwise clinically silent (e.g., some occipital pathology) may present first to the ophthalmologist.

The patient will usually be vague about the problem with his/her vision, and even a dense hemianopia may be missed unless visual fields are routinely assessed (e.g., by confrontational testing).

Clinical features

Optic tracts

● Incongruous homonymous hemianopia, optic atrophy, contralateral RAPD, larger pupil on the side of the hemianopia (Behr pupil), pupillary hemiakinesia (Wernicke's pupil).

Lateral geniculate nucleus

● Incongruous homonymous hemianopia, normal pupils; often associated with thalamic and corticospinal signs (mild hemiparesis).

Optic radiations

Parietal lesions

● Inferior incongruous homonymous defect, usually sparing fixation (macula fibers pass between parietal and temporal lobes); may be associated with damage to the posterior limb of the internal capsule (contralateral hemiparesis + hemianesthesia), injury to the pursuit pathways (patient fails to pursue to the side of the lesion; cannot follow an optokinetic nystagmus (OKN) drum rotated to the side of the lesion), and Gerstmann's syndrome (dominant parietal lobe only).

Temporal lesions

● Superior incongruous homonymous defect ("pie in sky"), usually sparing central vision. They may be associated with memory loss, hallucinations (olfactory, gustatory, auditory), and receptive dysphasia.

Calcarine cortex (occipital) lesions

● Congruous homonymous defect; variants include sparing of the temporal crescent (represented anteriorly), sparing of the macula (represented posteriorly), or a congruous homonymous macular lesion (selective injury to the occipital tip). These may be associated with visual hallucinations (usually in the hemianopic field) and denial of blindness (Anton's syndrome).

Investigations

● *Urgent neuroimaging:* MRI (gadolinium enhanced) is preferable, although CT may be adequate for many lesions and may be advantageous in the presence of extensive hemorrhage.

● Further investigations will be directed by the nature of the lesion found.

Treatment

After diagnosis, the main role of the ophthalmologist is to refer for appropriate treatment of the underlying cause (e.g., to stroke unit, neurosurgery, oncology). A secondary role is coordination of visual rehabilitation and support (which may include visual impairment registration).

Migraine

Migraine is a very common condition that may be severely disabling. Its prevalence is estimated at up to 20% for men and 40% for women. Around 25% of cases present before the age of 10 years, and 90% present before age 40. Overall, it is more common in women, but under 12 years of age it is slightly more common in boys.

It is classified as migraine without aura ("common migraine") or migraine with aura ("classic migraine"); migraine without aura is three times as common as migraine with aura. A first-degree relative confers a relative risk of 3.8 for classic migraine and 1.9 for common migraine.

The mechanism is uncertain: patients with migraines appear to have an inherited susceptibility to environmental factors that trigger noradrenaline and serotonin release. These cause constriction of cortical vessels (spreading neuronal depression aura) and dilation of extracranial vasculature (perivascular pain receptors → headache).

Clinical features

Migraine without aura

- *Prodrome:* mood and autonomic system disturbance (e.g., fatigue, hunger, irritability).
- *Headache:* unilateral (may generalize), throbbing, moderate to severe intensity, worsens over 1–2 hours, usually subsides over 4–8 hours but may last 1–3 days. It may be associated with nausea, photophobia, and sensitivity to noise (phonophobia).
- Termination and postdrome phase: recovery stages marked by fatigue.

Migraine with aura

This variant is characterized by an aura that usually precedes the headache phase, but may coincide with or follow it. The aura is most often visual but may be somatosensory, motor, or speech.

- *Visual* (99% of patients): typically starts paracentrally and expands temporally; the advancing edge forms a positive scotoma (flickering, shimmering, zigzag, multicolored lights), whereas the trailing edge is negatively scotomatous. Other visual phenomena include foggy vision, heat waves, tunnel vision, and complete loss of vision (see Box 16.4).
- *Somatosensory* (40%): hemisensory paresthesia/anesthesia.
- *Motor* (18%): hemiparesis.
- *Speech* (20%): dysphasia.

Other migraine variants (see Table 16.16)

Investigation

Migraine (with or without aura) may be diagnosed on the basis of a typical history in the presence of a normal neurological examination. Atypical features in the history (e.g., age >55 years, occipitobasal headache) or persistent neurological deficits require further assessment by a neurologist which may include neuroimaging, carotid Doppler scan, ECG, echocardiography, and vasculitis screen).

Treatment
- *Prophylactic:* avoid trigger factors (e.g., cheese, chocolate, coffee, citrus, cola, Chinese food/MSG, contraceptive pill); medical treatment is considered if there are ≥2 disabling attacks per month (e.g., propranolol, amitriptyline, sodium valproate).
- *Therapeutic:* relax in a dark quiet room; aspirin, NSAIDs, or combination analgesics. Consider 5HT1 agonist (e.g., sumatriptan 50 mg PO or 10 mg nasally stat) for more severe attacks.

Box 16.4 Ophthalmic complications of migraine

- Visual aura
- Retinal migraine
- Ophthalmoplegic migraine
- Retinal arterial occlusion
- Anterior ischemic optic neuropathy
- Posterior ischemic optic neuropathy
- Benign unilateral episodic mydriasis
- Adies pupil
- Increased risk of normal tension glaucoma

Table 16.16 Migraine classification

Migraine without aura	
Migraine with aura	
Migraine with typical aura	Aura <60 min and typical; full recovery
Migraine with prolonged aura	Aura >60 min; full recovery
Familial hemiplegic migraine	Familial (AD, Ch19), hemiparesis ± sensory, visual, speech, cerebellar aura; rare
Basilar migraine	Bilateral visual disturbance + brainstem or cerebellar aura (collapse, diplopia, ataxia, vertigo, dysarthria)
Migraine aura without headache	"Acephalgic migraine"; more common over age 40 years; must be differentiated from TIAs
Ophthalmoplegic migraine	Transient paresis of either CN III, IV, or VI occurring during migraine and lasting for days to weeks; usually full recovery; rare
Retinal migraine	Recurrent monocular visual disturbance; variable scotoma (dark, light, scintillating; focal, altitudinal, complete); 5–15 min duration; retinal vessel narrowing during attack
Childhood periodic syndromes	E.g., abdominal migraine
Complications of migraine	Migrainous infarction: aura >1 week or ischemia on scan
Atypical migraine	Migraine that does not fulfill above criteria

Supranuclear eye movement disorders (1)

Eye movements serve to either bring an object of interest on to the fovea (saccades, quick phase of nystagmus) or maintain it there (vestibular, optokinetic, pursuit, vergences). Movement of the globe requires sufficient contraction of the extraocular muscles to first overcome orbital viscosity and then to sustain the new position against the elastic restoring force. The ocular motor neurons (originating from III, IV, VI nuclei; see Table 16.17) achieve this by pulse-step innervation whereby they generate first a phasic and then a tonic stimulus. For example, in saccades, a high-frequency signal from excitatory burst neurons excites the ocular motor nucleus directly (resulting in a pulse) but also indirectly via neural integrators (which mathematically integrate the signal to give a step).

Pause cells act as dampers to prevent unwanted saccadic activity. Supranuclear pathways control this activity.

Horizontal conjugate gaze requires the CN VI nucleus to simultaneously drive ipsilateral LR, drive contralateral MR (via the MLF to contralateral CN III nucleus), and inhibit the contralateral LR (via inhibitory burst cells to contralateral CN VI nucleus).

Saccades originate in the contralateral frontal eye field (FEF). Pursuit eye movements originate in the ipsilateral parieto-occipito-temporal (POT) junction. Vestibular input (e.g., for vestibulo-ocular reflex [VOR]) is from the contralateral vestibular nuclei. Convergence input is directly to both CN III nucleus complexes, avoiding the MLF (Fig. 16.2).

Control of vertical eye movements is more complex, since the system is effectively a torsional one that has been subverted to allow vertical movements.

Table 16.17 Location of ocular premotor and motor neurons

Pause cell	Nucleus raphe interpositus
Horizontal burst cell	Paramedian pontine reticular formation (PPRF)
Horizontal inhibitory burst cell	Nucleus paragigantocellularis dorsalis
Horizontal integrator	Medial vestibular nucleus
	Nucleus prepositus hypoglossi
Horizontal ocular motor nucleus	CN VI nucleus
Vertical burst cell	Rostral interstitial nucleus of MLF
Vertical inhibitory burst cell	Rostral interstitial nucleus of MLF (probable)
Vertical integrator	Interstitial nucleus of Cajal
Vertical ocular motor nuclei	CN III nucleus, CN IV nucleus

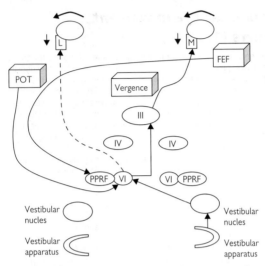

Figure 16.2 Supranuclear inputs for horizontal eye movements. Connections are shown for eye movements to the left (including saccades from FEF, smooth pursuit from POT, and vestibulo-ocular reflex from vestibular nucleus). For convergence movements, the CN III nuclei are innervated directly to drive both MR. For further explanation, see text.

Disorders of horizontal gaze

Horizontal gaze palsy
Lesions of the paramedian pontine reticular formation (PPRF) or CN VI nucleus result in failure to move the eyes beyond the midline to the side of the lesion. The VOR is preserved in a PPRF lesion but is lost in a CN VI nucleus lesion.

Internuclear ophthalmoplegia (INO)
Lesions of the MLF result in failure of ipsilateral adduction and overshoot of the contralateral eye (ataxic nystagmus), which are best demonstrated on saccadic movements. It may be associated with upbeat and torsional nystagmus, loss of vertical smooth pursuit, abnormal VOR, and skew deviation. Convergence is preserved.

One-and-a-half syndrome
Lesions of the MLF and the PPRF (or CN VI nuc) on the same side result in an ipsilateral gaze palsy and a contralateral INO. There is loss of horizontal movements other than abduction of the contralateral eye.

Tonic gaze deviation

Destructive lesions of the FEF (e.g., acute strokes) cause loss of gaze initiation to the contralateral side, with the result that the eyes deviate to the side of the lesion. Irritative lesions (e.g., trauma, tumor) cause transient deviations to the contralateral side.

Locked-in syndrome

Large lesions of the ventral pons may destroy bilateral PPRF and the corticospinal pathways, resulting in loss of all voluntary motor activity except lid movements and vertical eye movements (cf. coma where all voluntary movements are lost).

Selective loss of pursuits

Lesions of the POT junction cause failure of pursuit to the side of the lesion. This can also be demonstrated by inability to follow an OKN drum rotated to the side of the lesion. It is often associated with a contralateral homonymous field defect (usually superior).

Selective loss of saccades

Selective saccadic loss may occur in congenital or acquired ocular motor apraxia. In the congenital form, the child learns after a few months to compensate by 'head thrusts' (± blinks) beyond the target; these become less noticeable with age. In the acquired form, head thrusts are not a major feature; it may occur in bilateral frontoparietal injuries or diffuse cerebral disease.

Supranuclear eye movement disorders (2)

Vertical gaze palsies

Parinaud dorsal midbrain syndrome

Lesions of the posterior commissure and pretectal area result in supranuclear upgaze palsy (saccades affected first, then pursuits, and finally VOR), light-near dissociation, lid retraction, and convergence retraction nystagmus. Causes include hydrocephalus, tumor, trauma, arteriovenous malformations (AVMs), cerebrovascular accident (CVA), and demyelination.

Progressive supranuclear palsy (Steele–Richardson–Olszewski syndrome)

In this neurodegenerative disease of the elderly, there is supranuclear vertical gaze palsy (downgaze affected first, then upgaze, and finally horizontal movements; saccades are affected before pursuits) and lid apraxia (usually seen as failure to blink). Other features include postural instability, Parkinsonism, pseudobulbar palsy, and dementia.

Other supranuclear gaze palsies

Selective upgaze palsy may occur in Wilson's disease. Selective downgaze palsy with athetosis and ataxia occurs in Niemann–Pick's disease type C.

Tonic gaze deviation

Raised intracranial pressure or thalamic hemorrhage may cause forced downgaze ("sunset sign"), although it may occur as a transient phenomenon in healthy neonates.

Selective loss of saccades

In Huntington's disease, there is selective loss of saccades (vertical more than horizontal) which may be compensated for by head thrusts and blinks.

Skew deviation

This is a vertical deviation that is usually concomitant and associated with torsion. Incomitant skews may be confused with CN IV (or CN III) palsies. Skew deviations are usually caused by lesions of the pons or lateral medulla (e.g., CVA, demyelination).

Third nerve disorders

A third nerve palsy may be the first sign of an aneurysm of the posterior communicating artery. Unfortunately, it may also be the last sign before the aneurysm ruptures, causing subarachnoid hemorrhage and often death.

Diagnosis may be difficult: a partial palsy may simulate a number of other conditions. Classical teaching associates painful, pupil-involving, progressive palsies with compressive disease (e.g., an expanding aneurysm). However, the differentiation of a compressive from an ischemic third nerve palsy may not be possible on clinical grounds alone.

Classification

Accurate localization greatly assists diagnosis. Identify whether it is

- Complete vs. partial (including aberrant regeneration).
- Pupil-sparing vs. pupil-involving.
- Nuclear, fascicular, or peripheral (nerve palsy).
- Isolated or complex (other neurological defects).

Clinical features

Headache and pain

A severe headache ("worst pain in my life," "like someone kicked me in the back of the head") in this context should be assumed to be due to subarachnoid hemorrhage until proven otherwise. Pain is classically associated with compressive lesions but may also occur in ischemia.

Complete

- Diplopia (horizontal and often vertical).
- Complete ptosis, eye abducted, and usually depressed.

Partial

- Any of the above features from near-complete involvement to single muscle paresis (rare).
- Aberrant regeneration is usually associated with long-standing compressive lesions. In lid-gaze dyskinesia, there is lid elevation on adduction ("inverse Duane's") or on depression ("pseudo von Grefe"). In pupil-gaze dyskinesia, there is pupil constriction on adduction or depression. Pure eye movement dyskinesias may also occur (e.g., elevation when trying to adduct).

Pupil involving (cf. pupil sparing)

There is also mydriasis (no light or near response) and difficulty focusing.

Nuclear, fascicular, or peripheral (nerve palsy)

Certain patterns of CN III disorder are localizing (Box 16.5, Table 16.18)

Isolated or complex

Check for involvement of all other cranial nerves, including CN II (especially fields, discs), CN VI (abduction), CN IV (intorsion), cerebellum, and peripheral nervous system (PNS). Other neurological signs may be local (e.g., compressive lesion) or disseminated (e.g., demyelination).

Box 16.5 Causes of CN III palsy

- Aneurysms (usually of the posterior communicating artery)
- Microvascular infarction
- Tumor (e.g., parasellar)
- Trauma
- Demyelination
- Vasculitis
- Congenital

Table 16.18 Nuclear and fascicular CN III syndromes

Nuclear	
Definitely nuclear	Unilateral palsy with contralateral SR paresis and bilateral partial ptosis
	Bilateral palsy without ptosis

Fascicular	
Red nucleus (paramedian midbrain)	Ipsilateral CN III palsy
	Contralateral intention tremor + ataxia ± contralateral anesthesia (Benedikt's syndrome)
Cerebral peduncle (anterior midbrain)	Ipsilateral CN III palsy
	Contralateral hemiparesis (Weber's syndrome)

Investigation

Pupil-involving or partial CN III palsies (often compressive)

Use emergency neuroimaging (MRI with MRA or high-resolution CTA). If normal, consider further investigation, such as LP (CSF for oligoclonal bands, glucose, protein, xanthochromia, microscopy, culture, and sensitivities [MC&S], cytology).

Pupil-sparing complete CN III palsies (usually ischemic)

Assess vascular risk factors (atherosclerosis or arteritis; BP, glucose, lipids, ESR, CRP, CBC) and monitor closely for the first week (e.g., every 2 days) to ensure there is no developing pupil involvement. The likelihood of ischemic etiology is increased if there is age >40 years, known vasculopathy, acute onset, nonprogressive characteristic(s), and no additional neurological abnormality.

If there is no recovery at 3 months, investigate further (including MRI).

Monitor in conjunction with orthoptists (including Hess/Lees charts and fields of BSV).

Treatment

This depends on the underlying cause. Posterior communicating artery aneurysms require immediate transfer to a neurosurgical unit for open (clips) or endovascular (coils, balloons) treatment. Other pathologies may require referral to neurology, neurosurgery, oncology, or medicine.

Diplopia may be relieved by intrinsic ptosis or occlusion (patch or contact lens). Surgery is dictated by any residual function and may comprise staged lid and muscle procedures. While this may improve cosmesis, its effect on the field of BSV is less predictable; it may even worsen diplopia.

Prognosis

Untreated posterior communicating artery aneurysms rupture in two-third of cases, of which half are fatal. Treatment reduces the mortality rate to <5%. After surgery, compressive CN III palsies usually recover (at least partially) over 6 months. Ischemic CN III palsies usually spontaneously recover over 4 months.

Fourth nerve disorders

Superior oblique weakness secondary to CN IV palsy is a common cause of vertical strabismus. One third of cases are congenital, but they may not present until adulthood. Acquired cases are commonly traumatic or due to microvascular infarction. Bilateral CN IV palsy is most commonly due to head injury (see Box 16.6).

Clinical features

- Diplopia (vertical and torsional; worse on downgaze), head tilt (to opposite side), esthenopia.
- Ipsilateral hypertropia/phoria worse on downgaze or on ipsilateral head tilt; compensatory head tilt to opposite side; limited depression in adduction; extorsion (examine fundus: normal foveal position is level with lower third of disc; measure angle with double Maddox rod); may have V pattern.
- Park's three-step test (p. 32).

Congenital or acquired

A large vertical prism fusion range and high concomitance suggest that the paresis is either congenital or, if acquired, a long-standing lesion.

Unilateral or bilateral

Bilateral palsy is fairly common (particularly after head injury) but may be asymmetric. Typically, there is a reversing hypertropia with L/R on right gaze and R/L on left gaze, a prominent V pattern, and significant excyclotorsion. See Box 16.7.

Isolated or complex

Check for involvement of all other cranial nerves, including CN II (especially fields, discs), CN III, V, and VI, pupils (Horner's, RAPD), cerebellum, and peripheral nervous system (see Table 16.19). Other neurological signs may be local (e.g., orbital apex lesion) or disseminated (e.g., demyelination).

Investigation

A history of abnormal head posture (check old photographs) or recent trauma may identify the cause. Assess vascular risk factors (atherosclerosis or arteritis; BP, glucose, lipids, ESR, CRP, CBC). The likelihood of ischemic etiology is increased if there is age > 40 years, known vasculopathy, acute onset, nonprogressive characteristic(s), and no additional neurological abnormality.

   If etiology is unclear or there is no recovery at 3 months, then investigate further (including MRI). Monitor in conjunction with orthoptist (including Hess/Lees charts and fields of BSV).

Treatment

Orthoptic intervention with a vertical prism (or occlusion) may satisfactorily control diplopia. Surgical options include ipsilateral IO weakening (disinsertion or recession), contralateral IR recession, SO tuck, and modified Harada-Ito. SO tuck carries a significant risk of inducing an iatrogenic Brown's syndrome.

Box 16.6 Causes of CN IV palsy

- Trauma
- Microvascular infarction
- Tumor (e.g., pinealoma, tentorial meningioma)
- Demyelination
- Vasculitis
- Meningitis
- Cavernous sinus lesions
- Tolosa–Hunt syndrome
- Neurosurgery
- Herpes zoster ophthalmicus
- Congenital

Box 16.7 Features suggestive of bilateral CN IV palsy

- Chin-down head posture (without much tilt)
- Reversing hyperdeviation
- Excyclotorsion >10'
- Prominent V pattern
- Bilateral failure of adduction in depression

Table 16.19 Nuclear and fascicular CN IV syndromes

Sympathetic pathways	Ipsilateral Horner's syndrome Contralateral SO palsy
Medial longitudinal fasciculus	Ipsilateral INO Contralateral SO palsy
Superior cerebellar peduncle	Ipsilateral ataxia, intention tremor Contralateral SO palsy

Sixth nerve disorders

Sixth nerve palsy is the most common cause of neurogenic strabismus (for causes of CN VI palsy see Box 16.8). Although CN VI palsy results in an easily recognized abduction deficit, other pathologies may give a similar picture, notably Duane's syndrome, medial wall orbital fracture, and thyroid eye disease (Box 16.9).

Clinical features

- Diplopia (horizontal; worse for distance and on looking to the side of the lesion), head turn (to same side).
- Esophoria/tropia (worse for distance and on ipsilateral gaze); ipsilateral abduction deficit (ranges from saccadic slowing only, to complete loss of all movement beyond the midline).

Isolated or complex

Check for involvement of all other cranial nerves, including CN II (especially fields, discs), CN III, IV, V, and VII, pupils (Horner's), cerebellum, and peripheral nervous system (see Table 16.20). Other neurological signs may be local (e.g., the now very rare Gradenigo's syndrome), disseminated (e.g., demyelination), or reflect ↑ICP (if CN VI palsy is a false localizing sign).

Investigation

Assess vascular risk factors (atherosclerosis or arteritis; BP, glucose, lipids, ESR, CRP, CBC). The likelihood of ischemic etiology is increased if there is age >40 years, known vasculopathy, acute onset, nonprogressive characteristic(s), and no additional neurological abnormality.

If etiology is unclear or there is no recovery at 3 months, then investigate further (including MRI). Monitor in conjunction with orthoptists (including prism cover test, Hess charts, and fields of BSV).

Treatment

Orthoptic intervention with a base-out prism (or occlusion) may satisfactorily control diplopia. Botulinum toxin injection into ipsilateral MR has both a therapeutic and diagnostic role. It may restore BSV and, if only temporary, may be repeated. In any event, it reveals any residual CN VI function that might be augmented by an LR resection/MR recession.

If there is no residual function, then vertical muscle transposition would be required.

Box 16.8 Causes of CN VI palsy

- Microvascular infarction
- Tumor (e.g., clivus, cerebellopontine angle, pituitary, nasopharyngeal)
- ↑ICP
- Trauma (basal skull fracture)
- Demyelination
- Vasculitis
- Meningitis
- Cavernous sinus thrombosis
- Carotid–cavernous fistula
- Congenital

Box 16.9 Differential diagnosis of abduction deficit

- Duane's syndrome
- Convergence spasm
- Thyroid eye disease
- Myasthenia
- Myositis
- Medial wall fracture
- Distance esotropia of high myopia

Table 16.20 Nuclear and fascicular CN VI syndromes

Nuclear	
PPRF (dorsal pons)	Ipsilateral gaze palsy
PPRF + MLF (dorsomedial pons)	Ipsilateral gaze palsy Contralateral INO (one-and-a-half syndrome)
AICA territory (dorsolateral pons)	Ipsilateral gaze palsy Ipsilateral CN VII palsy Ipsilateral CN V palsy Contralateral hemianesthesia (Foville syndrome)
Fascicular	
Corticospinal tract (ventral pons)	Ipsilateral CN VI palsy Contralateral hemiparesis (Raymond's syndrome)
Facial colliculus (dorsal pons)	Ipsilateral CN VI palsy Ipsilateral CN VII palsy (Millard–Gubler syndrome)

AICA, anterior inferior cerebellar artery.

Horner's syndrome

The ocular sympathetic supply may be damaged anywhere along its route (see Table 16.21). The extent of sympathetic dysfunction, associated neurological signs, and pharmacological tests may help identify the location of the injury.

Clinical features
- The pupil is miotic with normal light and near reaction.
- Anisocoria is most marked in dim conditions.
- Also ptosis, apparent (but not true) enophthalmos, conjunctival injection; facial anyhydrosis suggests a lesion of the first or second-order neuron. Iris hypochromia suggests a congenital lesion but may be a longstanding acquired lesion.

Isolated or complex
Check for involvement of all other cranial nerves, including CN II (especially fields, discs), CN III, IV, V and VI, cerebellum, and peripheral nervous system. Other neurological signs may be local (e.g., cavernous sinus pathology) or disseminated (e.g., demyelination).

Also check for history of pain (headache, neck pain, arm pain), trauma or surgery, and any other physical signs, e.g., scars and masses (lung apices, neck, thyroid).

Investigation
Confirm diagnosis
Administer 4% cocaine to both eyes; repeat at 1 min. At 0 and 60 min, measure pupil sizes when fixing on a distant target in identical ambient lighting conditions. A positive test for Horner's is if there is no or poor dilation to cocaine (blocks reuptake of NorA at the dilator papillae neuromuscular junction).

Identify level
Administer 1% hydroxyamphetamine to both eyes. If there is a first- or second-order neuron lesion, there will be normal dilation; if a third-order neuron lesion, there will be no or poor dilation. This test is seldom performed in clinical practice.

Topical hydroxyamphetamine is expensive and may not be readily available. The test is not reliable if performed within 48 hours of a cocaine test.

Identify etiology
Further investigation is directed by the likely cause and level of lesion (Table 16.22).

Treatment and prognosis
This is dependent on the underlying etiology and may involve urgent referral to neurosurgery, neurology, vascular surgery, or ENT. Any recovery of a Horner's syndrome also depends on the underlying cause and treatment. In cases associated with cluster headaches (Reder's syndrome), recovery may occur within a few hours. Invasive tumors may cause relentless irreversible progression.

Table 16.21 Causes of Horner's syndrome

Lesion type	Location	Cause
Central	Brainstem	CVA
		Tumor
		Demyelination
	Spinal cord	Tumor
		Syringomyelia
		Trauma
Preganglionic	Lung apex	Pancoast tumor
		Trauma
	Neck	Trauma
		Surgery
		Tumor (thyroid, cervical LN)
		CCA dissection
Postganglionic	ICA	ICA dissection
	Middle ear	Otitis media
		Herpes zoster
	Cavernous sinus	Thrombosis
		Tumor
	Orbit	Tolosa–Hunt
		Tumor
		Cluster headache

Many acquired and congenital cases are idiopathic.

CCA, common carotid artery; ICA, internal carotid artery; LN, lymph node.

Table 16.22 Investigations of Horner's syndrome

Lesion type	Investigations
Central	MRI brain/spinal cord
Preganglionic	CXR
	CT thorax
	Carotid Doppler
	MRI or MRA head/neck
	LN biopsy
Postganglionic	Carotid Doppler
	MRI or MRA head/neck
	MRI orbits
	ENT assessment

Adie's tonic pupil

In Adie's pupil, the parasympathetic supply from the ciliary ganglion to the iris and ciliary muscle is abnormal. It is thought that this arises from acute viral denervation and aberrant regeneration. It is most commonly unilateral (80%), occurring in otherwise healthy young women.

Clinical features

- Classically, the pupil is mydriatic and has poor response to light with vermiform movements seen at the slit lamp and exaggerated but slow and sustained (tonic) response to near; there is light-near dissociation.
- *Variants*: early lesions may show no response to light or near; late lesions are usually miotic; segmental lesions are common. There may be additional absence of deep tendon reflexes (Holmes–Adie syndrome) or patchy hypohidrosis (Ross's syndrome). With time, the pupil becomes miotic.

Investigations

Confirm diagnosis: administer 0.125% pilocarpine to both eyes. At 0 and 30 min, measure pupil size when fixing on a distant target in identical dim lighting conditions. In Adie's pupil, the response is greater in the affected eye (denervation hypersensitivity of sphincter pupillae).

Treatment

- Reassure patient.
- Weak-strength pilocarpine (e.g., 0.1% as often as required) may help treat mydriatic blurring and accommodative problems. Mydriasis may also be helped by a painted contact lens acting as an artificial pupil. Reading glasses may also help with the accommodative dysfunction.

Nystagmus (1)

Nystagmus, oscillations, and saccadic intrusions are a group of involuntary abnormalities of fixation. In nystagmus there is an abnormal, slow movement away from fixation that is then corrected by a fast movement (jerk nystagmus) or by another slow movement (pendular nystagmus).

In oscillations and intrusions, there is an abnormal saccade away from fixation, followed by a corrective saccade (i.e., both movements are fast). The corrective saccade may be immediate (oscillation) or delayed (intrusion).

Classification

Analyze the movement disorder in a logical manner:

- History: early or late onset; presence of oscillopsia.
- Abnormal movement away from fixation: slow or fast.
- Corrective movement: slow or fast.
- Direction: horizontal, vertical, or rotatory.
- Symmetry: conjugate or disconjugate.
- Effect on direction and amplitude of time, direction of gaze, fixation, and head position.
- Visual acuity.
- Associated involuntary movements: palate, head, and neck.

Early-onset nystagmus

Early-onset or congenital nystagmus is not associated with oscillopsia, but other ophthalmic abnormalities are common (Table 16.23).

Idiopathic congenital

Conjugate horizontal (usually) jerk nystagmus worsens with fixation but improves within "null zone" and on convergence. The null zone is a direction of gaze in which the nystagmus is dampened down. It has a very early onset (usually by 2 months of age) and may initially be pendular. It can occasionally be vertical or rotatory. There is usually only mild ↓VA; strabismus is common. It may be inherited (AD, AR, X-linked).

Sensory deprivation

There is an erratic waveform ± roving eye movements; moderate to severe ↓VA is due to ocular or anterior visual pathway disease.

Manifest latent

Conjugate horizontal jerk nystagmus with fast phase toward the fixing eye worsens with occlusion of the nonfixing eye and with gaze toward fast phase, but improves with gaze toward slow phase. It alternates if the opposite eye takes up fixation; this is often associated with infantile esotropia.

Table 16.23 Early-onset nystagmus

Waveform	Effect of occlusion	Nystagmus type
Horizontal jerk	Already evident	Idiopathic congenital
	Becomes manifest	Manifest latent
Erratic ± roving	No effect	Sensory deprivation

Nystagmus (2)

Late-onset nystagmus—conjugate

Late-onset or acquired nystagmus is usually associated with oscillopsia and is often associated with other neurological abnormalities (Table 16.24).

Gaze-evoked nystagmus (GEN)

- Conjugate horizontal (usually) jerk nystagmus on eccentric gaze with fast phase toward direction of gaze. It occurs at smaller angles than physiological end-point nystagmus (i.e., <45°).

Asymmetric gaze-evoked nystagmus usually indicates failure of ipsilateral neural integrator/cerebellar dysfunction (p. 543). Symmetric GEN may be due to CNS depression (fatigue, alcohol, anticonvulsants, barbiturates) or structural pathology (e.g., brainstem, cerebellum).

Periodic alternating nystagmus (PAN)

- Conjugate horizontal jerk nystagmus present in primary position with waxing–waning nystagmus lasting for 90 sec in each direction with a 10 sec gap or "null" period.

PAN is usually due to vestibulocerebellar disease (e.g., demyelination, Arnold–Chiara malformation). An alternating nystagmus without such regular periodicity may also be seen in patients with severe ↓VA.

Peripheral vestibular nystagmus

- Conjugate horizontal jerk nystagmus, improves with fixation and with time since injury, worsens with gaze toward fast phase (Alexander's law) or change in head position.

Nystagmus with fast phase away from the lesion is associated with destructive lesions of the vestibular system (e.g., labyrinthitis, vestibular neuritis), whereas nystagmus to the same side may be seen in irritative lesions (e.g., Meniere's disease). It may be associated with vertigo, deafness, or tinnitus.

Central vestibular, cerebellar, or brainstem nystagmus

- Conjugate jerk (usually) nystagmus that may be horizontal, vertical, or torsional and that does not improve with fixation.

Horizontal central vestibular nystagmus is usually due to lesions of the vestibular nuclei, the cerebellum, or their connections.

Upbeat nystagmus in primary position is usually due to cerebellar or lower brainstem pathology (e.g., demyelination, infarction, tumor, encephalitis, Wernicke's syndrome).

Downbeat nystagmus in primary position is usually due to pathology of the craniocervical junction (e.g., Arnold–Chiari malformation, spinocerebellar degenerations, infarction, tumor, demyelination).

Table 16.24 Late-onset nystagmus—conjugate

Effect of gaze	Effect of time	Direction	Effect of fixation	Nystagmus type
Present in primary position	Sustained	Horizontal	Improves	Peripheral vestibular
			Worsens	Central vestibular
		Vertical	N/A	Upbeat Downbeat
	Periodic	Horizontal	N/A	Periodic alternating
Only present in eccentric gaze	N/A	Usually horizontal	N/A	Gaze evoked

Table 16.25 Late-onset nystagmus—disconjugate

Extent	Waveform	Nystagmus type
Unilateral	Torsional Horizontal in abducting eye	Superior oblique myokymia Internuclear ophthalmoplegia associated
Bilateral	Pendular Seesaw	Acquired pendular Seesaw

Late onset nystagmus—disconjugate (Table 16.25)

Acquired pendular nystagmus

* Usually disconjugate with horizontal, vertical, torsional components.

This is associated with brainstem and cerebellar disease, including toluene abuse. It also may be associated with involuntary repetitive movement of palate, pharynx, and face (oculopalatal myoclonus).

Superior oblique myokymia

* Unilateral high-frequency low-amplitude torsional nystagmus.

It may cause occasional diplopia but is rarely associated with underlying disease.

Internuclear ophthalmoplegia

* Nystagmus of the abducting (and occasionally adducting) eye.

The mechanism is uncertain; it is possibly due to gaze paresis or ataxia.

Seesaw nystagmus

* Vertical and torsional components with one eye elevating and intorting while the other depresses and extorts.

This usually has a slow pendular waveform, although a jerk seesaw nystagmus may also be seen. In the congenital form, the torsional element is reversed (i.e., the elevating eye extorts).

Treatment

Treatment of nystagmus is difficult and often disappointing. Treatment options depend on visual potential, presence of visual symptoms (oscillopsia), and the location of a null position.

Drug treatment includes GABA-ergics (e.g., gabapentin) and anticholinergics (e.g., scopolamine).

Optical devices aim to stabilize (e.g., high plus spectacle lens with high minus contact lens) or optimize the null position (e.g., prisms to move null position towards the primary position).

Surgical procedures may generally stabilize (e.g., bilateral weakening procedures—usually only a transient benefit) or move the null position (Kestenbaum procedure).

Retrobulbar botulinum toxin causes general dampening of ipsilateral nystagmus; however, induced diplopia may require occlusion of other eye.

Saccadic oscillations and intrusions

In oscillations and intrusions, there is an abnormal saccade away from fixation, followed by a corrective saccade, i.e., both movements are fast. The corrective saccade may be immediate (oscillation) or delayed (intrusion).

Saccadic oscillations

Ocular flutter

- Bursts of moderate-amplitude horizontal saccades without intersaccadic interval.

It is associated with cerebellar and brainstem disease.

Opsoclonus

- Bursts of large-amplitude multidirectional saccades without intersaccadic interval.

This is associated with loss of pause-cell activity, which may be caused by viruses, myoclonic encephalopathy, paraneoplastic syndromes (neuroblastoma in children, small cell lung cancer in adults), and demyelination.

Saccadic intrusions

Small, infrequent square-wave jerks may be physiological. However, other intrusions are usually pathological, most commonly from cerebellar disease.

Square-wave jerks and macrosquare-wave jerks

- Horizontal 1–5' (square wave) or 10–40' (macro) excursions from fixation and back again.

Macrosaccadic oscillations

- Series of hypermetric saccades attempting to narrow in on the target; ocular past-pointing.

Coma-associated eye movements

Ocular bobbing

- Conjugate fast downward movements with slow drift upward.

Ocular bobbing may be caused by large lesions of the pons, metabolic encephalopathies, or hydrocephalus.

Ocular dipping

- Conjugate slow downward movements with fast saccade upward.

This and other variants of ocular bobbing are fairly nonspecific.

Ping-pong gaze

- Conjugate horizontal movements alternating side every few seconds.

This is associated with bilateral cerebral hemispheric lesions.

Neuromuscular junction disorders

Myasthenia gravis

Myasthenia gravis (MG) is an uncommon autoimmune disease character-ized by weakness and fatiguability of skeletal muscle. Antibodies against postsynaptic acetylcholine receptors (AChR) cause loss of receptors and structural abnormalities of the neuromuscular junction. Its prevalence is estimated as up to 1 in 10,000.

It may occur at any age but has a bimodal distribution with peaks at around 20 years and 60 years. There is a female bias (3:2 F:M). It may be associated with thymic hyperplasia and other autoimmune disease (e.g., Graves' disease in 4–10%).

Clinical features

MG is a great mimic. Consider this diagnosis when confronted with ocular motility abnormalities that do not fit, particularly when these seem to be highly variable. Ocular signs are the presenting feature in 70% and are present at some point in 90% of MG. Ocular MG becomes generalized in 80% of patients (usually within 2 years).

Ocular

- Variable diplopia or ptosis (usually worsening toward evening or with exercise).
- Variable and fatiguable ptosis or ocular motility disturbance (any pattern); sustained eccentric gaze of ≥1 min or repeated saccades demonstrates fatigue, e.g., attempted prolonged upward gaze demonstrates fatigue of LPS and elevators; Cogan's twitch (ask patient to look down for 20 sec and then at object in the primary position: positive if lid overshoots). Spontaneous twitching is a sign of severe fatigue.

Systemic

- Fatiguable weakness of limbs, speech, chewing, swallowing, breathing. Take breathlessness seriously, as fatal respiratory failure may occur.

Investigations

- *Ice-pack test:* measure ptosis; place ice wrapped in a towel or glove on the closed eyelid for 2 min. Remeasure ptosis. The test is significantly positive if ≥2 mm.
- *Tensilon (edrophonium) test:* ensure that IV atropine (0.5–1 mg), resuscitation equipment, and trained staff are on hand. Cardiac monitoring is essential. Give 2 mg edrophonium IV (test dose); if there are no ill effects at 30 sec, give further 8 mg edrophonium IV (slow injection). Compare pre- and post-test ptosis or motility disturbance (consider Hess chart).
- *Serum antibodies:* anti-AChR is present in ≤95% patients with generalized myasthenia but only 50% of ocular myasthenia. Anti-skeletal muscle is present in 85% of patients with thymoma. Anti-thyroid antibodies and ANA may detect associated disease.
- *EMG:* repetitive supramaximal stimuli demonstrate reduction in action potential amplitude; also jitter (the EMG equivalent of twitch).

Treatment

Anticholinesterases

- Pyridostigmine: start 30–60 mg PO 1–2×/day, gradually increasing if required to maximum of 450 mg/day. Gastrointestinal disturbance is common but can be treated by propantheline.

Immunosuppression

If there is generalized disease, refer to a physician for further assessment and immunosuppression. This may include corticosteroids, azathioprine, IV immunoglobulin, plasmaphoresis, and thymectomy. Thymectomy is associated with remission of MG in 80% of nonthymoma patients but only 10% of thymoma patients.

Prognosis

Fatal cardiorespiratory failure may rarely occur, usually during the first year of disease. Prognosis is worse for those with thymoma and with a late onset of disease. Most patients are well controlled on treatment; some spontaneously remit.

Other neuromuscular junction disorders

Less commonly, disorders of the neuromuscular junction occur as a para-neoplastic or toxic phenomena (see Table 16.26).

Table 16.26 Neuromuscular junction disorders

Syndrome	Pathogenesis	Ocular features	Systemic features
Inhibitory syndromes			
MG	Antibodies to postsynaptic AChR	Fatiguable ptosis, abnormal motility	Fatigue of limbs, bulbar function, respiratory failure
LEMS	Paraneoplastic presynaptic ↓ACh release	↓Lacrimation, tonic pupils, abnormal motility	Proximal weakness Autonomic dysfunction
Botulism	Toxin presynaptic ↓ACh release	Ptosis, tonic pupils, abnormal motility	Weakness of bulbar function Autonomic dysfunction
Excitatory syndromes			
Organophosphate	Toxin inhibits ACh-esterase	Miosis	Respiratory failure Fasciculation Paralysis
Scorpion toxin	Toxin presynaptic ↑ACh release	↓VA, abnormal motility	Respiratory failure Mental disturbance

Lambert–Eaton myasthenic syndrome (LEMS)

This is a disorder of the presynaptic calcium channels, causing impaired release of ACh. It is usually associated with malignancy (e.g., small cell lung cancer) but may be an isolated autoimmune disorder. The main ocular feature is decreased lacrimation, although ocular motility abnormalities and tonic pupils may occur. In contrast to MG, repeated or sustained testing may cause improvement in any abnormalities.

Toxins

Toxins may act presynaptically to either impair ACh release (botulism, tick paralysis) or increase its release (black widow spider, scorpion bite). Organophosphates (fertilizers, nerve gas) act within the cleft to inhibit acetylcholinesterase.

Treatment includes supportive measures, antitoxin (if available), and, for the excitatory syndromes, atropine blockade.

Myopathies

Inherited myopathies are rare, insidious, and easily missed in their early stages. Diplopia is uncommon and patients may adopt exaggerated head movement. It is important to consider the diagnosis in all patients with bilateral ptosis, partly because a more cautious approach to lid surgery is necessary.

Acquired myopathies due to orbital inflammation or infiltration (e.g., thyroid eye disease and myositis, pp. 475–482) are much more common. Florid cases are easily recognized, but early cases may cause a nonspecific restrictive pattern.

Chronic progressive external ophthalmoplegia (CPEO)

This is a rare group of conditions in which there is progressive failure of eye movement. Mutations of mitochondrial DNA lead to abnormalities of oxidative phosphorylation and consequent muscle and CNS injury.

Clinical features

- Bilateral ptosis, ↓smooth pursuits, saccades, reflex eye movements (downgaze usually affected last; diplopia uncommon); weakness of orbicularis oculi and facial muscles.

Variants

- *Kearns-Sayre syndrome:* CPEO, pigmentary retinopathy (granular pigmentation, peripapillary atrophy), and heart block; usually presents before age 20.
- *MELAS syndrome:* mitochondrial encephalopathy, lactic acidosis, stroke-like episodes; also CPEO, hemianopia, cortical blindness.

Investigations

- ECG: check for conduction abnormalities.
- Consider skeletal muscle biopsy (ragged red fibers with peripheral concentration of mitochondria); peripheral blood (mitochondrial DNA analysis: fasting sample for glucose, lactate, pyruvate, pH); MRI, and EMG (to rule out other diagnoses).

Treatment

Symptomatic ptosis or diplopia may be relieved by cautious surgery (be aware of weak orbicularis oculi and poor Bell's phenomenon). Conduction abnormalities may require pacemaker insertion. Coenzyme Q10 has some benefit on the systemic features of Kearns–Sayre syndrome.

Oculopharyngeal dystrophy

This rare autosomal dominant (occasionally sporadic) condition is associated with an expanded GCG repeat in the poly(A) binding protein 2 gene. It typically presents in the sixth decade and has been identified in a large French-Canadian pedigree.

It is a form of myotonia (i.e., there is a delay in muscle relaxation post-contraction). The condition progresses from dysphagia to bilateral ptosis to external ophthalmoplegia and orbicularis weakness.

Myotonic dystrophy

This uncommon autosomal dominant dystrophy results from an expanded CTG repeat in the dystrophica myotonica protein kinase (DMPK) gene (Ch19q). Anticipation occurs whereby the triplet expansion increases in successive generations, leading to earlier and more severe disease.

Prevalence is estimated at around 5/100,000, being highest among French-Canadians. It is characterized by a failure of muscle relaxation after contraction.

Clinical features

Ocular

- Bilateral ptosis, cataracts (polychromatic "Christmas tree cataracts" or posterior subcapsular), orbicularis oculi weakness; rarely, pigmentary retinopathy ("butterfly" pigmentation centrally, reticular at mid-periphery, and atrophic far periphery), and myotonia of extraocular muscles.

Systemic

- Mournful facies, dysphasia, dysphagia, muscle weakness with delayed relaxation ("myotonic grip"), testicular atrophy, frontal baldness, ↓IQ, cardiac myopathy, and conduction abnormalities (may lead to fatal cardiac failure).

Investigations

- *DNA analysis* is used to confirm the diagnosis.
- *ECG* should be performed annually for conduction abnormalities; these may occur in otherwise minimally affected individuals.

Treatment

Multidisciplinary management may include neurology, cardiology, physiotherapy, occupational therapy, and speech therapy. Offer genetic counseling, annual influenza vaccination, and cataract surgery (when symptomatic). General anesthetics may unmask subclinical respiratory failure, leading to problems of ventilatory weaning.

Blepharospasm and other dystonias

Blepharospasm is a relatively common condition that, in its severe form, can be very disabling in terms of both vision and social function. It is more common in women (F:M 2:1) and increases with age. It is a type of focal dystonia in which there is tonic spasm of the orbicularis oculi.

The condition may be idiopathic (essential blepharospasm) or secondary to ocular or periocular disease (see Table 16.27). Blepharospasm may be associated with dystonias involving other facial muscles.

Essential blepharospasm

Clinical features

- Bilateral involuntary lid closure, increase frequency of lid closure (normal is around 10–20×/min); may be precipitated by stress, fatigue, social interactions; may be relieved by relaxation or distraction, e.g., touching face or whistling. There are often marked fluctuations from day to day, but the condition generally worsens over years.
- Associated ocular disease may include underlying precipitants (particularly lid and ocular surface) and secondary anatomical changes of the lid (ptosis or entropion) or brow (brow-ptosis or dermatochalasis).

Investigations

Typical isolated blepharospasm does not usually require investigation. If atypical (e.g., associated weakness or any other neurological abnormality), consult with a neurologist and consider imaging (e.g., MRI) and other tests (e.g., EMG).

Treatment

- Botulinum toxin (A) is usually given as multiple injections of the upper and lower lid; it has high rate of success in the short term (up to 98%) but generally only lasts for 3 months. Complications include ptosis, epiphora, keratitis, dry eyes, and ocular motility disorders (diplopia).
- Treat any underlying ocular disease.
- Other treatment options include medical (e.g., benzodiazepines) and surgical (myectomy or chemomyectomy with doxorubicin) ones.

Table 16.27 Causes of blepharospasm

Type	Cause
Essential	Idiopathic
Secondary	*Common*
	Blepharitis
	Trichiasis
	Dry eyes/keratoconjunctivitis sicca
	Other chronic lid disease
	Other chronic ocular surface disease
	Rare
	Glaucoma
	Uveitis

Other dystonias of the face and neck
- *Meige's syndrome:* blepharospasm with midfacial spasm; regarded as a spillover of essential blepharospasm to involve the midfacial musculature. It may compromise speech and eating and drinking.
- *Torticollis:* tonic spasm of sternocleidomastoid causes sudden sustained movement of the head to one side.

Other involuntary facial movement disorders
- *Hemifacial spasm:* tonic-clonic spasm of facial musculature that, unlike blepharospasm or Meige's syndrome, is unilateral, may occur during sleep, and typically affects a younger age group. It suggests irritation of the root of the CN VII by a compressive lesion (usually an abnormal vessel, but needs imaging to rule out a posterior fossa tumor).
- *Facial myokymia:* fleeting movements of facial musculature that may be associated with caffeine, stress, MS, or rarely tumors of the brainstem
- *Facial tic:* brief, repetitive stereotypic movements that are suppressible (at least initially). It may be associated with Gilles de la Tourette syndrome.

Lid apraxia

Normal blinking requires both the inhibition of levator palpebre superioris and the activation of orbicularis oculi. In lid-opening apraxia, there is total inhibition of LPS with no activation of orbicularis oculi (OO). This results in sustained lid closure with difficulty in initiating lid opening. It is associated with extrapyramidal diseases (e.g., Parkinson's disease, progressive supranuclear palsy, Huntington's disease, Wilson's disease).

Lid retraction and poor initiation of lid closure may also be seen in Parkinson's disease, progressive supranuclear palsy, and Parinaud's syndrome.

Functional visual loss

Functional visual loss (also called nonorganic visual loss, psychogenic visual impairment) is a diagnosis of exclusion. It can often coexist with genuine pathology.

Suspecting functional visual loss

Consider this diagnosis when the patient reports poor vision but some of the following features are present.

Visual function and history

- Visual functioning obviously does not correlate with history (e.g., patient reported blindness but was able to navigate around the hospital, waiting room, or examination room).
- Patient cannot perform tasks that he/she may consider to be visual but actually are not (e.g., signing name).
- Recent stressful event elicited in history (e.g., impending exams).

Normal examination

- No apparent pathology after *detailed* examination
- Absence of RAPD in the context of profound reported asymmetrical visual loss. Bilateral symmetrical pathology may give slow (sluggish) pupillary light responses but no RAPD.
- Retinoscopy and subjective refraction shows absence of uncorrected refractive error.
- Optokinetic nystagmus is demonstrable using field stimulus that patient reports not being able to discern.

Inconsistent abnormalities in the examination

- *Goldman perimetry features:* Spiraling isopters regress toward fixation as the test progresses; crossed isopters show that a dimmer or smaller target is surprisingly seen further in the periphery than a brighter or larger target. Crowded isopters show that targets of greatly differing size or brightness are suddenly seen when they reach about the same eccentricity within the visual field.
- *Ishihara plates:* patient may give inconsistent responses (e.g., recognize "12" but no other numbers, yet repeatedly trace the plates correctly). It is important to exclude defective color vision in the normal eye to validate RAPD observations.

Diagnosing functional visual loss

Diagnose functional visual loss only when the patient has demonstrated normal vision. This requires an encouraging, empathic approach and an adroit examination. Consider the following methods.

Tests of stereoacuity

Normal stereoacuity implies normal visual acuity.

The crossed-cylinder technique

- Fog good eye with +6D lens in trial frame, +0.25 before "blind" eye.
- Rotate a crossed +3D cyl before a −3.0 cyl.
- See if the patient can be encouraged to read with the "blind" eye when the cylinders are superimposed to negate each other.

Tests of reading vision
In some cases, normal reading vision can be demonstrated, proving normal visual potential despite apparently impaired Snellen acuities.

Tests of color vision
If the patient gives normal Ishihara plate responses, then his/her visual acuity is at least 20/80. For those with congenital red-green color blindness, the presence of a red filter should enable them to read the plates, provided they have an acuity of at least 6/24.

Etiologies
- *Conversion disorder*: visual loss may be a manifestation of psychological or social difficulties.
- *Malingering*: feigned visual loss for other (usually material) benefit.

Management
Patients suspected of functional visual loss will often need encouragement, reassurance, and follow-up. If the diagnosis remains uncertain, use a term such as *visual loss of unknown cause* in the notes.

Referral to an ophthalmologist familiar with unexplained visual loss (e.g., neuro-ophthalmologist or pediatric ophthalmologist) may avoid unnecessary investigations.

Investigations
Investigation is mandatory when there is diagnostic uncertainty. Consider the following:
- Electrodiagnostic testing (EDT): normal VEP results support reasonable vision but abnormal results can be found in the absence of genuine pathology. EDT may identify early Stargardt's disease or cone dystrophy.
- Neuro-imaging, e.g., contrast-enhanced MRI of visual pathway.
- Investigation as a chronic optic neuropathy of unknown etiology (e.g., for Leber's mutations).
- In exceptional circumstances (when cortical injury is suspected), positron emission tomography (PET) can reveal organic disease when other imaging techniques give normal results.

Treatment
When functional visual loss is diagnosed, the patient should be counseled carefully. The physician faces the unusual situation of contesting the patient's symptoms. However, an adversarial scenario can be both disagreeable and entirely counterproductive. The patient can be reassured that he/she has healthy eyes and that the return of normal visual functioning is expected.

With support, patience, and reassurance, the patient can be allowed to resolve his/her visual functioning. The underlying problem may be far beyond the scope of most ophthalmologists' expertise. In some cases, a clinical psychologist may be helpful.

Strabismus

Anatomy and physiology (1)

Extraocular muscles

The orbit forms a pyramid in which the lateral and medial walls are at 45° to each other, and the central axis is thus at 22.5° (approximated to 23°). The four rectus muscles originate from the annulus of Zinn (Table 17.1).

The superior oblique (SO; like the levator palpebrae superioris) originates from the orbital apex outside the annulus; in contrast, the inferior oblique (IO) arises from the nasal orbital floor. The obliques lie inferior to their corresponding rectus (R) muscle (i.e., SO lies inferior to SR and IO inferior to IR) (see Figs. 17.1 and 17.2).

The spiral of Tillaux describes the way the recti insert increasingly posterior to the limbus (MR, IR, LR, then SR). Innervation is by CN III for SR, MR, IR, IO; by CN IV for SO; and by CN VI for LR.

Table 17.1 Anatomy of extraocular muscles

	Origin	Muscle length	Tendon length	Insertion (mm from limbus)
MR	Annulus of Zinn	40 mm	3.6 mm	5.5 mm
LR	Annulus of Zinn	40 mm	8.4 mm	6.9 mm
SR	Annulus of Zinn	41 mm	5.4 mm	7.7 mm
IR	Annulus of Zinn	40 mm	5.0 mm	6.5 mm
SO	Sphenoid	32 mm	From 10 mm pretrochlea	Posterior superotemporal
IO	Orbital floor	34 mm	Minimal	Posterior temporal

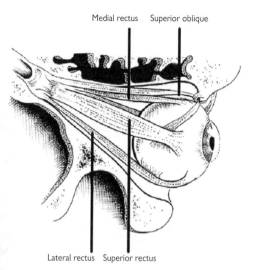

Figure 17.1 Superior view of the right globe showing muscle insertions (LPS removed).

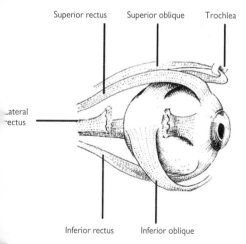

Figure 17.2 Lateral view of the right globe showing muscle insertions (LR partly removed).

Anatomy and physiology (2)

Eye movements

Eye movements may be monocular (ductions) or binocular (versions and vergences). Versions are conjugate eye movements, i.e., both eyes move in the same direction, whereas vergences are disconjugate, i.e., both eyes move in opposite directions. Eye movements may be described as rotations of the globe around horizontal (x), anteroposterior (y), and vertical (z) axes—the axes of Fick.

Ductions comprise abduction (outward), adduction (inward), supraduction (upward), infraduction (downward), intorsion (superior limbus moves inward), and extorsion (superior limbus moves outward) (Table 17.2).

Versions include dextroversion (right gaze), levoversion (left gaze), supraversion (upgaze), infraversion (downgaze), dextrocycloversion (superior limbus moves right), and levocycloversion (superior limbus moves left) (Fig. 17.3). Vergences include convergence (inward) or divergence (outward).

The extraocular muscles do not act in isolation. Each agonist (e.g., LR) has an antagonist that acts in the opposite direction in the same eye (i.e., ipsilateral MR). Increased innervation of the agonist is accompanied by decreased innervation of its antagonist (Sherrington's law). Each agonist also has a yoke muscle that acts in the same direction in the other eye (i.e., contralateral MR in this example). During conjugate movement yoke muscles receive equal and simultaneous innervation (Hering's law).

Table 17.2 Actions of extraocular muscles

	In primary position (subsidiary actions)	In abduction	In adduction
MR	Adduction	Adduction	Adduction
LR	Abduction	Abduction	Abduction
SR	Elevation (intorsion, adduction)	Elevation (isolated at 23° abduction)	Intorsion (isolated at 67° adduction)
IR	Depression (extorsion, adduction)	Depression (isolated at 23° abduction)	Extorsion (isolated at 67° adduction)
SO	Intorsion (depression, abduction)	Intorsion (isolated at 39° abduction)	Depression (isolated at 51° adduction)
IO	Extorsion (elevation, abduction)	Extorsion (isolated at 39° abduction)	Elevation (isolated at 51° adduction)

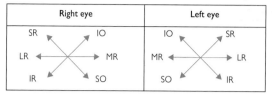

Figure 17.3 The six cardinal positions of gaze (from observer's perspective).

Amblyopia

Amblyopia is a developmental defect of central visual processing leading to reduced visual form sense. Effectively, this means that during the first 8 to 10 years of life, our capacity for high-level vision is vulnerable. Anything less than perfect, balanced foveal images from both eyes can lead to loss of vision in one or both eyes.

With increasing age, this is harder to reverse and by about 10–12 years of age is usually permanent. However, some recent studies have shown success of amblyopia treatment even in older children.

Causes of amblyopia

No or reduced image

Deprivation amblyopia

Constant monocular occlusion for >1 week/year of life is very likely to lead to amblyopia in those <6 years. Significant unilateral congenital cataracts require urgent removal with optical correction in the first few weeks of life; significant bilateral congenital cataracts should be removed in the first 6–8 weeks of life.

Image blurring from refractive error

- *Anisometropic amblyopia*: there is significant risk with difference of refraction of >2.5D, and increased risk if present >2 years. This is a highly amblyogenic stimulus.
- *Ametropic amblyopia*: significant risk if refractive error is greater than +5.00D or –10.00D; bilateral amblyopia may occur if uncorrected.
- *Astigmatic/meridional amblyopia*: significant risk if >0.75D cylinder; risk is increased if there is a different axis and/or magnitude between the two eyes.

Abnormal binocular interaction

- *Strabismic amblyopia*: significant risk if one eye is preferred for fixation; if it is freely alternating, then there is low risk. This is more common in esotropia than in exotropia.

Clinical features

- Reduced visual acuity in the absence of an organic cause and despite correction of refraction.
- Exaggeration of the crowding phenomenon (better visual acuity with single optotypes).
- Tolerance of a neutral density filter (for a specific filter, VA is reduced significantly less in amblyopia than in organic lesions).

Treatment

The critical period during which visual development may be influenced i up to 10 years. Newer research shows promise at up to 12 or more year of age, but with less effect.

At younger ages, there is more rapid reversal of amblyopia but increase risk of inducing occlusion amblyopia in the covered eye.

Occlusion

Adjust for age, acuity, and social factors. Practice is very variable, but longer episodes (time per day) and longer treatment (weeks of patching) are required for older patients and those with worse VA. This may range from 10 min/day in a 6-month-old to full-time in a 6-year-old. Most often, 1 to hours of patching per day is prescribed.

Penalization

Atropinization may reduce the VA in the better eye to around 20/80. This is only effective if the amblyopic eye has VA >20/80.

Binocular single vision

Binocular single vision (BSV) is the ability to view the world with two eyes, form two separate images (one for each eye), and yet fuse these centrally to create a single perception.

The development of BSV depends on correct alignment and similar image clarity of both eyes from the neonatal period. This permits *normal retinal correspondence* in which an image will stimulate anatomically corresponding points of each retina and subsequent stimulation of functionally corresponding points in the occipital cortex to produce a single perception.

The points in space that project onto these corresponding retinal points lie on an imaginary plane. The *horopter. Panum's fusional area* is the narrow plane in front and behind the horopter in which, despite disparity, points will be seen as single.

Levels of binocular single vision

Binocular vision may be graded as follows:

1. *Simultaneous perception:* simultaneously perceives an image on each retina;
2. *Fusion:* stimulation of corresponding points allows central fusion of image;
3. *Stereopsis:* images are fused but slight horizontal disparity gives a perception of depth.

Fusion has sensory and motor components. Whereas sensory fusion generates a single image from corresponding points, motor fusion adjusts eye position to maintain sensory fusion. Fusional reserves (also called fusional amplitudes) indicate the level at which these mechanisms break down (usually seen as diplopia) (Table 17.3).

Abnormalities of BSV

Confusion and diplopia

These are abnormalities of simultaneous perception.

- *Confusion* is the stimulation of corresponding points by dissimilar images (i.e., two images appear superimposed in the same location).
- *Diplopia* is the stimulation of noncorresponding points by the same image (i.e., double vision).

Adaptive mechanisms

Adaptive mechanisms include suppression, abnormal retinal correspondence, and abnormal head posture.

- *Suppression* is a cortical mechanism to ignore one of the images causing confusion (central suppression at the fovea) or diplopia (peripheral suppression). Monocular suppression leads to amblyopia if not treated; alternating suppression (between the two eyes) does not, but depth perception and stereopsis will be decreased. The size and density of the suppression scotoma is also variable.

Table 17.3 Fusional reserves (approximate values)

Horizontal	Near	Convergent	32Δ BO
		Divergent	16Δ BI
	Distance	Convergent	16Δ BO
		Divergent	8Δ BI
Vertical			2–3Δ

- *Abnormal retinal correspondence (ARC)* is a cortical mechanism to allow anatomically noncorresponding points of each retina to stimulate functionally corresponding points in the occipital cortex to produce a single perception. This allow a degree of BSV despite a manifest deviation.
- *Abnormal head posture* is a behavioral mechanism that usually brings the object into the field of single vision.

Microtropia

The advantages of the above adaptive mechanisms are seen in a microtropia. This is a small manifest deviation with a degree of BSV permitted by variable combinations of ARC, eccentric fixation, and central suppression scotoma.

There is usually no movement on cover test (microtropia with identity), unless the eccentric fixation is not absolute (microtropia without identity).

Strabismus: assessment

Although the patient's (or parents') primary concern is likely to be the ocular misalignment (strabismus), it is imperative to step back and consider the whole child, their visual development, and their ophthalmic status. Proper assessment requires taking a history (visual, birth, developmental; see Table 17.4), appropriate measurement of vision, refraction and ophthalmic examination (Table 17.5), and consideration of any amblyopic risk.

Strabismus may be the first presentation of a serious ocular pathology (e.g., retinoblastoma, cataract), thus careful ophthalmic examination (including dilated fundoscopy) is essential.

The general ophthalmic approach to examining the child (p. 606) must be adapted to include orthoptic examination and refraction. Turn the examination into a game whenever possible. Efficient examination helps reduce patient (and examiner) fatigue. When there is concern over possible systemic abnormalities, refer the child to a pediatrician.

The individual tests are discussed as part of clinical methods (pp. 29–32).

History

Table 17.4 An approach to assessing strabismus— history

Visual symptoms	Duration, variability, and direction of strabismus; precipitants, fatigability, associations (visual acuity and development, diplopia, abnormal head position)
POH	Previous or current eye disease; refractive error; any previous surgery, especially on extraocular muscles
PMH	Obstetric or perinatal history; developmental history
Review of systems	Any other systemic (especially CNS) abnormalities
SH	Family support (for children)
FH	Family history of strabismus or other visual problems
Drug history	Drugs
Allergy history	Allergies

Examination

Table 17.5 An approach to assessing strabismus—examination

Observation	Whole patient (e.g., dysmorphic features, use of limbs, gait), face (e.g., asymmetry), abnormal head posture, globes (e.g., proptosis), lids (e.g., ptosis), alignment of the eyes
Visual acuity	Use age-appropriate test (p. 9) when quantitative not possible, qualitatively grade ability to fix and follow (i.e., is it central, steady, and maintained?)
Visual function	Check for RAPD
Cover test	Near, distance, far distance
Deviation	Measure with prism cover test or estimate with Krimsky or Hirschberg test; may be measured with synoptophore
Fusional reserves	Measure prism (horizontal and vertical) tolerated before diplopia or blurring
Motility	Ductions and versions (9 positions of gaze)
	Convergence
	Saccades
	Doll's eye movements
Accommodation	AC/A ratio, deviation with correction of refractive error
Fixation	Fixation behavior, normal vs. eccentric, visuscope
Binocularity	Check for simultaneous perception with Worth 4-dot test or Bagolini glasses
Suppression	Detect with Worth 4-dot test, 4Δ base-out prism test, or Bagolini glasses
Correspondence	Detect anomalous retinal correspondence with Worth 4-dot, Bagolini glasses, or after-image test
Stereopsis	Measure level with Titmus, TNO, Lang, or Frisby tests, or with synoptophore
Refraction	Cycloplegic refraction (for children)
Ophthalmic	This should include dilated funduscopy. Identify any cause of ↓ VA or associated abnormalities (p. 611)
Systemic review	Notably cranial nerves; sensory, motor, cerebellar function; speech; mental state

Strabismus: outline

Esodeviations: the eye that turns in

Is there a deviation?

Abnormalities of the face, globe, or retina may simulate an esodeviation.

Table 17.6 Causes of pseudo-esotropia

Specific	Epicanthic folds
	Narrow interpupillary distance
	Negative angle kappa
General	Face—asymmetry
	Globe—proptosis, enophthalmos
	Pupils—miosis, mydriasis, heterochromia

Esophoria vs. esotropia

Phorias are latent deviations that are controlled by fusion. In certain circumstances (specific visual tasks, fatigue, illness, etc.), fusion can no longer be maintained and the eyes deviate.

Tropias are manifest deviations (Table 17.7). Some individuals may be phoric in one situation (e.g., for distance) and tropic in another (e.g., for near).

Table 17.7 Esotropia

Primary			
Accommodative	Varies with accommodation	Normal AC:A ratio Resolves with hypermetropic correction	Fully accommodative esotropia
		Normal AC:A ratio Improves with hypermetropic correction	Partially accommodative esotropia
		High AC:A ratio	Convergence excess
Nonaccommo-dative	Constant	Starting <6 months	Infantile esotropia
		Starting >6 months	Basic esotropia
	Varies with fixation distance despite relief of accommodation	Near fixation only	Near esotropia (nonaccommodative convergence excess)
		Distance fixation only	Distance esotropia (divergence insufficiency)
	Varies with time	Cyclic	Cyclic esotropia
Secondary		Organic ↓VA (e.g., media opacities)	Secondary esotropia(sensory)
Post-exotropia		Previous surgery for exotropia	Consecutive esotropia

Exodeviations: the eye that turns out

Is there a deviation?

As with esodeviations, structural abnormalities may simulate an exodeviation. Angle kappa (the difference between the pupillary axis and the optical axis) is usually slightly positive. An abnormally large positive angle kappa simulates an exodeviation.

A negative angle occurs from abnormal nasal positioning of the fovea (high myopia, traction, etc.). This simulates esodeviation.

Table 17.8 Causes of pseudo-exotropia

Specific	Wide interpupillary distance
	Postive angle kappa
General	Face—asymmetry
	Globe—proptosis/enophthalmos
	Pupils—miosis/mydriasis/heterochromia

Exophoria vs. exotropia

Exophorias are latent deviations that are generally asymptomatic. However, when fusion can no longer be maintained, they decompensate with symptoms of asthenopia (eye strain), blurred vision, or diplopia. Exotropias are manifest deviations that may be variable or constant (Table 17.9).

Table 17.9 Exotropia

Primary	Constant	Starting <6 months	Infantile exotropia
		Starting >6 months	Basic exotropia
	Variable	Worse for near	Convergence weakness
		Worse for distance High AC:A ratio	Simulated divergence excess
		Worse for distance Normal AC:A ratio	True divergence excess
Secondary		Organic ↓ VA (e.g., media opacities)	Secondary exotropia
Post-esotropia		Develops with time in absence of fusion	Consecutive exotropia

Comitant strabismus: esotropia

Esotropia is a manifest inward deviation of the visual axes relative to each other. It is the most common form of strabismus. The condition may be primary, secondary (most commonly due to poor vision), or consecutive (after surgery for an exodeviation). Primary esotropias are classified as accommodative or nonaccommodative.

As with all strabismus, the assessment should include refraction, full ophthalmic examination, and addressing of amblyopic risk. It is essential to detect or rule out underlying pathology (e.g., intraocular tumor, cataract) at the outset.

Accommodative esotropia

Accommodative esotropia usually presents between 1 and 5 years of age. It may be refractive or nonrefractive. In the refractive group, increased accommodation tries to compensate for uncorrected hypermetropia and is accompanied by excessive convergence.

In the nonrefractive group, there is an abnormal accommodative convergence–accommodation (AC:A) ratio. There may be overlap between these groups.

Refractive: fully accommodative esotropia
- Esotropia fully corrected for distance and near by hypermetropic (usually +2 to +7D) correction; normal AC:A ratio; normal BSV if corrected; often intermittent initially (e.g., with fatigue, illness).

Treatment

Full hypermetropic correction is needed; treat any associated amblyopia. Orthoptic exercises may overcome suppression or improve fusion range.

Refractive: partially accommodative esotropia
- Esotropia only partially corrected by hypermetropic correction; BSV absent, or limited with ARC; ± bilateral IO overaction.

Treatment

Full hypermetropic correction is needed; treat amblyopia. Consider surgery if there is potential for BSV (aim to convert to a fully accommodative esotropia) or cosmesis (if cosmetically unacceptable despite glasses).

Nonrefractive: convergence excess esotropia
- Esotropia for near due to high AC:A ratio; ortho- or esophoric for distance; ↓BSV for near, normal BSV for distance; usually hypermetropic.

Treatment

Treat any associated hypermetropia or amblyopia. Consider surgery (bilateral MR recession ± posterior fixation sutures), orthoptic exercises, executive bifocal glasses, or miotics.

Nonaccommodative

The most common esotropia is the nonaccommodative infantile esotropia (also called congenital esotropia). This is a large-angle esotropia presenting before 6 months, with poor BSV potential and near-normal refraction. Fixation often alternates between the eyes.

Other nonaccommodative esotropias usually present later (i.e., after 6 months of age).

Infantile esotropia

- Esotropia presenting before 6 months, large angle (>30Δ), cross-fixation is common (if present, low risk of amblyopia), poor BSV potential; often emmetropia/mild hypermetropia; ± dissociated vertical deviation (DVD: upward deviation on occlusion with recovery on removal of cover and no movement of other eye); ± manifest latent nystagmus (p. 557).

Treatment

Treat any associated amblyopia (e.g., occlusion of better eye if not freely alternating); correct hypermetropia if >2D. The aim of surgery ocular alignment by 12 months (with better potential BSV) and usually comprises symmetrical MR recessions (± LR resection).

Additional IO-weakening procedures should be used with caution. Botulinum toxin may be used as an alternative to surgery.

Other nonaccommodative esotropias

- *Basic esotropia:* constant esotropia for near and distance; treat surgically.
- *Near esotropia* (nonaccommodative convergence excess): esotropia for near, ortho- or esophoria for distance but with normal AC:A ratio. Treatment, if any, is surgical (medial recti > lateral recti).
- *Distance esotropia* (divergence insufficiency): esophoria (or small esotropia) for near, larger esotropia for distance; associated with poor fusional divergence. Rule out bilateral CN VI palsies.
- *Cyclic esotropia:* rare, periodic (e.g., alternate days), may proceed to constant esotropia.

Secondary esotropias

Esotropia may arise secondary to ↓VA, thus full ocular examination is vital in all cases with esotropia. Some esotropic syndromes may arise secondary to intracranial pathology.

- *Sensory deprivation:* secondary to unilateral/bilateral ↓VA.
- *Divergence paralysis:* secondary to tumor, trauma, or stroke. Unlike a bilateral CN VI palsy, the esodeviation remains constant or even decreases on lateral gaze.
- *Convergence spasm:* usually functional. The esotropia is intermittent and is associated with miosis and accommodative spasm resulting in pseudomyopia. Ductions are normal. Treat with cycloplegia and full hypermetropic correction.

Pseudoesotropia

Various conditions may mimic an esotropia (see Table 17.6).

Comitant strabismus: exotropia

Exotropia is a manifest outward deviation of the visual axes relative to each other. It may be primary, secondary (associated with poor vision), or consecutive (may follow an esotropia with time or after surgical correction).

Primary exotropias may be constant or intermittent. Intermittent exotropias range according to ease of dissociation. Exotropias that are difficult to dissociate may be regarded as being at the exophoria end of the spectrum.

As with all strabismus, the assessment should include refraction, full ophthalmic examination, and addressing of amblyopic risk. It is essential to detect and rule out underlying pathology (e.g., intraocular tumor, cataract) at the outset.

Constant exotropia

Infantile (or congenital) exotropia
- Constant large-angle exotropia presenting at 2–6 months of age; often associated with ocular/CNS abnormalities. Rarely, exotropia is present at birth (congenital exotropia).

Treatment is usually surgical (e.g., bilateral LR recessions ± MR resection).

Basic constant exotropia
- Constant exotropia with same angle for near and distance, presenting after 6 months of age.

Treatment is usually surgical.

Intermittent exotropia

This is the most common form of exotropia, and usually presents at 2–5 years of age.

Basic
- Exotropia is the same for distance and near.

True divergence excess
- Exotropia is worse for distance, with normal AC:A ratio; it is rare.

Simulated divergence excess
- Exotropia is worse for distance since an ↑AC:A ratio (and fusional reserves) fully or partially corrects for near. This is much more common than true divergence excess.

Treatment
Correct any myopia, astigmatism >0.75D, and high hypermetropia; treat amblyopia; use orthoptic exercises. Consider prisms, minus lenses, botulinum toxin, or surgery for more severe cases. Surgery is generally performed before 5 years of age.

Traditionally, bilateral LR recession was used when the angle was worse at distance, and unilateral LR recession /MR resection if equal or worse at near.

Convergence weakness
- Exotropia worse for near, often exophoric for distance; more common in young adults who report asthenopia or diplopia for reading. It may be associated with myopia.

Treatment
Correct any myopia, astigmatism >0.75D, and high hypermetropia. Consider surgical treatment (e.g., bimedial MR resection).

Convergence insufficiency
This is not an exotropia but is considered here as an important differential diagnosis.
- Near point of convergence is more distant; no manifest deviation but usually exophoria at near. It is more common in teenagers who report asthenopia.

Treatment
Full myopic correction is needed. Convergence exercises (e.g., pencil push-ups) are effective (rarely necessary to consider prisms, botulinum toxin, or surgery for more severe cases).

Secondary exotropia
Exotropia is the most common strabismic outcome of ipsilateral ↓VA, although sensory esotropia may occur in young children (p. 585). Full ocular examination is vital in all cases.

Consecutive exotropia
With time, an esotropia in which fusion has not been established may become an exotropia. Surgical correction may also cause a consecutive exotropia.

Pseudoexotropia
Various conditions may mimic an exotropia (see Table 17.8).

Incomitant strabismus

In incomitant strabismus, the angle of deviation of the visual axes changes according to the direction of gaze. Incomitant strabismus is often grouped into neurogenic or mechanical types. In neurogenic strabismus, the abnormality may occur in the nucleus, nerve, neuromuscular junction, muscle, or orbit.

In incomitant strabismus, the aims are to identify the pattern and cause of the strabismus and address any actual or potential complications, such as amblyopia, diplopia, or poor cosmesis.

Neurogenic strabismus

There is underaction with slowing of saccades in the direction of paretic muscle (underaction may be more marked for versions than ductions). It may develop full sequelae with time (see Table 17.10).

Investigations

- *Hess/Lancaster charts:* inner and outer fields are differently affected, as strabismus tends to be incomitant if neurogenic. Full sequelae may develop if longstanding.
- *Forced duction test:* full passive movement, unless chronic contracture of antagonist
- Further investigation and treatment are according to cause (third nerve palsy, p. 547; fourth nerve palsy, p. 550; sixth nerve palsy, p. 552).

Mechanical strabismus

There is underaction in the direction away from restricted muscle (equal for ductions and versions). Saccades are of normal speed, but with sudden early stop due to restriction. Globe retraction and IOP increase in the direction of limitation (see Table 17.10).

Investigations

- *Hess/Lancaster charts:* inner and outer fields are compressed in the direction of limitation; outer is affected more than inner. Sequelae are limited to overaction of contralateral synergist.
- *Forced duction test:* reduced passive movement is in the direction of limitation. Further investigation and treatment are according to cause (thyroid eye disease, p. 475; orbital fracture, p. 87; Duane's and other restrictive syndromes, p. 590).

Myasthenic strabismus

Variable and fatiguable ocular motility disturbance (any pattern) is often associated with ptosis. Sustained eccentric gaze of ≥1 min or repeated saccades demonstrate fatigue. Cogan's twitch can occur (ask patient to look down for 20 sec and then at an object in the primary position: the test is positive if the lid overshoots).

Patients may have systemic involvement (e.g., speech, breathing).

Investigations

- *Hess/Lancaster charts:* range from normal to highly variable and frustrating for operator. Results may follow any pattern.
- *Forced duction test:* full passive movement.
- *Ice-pack test:* measure ptosis; place ice wrapped in a towel or glove on the closed eyelid for 2 min; remeasure ptosis. The test is significantly positive if ≥2 mm.

For further investigation (including Tensilon test, serum antibodies, and EMG) and treatment, see p. 562.

Myopathic strabismus

Gradual, symmetrical nonfatiguable loss of movement associated with ptosis is seen in the inherited myopathies (e.g., chronic progressive external ophthalmoplegia [CPEO]). Acquired myopathies (e.g., thyroid eye disease and myositis) may be regarded as causing a mechanical strabismus pattern.

Investigations

- *Hess/Lancaster charts:* symmetrical and proportional reduction in inner and outer fields.
- Further investigation and treatment are according to etiology (p. 565).

Table 17.10 Features of neurogenic and mechanical incomitant strabismus

	Neurogenic	Mechanical
Ductions/ versions	Ductions > versions	Ductions = versions; May be painful
Saccades	Slow in paretic direction	Normal speed with sudden stop
Sequelae	Full sequelae with time	Sequelae limited to overaction of contralateral synergist
IOP change	IOP ± constant	IOP increases in the direction of limitation
Globe	No change	May retract on movement in direction of limitation
Hess/Lees	Inner and outer fields are proportional. The smaller field is of the affected eye (but sequelae reduce this effect with time)	Inner and outer fields are compressed in direction of limitation
Forced duction testing	Full passive movement (but antagonist contracture with time)	Reduced passive movement in direction of limitation

Restriction syndromes

Syndromic patterns of mechanical restriction are uncommon causes of strabismus. They are usually congenital, although later presentations may occur.

Duane syndrome

This is thought to arise from aberrant co-innervation of LR and MR by CN III, which may be associated with CN VI nucleus hypoplasia (can be seen on MRI; imaging is not necessary for diagnosis). It is usually sporadic but may be autosomal dominant.

The most common form (type I) preferentially affects girls (60%) and the left eye (60%). It is bilateral (usually asymmetric) in at least 20%.

Clinical features
• Retraction of globe (with reduction in palpebral aperture) on attempted adduction; ± up- or down-shoots or attempted adduction; additional features according to classification type (Tables 17.11a, 17.11b).
• Systemic associations (30%): deafness, Goldenhar's syndrome, Klippel–Feil syndrome, Wildervanck syndrome (Duane, Klippel–Feil, and deafness).

Table 17.11a Brown's classification of Duane syndrome

Type	Feature
A	↓Abduction (less ↓adduction)
B	↓Abduction (normal adduction)
C*	↓ Adduction > ↓abduction

*Gives rise to divergent deviation and a head posture in which the face is turned away from the side of the affected eye.

Table 17.11b Huber's classification of Duane syndrome (based on EMG)

Type	Frequency	Primary position	Primary feature	Globe retraction
I	85%	Eso or ortho	↓ Abduction	Mild
II	14%	Exo or ortho	↓ Adduction	Severe
III	1%	Eso or ortho	↓ Abduction and ↓ adduction	Moderate

Treatment

Assess and treat for refractive error and potential amblyopia. Reassure the patient if he/she is managing well with minimal or mild compensatory head posture. Consider prisms for comfort or to improve head position.

Consider surgery to improve BSV and improve head position. Usual practice is uni- or bilateral MR recession for esotropic Duane syndrome and uni- or bilateral LR recession (±MR resection) for exotropic Duane syndrome. Avoid LR resection as it increases retraction more than improving abduction.

Brown syndrome

This is a mechanical restriction syndrome, which Brown attributed to the superior oblique tendon sheath. It appears to arise from structural or developmental abnormalities of the SO trochlear–tendon complex, leading to limitation in the direction of its antagonist (IO). This results in limited or absent elevation in adduction.

In most cases, it is congenital (or at least infantile) and usually improves or resolves by 12 years of age. Acquired cases may result from trauma, surgery (e.g., SO tuck, scleral buckling, orbital), or rarely inflammation (e.g., juvenile idiopathic arthritis [JIA], sinusitis).

Clinical features

- Limited elevation in adduction ± pain/click (click often occurs during resolution); limited sequelae (i.e., overaction of contralateral SR only); V pattern; may down-shoot in adduction; positive forced duction test.

Treatment

Reassure patient if managing well with minimal or mild compensatory head posture: it usually improves with age and upgaze is less of an issue with increased height. Consider surgery if there is significantly abnormal head posture or if strabismus is in the primary position. The aim is to release the restriction until a repeated traction test demonstrates free rotation of the globe.

Complications of SO tenotomy include SO palsy, and results are often disappointing. The preferred surgical procedure is graded SO weakening using a silicone spacer or suture, which avoids this complication.

Möbius syndrome

This rare sporadic congenital syndrome includes bilateral CN VI and CN VII nerves palsies and often other neurological abnormalities. It is included here because it may be associated with bilateral tight MR, causing restriction in addition to the horizontal gaze palsy.

Clinical features

Bilateral failure of abduction; may be pure gaze palsy, or bilateral tight MR can lead to esotropia and positive forced duction test.
Systemic associations: bilateral CN VII palsy (expressionless face), bilateral CN XII palsy (atrophic tongue), ↓IQ, digital abnormalities.

Congenital fibrosis of the extraocular muscles (CFEOM)

This rare congenital syndrome probably arises from abnormal development of the oculomotor nuclei. Classic CFEOM (CFEOM1) is autosomal dominant (Ch12).

There is bilateral restrictive ophthalmoplegia and ptosis, with an inability to elevate the globes above midline. CFEOM2 is autosomal recessive (Ch11). There is bilateral ptosis, large-angle exotropia, and severe limitation of horizontal and vertical movements. In CFEOM3 (Ch16), there are more variable motility defects.

Strabismus fixus

In this very rare sporadic congenital syndrome, the eyes are firmly fixed in adduction or occasionally in abduction. The eyes appear to be anchored both by fibrosis of the rectus muscles and additional fibrous cords. It may be associated with pathological myopia.

Alphabet patterns

Horizontal deviations may vary in size according to vertical position. The deviation is measured at 30° upgaze, primary position, and 30° downgaze while fixing on a distance target. Significant incomitance is described according to the following alphabet patterns.

V pattern

Clinically significant V-pattern is defined as a horizontal deviation, which is 15Δ more divergent (or less convergent) in upgaze than in downgaze.

Clinical features

- V-pattern esotropia usually arises from IO overaction or SO palsy (Table 17.12). It is also associated with antimongoloid palpebral fissures (seen in patients with, e.g., Crouzon or Apert syndrome; altering the rectus insertions). Patients often adopt a chin-down posture.
- V-pattern exotropia usually arises from IO overaction. Patients adopt a chin-up posture.

Treatment

Surgical treatment for significant V patterns may require IO weakening (if overacting), vertical transposition of the horizontal rectus (upward for LR, downward for MR), and correction of the horizontal component (e.g., MR recession for esotropia; LR recession for exotropia).

For both A and V patterns, the acronym *MALE* identifies the direction of vertical translation: MR to Apex, LR to Ends.

A pattern

Clinically significant A-pattern is defined as a horizontal deviation, which is 10Δ less divergent (or more convergent) in upgaze than in downgaze.

Clinical features

- A-pattern esotropia usually arises from SO overaction (Table 17.12). It may also be associated with mongoloid palpebral fissures. Patients often adopt a chin-up posture.
- A-pattern exotropia usually arises from SO overaction. Patients adopt a chin-down posture.

Treatment

Surgical treatment for significant A-patterns may require cautious SO weakening (if overacting), e.g., SO silicone spacer, vertical translations of the horizontal rectus muscles (upward for MR, downward for LR), and correction of the horizontal component (e.g., MR recession for esotropia; LR recession for exotropia).

Other patterns

- *Y-pattern:* exotropia in upgaze only. It is usually due to IO overaction, in which case it can be treated by IO weakening alone.
- *λ-pattern:* exotropia in downgaze only. It may be treated by downward translation of both LR.
- *X-pattern:* exotropia in upgaze and downgaze but straight in the primary position. It usually arises in a longstanding exotropia with overaction of all four oblique muscles.

Table 17.12 Causes of alphabet patterns

A pattern	Overaction of SO
	Underaction of IO, IR, LR
V pattern	Brown syndrome
	Overaction of IO, SR, or LR
	Underaction of SO

Strabismus surgery: general

Strabismus surgery should only be performed after full assessment and treatment of causative factors (e.g., refractive error) and consideration of nonsurgical alternatives (e.g., prisms, botulinum toxin). The main role for surgery is when a significant deviation remains despite appropriate refraction, when the deviation is stable over time, and when further improvement is not anticipated.

Surgical options involve weakening, strengthening, or transposing the extraocular muscles (see Table 17.13). These procedures adjust the effective pull of the muscle (by changing stretch and torque) and/or direction of action.

The aim is to produce eyes that are straight in the primary position and downgaze while keeping the largest possible field of BSV. It may be necessary to sacrifice BSV in lower-priority gaze positions (e.g., upgaze) to achieve this goal.

General principles

- Identify 1) direction of overaction, 2) any incomitance, and 3) any oblique muscle dysfunction.
- Weaken overacting muscle and strengthen its antagonist.
- Balance these procedures to prevent induced incomitance or to treat pre-existing incomitance.
- Reduce oblique muscle overaction or underaction.

Adjustable sutures

Surgical results are improved by the use of adjustable sutures. These can be used in conjunction with recessions, resections, and advancements. They are of particular value in repeat operations, mechanical strabismus, and when there is a significant risk of postoperative diplopia.

Complications

Complications include suture granuloma, scleral perforation (0.5%), slipped or lost muscle, anterior segment ischemia, consecutive strabismus, and postoperative diplopia. Rarely there is cellulitis or endophthalmitis.

Table 17.13 Overview of common strabismus operations

Operation	Muscles	Procedure
Weakening		
Recession	Recti or IO	Moves insertion posteriorly
Myectomy/ disinsertion	IO	Removal of part of muscle in combination with disinsertion
Myotomy	Recti	Two alternate incisions of around 80% width weakens muscle without changing insertion
Faden procedure	SR, IR, or MR	Postequatorial fixation suture (nonabsorbable) weakens muscle without affecting primary position
Strengthening		
Resection	Recti	Shortens or stretches muscle
Advancement	Recti	Moves insertion anteriorly (often of previously recessed muscle)
Tuck	SO	Loop of lax tendon sutured to sclera
Transposition		
To improve abduction		
Hummelsheim	SR and IR	Lateral half of SR, and IR disinserted and attached adjacent to LR insertion; MR may also be weakened
Jensen	LR, SR, and IR	Split LR, SR, and IR; suture neighboring parts of LR + SR, and LR + IR together
To improve elevation		
Knapp	LR and MR	LR and MR disinserted and attached adjacent to SR insertion
To improve depression		
Inverse Knapp	LR and MR	LR and MR disinserted and attached adjacent to IR insertion
To improve intorsion		
Harado-Ito	SO	Split SO; move insertion of anterior part forward to the superior margin of LR

Strabismus surgery: horizontal

The most common deviations (esotropia and exotropia) are horizontal and are therefore generally amenable to surgery on the horizontal recti (Table 17.14). The most common procedure is a unilateral "recess/resect," although the options range from single-muscle procedures to bilateral (simultaneous or staged) surgery involving multiple muscles.

Recess/resects

An MR recession/LR resection will reduce convergence, whereas an LR recession/MR resection will reduce divergence. Estimation of the amount of surgical correction (in mm) required for the size of strabismus (in Δ) may be assisted by use of surgical tables (e.g., Table 17.15).

However, such tables are only a guide and should be modified by each surgeon according to their own individualized outcomes.

Table 17.14 Outline of horizontal muscle surgery

Recession	• Local conjunctival peritomy
	• Identify and expose muscle
	• Free muscle from Tenon's layer
	• Place two locking bites of an absorbable suture through the outer quarters of the muscle
	• Disinsert tendon and measure recession
	• Suture in new position: either directly to adjacent sclera or to the insertion (hang back technique)
	• Close conjunctiva
Resection	• Local conjunctival peritomy
	• Identify and expose muscle
	• Free muscle from Tenon's layer
	• Measure and place two locking bites of an absorbable suture posterior to intended resection
	• Resect desired length of muscle
	• Suture remaining muscle to insertion
	• Close conjunctiva

Table 17.15 Absolute maximum surgical adjustments for rectus muscles

	Resect	Recess
LR	10 mm	8–12 mm
MR	8 mm	8 mm
IR	5 mm	5 mm
SR	5 mm	5 mm

Pediatric ophthalmology

Related pages:

Embryology (1)

The normal eye forms from an outpouching of the embryonic forebrain (neuroectoderm) with contributions from neural crest cells, surface ectoderm, and, to a lesser extent, mesoderm. The interactions between these layers are complex; failure may result in serious developmental abnormalities (p. 635).

General

The developing embryo comprises three germinal layers: ectoderm, mesoderm, and endoderm. The ectoderm differentiates into outer surface ectoderm and inner neuroectoderm.

The neuroectoderm continues to develop, forming first a ridge (neural crest), then a cylinder (neural tube), and finally vesicles within the cranial part of the tube to form the fore-, mid-, and hindbrain (prosencephalon, mesencephalon, telencephalon). The neural crest cells also migrate to contribute widely to ocular and orbital structures.

The globe

The optic vesicle develops as a neuroectodermal protrusion of the prosencephalon. It induces the overlying surface ectoderm to thicken into the lens placode. Then (week 4) both these structures invaginate to form a double-layered optic cup and lens vesicle, respectively. The cup is not complete but retains a deep inferior groove (optic fissure) in which mesodermal elements develop into the hyaloid and other vessels.

Closure starts at the equator (week 5) and proceeds anteroposteriorly; failure of closure results in colobomata (p. 635).

Anterior segment

Lens

The lens placode forms from surface ectoderm and invaginates to form the lens vesicle (week 5). At this point, the anterior lens epithelium is a unicellular layer surrounded by a basement membrane (the future capsule). This layer continues to divide throughout life.

The posterior cells elongate and differentiate into primary lens fibers. The anterior cells migrate to the equator and elongate forming the secondary lens fibers. These meet at the lens sutures.

Cornea

After separation of the lens vesicle, the surface ectoderm reforms as an epithelial bilayer with basement membrane. It is joined by three waves of migrating neural crest cells: the first wave (week 6) forms the corneal and trabecular endothelium; the second (week 7) forms the stroma; the third (also week 7) forms the iridopupillary membrane.

Sclera

The sclera develops from a condensation of mesenchymal tissue situated at the anterior rim of the optic cup. This begins at the limbus (week 7) and proceeds posteriorly to surround the optic nerve (week 12).

Iris, trabecular meshwork, and angle

The optic cup grows around the developing lens such that the cup rims meet the iridopupillary membrane. The optic cup rims give rise to the epithelial layers of the iris, which are therefore continuous with the ciliary body and retina/RPE layers.

The iridopupillary membrane (neural crest) develops into the iris stroma. The dilator and sphincter muscles are both neuroectodermal.

The trabecular meshwork and Schlemm's canal arises from first-wave neural crest tissue located in the angle (week 5).

Ciliary body

The ciliary body forms as a kink in the optic cup rim (contributing an epithelial bilayer) and associated neural crest tissue (ciliary muscles and vasculature). The longitudinal musculature appears first (month 3); the circular musculature continues to develop after birth (year 1 postnatal).

Embryology (2)

Posterior segment

Retina

All retinal tissues develop from the optic cup (neuroectoderm). The inner layer of the cup divides into two zones: a superficial non-nucleated marginal zone and a deeper nucleated primitive zone. Mitosis and migration from the primitive zone leads to the formation of an inner neuroblastic layer (in which Müller cells, ganglion cells, bipolar cells, horizontal cells, and amacrine cells develop) and an outer neuroblastic layer (giving rise to primitive photoreceptor cells).

Familiar retinal organization starts with the formation of the ganglion cell layer and continues at the deeper levels with both cellular and acellular zones (nuclear and plexiform layers). This wave of retinal development starts at the posterior pole and proceeds anteriorly.

The photoreceptors arise from the outermost cells of the inner layer. Originally ciliated, these are replaced by distinctive outer segments. Cones develop first (months 4–6), rods later (month 7 on). These photoreceptor cells project toward the outer layer of the cup. The outer layer (the retinal pigment epithelium) thins to become one cell thick and becomes pigmented, the first structure in the body to do so.

Retinal vasculature develops from the hyaloid circulation and spreads in an anterior wave, reaching the nasal periphery before the temporal periphery (month 9); it may not be fully developed in premature infants.

Choroid

This vascular layer arises from endothelial blood spaces around the optic cup; the extension of posterior ciliary arteries to join the primitive choroidal vasculature; and the consolidation of venous networks to form the four vortex veins.

Optic nerve

Vacuolization of cells within the optic stalk allows ganglion cell axons to grow through from the retina. The appearance of crossed and uncrossed fibers results in the formation of the chiasm (months 2–4).

Myelination proceeds anteriorly from the lateral geniculate nucleus (LGN, month 5) to the lamina cribrosa (month 1 postnatal). The inner layer of the stalk develops supportive glial cells, which separate the nerve fibers into bundles; the outer layer gives rise to the lamina cribrosa.

Vitreous

The primary vitreous (week 5) forms in the retrolental space. It contains collagen fibrils, mesenchymal elements, and the hyaloid vasculature (which forms the tunica vasculosa lentis). Later (week 6) this is surrounded by the secondary vitreous and effectively forms Cloquet's canal.

The secondary vitreous is avascular, transparent, and composed of very fine organized fibers. Failure of the vascular system to regress causes Mittendorf's dot, Bergmeister's papilla, persistent hyaloid artery, and persistent fetal vasculature (PFV; formerly known as persistent hyperplastic primary vitreous, PHPV).

Traditionally, *tertiary vitreous* was used to describe a relatively anterior condensation associated with the formation of lens zonules (which arise from the ciliary body).

Nasolacrimal drainage system

This develops from a cord of surface ectoderm, which is met by proliferating cords of cells from the lids above and from the nasal fossa below (see Table 18.1). Cannulation of the cord may be delayed distally, causing congenital obstruction. More commonly there is simply an imperforate mucus membrane at the valve of Hasner, which most often resolves spontaneously within the first year (year 1 postnatal).

Table 18.1 Summary of germinal layers

Ectoderm	Neuroectoderm	Iris epithelium
		Iris sphincter and dilator
		Ciliary body epithelium
		Neural retina
		RPE
		Optic nerve (axons and glia)
	Neural crest	Corneal stroma
		Corneal endothelium
		Trabecular meshwork
		Ciliary musculature
		Sclera
		Choroidal stroma
	Surface ectoderm	Skin and lids
		Conjunctival epithelium
		Corneal epithelium
		Lacrimal gland
		Nasolacrimal duct
		Lens
Mesoderm		Extraocular muscles
		Ocular vasculature

Genetics

Genetic disorders may result from an abnormal karyotype (abnormal number of chromosomes, e.g., trisomies), an abnormal region of the chromosome (e.g., deletions, duplications), abnormal gene(s) at a single locus (autosomal or X-linked), abnormal mitochondrial DNA, or the interaction of a number of genes with the environment.

Single-gene autosomal disorders obey the laws of segregation and independent assortment noted by Mendel. This results in predictable patterns of inheritance (Table 18.2). More complex patterns arise from X-linked and mitochondrial disease. Most common conditions appear to be polygenic with additional contributions from environmental factors.

Even for single-gene disorders, the pattern of disease may be unpredictable. Such conditions may have incomplete *penetrance* (i.e., genotype present without the phenotype) or variable *expressivity* (i.e., wide range within the phenotype). In some conditions, *anticipation* may occur, where succeeding generations develop earlier and more severe disease. This is due to triplet repeats in which the number of repeats of a particular codon (e.g., GCT in the myotonic dystrophy gene) increases from generation to generation.

Inheritance patterns

Table 18.2 Inheritance patterns for single-gene defect with 100% penetrance

Autosomal dominant	One parent carries the mutation (and usually has the phenotype).
	50% chance of inheriting gene and of developing the phenotype
Autosomal recessive	Both parents carry the mutation, but neither has the phenotype.
	50% chance of inheriting one copy of gene (i.e., carrier without the phenotype)
	25% chance of inheriting two copies of gene and of developing the phenotype
X-linked	*If mother carries the mutation:*
	50% chance of inheriting gene and developing the phenotype for a son
	50% chance of inheriting gene and becoming a carrier for a daughter
	If father carries the mutation:
	100% chance of inheriting gene and becoming a carrier for a daughter
	0% chance of inheriting gene for a son
Mitochondrial	The mother carries the mutation
	Variable probability of inheritance dependent on proportion of abnormal mitochondria in oocyte that becomes fertilized (heteroplasmy)

Table 18.3 Chromosomal locations of genes involved in ophthalmic disease (selected)

1	Schnyder dystrophy Stargardt/fundus flavimaculatus (ABCR4)
2	Oguchi disease (arrestin) Waardenburg syndrome (PAX3)
3	VHL (*VHL* gene) CSNB1(transducin (α))
4	Anterior segment dysgenesis (PITX2)
5	Reis–Bücklers, Thiel–Behnke, granular, lattice I (keratoepithelin, BIGH3)
6	Tritanopia (S opsin) Anterior segment dysgenesis (FOXC1)
7	
8	Retinitis pigmentosa (RP1, and numerous others)
9	Tuberous sclerosis (TSC1, harmartin) Oculocutaneous albinism (OCA III, TRP1)
10	Gyrate atrophy (OAT)
11	Best's disease (bestrophin) Aniridia, Peter's anomaly (PAX6) Oculocutaneous albinism (OCA1, tyrosinase)
12	Meesmann (K3, keratin) Chronic fibrosis of extraocular muscles (CFEOM1)
13	Wilson disease
14	
15	Marfan syndrome (FBN1, fibrillin) Oculocutaneous albinism (OCAII, p)
16	Tuberous sclerosis (TSC2, tuberin)
17	Neurofibromatosis-1 (NF1, neurofibromin) Meesmann (K12, keratin)
18	
19	Myotonic dystrophy (DMPK)
20	
21	Homocystinuria type 1 (cystathionine synthetase)
22	Neurofibromatosis-2 (NF2, merlin) Sorsby fundus dystrophy (TIMP)
X	Ocular albinism (OA1) X-linked RP (RP2) X-linked juvenile retinoschisis (RS1) Choroideremia (REP1)

Pediatric examination

The assessment of children (see Tables 18.4 and 18.5) requires a flexible and often undignified approach. The goal is to keep everyone—patient, parents, and extended family—on the same side. Without this it is very difficult to achieve an adequate clinical assessment and impossible to institute treatment.

The awake child

Attempt to entertain the child during history taking (e.g., with a toy) and turn the examination into a game. Explain what you are about to do (e.g., with drops) and why.

Examine opportunistically and be patient. Surprisingly, young children may be happy to be examined at the slit lamp (standing, kneeling on the chair, or sitting on caregiver's knee). If this is impossible, consider a portable slit lamp for the anterior segment, the indirect ophthalmoscope for the fundus, and the direct ophthalmoscope for higher magnification of the macula and disc. Applanation tonometry and gonioscopy may only be possible by examination under anesthesia (EUA).

Keeping the child happy usually keeps the adults happy. Good communication is essential.

The anesthetized child (EUA)

An EUA may be indicated if detailed examination is impossible with the child awake. It may be performed when the child is being anesthetized for a different procedure, thus coordinated care with other specialists involved with the child is essential. The anesthesiologist should have appropriate experience with pediatric anesthesia.

The presence of the speculum may affect IOP and refraction. It is thus recommended that tonometry (Tonopen or Perkins) and retinoscopy be performed early in the examination and before insertion of the speculum.

Examine the anterior segment with the portable slit lamp, the operating microscope, and gonioscopy lens. Examine the posterior segment with the direct and indirect ophthalmoscope. Consider A- and B-scan ultrasonography.

Table 18.4 Visual milestones

6 weeks	Can fix and follow a light source, face or large, colorful toy, smiling responsively
3 months	Fixation is central, steady and maintained, can follow a slow target, and converge
6 months	Reaches out accurately for toys
2 years	Picture matching
3 years	Letter matching of single letters (e.g., Sheridan Gardiner)
5 years	Snellen chart by matching or naming

Table 18.5 A systematic approach to examining children

Visual symptoms	History of poor visual behavior for their age, strabismus, nystagmus, head nodding, red eye, epiphora, photophobia, asymmetry of pupils, corneas, globes, or red reflexes
POH	Previous or current eye disease; refractive error
PMH	Obstetric and perinatal history; developmental history
Systemic conditions	Any other systemic (especially CNS) abnormalities
SH	Family support
FH	Family history of strabismus/other visual problems
Drug history	Drugs
Allergy history	Allergies
Visual acuity	Select test according to age (p. 9); when quantitative testing is not possible, grade ability to fix gaze and follow (i.e., is it central, steady, and maintained?)
Visual function	Check for RAPD, binocularity, stereopsis, suppression and retinal correspondence (pp. 9–10)
Cover test	Near/distance/prism cover test
Motility	Ductions, versions, convergence, saccades, doll's eye movements
Accommodation	
BSV	Level of BSV
Fixation	Fixation behavior, visuscope
Refraction	Cycloplegic refraction
Orbit	Proptosis, inflammation, masses
Lids	Lid crease, additional skin folds, puncta
Conjunctiva	Inflammation, adhesions
Cornea	Diameter, thickness, opacity, staining
AC	Flare, cells
Gonioscopy	(may require EUA) Angle, dysgenesis
Iris	Coloboma, anisocoria, polycoria, corectopia
Lens	Lens opacity, shape, position
Tonometry	Applanation (may require EUA); digital
Vitreous	Hyaloid remnants, inflammation, empty
Optic disc	Size, cup, congenital anomaly, edema
Fundus	Macula, vessels, retina (e.g., tumors, inflammation, dystrophies, exudation)
Systemic review	For dysmorphic features (including face, ears, teeth, hair) or any other systemic abnormalities

The child who does not see

Worldwide, there are over 1.5 million children who are blind or severely visually impaired. Major causes include inherited abnormalities (e.g., cataracts, glaucoma, retinal dystrophies), intrauterine insults (e.g., infection) and acquired problems (e.g., retinopathy of prematurity, trauma).

The ophthalmologist's primary aim—the best possible vision for the child—must be seen in the context of the child's overall health, quality of life, and family support. Likewise, the ophthalmologist's contribution should be seen in the context of the multidisciplinary team, which may include pediatricians, optometrists, orthoptists, primary care physicians, specialist nurses, social workers, and teachers. The challenge to provide the best possible care for the child (and family) will depend on the following factors.

Disability

Is the visual impairment the only problem, or are there associated disabilities? These may range from mild developmental delay (e.g., motor, speech, social) to profound neurological or systemic abnormalities. In some severe diseases, life expectancy may also be considerably reduced.

Such children require the full benefit of the multidisciplinary team, usually coordinated by the pediatrician.

Treatment

What treatment might be possible now or in the future? Be realistic about what is and what is not currently possible. Ensure best visual potential with refraction, visual aids, and other supportive measures.

When more invasive treatment is indicated, ensure that the parents are fully aware of the risks, realistic outcome, and the extent of care that they will need to give in the perioperative period (e.g., drops, contact lens, frequent clinic visits).

Equipment

What equipment will help the child function best at home and at school? Reading may require Braille (it is important to start early) or large-print books (usually beneficial if reading vision is worse than N10).

Normal-sized print may be read by closed-circuit television (CCTV) magnification or by a scanner attached to a computer that has a magnified display facility or has optical character recognition with a speech synthesizer. The ease of use of standard computer systems has been revolutionized since accessibility options became a standard feature of computer operating systems (e.g., Windows®).

Schooling

Will the child manage best in a specialist school (for the blind or partially sighted) or in a mainstream school (with specialist teacher support)? This is usually determined by the level of visual impairment, any associated disabilities, and the availability of resources locally.

Resources
How much assistance (practical and financial) is the family and/or social services able to provide? Social workers should ensure that parents are receiving appropriate financial benefits. Community-based pediatricians may be invaluable in coordinating local resources. Nonprofit, governmental organizations often provide help, including advice and emotional support for the parents.

Social
Is the disability accepted by the family and community? The diagnosis may stretch family relationships to a breaking point. Siblings may become jealous of the extra attention the child needs.

In some communities, blindness is regarded as a stigma. This may adversely affect family dynamics and hinder the child's wider social interactions.

Implications
Are other family members or future siblings at risk of developing the disease, or of being carriers? Initial knowledge of related genetic disease may produce strong emotions; counseling requires time, patience, and often multiple consultations. The parents may feel guilty about passing on an inherited disease to their child.

Prognosis
Is the visual impairment stationary or progressive? Parents may want to know the probable impact on navigation, education, work, and driving. Whenever possible, balance the negative (what they won't be able to do) with the positive (what they will be able to do). Stress that medical knowledge is limited and that such prognoses are a best guess.

Child abuse

The physician has a legal duty of care toward any child he or she sees. This means that if there is any concern or suspicion of possible abuse, it is the physician's responsibility to act in the child's best interest.

Concern might relate to injuries that are inconsistent with the mobility of the child or with the reported mechanism, histories that are inconsistent with each other or evolve with time, or an unusual relationship between the caregiver and child. Appropriate action may include discussion with a senior ophthalmologist, referral for a pediatric opinion, direct referral to social services, or consultation with the child's teacher. It is not acceptable to ignore concerns or to assume someone else will act.

On occasion, the ophthalmologist may be asked to examine a child as part of child protective services investigations. This should be performed by the most senior ophthalmologist available in the care pediatric pateints. It is important to complete as full an examination as possible and for it to be carefully documented.

Photographs may be helpful: if a digital system is used, an unmodified printout should be made at the time and signed by two witnesses. If a report is required, this should be phrased in terms comprehensible to an educated lay public and include the examiner's full name, qualifications, and the situation in which he or she saw the child.

Retinal hemorrhages and shaken baby syndrome

Shaken baby syndrome (SBS)

Retinal hemorrhages in the absence of bony injury or external eye injury may arise from severe shaking of young children (shaken baby syndrome). They are not diagnostic of abuse and must be taken in the context of the whole patient.

Alternative mechanisms

Additional consideration for other putative mechanisms of retinal and intracranial hemorrhage include the following:

- *Normal handling* (e.g., vigorous play): it is highly unlikely that the forces required to produce retinal hemorrhage in a child <2 years of age would be generated by a reasonable person during the course of vigorous (even rough) play.
- *Short-distance falls:* in a child with retinal hemorrhages and subdural hemorrhages who has not sustained a high-velocity injury and in whom other recognized causes of such hemorrhages have been excluded, child abuse is the most likely explanation; rarely, accidental trauma may give rise to a similar picture.
- *High cervical injuries:* cervical injuries alone do not result in retinal bleeding, unless combined with circulatory collapse.
- *Hypoxia:* acute hypoxia from transient apnea has not been shown to result in the SBS picture, unless combined with circulatory collapse.
- *Intracranial bleeding:* Terson syndrome (retinal hemorrhages secondary to intracranial bleeding) is rare in children and any hemorrhages tend to be concentrated around the optic disc.

Common clinical presentations: vision and movement

The following discussion outline common reasons for parents to seek ophthalmic advice. The underlying diseases range from the innocuous to the blinding and/or fatal. A complete ophthalmic (and usually systemic) examination should be performed in all cases.

Tables 18.6, 18.7, and 18.8 indicate the main causes of these clinical presentations, their key features, and/or a cross-reference to further information.

The child who does not see

Unilateral visual loss may not be noticed by parents until picked up at screening or during investigation for an associated abnormality (usually strabismus). Bilateral visual loss will be apparent in the child's visual behavior. In addition, children who have bilateral poor vision from an early age often have nystagmus or roving eye movements, although this does not occur in patients with retrochiasmal lesions.

- *Examination*: orthoptic, refractive, ophthalmic, neurological ± systemic (as indicated) (Table 18.6).

Abnormal eye alignment

Strabismus is common, affecting around 2% of children. While many cases are detected by parents, significant deviations may be missed because of their size, intermittent nature, or compensatory head posture. Conversely, a number of factors may give the appearance of strabismus in a perfectly orthophoric child—pseudostrabismus.

- *Examination*: refractive, ophthalmic, neurological ± systemic (as indicated) (Table 18.7).

Abnormal eye movements

Abnormal supplementary eye movements may occur as an isolated phenomenon or secondary to ocular or systemic disease (usually CNS pathology). They may be broadly divided into nystagmus or saccadic abnormalities.

- *Examination*: refractive, ophthalmic, neurological ± systemic (as indicated) (Table 18.8).

Table 18.6 Poor vision: outline of causes

General	Specific
Refractive	Myopia, hypermetropia, astigmatism
Cornea	Opacity, edema, abnormal curvature, or size
Lens	Cataract, subluxation, lenticonus
Vitreous	Persistent fetal vasculature, inflammation, hemorrhage
Retina	Coloboma, ROP, detachment, dysplasia, dystrophy, albinism
Macula	Hypoplasia, dystrophy, edema, inflammation, scarring, traction
Optic nerve	Inherited optic atrophy, compression, infiltration, inflammation
CNS	Hypoxia, inflammation, hydrocephalus, compression, delayed visual maturation
Other	Amblyopia, delayed visual maturation, functional

Table 18.7 Abnormal ocular alignment: outline of etiologies and key features

Strabismus (p. 580)	Intermittent or manifest misalignment of eyes that may be horizontal, vertical, or torsional
Pseudostrabismus	Consider epicanthal folds, asymmetry of face, globes (proptosis/ enophthalmos) or pupils, abnormal interpupillary distance or abnormal angle kappa

Table 18.8 Abnormal eye movements: outline of etiologies and key features

Nystagmus (p. 557)	Slow movement away from fixation corrected by fast movement (jerk nystagmus) or another slow movement (pendular nystagmus)
Saccadic abnormalities (p. 561)	Fast movement away from fixation, corrected by fast movement immediately (oscillation e.g., opsoclonus, ocular flutter) or after delay (intrusion)

Common clinical presentations: red eye, watery eye, and photophobia

Red (Table 18.9) or watery eyes (Table 18.10) are among the most common ocular presentations in primary care. Often these are relatively benign conditions, many of which may be successfully treated by general practitioners.

However in the presence of atypical features (particularly visual symptoms), more serious diagnoses should be considered. The presence of photophobia is usually an indication of more severe ocular pathology (Table 18.11).

- *Examination*: ophthalmic ± refractive, neurological, systemic (as indicated).

Red eye(s)

Table 18.9 Red eye: etiologies and key features

Normal VA	
Conjunctivitis (infective, allergic, chemical)	Gritty, often itchy, discharge, diffuse superficial injection, ± lid papillae/follicles
Foreign body	FB sensation, FB visible or in fornix/subtarsal, local injection, linear corneal abrasions (if subtarsal FB)
Episcleritis	Mild local pain, sectoral superficial injection (constricted by phenylephrine)
Scleritis	Severe pain, deep often diffuse injection; complications may lead to ↓VA
Vascular malformation	Abnormal conjunctival blood vessels, usually chronic, ± systemic vascular abnormalities
↓VA	
Corneal abrasion/erosion	Photophobia, watery eye, sectoral/circumlimbal injection, epithelial defect
Keratitis	Photophobia, watery eye, circumlimbal injection, corneal infiltrate ± epithelial defect ± AC activity
Glaucoma (acute ↑IOP)	Photophobia, watery eye, corneal edema, ↑IOP ± anterior segment/angle abnormalities
Anterior uveitis (acute)	Photophobia, watery eye, keratic precipitates, AC activity, ± posterior synechiae
Endophthalmitis	Pain, floaters, watery eye, diffuse deep injection, inflammation (vitreous > AC), chorioretinitis, decreased vision (most common)

Photophobia

Table 18.10 Watery eye: etiologies and key features

Increased tears

Blepharitis (posterior)	Chronic gritty, irritable eyes, poor tear film quality, ± meibomitis
Conjunctivitis (infective, allergic, chemical)	Gritty, often itchy, discharge may be sticky, diffuse superficial injection, ± lid papillae/follicles
Foreign body	FB sensation, FB visible or in fornix/subtarsal, local injection, corneal lacerations (if subtarsal FB)
Corneal abrasion/erosion	Photophobia, sectoral/circumlimbal injection, epithelial defect
Keratitis	Photophobia, sectoral/circumlimbal injection, corneal infiltrate ± epithelial defect ± AC activity
Glaucoma (acute ↑IOP)	Photophobia, injection, corneal edema, ↑IOP ± anterior segment/angle abnormalities
Anterior uveitis	Photophobia, circumlimbal injection, keratic precipitates, AC activity, ± posterior synechiae

Decreased drainage

Nasolacrimal duct obstruction	Chronic watery eye (may have sticky discharge) without other ocular signs ± lacrimal sac swelling

Watery eyes

Table 18.11 Photophobia: etiologies and key features

Anterior segment disease

Corneal abrasion/erosion	Watery eye, sectoral/circumlimbal injection, epithelial defect
Keratitis	Watery eye, circumlimbal injection, corneal infiltrate ± epithelial defect ± AC activity
Anterior uveitis (acute)	Watery eye, circumlimbal injection, keratic precipitates, AC activity, ± posterior synechiae
Glaucoma (acute ↑IOP)	Watery eye, injection, corneal edema, ↑IOP ± anterior segment/angle abnormalities
Inadequate iris sphincter	Complete/partial absence of tissue (e.g., aniridia, coloboma), mydriasis or hypopigmentation (albinism)

Posterior segment disease

Endophthalmitis	Decreased vision, pain, floaters, watering, diffuse deep injection, inflammation (vitreous > AC), chorioretinitis
Retinal dystrophies	Cone deficiencies (achromatopsia, blue cone monochromatism) or later-onset dystrophies

CNS disease

Meningitis/encephalitis	Fever, headache, neck stiffness, altered mental state, neurological dysfunction, normal ocular examination

Common clinical presentations: proptosis and globe size

Abnormalities of the whole globe are usually congenital and represent developmental abnormalities. Abnormal protrusion of the eye (proptosis) usually represents an acquired, progressive disease.

Proptosis

Abnormal protrusion of the eye (proptosis) is uncommon, but usually signifies severe orbital pathology (Table 18.12). Acute onset in an ill child may represent orbital cellulitis, an ophthalmic emergency. Orbital tumors (Table 18.13) usually present with more gradual proptosis, although rhabdomyosarcoma is well known to present acutely, mimicking orbital cellulitis.

Table 18.12 Proptosis: etiologies and key features

Infection	
Orbital cellulitis	Febrile, illness, with acute pain, lid swelling, restricted eye movements, ± ↓VA
Inflammation	
Idiopathic orbital inflammatory disease	Acute pain, lid swelling, conjunctival injection ± intraocular inflammation and ↓VA; diffuse orbital disease vs. localized (e.g., myositis or dacroadenitis)
Thyroid eye disease	Pain, conjunctival injection, lid retraction, restrictive myopathy, ↓VA; usually older children
Vasculitis	Usually present acutely and are ill (e.g., Wegener's granulomatosis, PAN)
Tumors	
Acquired (e.g., rhabdomyosarcoma)	Proptosis ± pain, ↓VA, abnormal eye movements; usually gradual onset but some (e.g., rhabdomyosarcoma) may present acutely
Congenital (e.g., dermoid cysts)	Superficial lesions present early as a round lump, deep lesions may cause pain and gradual proptosis
Vascular anomalies	
Congenital orbital varices	Intermittent proptosis exaggerated by Valsalva maneuver or forward posture
Carotid–cavernous fistula	Arterialized conjunctival vessels, chemosis, ± bruit; usu. traumatic in children; orbital bruit on auscultation
Bony anomalies	
Sphenoid dysplasia	Pulsatile proptosis, encephalocele, associated with neurofibromatosis-1
Craniosynostosis	Premature fusion of sutures resulting in characteristic skull abnormalities
Other	
Pseudoproptosis	Consider ipsilateral large globe or lid retraction, contralateral enophthalmos or ptosis, facial asymmetry, shallow orbits

Table 18.13 Orbital tumors of childhood (selected)

Congenital	Examples
Choristoma	Dermoid cysts
Acquired	
Optic nerve	Glioma
Vascular	Capillary hemangioma, lymphangioma
Infiltrative	Myeloid leukemia, histiocytosis
Other	Rhabdomyosarcoma, teratoma
Metastases	Neuroblastoma, nephroblastoma, Ewing's sarcoma

Abnormal eye size

Abnormalities of globe size usually result from abnormalities of development, although it may arise secondary to ocular disease (e.g., buphthalmo in glaucoma) (Table 18.14). While severe forms may be obvious from simple observation, milder isolated aberrations of size may only be evident a an axial refractive error.

Table 18.14 Abnormal eye size: causes and key features

Abnormally large eye	
Axial myopia	Mild (physiological) to severe and progressive (pathological) ↑length; ± other ocular abnormalities
Buphthalmos	Diffusely large eye (with megalocornea) associated with glaucoma
Megalophthalmos	Diffusely large eye (with megalocornea) without glaucoma; ± other ocular abnormalities
Pseudo-large eye	Consider proptosis or abnormally small contralateral eye
Abnormally small eye	
Microphthalmos	Diffusely small eye (axial length 2 SD < normal) ± ocular or systemic anomalies
Nanophthalmos	Small eye with microcornea, normal-sized lens, and abnormally thick sclera
Phthisis bulbi	Acquired shrinkage of the eye due to chronic ocular disease
Pseudo-small eye	Consider ipsilateral ptosis or enophthalmos, or abnormally large contralateral eye

Common clinical presentations: cloudy cornea and leukocoria

Opacification of the cornea, lens, or posterior structures is usually associated with poor vision and may indicate serious, even life-threatening, pathology.

Cloudy cornea

Corneal opacities may be focal (either central or peripheral) or diffuse in nature (Table 18.15). They may be an isolated finding, associated with other ocular abnormalities, or part of an inherited syndrome. They may be congenital, acquired at birth, or develop during childhood.

Leukocoria

All patients with leukocoria (Table 18.16) must be urgently assessed for the possibility of retinoblastoma. Congenital cataracts are generally easily identified. Other conditions may be less readily differentiated from retinoblastoma, most commonly persistent fetal vasculature syndrome, Coats' disease, toxocara infection, and ROP.

Table 18.15 Corneal opacities: etiologies and key features

Diffuse	
Birth trauma	Forceps injury may induce ruptures in Descemet's membrane (usually unilateral with vertical break)
Keratitis (infective, allergic, exposure)	Photophobia, watery eye, circumlimbal injection, corneal infiltrate ± epithelial defect ± AC activity
Corneal dystrophies	Clinical pattern varies but may be evident from birth (e.g., congenital hereditary endothelial dysfunction)
Metabolic	Bilateral corneal clouding with systemic abnormalities in some mucopolysaccharidoses or mucolipidoses
Central	
Peter's anomaly	Congenital, usually bilateral central opacities ± adhesions to iris/lens (posterior ulcer of von Hippel)
Peripheral	
Sclerocornea	Bilateral (often asymmetric), peripheral opacification with vascularization ± other corneal/angle anomalies
Limbal dermoid	Solid white mass that may involve peripheral cornea; rarely bilateral and 360° around the limbus
Posterior embryotoxon	Peripheral opacity due to anteriorly displaced Schwalbe's line ± other angle/ocular abnormalities

Table 18.16 Leukocoria: etiologies and key features

Lens

Cataract	Lens opacity: stationary or progressive; isolated, or associated with other ocular or systemic abnormalities

Vitreous

Persistent fetal vasculature syndrome	Variable persistence of fetal vasculature/hyaloid remnants; often microphthalmic; usually unilateral
Inflammatory cyclitic membrane	Fibrous membrane behind the lens arising from the ciliary body due to chronic intraocular inflammation

Retina

Retinoblastoma	Retinal mass of endophytic, exophytic, or infiltrating type; tumor may spread to anterior segment, orbit. This is life threatening if untreated!
Coloboma	Developmental defect resulting in variably sized defect involving optic disc, choroid, and retina
Coats' disease	Retinal telangiectasia with exudation, →exudative retinal detachment in severe cases
Retinopathy of prematurity (ROP)	Early cessation of peripheral retinal vascularization due to prematurity causes fibrovascular proliferation
Familial exudative vitreoretinopathy	Early cessation of peripheral retinal vascularization due to inherited defect causes ROP-like picture in full-term infant
Incontinentia pigmenti	Abnormal peripheral retinal vascularization due to inherited defect causes ROP-like picture in girls (lethal in boys)
Retinal dysplasia	Gray vascularized mass from extensive gliosis (e.g., Norries disease, Patau syndrome)

Infection

Toxocara	Unilateral granuloma or endophthalmitis

Intrauterine infections

Congenital infections have a variable effect on morbidity and mortality dependent on the infecting organism and stage of gestation of the fetus. Overall, however, ocular morbidity is common.

These organisms can be screened by means of the TORCH screen for maternal antibodies to Toxoplasma, Other (e.g., syphilis), Rubella, Cytomegalovirus, and Herpes simplex.

Congenital toxoplasmosis

The impact of transplacental infection by toxoplasma is greatest early in pregnancy. The spectrum of disease ranges from an asymptomatic peripheral patch of retinochoroiditis (often an incidental finding of inactive scar years later) to a blinding endophthalmitis (Table 18.17).

Congenital syphilis

Previously in decline, syphilis has made a comeback in recent years. The early stage is characterized by inflammation (Table 18.18). Many of the late manifestations are direct sequelae of this process. Others (such as interstitial keratitis) may be an immunological phenomenon.

Congenital rubella

Incidence of rubella has declined since the advent of the rubella vaccination. The virus is well known for its teratogenic effects (especially with early infection). It also has ongoing pathogenicity with virus shedding for up to 2 years of age, interstitial pneumonitis and pancreatic inflammation within the first year, and panencephalitis as late as 12 years of age (Table 18.19).

Congenital CMV

Although commonly asymptomatic, congenital infection with CMV may cause severe systemic disease. Retinitis tends to be unifocal, more similar to toxoplasmosis than adult CMV retinitis (Table 18.20).

Congenital HSV

It is rare for HSV to be acquired at the intrauterine stage; more commonly, HSV may be acquired at birth from maternal genital HSV lesions (Table 18.21).

Table 18.17 Clinical features of congenital toxoplasmosis

Ocular	Retinochoroiditis (more commonly bilateral and affecting the macula than in acquired disease), cataract, microphthalmos, strabismus
Systemic	Hydrocephalus, intracranial calcification, hepatosplenomegaly

Table 18.18 Clinical features of congenital syphilis

Early disease (<2 years of age)	
Ocular	Chorioretinitis and retinal vasculitis (results in characteristic salt-and-pepper fundus) Conjunctivitis
Systemic	Mucocutaneous rash; periostitis and osteochondritis
Late disease (>2 years of age)	
Ocular	Interstitial keratitis (usually presents at 5–20 years of age) Optic atrophy
Systemic	Saddle nose, frontal bossing, saber shins, Hutchinson's teeth, scoliosis, hard palate perforation

Table 18.19 Clinical features of congenital rubella

Ocular	Nuclear cataract, microphthalmos, glaucoma (congenital or infantile), corneal clouding, retinitis
Systemic (early/late)	Congenital heart disease, sensorineural deafness, anemia, thrombocytopenia, bone abnormalities, hepatitis, CNS abnormalities (e.g., encephalitis)

Table 18.20 Clinical features of congenital CMV

Ocular	Retinitis (focal)
Systemic	IUGR, microcephaly, hydrocephalus, intracranial calcification, hepatosplenomegaly, thrombocytopenia

Table 18.21 Clinical features of congenital HSV

Ocular	Chorioretinitis
Systemic	Microcephaly, intracranial calcification

Ophthalmia neonatorum

Ophthalmia neonatorum is defined as a conjunctivitis occurring within the first month of life. Organisms are commonly acquired from the birth canal. The main risk factor is therefore the presence of sexually transmitted disease in the mother.

Ophthalmia neonatorum affects up to 12% of neonates in the Western world and up to 23% in developing countries. It is potentially sight threatening and may cause systemic complications. In some countries (including the United States), it is a reportable disease (within 12 hours).

Gonococcal neonatal conjunctivitis

Clinical features
- Hyperacute (within 1–3 days of birth), with severe purulent discharge, lid edema, chemosis, ± pseudomembrane, ± keratitis.

Investigation
- Prewet swab or conjunctival scrapings: immediate Gram stain (gram-negative diplococci), culture (chocolate agar), and sensitivities.

Treatment
- Ceftriaxone 50 mg/kg IV 1×/day 1 week; frequent saline irrigation of discharge until eliminated.
- After appropriate counseling, refer mother (with partner) to urogenital physician.

Chlamydial neonatal conjunctivitis

This is the most common cause of neonatal conjunctivitis. A papillary rather than follicular reaction is seen from delayed development of palpebral lymphoid tissue.

Clinical features
- Subacute onset (4–28 days after birth), mucopurulent discharge, papillae, ± preseptal cellulitis.
- Systemic (uncommon): rhinitis, otitis, pneumonitis.

Investigation
- Prewet swabs are usually for immunofluorescent staining, but cell culture, PCR, and ELISA may be used.
- Conjunctival scrapings: Giemsa stain.

Treatment
- Erythromycin 25 mg/kg 2×/day for 2 weeks.
- After appropriate counseling, refer mother (with partner) to urogenital physician.

Other bacterial neonatal conjunctivitis

Other bacterial causes include *Staphylococcus aureus*, *Streptococcus pneumoniae* (which require topical antibiotics only), and *Haemophilus* and *Pseudomonas* (which requires additional systemic antibiotics to prevent systemic complications).

Clinical features
- Subacute onset (4–28 days after birth), purulent discharge, lid edema, chemosis, ± keratitis (*Pseudomonas*)

Investigation
- Prewet swab or conjunctival scrapings: Gram stain, culture, sensitivities.

Treatment
- Gram-positive organisms: topical (e.g., erythromycin ointment 4x/day); adjust according to sensitivities.
- Gram-negative organisms: topical (e.g., tobramycin ointment 4x/day); adjust according to sensitivities.

HSV neonatal conjunctivitis

Although viral causes of neonatal conjunctivitis are uncommon, they may cause serious ocular morbidity and systemic disease.

Clinical features
- Acute onset (1–14 days), vesicular lid lesions, mucoid discharge ± keratitis (e.g., microdendrities), anterior uveitis, cataract, retinitis, optic neuritis (rare).
- Systemic (uncommon but may be fatal): jaundice, hepatosplenomegaly, pneumonitis, meningoencephalitis, disseminated intravascular coagulopathy (DIC).

Investigation
- Swab or conjunctival scrapings transported in viral culture medium; PCR.
- Newborns with ocular HSV infection must be evaluated for systemic infection. There should be a very low threshold for hospital admission and systemic antiviral treatment.

Treatment
- Acyclovir ointment 5x/day for 1week ± acyclovir IV 10 mg/kg 3x/day for 10 days.

Chemical conjunctivitis

Silver nitrate drops are commonly used in some parts of the world as a protective measure against ophthalmia neonatorum (Table 18.22). While effective against gonococcal disease, they are of limited use against other bacteria and are of no use against *Chlamydia* or viruses. In most neonates the drops cause red, watery eyes 12–48 hours after instillation.

Conjunctivitis in the older child

Children are commonly affected by infective and allergic conjunctivitis. In the older child, it behaves in a more similar manner to adult disease: viral (p. 142), bacterial (p. 140), chlamydial (p. 144), and allergic (p. 146).

Table 18.22 Timing of onset of ophthalmia neonatorum by etiology

Chemical	<2 days
Gonococcal	1–3 days
Other bacteria	2–5 days
HSV	1–14 days
Chlamydia	4–28 days

Orbital and preseptal cellulitis

Orbital cellulitis may cause blindness and even death. It requires emergency assessment, imaging, and treatment under the joint care of an ophthalmologist, ENT specialist, and pediatrician. Part of the ophthalmologist's role is to assist in differentiating orbital cellulitis from the more limited preseptal cellulitis.

Orbital cellulitis

Infective organisms include *Streptococcus pneumoniae*, *Staphylococcus aureus*, *Streptococcus pyogenes*, and *Haemophilus influenza* (previously common in younger children, but less likely if Hib vaccinated).

Risk factors

- *Sinus disease:* ethmoidal sinusitis (common), maxillary sinusitis.
- *Infection of other adjacent structures:* preseptal or facial infection, dacrocystitis, dental abscess.
- *Trauma:* septal perforation.
- *Surgical:* orbital, lacrimal, and vitreoretinal surgery.

Clinical features

- Fever, malaise, painful, swollen orbit.
- Inflamed lids (swollen, red, tender, warm), proptosis, painful restricted eye movements ± optic nerve dysfunction (↓VA, ↓color vision, RAPD).
- *Complications:* optic nerve compromise is the most important; also exposure keratopathy, ↑IOP, CRAO, CRVO.
- *Systemic:* meningitis, cerebral abscess, cavernous sinus thrombosis, orbital or periorbital abscess.

Investigation

- Temperature.
- CBC, blood culture.
- CT (dedicated CT for orbit and sinuses; possibly brain): diffuse orbital infiltrate with fat stranding, proptosis ± sinus opacity, orbital abscess.

Treatment

- Admit for intravenous antibiotics (e.g., either floxacillin 25 mg/kg 4×/day or cefuroxime 50 mg/kg 4×/day with metronidazole 7.5 mg/kg 3×/day).
- ENT specialist to assess for sinus drainage (required in up to 50%).

Preseptal cellulitis

Preseptal infection is much more common than orbital cellulitis. The main causative organisms are once again staphylococci and streptococci.

This is generally a less severe disease, at least in adults and older children (see Table 18.23). In younger children in whom the orbital septum is not fully developed, there is a high risk of progression, thus the disease should be treated similarly to orbital cellulitis.

Clinical features
- Fever, malaise, painful, swollen lid/periorbita.
- Inflamed lids but no proptosis, normal eye movements, normal optic nerve function.

Investigation

Investigation is not usually necessary unless there is concern about possible orbital or sinus involvement (Table 18.24).

Treatment
- Admit young or ill children; otherwise daily observation is sufficient until disease resolution.
- Treat with oral antibiotics (e.g., floxacillin and metronidazole).

Table 18.23 Differentiating features of orbital vs preseptal cellulitis

	Orbital	Preseptal
Proptosis	Present	Absent
Ocular motility	Painful + restricted	Normal
VA	↓ (in severe cases)	Normal
Color vision	↓ (in severe cases)	Normal
RAPD	Present (in severe cases)	Normal

Table 18.24 Development of paranasal sinuses

Sinus	Onset of development	Onset of adult configuration
Maxillary	In utero	Late childhood (12 years)
Sphenoidal	In utero	Puberty
Ethmoidal	In utero	Puberty
Frontal	Postnatal	Adulthood

Congenital cataract: assessment

Congenital cataract affects up to 1 in 4000 live births and is a significant cause of visual impairment in children. Since it is amblyopiagenic, that is likely to limit final visual outcome, this condition requires urgent expert assessment, with a view to early surgery.

Assessment

- *History:* observed visual function, intrauterine exposure (infections, drugs, toxins, radiation), medical history (e.g., syndromes), family history (approximately 50% of bilateral cataracts are hereditary, although severity can vary between family members).
- *Visual function:* clinical tests appropriate to age. Poor fixation, strabismus, and nystagmus suggest severe visual impairment.
- *Cataract density* is indicated by red reflex pre- to post-dilation and quality of fundus view with a direct or indirect ophthalmoscope. Risk to vision is worse if the cataract is posterior, dense, axial, and >3 mm in diameter.
- *Cataract morphology* may suggest underlying etiology.
- *Remainder of the eye:* visual potential (check pupil reactions and optic nerve and retina, as possible), associated ocular abnormalities (may require treatment, influence surgery, or suggest underlying cause).
- *Systemic:* numerous systemic conditions are associated with congenital cataracts (Table 18.25). Clinical examination will direct appropriate investigation.

Investigation

Coordinate with a pediatrician, but consider the following:

- Urinalysis (reducing substances in galactosemia and amino acids in Lowe syndrome—this affects boys).
- Serology: TORCH screen (toxoplasma, other [e.g., syphilis], rubella, CMV, HSV 1 and 2).
- Biochemical profile, including glucose, calcium, phosphate.
- Erythrocyte enzyme analysis, including galactokinase, G1PUT.
- Karyotyping and clinical geneticist referral, e.g., if child is dysmorphic.

Table 18.25 Causes of congenital and presenile cataracts

Isolated		AD, AR, XR
Chomosomal	Trisomies	Down(21), Edward(18), Patau(13) syndromes
	Monosomies	Turner syndrome
	Deletions	5p (Cri-du-chat syndrome), 18p, 18q
	Microdeletion	16p13- (Rubinstein–Taybi syndrome)
	Duplications	3q, 10q, 20p
Syndromic	Craniosynostosis	Apert syndrome Crouzon syndrome
	Craniofacial defects	Smith–Lemli–Opitz syndrome Hallerman–Streiff–Francois syndrome
	Dermatological	Cockayne syndrome, incontinentia pigmenti, hypohidrotic ectodermal dysplasia, ichthyosis, nevoid BCC syndrome, Rothmund–Thomson syndrome
	Neuromuscular	Alstrom disease, myotonic dystrophy, Marinesco–Sjogren syndrome
	Connective tissue	Marfan syndrome Alport syndrome Conradi syndrome Spondyloepiphyseal dysplasia
	AS dysgenesis	Peters anomaly Rieger syndrome
Metabolic	Carbohydrate	Hypoglycemia Galactokinase deficiency Galactosemia, Mannosidosis
	Lipids	Abetalipoproteinemia
	Amino acid	Lowe syndrome Homocysteinuria
	Sphingolipidoses	Niemann–Pick disease Fabry disease
	Minerals	Wilson disease Hypocalcemia
	Phytanic acid	Refsum disease
Endocrine		Diabetes mellitus Hypoparathyroidism
Infective		Toxoplasma Rubella Herpes group (CMV, HSV1 & 2, VZV) Syphilis Measles Poliomyelitis Influenza
Other		Trauma Drugs (steroids) Eczema Radiation

Congenital cataract: management

Timing of surgery

Remove visually significant cataracts as early as possible. Significant unilateral congenital cataracts require urgent removal with optical correction in the first 4–6 weeks of life; significant bilateral congenital cataracts should be removed in the first 8 weeks of life. If cataracts are bilateral, remove both consecutively within a few days of each other.

Procedure

Debate continues over the procedure of choice and when to use implantable lenses. In younger children (<2 years), it is most common to perform a mechanical lensectomy–vitrectomy. In older children, an anterior continuous curvilinear capsulorhexis may be performed with a view to implanting a lens.

Posterior capsular opacification is universal under the age of 6 years, so perform a posterior capsulorhexis and shallow anterior vitrectomy (anterior or pars plana approach). Suture (absorbable) to close the incisions.

There is considerable debate over the estimation of IOL power in children undergoing cataract surgery.

Postoperative care

Excellent postoperative care requires highly motivated parents, coordinated orthoptists and ophthalmologists, and regularly updated refractions.

While contact lenses have many theoretical advantages (particularly in aphakia), their use may be problematic, particularly in younger children. Increased implantation of IOLs results in smaller refractive errors that can be easily corrected by spectacles Older children (≥3 years) benefit from bifocal lenses with an add of +3.00 for near.

In unilateral cases, patching of the unaffected eye is essential. Aggressive patching improves the visual outcome in the operated eye but increases the amblyopic risk to the normal eye. Close monitoring is a priority whichever regimen is used. Parental education pre- and post-surgery is essential.

Postoperative complications

These include anterior uveitis, posterior capsular opacification, lens reproliferation (e.g., Soemmerring ring), secondary pupillary membranes, glaucoma (especially if aphakic), retinal detachment (often years later), contact lens problems, and unpredictable final refraction.

Uveitis in children

Although uveitis is much less common in children than in adults, it is still a significant cause of ocular morbidity. This is most marked in the context of the silent anterior uveitis of juvenile idiopathic arthritis, which accounts for up to 80% of all childhood uveitis. However, it is important to recognize that most other types of uveitis may also affect children.

Juvenile idiopathic arthritis (JIA)

JIA is defined as idiopathic arthritis of >6 weeks duration with onset before 16 years of age. It may be subclassified into systemic, oligoarthritis (≤4 joints), RF-negative polyarthritis (>4 joints), RF-positive polyarthritis, psoriatic, enthesitis-related, and other/overlap syndromes.

The term *juvenile idiopathic arthritis* replaces juvenile chronic arthritis (JCA) and juvenile rheumatoid arthritis (JRA). Of those with JIA, 20% will develop anterior uveitis, of which 70% will be bilateral and 25% will be severe sight-threatening disease. JIA is more common in females.

Clinical features

Ophthalmic
- Asymptomatic, rarely floaters, ↓VA from cataract.
- White eye, small KPs, AC cells/flare, posterior synechiae, vitritis, CME (rare); complications include band keratopathy, cataract, inflammatory glaucoma, or phthisis bulbi.
- *Arthritis:* oligoarthritis, polyarthritis, psoriatic type, or enthesitis related.
- *Systemic:* fever, rash, lymphadenopathy, hepatosplenomegaly, serositis.

Screening

Patients diagnosed with JIA should be seen as soon as possible by an ophthalmologist. If ophthalmic examination is normal, regular follow-up is indicated according to risk.

Treatment

The treatment goal is to control the uveitis with topical steroids and mydriatic; if systemic therapy is required, this should be done with the help

Table 18.26 Summary of recommendations for evaluation of JIA by ophthalmologists

Risk	Factors	Screening
High	Onset <6 years age Pauciarticular AND ANA+	Every 3 months for 1 year Every 6 months for next 5 years Every 12 months thereafter
Medium	Polyarticular AND ANA+ Pauciarticular AND ANA−	Every 6 months for 5 years Every 12 months thereafter
Low	Onset >11 years age Systemic onset HLA-B27+	Every 12 months

of a pediatrician or rheumatologist. NSAIDs and steroid-sparing agents such as methotrexate are commonly used to minimize side effects.

In long-standing uveitis chronic breakdown of the blood–aqueous barrier leads to persistent flare; AC cells are thus a better guide to disease activity.

Other causes of uveitis in children

The clinical features, investigation, and treatment of these conditions (Table 18.27) are discussed under Uveitis (pp. 313–372).

Treatment

While there are many similarities to adult disease, the following should be noted:

- Children are still growing: systemic steroids reduce growth rate and final height; topical steroids may have systemic side effects and also increase IOP and lead to cataract formation.
- Children are smaller: all treatments should be appropriately titrated to body size and weight.
- Children have longer to live: they are at higher risk of delayed complications (e.g., post-immunosuppression malignancies).

Table 18.27 Uveitis in children

Anterior	Juvenile idiopathic arthritis (JIA)	📖 p. 331
	HLA-B27 associated (e.g., psoriasis, ankylosing spondylitis, inflammatory bowel disease)	📖 p. 329
	Kawasaki disease	📖 p. 328
	TINU	📖 p. 327
	Idiopathic	📖 p. 325
Intermediate	Idiopathic/Pars planitis	📖 p. 333
	Toxocara	📖 p. 364
	Lyme disease	📖 p. 359
	Inflammatory bowel disease	📖 p. 330
Posterior	Toxoplasma	📖 p. 361
	Toxocara	📖 p. 364
	Congenital syphilis	📖 p. 357
	TB	📖 p. 354
	HIV associated (e.g., CMV retinitis)	📖 p. 352
	Sarcoidosis	📖 p. 337
	Behçet's disease	📖 p. 340
Vasculitis	Leukemia	📖 p. 450
	Cat-scratch disease	📖 p. 336
	Systemic vasculitis (e.g., SLE)	📖 p. 336
	Herpes group (e.g., HSV)	📖 p. 345
	HIV related (e.g., CMV)	📖 p. 352

Glaucoma in children

The childhood glaucomas are a significant cause of blindness in children but may be missed, being both rare and insidious. Unfortunately, the terms *congenital*, *infantile*, and *juvenile* are often used incorrectly and interchangeably, thereby rendering the nomenclature confusing. Classifying childhood glaucoma by etiology may therefore be more useful.

Causes

Primary (primary congenital glaucoma, trabeculodysgenesis)

In this rare syndrome (1/10,000 live births), angle dysgenesis causes reduced aqueous outflow. It is usually sporadic, but 10% of cases are familial. Genes identified include *GLC3A* (Ch2p), *GLC3B* (Ch1p), and *GLC3C* (Ch14q), all of which result in autosomal recessive disease.

Secondary

Anterior segment dysgenesis, (p. 635)

Developmental abnormalities of the anterior segment result in a spectrum of anterior segment anomalies, including Axenfeld–Rieger syndrome, and Peter's anomaly, and associated abnormalities of the drainage angle. Glaucoma occurs in about 50% of cases.

Aniridia

In aniridia (also called iridotrabeculodysgenesis), the iris tissue is abnormal or absent and is associated with glaucoma in up to 75% of patients.

Lens or surgery related

Surgery for congenital cataracts is associated with glaucoma in up to 40%, being highest for early total lensectomy.

Posterior segment developmental abnormalities

Persistent fetal vasculature syndrome and retinopathy of prematurity may cause glaucoma by a secondary angle-closure mechanism.

Tumor related

Tumors may cause ↑IOP by reduced aqueous outflow (mechanical, clogging of trabecular meshwork by cellular debris, or secondary hemorrhage). Tumors may be anterior (e.g., juvenile xanthogranuloma), posterior (e.g., retinoblastoma), or systemic (e.g., leukemia).

Phakomatoses

Sturge–Weber syndrome is associated with ipsilateral glaucoma in up to 50% of patients, being highest when the nevus flammeus involves both upper and lower lid. Neurofibromatosis also carries an increased risk, particularly in the presence of an ipsilateral neurofibroma.

Connective tissue disease

Marfan syndrome, homocystinuria, and Weill–Marchesani syndrome are associated with glaucoma. This may arise from abnormal trabecular meshwork or lens block.

Uveitis
Chronic uveitis of childhood (e.g., associated with JIA) may result in secondary glaucoma. This is usually of relatively late onset.

Clinical features

- Watery eye(s), photophobia, blepharospasm, enlarged eye(s), cloudy cornea.
- Corneal edema, enlargement of cornea or globe (if onset <4 years of age), breaks in Descemet's membrane (Haab striae), ↑IOP.

Additional features may indicate the cause of glaucoma:

- *Ophthalmic:* posterior embryotoxon, leukoma, anterior iris strands, iris hypoplasia, aniridia, iris cyst or tumor, iritis, cataract, ectopia lentis, aphakia, persistent fetal vasculature, ciliary body tumors, retinal masses.
- *Systemic:* nevus flammeus (Sturge–Weber syndrome), neurofibromatosis (NF-1 or -2), Marfanoid habitus (Marfan syndrome, homocystinuria), brachydactyly (Weill–Marchesani syndrome), abnormal dentition (Axenfeld–Rieger syndrome).

Treatment

Titrate antiglaucoma treatment on the basis of level of IOP, worsening disc appearance, and increasing corneal diameter. Medical treatment is usually not a satisfactory long-term solution but may be used while awaiting surgery. The preferred surgical technique depends on the type of glaucoma:

- *Primary congenital glaucoma* responds well to goniotomy (>90% IOP control at 5 years).
- *Secondary glaucomas* generally require more extensive procedures. Examples include the following:
  - *Anterior segment dysgenesis:* consider trabeculotomy or trabeculectomy.
  - *Aniridia:* consider antimetabolite-augmented trabeculectomy.
  - *Aphakia:* consider tube procedure; goniotomy or trabeculotomy if the angle looks abnormal.
  - *Sturge–Weber syndrome:* early onset: goniotomy; late onset: trabeculectomy.
  - *Connective tissue disease:* consider iridectomy or lens-related surgery.
  - *Uveitis:* consider antimetabolite-augmented trabeculectomy.

Retinopathy of prematurity

Retinopathy of prematurity (ROP) was first reported in 1942. By the 1950s it was the leading cause of childhood blindness. At this point, tight oxygen control was introduced, with a dramatic fall in ROP but a significant rise in neonatal death and neurological disability. Supplemental oxygen therapy is now considered a compromise between these conflicting results.

Risk factors
- Low gestational age ($\leq$31 weeks).
- Low birth weight (<1500 g).
- High or variable oxygen tension.

Classification (see Fig. 18.1)

Stages
- *Stage 1:* demarcation line: flat white line separating vascular from avascular zones.
- *Stage 2:* ridge: line becomes elevated, thickened, and may become pinkish.
- *Stage 3:* extraretinal fibrovascular proliferation: vascular tissue grows from the posterior margin onto the retina or into the vitreous.
- *Stage 4:* subtotal retinal detachment: extrafoveal (4A) or foveal (4B).
- *Stage 5:* total retinal detachment.
- *Plus disease:* these signs of vascular incompetence include arterial tortuosity and venous dilation (sometimes present: iris vessel dilation, pupil rigidity, and vitreous haze).

Location
- *Zone 1:* circle centered on the disc, with radius twice the disc–foveal distance.
- *Zone 2:* ring centered on the disc, extending from zone 1 to ora nasally and equator temporally.
- *Zone 3:* remaining temporal crescent.

Extent
- Measured in clock-hours.

Threshold disease
Originally an estimate of when progression and regression were equally likely, this is now used as the level at which treatment is indicated. Threshold disease is defined as stage 3 + disease in zones 1 or 2 and of 5 continuous or 8 noncontinuous clock-hours. Threshold ROP as a criterion to treat ROP has been replaced by type 1 vs. type 2 ROP.

Type 1 vs. type 2 ROP
The Early Treatment of ROP (ETROP) Study supported retinal ablative therapy for eyes with type 1 ROP, defined as zone 1, any stage ROP with plus disease; zone 1, stage 3 ROP without plus disease; or zone 2, stage 2 or 3 ROP with plus disease.

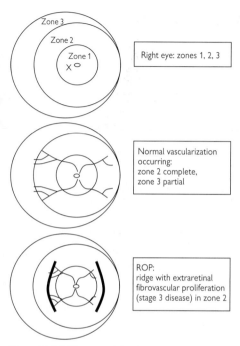

Figure 18.1 ROP zones and classification.

Right eye: zones 1, 2, 3

Normal vascularization
occurring:
zone 2 complete,
zone 3 partial

ROP:
ridge with extraretinal
fibrovascular proliferation
(stage 3 disease) in zone 2

Screening

Screening should be performed on those infants ≤31 weeks of age or <1500 g. This should start 42–49 days postnatally and continue at least every 2 weeks until 1) progression of retinal vascularization into zone 3 without zone 2 ROP, or 2) full vascularization has occurred.

Indirect ophthalmoscopy with a 28D lens permits a wide field of view. Dilate in advance (cyclopentolate 0.5% + phenylephrine 2.5%) and consider a lid speculum and scleral indentation as needed.

Treatment

Treatment is recommended for threshold disease and worse; however, recent evidence suggests that high-risk prethreshold disease may also benefit. Cryotherapy has been used for over 30 years but has largely been replaced by laser photocoagulation, which is more portable, better tolerated, and more effective for posterior disease. Photocoagulation should be nearly confluent (half burn-width separation), should extend from the ora up to the ridge, and should surround the full 360°.

Vitreoretinal surgery aims to repair or prevent progression of ROP-associated retinal detachment (stages 4A, 4B, and 5). Unfortunately, results are generally disappointing.

Other retinal disorders

ROP-like syndromes

Familial exudative vitreoretinopathy (FEVR)

This rare condition usually shows autosomal dominant inheritance (Ch11q). Clinical features include abrupt cessation of peripheral retinal vessels at the equator (more marked temporally) and vitreous bands in the periphery.

Complications include fibrovascular proliferation, macular ectopia, retinal detachment (similar to ROP), and subretinal exudation (similar to Coats' disease).

Incontinentia pigmenti (Bloch–Sulzberger syndrome)

This rare condition shows X-linked dominant inheritance being lethal in utero for male embryos. Clinical features include abnormal peripheral vasculature, gliosis, tractional retinal detachment, and systemic features such as abnormal teeth, cutaneous pigment whorls, and CNS anomalies.

Retinal dysplasia

A number of conditions are associated with more extensive retinal abnormalities, probably arising from abnormal development involving the inner wall of the optic cup. Clinical features include extensive retinal folds, retinal detachments, retinal hemorrhages, vitreous hemorrhages, retrolental gray mass, and phthisis bulbi.

Associated syndromes include Patau's syndrome (p. 638), Edward syndrome (p. 638), Norrie disease (retinal dysplasia, deafness, ↓IQ), and Walker–Warburg syndrome (retinal dysplasia, muscular dystrophy, Dandy–Walker malformation).

Other retinochoroidal disorders

Many stationary and progressive disorders of photoreceptors, RPE, choroid and retinal vasculature present in childhood. They are discussed elsewhere in this book: retinitis pigmentosa (p. 456), congenital stationary night blindness (p. 458), macular dystrophies (p. 459), choroidal dystrophies (p. 462), hereditary vitreoretinal degenerations (p. 389), albinism (p. 464), and Coats' disease (p. 452).

Developmental abnormalities

Anterior segment

Anterior segment dysgenesis results in a variety of abnormalities of variable severity (Box 18.1). The Axenfeld–Rieger spectrum tends to have autosomal dominant inheritance whereas Peters' anomaly is usually sporadic. All are associated with glaucoma.

Rieger's anomaly may be associated with systemic abnormalities (teeth small and fewer than normal, maxillary hypoplasia), when it is known as Rieger syndrome. More recently, all disorders falling into this spectrum have been grouped as Axenfeld–Rieger syndrome.

Box 18.1 Anterior segment dysgenesis

Posterior embryotoxon
    + anterior iris strands = Axenfeld's anomaly
        + iris hypoplasia = Rieger's anomaly
            + systemic abnormalities = Rieger's syndrome

Corneal opacity (leukoma)/posterior corneal defect = Peters' anomaly of
    + anterior iris strands   increasing
        + lens/corneal touch   severity

Optic fissure

A *coloboma* is a defect resulting from failure of closure of an embryological fissure. Within the eye, defects may occur anywhere from the optic disc to iris, and vary dramatically in size and severity. Colobomas may be blinding and may be associated with more extensive disease.

Vitreous

Abnormalities within the vitreous cavity include remnants of the hyaloid vascular system (Table 18.28), and abnormalities of the vitreous structure, e.g., type II collagen abnormalities resulting in Stickler syndrome).

Table 18.28 Hyaloid remnants

Glial remnant just posterior to lens	Mittendorf's dot
Glial remnant just anterior to disc	Bergmeister's papilla
Vascular remnant arising from disc	Persistent hyaloid artery
Vascular remnant and retrolental mass	Persistent fetal vasculature

Optic nerve anomalies

These include optic disc pits, optic disc hypoplasia, coloboma, and morning glory anomaly (p. 535). Although disc pits are often isolated findings, more severe disc abnormalities are often associated with systemic pathology.

Patients with bilateral optic disc hypoplasia should be evaluated for other cerebral midline abnormalities (e.g., septo-optic dysplasia) and pituitary dysfunction. Patients with morning glory anomaly have a higher incidence of intracranial vascular abnormalities, including moyamoya disease (arterial occlusive disorders).

Retina

Premature cessation of peripheral retina vascularization may occur as a result of an inherited defect (familial exudative vitreoretinopathy [FEVR] Ch11q) or acquired insult (retinopathy of prematurity). This results in fibrovascular proliferation, traction, exudation, and retinal detachment.

Retinal dysplasia may occur in isolation but is usually part of a syndrome such as Edward, Patau, Norrie, or Warburg syndrome or incontinentia pigmenti. Severe forms present with bilateral leukocoria and very poor vision.

Macular hypoplasia may occur in isolation or with syndromes such as albinism or aniridia. There is variable loss of the normal foveal reflex and in some cases, loss of the avascular zone.

Nasolacrimal duct

Cannulation of the nasolacrimal cord may be delayed distally, resulting in congenital obstruction. More commonly, there is simply an imperforate mucosal membrane at the valve of Hasner, which opens within the first year of life.

Overall, 90% spontaneously resolve by 1 year of age. In those that persist, a probing and irrigation carries a 90% success rate (see Box 18.2). In older children or those with more complex pathology, intubation or balloon dacryoplasty (using Lacricath®) should be considered as the primary procedure. Where blockage is sufficient to prevent the passage of the probe, a DCR is usually required.

Box 18.2 Outline of syringe and probe for congenital nasolacrimal obstruction

- Anesthesia (usually GA)
- Introduce nasolacrimal cannula into the lower or upper canaliculus.
- Inject fluorescein-stained saline solution to confirm nasolacrimal obstruction.
- Pull the lower lid laterally and introduce probe into the inferior punctum and then medially to the sac.
- Turn the probe 90° so as to direct it inferiorly down the nasolacrimal duct to perforate membrane.
- Repeat syringing to confirm patency of nasolacrimal duct with recovery of fluorescein from the nose.

Hamartomas and choristomas

Hamartomas (congenital tumors of tissues normal to that location) include the common capillary hemangioma. These bright red tumors usually appear before 2 months of age, reach full size by 1 year, and involute by 6 years.

When located on the lid, they may obscure the visual axis or cause astigmatism, resulting in amblyopia. In these cases, treatment may be indicated (systemic steroids or propranolol; for the latter, cooperation with a pediatric cardiologist is mandatory).

Choristomas (congenital tumors of tissues abnormal to that location) include dermoids, which probably represent surface ectoderm trapped at lines of embryonic closure and suture lines. These are most commonly located on the superotemporal orbital rim but may extend deceptively far posteriorly.

Chromosomal syndromes

Trisomy syndromes

Down syndrome

Down syndrome (trisomy 21) is the most common autosomal trisomy, with an incidence of 1 in 650 live births. It is also the most common genetic cause of learning difficulties (see Table 18.29). Most cases arise by nondisjunction (94%), some by translocation (5%), and rarely by mosaicism (1%). Mosaic cases usually have a milder phenotype.

Edwards syndrome

Edwards syndrome (trisomy 18) (Table 18.30) is the second most common autosomal trisomy at 1: in 8000 live births. Life expectancy is <1 year.

Patau syndrome

Patau syndrome (trisomy 13) (Table 18.31) is the third most common autosomal trisomy at 1 in 14,000 live births. Life expectancy is <3 months.

Deletion syndromes

Turner syndrome

Turner syndrome (XO) (Table 18.32) occurs in 1 in 2000 live female births. Only half are XO (also known as 45, X), with 15% being mosaics and the remainder having partial deletions or other abnormalities. The Turner phenotype arises from X-linked genes that escape inactivation (e.g., the SHOX, short stature homeobox gene).

Other deletion syndromes

Although microdeletions are probably fairly common, macrodeletions other than Turner syndrome are rare. Syndromes with ophthalmic features include the cri-du-chat syndrome (5p-), DeGrouchy syndrome (18q-), and the 13q- deletion syndrome. Common features are hypertelorism and epicanthal folds. In addition, in 13q-, there is a significantly increased risk of retinoblastoma.

Table 18.29 Clinical features of Down syndrome

Ocular	• Mongoloid palpebral fissures, hypertelorism, epicanthic folds, ectropia, blepharoconjunctivitis
	• Myopia, astigmatism
	• Strabismus, nystagmus
	• Keratoconus, Brushfield spots, cataracts
	• Hypoplastic optic disc
Systemic	• Short stature, macroglossia, flat nasal bridge, broad hands, single palmar crease, clinodactyly, sandal-gap toes, hypotonia
	• Congenital heart disease (ASD, VSD), duodenal atresia, hypothyroidism, diabetes mellitus, ↑risk of leukemia
	• ↓IQ and early Alzheimer's dementia

Table 18.30 Clinical features of Edwards syndrome

Ocular	• Epicanthal folds, blepharophimosis, ptosis, hypertelorism
	• Microphthalmos, corneal opacities, congenital glaucoma, cataracts
	• Uveal colobomas
Systemic	• Failure to thrive
	• Small chin, low-set ears, overlapping fingers, rocker-bottom feet
	• Congenital heart defects, renal malformations

Table 18.31 Clinical features of Patau syndrome

Ocular	• Cyclopia, microphthalmos, colobomas
	• Corneal opacities, cataracts, intraocular cartilage, retinal dysplasia, optic nerve hypoplasia
Systemic	• Failure to thrive
	• Microcephaly, scalp defects, hernias, polydactyly
	• Congenital heart defects, renal malformations, apneas

Table 18.32 Clinical features of Turner syndrome

Ocular	• Antimongoloid palpebral fissures, epicanthus, ptosis, hypertelorism
	• Strabismus, convergence insufficiency
	• Cataracts
	• Male levels of X-linked recessive disease (e.g., red-green color blindness)
Systemic	• Neonatal lymphedema of hands and feet
	• Short stature, webbed neck, low posterior hairline, wide carrying angle, broad chest with apparent wide-spaced nipples
	• Congenital heart defects (notably coarctation of the aorta)
	• Primary gonadal failure
	• Normal IQ, sensorineural deafness, delayed motor skills

Metabolic and storage diseases (1)

Although individually these conditions are rare (or very rare), as a group they feature regularly in the pediatric clinic. The ophthalmologist has an important role in both the diagnostic process and the ongoing management of affected patients.

Table 18.33 Disorders of carbohydrate metabolism

Syndrome	Deficiency	Ocular features	Systemic features
Galactosemia	Galactose-1-phosphate uridyl transferase	Cataracts (oil droplet)	↓IQ Failure to thrive
Galactokinase deficiency	Galactokinase	Cataracts	Normal
Mannosidosis	α-mannosidase	Cataracts (spoke-like)	↓IQ MPS-like changes but clear corneas

All of the above conditions are autosomal recessive.

Table 18.34 Disorders of amino acid metabolism

Homocystinuria (I–III)	Cystathionine synthetase (I)	Ectopia lentis Myopia Glaucoma	↓IQ Marfanoid habitus Thromboses Fine, fair hair
Cystinosis	Lysosomal transport protein	Crystalline keratopathy	Renal failure Failure to thrive
Lowe syndrome	Phosphatidylinositol 4,5-bisphosphate 5-phosphatase deficiency	Microphakia Cataracts Blue sclera AS dysgenesis Glaucoma	↓IQ Failure to thrive Rickets (vitamin D resistant)
Zellweger syndrome	Peroxysome biogenesis (several genes)	Flat brows ON hypoplasia Pigmentary retinopathy Glaucoma	Dysgenesis of brain, liver and kidneys Metabolic acidosis
Albinism	p. 464	p. 464	p. 464
Alkaptonuria	Homogentisic acid dioxygenase	Scleral darkening	Ochronosis Arthritis
Sulfite oxidase deficiency	Molybdenum cofactor	Spherophakia Ectopia lentis	Neurodegeneration LE <2 years
Tyrosinemia (II)	Tyrosine transaminase	Herpetiform corneal ulcers	↓IQ (some) Hyperkeratosis of palms and soles
Gyrate atrophy	Ornithine 5-aminotransferase	p. 462	p. 462

All of the above conditions are autosomal recessive, except for Lowe's syndrome and ocular albinism, which are X-linked. LE, life expectancy.

Table 18.35 Disorders of lipid metabolism

Syndrome	Deficiency	Ocular features	Systemic features
Lipoproteins			
Abetalipo-proteinemia	Triglyceride transfer protein	Cataract Pigmentary retinopathy	Spinocerebellar degeneration LE <50 years
Sphingolipids			
G$_{M1}$ gangliosidosis	β-galactosidase	Cloudy cornea Cherry-red spot Optic atrophy	Neurodegeneration (types 1 and 2) Visceromegaly (1) LE 1 <4 years LE 2 <40 years
Tay–Sachs disease	Hexosaminidase A	Cherry-red spot Optic atrophy	Visceromegaly LE <3 years
Sandhoff disease	Hexosaminidase A Hexosaminidase B	Cherry-red spot Optic atrophy	Visceromegaly Neurodegeneration LE <3 years
Gaucher's disease (I–III)	β-glucosidase	Supranuclear gaze palsy (type IIIb)	Visceromegaly ± neurodegeneration LE I (old), II (2), III (15)
Niemann–Pick (type A) disease	Sphingomyelinase	Cherry-red spot Optic atrophy	Visceromegaly Neurodegeneration LE <3 years
Fabry disease	α-galactosidase	Vortex kerat- opathy Cataract Tortuous vessels	Angiokeratomas Painful episodes Renal failure Vascular disease LE = middle age
Metachromatic leukodystrophy	Arylsulphatase-A	Optic atrophy Nystagmus	Neurodegeneration LE α-type
Krabbe disease	Galacto-cerebrosidase	Optic atrophy	Neurodegeneration LE α-type
Farber disease	Ceramidase	Macular pigmentation	Granulomas Arthopathy
Other			
Neuronal ceroid lipofuscinosis (Batten disease)	Unknown	Macular discoloration RP-like changes Optic atrophy	Neurodegeneration LE α-type
Refsum syndrome	Phytanic acid α-hydrolase	Pigmentary retinopathy	Neuropathy Ataxia Deafness Ichthyosis

All of the above conditions are autosomal recessive, except for Fabry disease, which is X-linked. LE, life expectancy.

Metabolic and storage diseases (2)

Table 18.36 Disorders of glycosaminoglycan metabolism (mucopolysaccharidoses)

Syndrome	Deficiency	Ocular features	Systemic features
MPSI (Hurler/ Scheie/ Hurler–Scheie)	α-iduronidase	Cloudy cornea Pigmentary retinopathy Optic atrophy	Skeletal/facial dysmorphism ↓IQ Severity α-type: H > H/S > S
MPSII (Hunter)	Iduronate sulphatase	Pigmentary retinopathy Optic atrophy	Variable ↓IQ and dysmorphism
MPSIII (A-C) (Sanfillipo)	Heparan-N-sulphatase (A)	Pigmentary retinopathy Optic atrophy	Neurodegeneration Hyperactivity Mild dysmorphism
MPSIV (A-B) (Morquio)	Galactose-6-sulphatase (A)	Cloudy cornea	Skeletal dysplasia Normal facies/IQ
MPSVI (Maroteaux-Lamy)	N-acetyl-galactosamine-4-sulfatase	Cloudy cornea	Skeletal/facial dysmorphism Normal IQ
MPSVII (Sly)	β-glucuronidase	Cloudy cornea	Skeletal/facial dysmorphism ↓IQ

All of the above conditions are autosomal recessive, other than Hunter's, which is X-linked.

Table 18.37 Disorders of mineral metabolism

Wilson disease	Cu binding protein	Kayser–Fleischer ring Cataract	Neurodenereation Ataxia
Menkes syndrome	Cu transport protein	Optic atrophy	Kinky hair Neurodegeneration Ataxia

The above conditions are autosomal recessive.

Table 18.38 Disorders of connective tissues

Syndrome	Deficiency	Ocular features	Systemic features
Marfan syndrome	Fibrillin	Ectopia lentis glaucoma Blue sclera Keratoconus	Long-limbed arachnodactyly High-arched palate aortic dissection
Osteogenesis imperfecta	Collagen I	Blue sclera Keratoconus	Brittle bones
Stickler syndrome	Collagen II	Myopia Liquefied vitreous Retinal detachments	Arthropathy Midfacial flattening Cleft palate
Ehlers–Danlos syndrome (>10 types)	Collagens I and III	Blue sclera Keratoconus Angioid streaks	Hyperflexible joints Hyperelastic skin Vascular bleeds
Pseudoxanthoma elasticum	Elastin fragility	Angioid streaks	"Chicken" skin GI bleeds
Weill–Marchesani syndrome		Ectopia lentis microspherophakia	Short stature brachydactyly ↓IQ

Marfan's, and Stickler's are autosomal dominant; Weill–Marchesani is autosomal recessive; Ehlers–Danlos, pseudoxanthoma elasticum, and osteogenesis imperfecta have dominant and recessive forms.

Phakomatoses

The phakomatoses are a group of conditions with neurological, ocular, and cutaneous features and a tendency to develop tumors, usually of a hamartomatous type. There is considerable debate about which conditions to include, but neurofibromatosis, tuberous sclerosis, and von Hippel–Lindau syndrome are generally considered to be the archetypes.

Neurofibromatosis

Neurofibromatosis-1 (Table 18.39) is the most common of all the phakomatoses (prevalence 1/4000) and arises from mutations in the neurofibromin gene (Ch17q). Neurofibromatosis-2 (Table 18.40) is much less common (1/40,000) and the gene has been located to Ch22q. Both are autosomal dominant but with variable expressivity.

Tuberous sclerosis (TS)

Tuberous sclerosis (Table 18.41) has a prevalence of 1/6000. It arises from mutations in TSC1 (Ch9q) or TSC2 (Ch16p), which code for hamartin and tuberin respectively. It is autosomal dominant with variable expressivity; however, 50% of cases of TS are from new mutations.

Table 18.39 Features of neurofibromatosis-1

Ocular	Systemic
Optic nerve glioma*	Café-au-lait spots (≥6; each >0.5 cm pre-puberty or >1.5 cm post-puberty)*
Lisch nodules (≥ 2)*	
Lid neurofibroma	Axillary/inguinal freckling*
Choroidal nevi	Neurofibromas (≥1 plexiform type or ≥2 any type)*
Retinal astrocytoma	
	Characteristic bony lesion (sphenoid dysplasia which may →pulsatile proptosis; long bone cortex thinning/dysplasia)*
	First-degree relative with NF-1*

Diagnosis requires two or more of the features with asterisk (*).

Table 18.40 Features of neurofibromatosis-2

Ocular	Systemic
Early-onset posterior subcapsular or cortical cataracts	Acoustic neuroma
Combined hamartoma of RPE and retina	Meningioma
	Glioma
	Schwannoma
	First-degree relative with NF-2

- *Definite NF-2:* bilateral acoustic neuroma OR first-degree relative with NF-2 AND either unilateral acoustic neuroma (at <30 years) or two of the other diagnostic features.
- *Probable NF-2:* unilateral acoustic neuroma (at <30 years) AND one of the other diagnostic features; OR multiple meningiomas AND one of the other diagnostic features.

Von Hippel–Lindau syndrome

This rare condition (Table 18.42) arises from mutations in the *VHL* gene (Ch3p), which appears to be involved in vascular proliferation.

Sturge–Weber and Wyburn–Mason syndrome

These rare syndromes of vascular abnormalities differ from the above "true" phakomatoses in that they occur sporadically and the tumors (or AV malformations for Wyburn–Mason) are present from birth (see Tables 18.43 and 18.44).

Table 18.41 Features of tuberous sclerosis

Ocular	Systemic
Retinal astrocytoma, glaucoma	Adenoma sebaceum
	Ash-leaf spots
	Shagreen patches
	Subungual fibromas
	Cerebral astrocytomas (with epilepsy and ↓IQ)
	Visceral hamartomas (e.g., renal angiomyolipoma, cardiac rhabdomyoma)
	Visceral cysts
	Pulmonary lymphangioleiomyomatosis

Table 18.42 Features of von Hippel–Lindau syndrome

Ocular	Systemic
Retinal capillary hemangioma	Hemangioblastoma of cerebellum, spinal cord or brainstem
	Renal cell carcinoma
	Pheochromocytoma
	Islet cell carcinoma
	Epididymal cysts/adenomas
	Visceral cysts

Table 18.43 Features of Sturge–Weber syndrome

Ocular	Systemic
Episcleral hemangioma	Nevus flammeus of the face (port wine stain)
Ciliary body/iris hemangioma	CNS hemangioma
Choroidal hemangioma (diffuse)	
Glaucoma	

Table 18.44 Features of Wyburn–Mason syndrome

Ocular	Systemic
Retinal AVM	Cerebral/brainstem AVM
Orbital/periorbital AVM	

Aids to diagnosis

Acute red eye

Normal/near normal vision

Painful/discomfort

Diffuse superficial redness

- *Conjunctivitis:* infective, allergic, or chemical; gritty/itchy; watery, mucoid, mucopurulent, or purulent exudate; papillae or follicles.

Diffuse deep redness

- *Anterior scleritis:* severe pain; diffuse deep injection that does not blanch with vasoconstrictors (e.g., phenylephrine 10%), scleral edema; scleral thinning; lid edema; globe tenderness, pain with eye movement.

Circumlimbal redness

- *Keratitis:* photophobia, watery eye, circumlimbal injection, corneal infiltrate ± epithelial defect ± AC activity.
- *Anterior uveitis:* photophobia, watery eye, keratic precipitates, AC activity, ± posterior synechiae.
- *Corneal foreign body:* appropriate history, FB sensation, visible FB, rust ring.

Sectoral redness

- *Episcleritis:* mild discomfort; may be recurrent; sectoral (occasionally diffuse) redness that blanches with topical vasoconstrictor (e.g., phenylephrine 10%); globe nontender.
- *Marginal keratitis:* photophobia, watery eye, marginal corneal infiltrate ± epithelial defect in large persistent keratitis.

Painless

- *Subconjunctival hemorrhage:* well-defined confluent area of hemorrhage

Reduced vision

Normal IOP

Abnormal corneosclera

- *Corneal abrasion:* photophobia, watery eye, sectoral/circumlimbal injection, epithelial defect.
- *Keratitis:* photophobia, watery eye, circumlimbal injection, corneal infiltrate ± epithelial defect ± AC activity ± mucopurulent discharge.

Abnormal uvea

- *Anterior uveitis:* photophobia, watery eye, keratic precipitates, AC activity, ± posterior synechiae.
- *Endophthalmitis:* pain, floaters, watery eye, diffuse deep injection, inflammation (vitreous > AC), chorioretinitis, hypopyon.

↑IOP

- *Acute glaucoma:* usually due to angle closure; photophobia, watery eye, corneal edema, ± anterior segment/angle abnormalities such as rubeosis
- *Hypertensive uveitis:* anterior chamber cells and flare ± corneal involvement; often due to herpes group of viruses with sectoral iris atrophy.

Sudden or recent loss of vision

Painless

Few seconds duration

Unilateral

- *Giant cell arteritis:* usually age >55 years, weight loss, fatigue, jaw or tongue claudication, pulseless, tender, or thickened temporal artery, raised ESR, CRP.
- *Papilledema:* bilateral optic disc swelling, loss of spontaneous venous pulsation (SVP), peripapillary hemorrhages, features of raised ICP.
- *Impending central retinal vein occlusion:* dilated, tortuous retinal veins, hemorrhages.
- *Ocular ischemic syndrome:* veins dilated and irregular but not tortuous, midperipheral hemorrhages; ± NVD, ↓IOP, carotid bruits.

Bilateral

- *Papilledema:* see above.

Few minutes duration

Unilateral

- *Amaurosis fugax:* curtain across vision ± evidence of emboli, atrial fibrillation, carotid bruits.
- *Giant cell arteritis:* see above.

Bilateral

- *Vertebrobasilar artery insufficiency:* recurrent episodes ± ataxia, dysphasia, dysarthria, hemiparesis, hemisensory disturbance.

Up to 1 hour duration

- *Migraine:* fortification spectra, transient VF defects, unilateral headache, nausea/vomiting, photophobia, aura, family history.

Persistent

Abnormal cornea

- *Hydrops:* acute corneal edema associated with underlying disease such as keratoconus.

Abnormal vitreous

- *Vitreous hemorrhage:* varies from microscopic level to completely obscuring the fundus.

Abnormal fundus

- *Central retinal artery occlusion:* RAPD, attenuated arterioles, box carring of retina vessels, pale fundus, cherry-red spot.
- *Central retinal vein occlusion:* dilated tortuous veins, hemorrhages in all four quadrants, ± cotton wool spots, retinal edema, RAPD. Branch retinal vein occlusions may give symptomatic altitudinal defects, particularly if on temporal arcade.
- *Rhegmatogenous retinal detachment:* flashes/floaters, tobacco dust, corrugated elevated retina with (multiple) break(s).

- *Exudative retinal detachment:* convex elevated retina with shifting fluid, no break; tractional: concave elevated retina with tractional membranes.
- *Intermediate uveitis:* floaters, vitritis, snowballs/banking ± macular edema, optic nerve edema.
- *Posterior uveitis:* floaters, significantly reduced vision; vitritis, retinal/choroidal infiltrates, macular edema, vascular sheathing or occlusion, hemorrhages.

Abnormal optic disc
- *Anterior ischemic optic neuropathy:* RAPD, pale edematous disc ± flame-shaped hemorrhages; may have altitudinal field defect; may be arteritic (with signs of giant cell arteritis) or nonarteritic (usually sectoral).

Abnormal macula
- *Choroidal neovascular membrane:* distortion ± positive scotoma, drusen, subretinal membrane ± hemorrhage, exudate.
- *Central serous retinopathy:* color desaturation, micropsia, serous detachment of neurosensory retina.

Normal fundus
- *Cortical blindness:* ± denial, small residual field; normal pupil reactions; abnormal CT/MRI head.
- *Functional:* inconsistent acuity between different tests and at different times, normal ophthalmic examination, normal electrodiagnostic tests.

Painful

Abnormal cornea
- *Acute angle closure glaucoma:* usually hypermetropic, halos, frontal headache, vomiting; injected, corneal edema, fixed semidilated pupil, shallow anterior chamber with closed angle, raised IOP.
- *Bullous keratopathy:* thickened, hazy cornea, stromal or subepithelial edema, bullae, evidence of underlying pathology (e.g., ACIOL, Fuchs' endothelial dystrophy).
- *Keratitis:* photophobia, watery eye, circumlimbal injection, corneal infiltrate ± epithelial defect ± AC activity.

Abnormal optic disc
- *Optic neuritis:* usually age 18–45 years, with retro-orbital pain, especially on eye movement, RAPD, reduced color vision, visual field defects, swollen optic disc ± peripapillary flame-shaped hemorrhages. It may also be painless.

Abnormal uvea
- *Anterior uveitis:* anterior: pain, photophobia, mildly reduced vision, circumlimbal injection, anterior chamber cells and flare, keratic precipitates.

Normal fundus
- *Retrobulbar neuritis:* as for optic neuritis but with a normal optic disc. It may also be painless.

Gradual loss of vision

Generalized

Abnormal cornea

- *Corneal dystrophies:* corneal clouding (deposition/edema); usually bilateral but may be asymmetric. Common types include Fuchs' endothelial dystrophy in the elderly, and Reis–Buckler's dystrophy in young adults.
- *Keratoconus:* refractive error from progressive astigmatism; corneal edema and scar from acute hydrops; usually bilateral but may be asymmetric.

Abnormal lens

- *Cataract:* uni- or bilateral opacification of the lens; cloudy, misty; glare. This is most common in the elderly.

Central

Abnormal macula

Macular disease usually leads to distortion ± micropsia and early ↓VA; pupillary responses and color vision are relatively preserved. Common causes include the following:

- *Age-related macular degeneration:* very common bilateral disease of the elderly. The most common type involves dry changes, which are associated with gradual patchy central loss.
- *Macular dystrophies:* group of diseases with specific patterns occurring in younger age group; bilateral disease. Patients may have a family history of it, and genetic testing is sometimes possible.
- *Diabetic maculopathy:* ischemia may lead to gradual ↓VA; edema may lead to more acute distortion/↓VA. It is associated with other diabetic changes.
- *Cystoid macular edema:* edema resulting in distortion/↓VA may be associated with surgery, inflammation, or vascular disease.

Abnormal optic disc or nerve

Optic nerve disease usually leads to dimness and darkening of colors. Although commonly affecting central vision, it may lead to peripheral or generalized loss of vision. Pupillary responses, color vision, and brightness testing are all reduced. Important causes include the following:

- *Compressive optic neuropathy:* progressive ↓VA, optic disc pallor ± pain, involvement of other local structures.
- *Leber's hereditary optic neuropathy:* severe sequential ↓VA over weeks or months, telangiectatic vessels around disc (acutely); usually young adult males; family history mitochondrial inheritance.
- *Toxic or nutritional optic neuropathies:* slowly progressive symmetrical ↓VA with central scotomas; relevant nutritional, therapeutic, or toxic history.

- *Inflammatory optic neuropathies:* associated with systemic disease (e.g., sarcoid, vasculitis, and syphilis). They are often very steroid sensitive.
- *Chronic papilledema:* sustained optic disc swelling due to raised intracranial pressure may cause permanent optic nerve dysfunction, including ↓VA and field defects, and optic disc pallor.

Peripheral or patchy

Abnormal choroid/retina
- *Posterior uveitis:* floaters, patchy loss of vision ± central distortion/↓VA from CME; may include chorioretinitis, vitritis, retinal vasculitis.
- *Retinitis pigmentosa:* bilateral concentric peripheral field loss, peripheral "bone-spicule" pigmentation, retinal arteriole attenuation, and optic disc pallor.

Abnormal optic disc
- *Glaucoma:* asymptomatic peripheral field loss; usually bilateral but often asymmetric; characteristic optic disc cupping and other disc changes; often associated with ↑IOP.

The watery eye

Increased tear production

Basal increase
- *Increased parasympathetic drive:* from prosecretory drugs (e.g., pilocarpine) or autonomic disturbance.

Reflex increase
- *Local irritants:* e.g., foreign bodies, trichiasis.
- *Chronic ocular disease:* e.g., blepharitis, keratoconjunctivitis sicca.
- *Systemic disease:* e.g., thyroid eye disease.

Lacrimal pump failure

Lid tone
- *Lid laxity:* common involutional change in the elderly.
- *Orbicularis weakness:* associated with CN VII palsy.

Lid position
- *Ectropion:* most commonly an involutional change in the elderly but may also be cicatricial, mechanical, or congenital.

Decreased drainage

Punctal obstruction
- *Congenital:* punctal atresia.
- *Acquired:* punctal stenosis is most commonly idiopathic but may arise secondary to punctal eversion, post-HSV infection, or with any scarring process (e.g., post-irradiation, trachoma, cicatricial conjunctivitis).

Canalicular obstruction
- *Acquired:* canalicular fibrosis is most commonly idiopathic but may arise secondary to HSV infection, chronic canaliculitis (usually actinomycosis), chronic dacrocystitis, cicatricial conjunctivitis, and 5-FU administration.

Nasolacrimal duct obstruction
- *Congenital:* delayed canalization.
- *Acquired:* stenosis is most commonly idiopathic but may arise secondary to trauma (nasal or orbital fracture), post-irradiation, Wegener's granulomatosis, tumors (e.g., nasopharyngeal carcinoma), and other nasal pathology (chronic inflammation or polyps).

Flashes and floaters

Flashes only

Retinal traction
This involves vitreoretinal traction, proliferative diabetic retinopathy, sickle cell retinopathy, and retinopathy of prematurity.

Pseudoflashes
Ocular
- *Photophobia:* discomfort commonly associated with anterior segment inflammation or retinal hypersensitivity.
- *Glare:* visual symptom commonly associated with media opacities.
- *Halos:* ring effect associated with corneal edema and some media opacities.

CNS
- *Papilledema:* transient, associated with straining or change in posture.
- *Migraine:* classic enlarging zig-zag fortification spectra moving central to peripheral, usually followed by headache.
- *Occipital lobe lesions* (tumors, AVMs): colored shapes and blobs.
- *Other visual hallucinations:* bilateral severe visual loss may result in more complex visual hallucinations (Charles Bonnet syndrome).

Floaters only
- *Posterior vitreous detachment:* partial or complete Weiss ring overlying the optic disc ± visible posterior vitreous face.
- *Vitreous condensations:* degenerative changes within the vitreous lead to translucent opacities.
- *Vitreous hemorrhage:* red cells in the vitreous, varies from minor bleed (spots in vision, fundus easily visualized) to severe (profound ↓VA, no fundus view); may be followed by synchysis scintillans (golden particles that settle with gravity).
- *Vitritis:* white cells in the vitreous, may be bilateral and associated with features of intermediate or posterior uveitis.
- *Asteroid hyalosis:* small yellow-white particles that move with the vitreous (rather than settling with gravity), usually innocuous.
- *Amyloidosis:* sheet-like opacities, usually bilateral; most commonly seen with familial systemic amyloidosis.
- *Tumors* (e.g., choroidal melanoma, lymphoma): vitritis of inflammatory and/or tumor cells may be seen.

Flashes and floaters
- *Posterior vitreous detachment:* partial or complete Weiss ring overlying the optic disc ± visible posterior vitreous face.
- *Retinal tear:* usually horseshoe tear and pigment in the vitreous. It may be associated with vitreous hemorrhage or retinal detachment.
- *Retinal detachment:* usually rhegmatogenous (associated with a tear) resulting in elevated retina with subretinal fluid.
- *Tumors:* visual phenomena include slow moving ball of light and floaters secondary to tumor cells or inflammation associated with a choroidal or retinal mass.

Headache

Swollen optic discs

Bilateral

Serious or life-threatening headaches

- *Raised intracranial pressure:* worsening headache on lying flat, coughing, sneezing, or Valsalva maneuver; visual obscurations; diplopia, disc swelling with loss of SVP; blind spot enlargement; CN VI palsy. Causes include the following:
  - Cerebral tumor, idiopathic intracranial hypertension, venous sinus thrombosis, meningitis, encephalitis, brain abscess, congenital ventricular abnormalities, cerebral edema.
  - Subarachnoid hemorrhage: thunderclap headache, meningismus, altered consciousness.
- *Accelerated hypertension:* hypertensive retinopathy including cotton-wool spots (CWS), retinal hemorrhages, exudates, optic nerve edema, arterial occlusion and capillary closure.

Unilateral

Serious or life-threatening headaches

- *Giant cell arteritis:* usually age >55 years; visual loss, scalp tenderness (± necrosis), jaw or tongue claudication, limb girdle pain and weakness, fevers, weight loss; nonpulsatile, tender, thickened temporal arteries. AION results in unilateral or, less commonly, bilateral optic disc swelling.

No optic disc swelling

Serious or life-threatening headaches

- *Raised intracranial pressure* may occur in the presence of nonswollen discs (e.g., myopic discs, atrophic discs, anomalies of the optic nerve sheath).
- Giant cell arteritis: see above.
- Pituitary adenoma: endocrine dysfunction (amenorrhea, galactorrhea, infertility, acromegaly, Cushing's disease; optic atrophy; bitemporal field loss).
- Pituitary apoplexy: recent major hypotensive episode (e.g., surgery, postpartum hemorrhage); acute ↓VA, meningism, ↓LOC.

Headache syndrome

- *Tension headache:* very common; tightness, bifrontal, bioccipital, or band-like; may radiate to neck; headache-free intervals; no neurological or systemic features. This may be associated with cervical spondylosis.
- *Migraine:* common; prodrome, headache (usually hemicranial), nausea, photophobia, phonophobia. Visual phenomena include scintillating visual aura (starts paracentral and expands as it moves peripherally), transient visual loss (unilateral or homonymous hemifield), or ophthalmoplegia.
- *Cluster headache:* sudden oculotemporal pain, no prodrome, may have transient lacrimation, rhinorrhea, and Horner's syndrome.

Facial pain
- *Trigeminal neuralgia:* sudden stabbing pains in trigeminal branch distribution. Precipitants include touch, cold, and eating.
- *Ophthalmic shingles:* hyperesthesia in acute phase followed by neuralgic-type pain.

Sinus pain
- *Acute sinusitis:* coryza or upper respiratory tract infection (URTI) symptoms, tender over paranasal sinuses. Proptosis, diplopia, or optic neuropathy warrants urgent exclusion of orbital involvement.

Ocular pain
- *Generalized:* includes acute-angle closure glaucoma, anterior uveitis, keratitis, scleritis, ocular ischemia.
- *Retrobulbar:* includes optic neuritis, orbital pathology (e.g., infection, infiltration, neoplasm, thyroid eye disease).
- *On eye movement:* includes optic neuritis and posterior scleritis.

Asthenopia (eyestrain)
- Usually worsens with reading or fatigue; ametropia (especially hypermetropia), astigmatism, anisometropia, decompensating phoria, convergence insufficiency, etc.

Diplopia

Monocular

Abnormal refraction

- *High ametropia, astigmatism, or edge effect* from corrective lenses: usually correctable with appropriate refraction. Contact lenses may be more effective than glasses.

Abnormal cornea

- *Opacity:* associated with scarring (e.g., trauma, infection), edema (e.g., ↑IOP, decompensation), deposition (e.g., corneal dystrophies).
- *Shape:* peripheral thinning associated with ectasias (e.g., keratoconus), peripheral ulcerative keratitis, and other marginal disease.

Abnormal lens

- *Opacity:* cataract.
- *Shape:* lenticonus.
- *Position:* subluxation of lens (ectopia lentis) or implant (especially if complicated surgery).

Abnormal iris

- *Defect:* polycoria due to trauma (e.g., IOFB), peripheral iridotomy (laser or surgical), or disease (e.g., ICE syndrome).

Normal examination

- *Not diplopia:* "double vision" may be used by the patient to describe other visual anomalies (e.g., ghosting or blurring).
- *Functional:* this is a diagnosis of exclusion.

Binocular

Intermittent or variable

- *Decompensating phoria:* intermittent but usually predictable (e.g., when fatigued) with a constant pattern (e.g., only for distance, only horizontal); underlying phoria with variable to poor recovery.
- *Myasthenia gravis:* intermittent diplopia of variable orientation and severity that worsens with fatigue. It may be associated with ptosis progressive generalized muscular fatigue.
- *Internuclear ophthalmoplegia:* diplopia may only be noticed during saccades when the adducting eye is slower to refixate.
- *Giant cell arteritis:* intermittent diplopia may occur due to ischemia; may progress to become permanent.

Persistent

Neurogenic

In neurogenic lesions, the diplopia is worst when looking in the direction of the paretic muscle(s). Saccades are slowed in this direction; full sequelae will evolve with time. Forced duction test shows normal passive movements.

- *Horizontal only:* typically CN VI palsy → underaction of LR → ipsilateral reduced abduction ± convergent.

- *Vertical/torsional only:* typically, CN IV palsy with underaction of SO with ipsilateral hypertropia, extorsion, and reduced depression in adducted position.
- *Mixed ± ptosis/pupillary abnormalities:* typically, CN III palsy with underaction of any or all of LPS, SR, MR, IR, IO, and sphincter pupillae, resulting in anything from single-muscle involvement (rare) to complete ptosis obscuring a hypotropic divergent eye.
- *Complex:* unusual patterns may be due to brainstem lesions causing nuclear or supranuclear gaze palsies (often associated with other neurological signs), orbital pathology, or disorders of the neuromuscular junction (e.g., myasthenia gravis).

Mechanical

In mechanical lesions, the diplopia is worst when looking away from the restricted muscle(s); signs of restriction may include IOP increase, globe retraction, and pain when looking away from the restricted muscle(s). Ductions and versions are equally reduced but saccades are of normal speed. Sequelae are limited to underaction of contralateral synergist. Forced duction test shows restriction of passive movements.

- *Congenital:* these rarely give rise to diplopia unless progressive or decompensating.
- *Acquired:* associated with inflammation (e.g., thyroid eye disease, myositis, idiopathic orbital inflammatory disease), trauma (orbital wall/floor fracture), or infiltration.

Anisocoria

Anisocoria greatest in bright light

This implies that the larger pupil is the abnormal one.

Abnormal iris appearance (slit-lamp examination)

Vermiform movements

- *Adie's pupil:* pupil is initially dilated, later abnormally constricted. Response to light is poor, response to near is initially poor, later tonic (exaggerated but slow), i.e., there is light-near dissociation. It will constrict with 0.1% pilocarpine because of denervation hypersensitivity.

Structural damage

- *Iris trauma:* dilated pupil (often irregular) due to a torn sphincter with associated anterior segment damage (e.g., transillumination defects).
- *Iris inflammation:* dilated pupil (often irregular) due to sectoral iris atrophy (typically with herpes group of viruses) or stuck down by posterior synechiae.

Normal iris appearance

Constricts to pilocarpine 1%

- *Third nerve palsy:* dilated pupil associated with other features of a CN III palsy (e.g., ptosis, oculomotor abnormality). It will constrict with 1% pilocarpine.

Does not constrict to pilocarpine 1%

- *Pharmacological:* dilated pupil resulting from anticholiergic mydriatics such as atropine (rather than adrenergics).
- *Iris ischemia:* dilated pupil occurring after angle-closure glaucoma or intraocular surgery (e.g., Urrets–Zavalia syndrome).

Anisocoria greatest in dim light

This implies that the smaller pupil is the abnormal one.

Abnormal iris appearance (slit-lamp examination)

Structural damage

- *Iris inflammation:* constricted pupil (may be irregular) stuck down by posterior synechiae.

Normal iris appearance

Dilates at normal speed in dim light

Both pupils dilate equally quickly when ambient light is dimmed.

- *Physiological anisocoria:* anisocoria is usually mild (≤1 mm) and only marginally worse in dim rather than bright light. Responses to light and near are normal. The degree of anisocoria varies from day to day and may reverse; pupil will dilate with 4% cocaine (cf. Horner's syndrome).

Dilates in dim light but slowly (i.e., dilatation lag)

The smaller pupil is slower to dilate when ambient light is dimmed.

- *Horner's syndrome:* constricted pupil, with mild ptosis. Iris hypochromia suggests congenital or very long-standing lesion; confirm with 4% cocaine test (a Horner's pupil will not dilate).

Dilates with hydroxyamphetamine 1%
- *Central or preganglionic Horner's syndrome:* constricted pupil, mild ptosis, facial anhidrosis; may have other features related to level of lesion (brainstem, spinal cord, lung apex, neck).

Does not dilate with hydroxyamphetamine 1%
- *Postganglionic Horner's syndrome:* constricted pupil, mild ptosis; may have other features related to level of lesion (neck, cavernous sinus, orbit).

Does not dilate in dim light
- *Pharmacological:* constricted pupil may be due to cholinergic miotics, such as pilocarpine.

Nystagmus

Early onset

Horizontal jerk

- *Idiopathic congenital:* very early onset (usually by 2 months of age); worsens with fixation; improves within null zone and on convergence; mild ↓VA.
- *Manifest latent:* fast phase toward fixing eye; worsens with occlusion of nonfixing eye, and with gaze toward fast phase; alternates if opposite eye takes up fixation; often associated with infantile esotropia.

Erratic

- *Sensory deprivation:* erratic waveform ± roving eye movements; moderate to severe ↓VA due to ocular or anterior visual pathway disease.

Late onset

Conjugate

Present in primary position

Sustained

- *Peripheral vestibular:* conjugate horizontal jerk nystagmus, improves with fixation and, with time, since injury; worsens with gaze toward fast phase (Alexander's law) or change in head position.
- *Cerebellar, central vestibular, or brainstem:* conjugate jerk nystagmus that does not improve with fixation. It may be horizontal, vertical, or torsional:
  - *Horizontal type:* e.g., lesions of the vestibular nuclei, the cerebellum, or their connections.
  - *Upbeat type:* usually cerebellar or lower brainstem lesions (e.g., demyelination, infarction, tumor, encephalitis, Wernicke's syndrome).
  - *Downbeat type:* usually craniocervical junction lesions, (e.g., Arnold–Chiari malformation, spinocerebellar degenerations, infarction, tumor, demyelination).

Periodic

Periodic alternating: conjugate horizontal jerk nystagmus with waxing–waning nystagmus; 90 sec in each direction with a 10 sec null period; usually associated with vestibulocerebellar lesions.

Present only in eccentric gaze

Gaze evoked nystagmus (GEN): conjugate horizontal jerk nystagmus on eccentric gaze with fast phase toward direction of gaze.

- *Asymmetric type:* evoked nystagmus usually indicates failure of ipsilateral neural integrator or cerebellar dysfunction.
- *Symmetric type:* due to CNS depression (e.g., fatigue, alcohol, anticonvulsants, barbiturates) or structural pathology (e.g., brainstem, cerebellum).

Disconjugate
Unilateral
- *Internuclear ophthalmoplegia:* nystagmus of the abducting (and occasionally adducting) eye.
- *Superior oblique myokymia:* unilateral high-frequency and low-amplitude torsional nystagmus.

Bilateral
- *See-saw nystagmus:* vertical and torsional components with one eye elevating and intorting while the other depresses and extorts; slow pendular or jerk waveform.
- *Acquired pendular nystagmus:* usually disconjugate with horizontal, vertical, and torsional components; may be associated with involuntary repetitive movement of palate, pharynx, and face.

Ophthalmic signs: external

The patient

Consider the whole patient. Simple observation of the patient provides a vast amount of additional information and should be performed in all cases. Observe that the patient with juvenile cataracts and ↑IOP has severe facial eczema—he/she may not have thought to mention their topical corticosteroids when asked about their medication.

Note the rheumatoid hands of the patient in whom scleritis is suspected. Such information will also help with management (e.g., patient needs assistance with topical medication). Further hands-on systemic examination is directed according to clinical presentation.

Globe

Table 19.1 Ophthalmic signs—the globe

Sign	Causes
Proptosis	• Infection: orbital cellulitis
	• Inflammation: thyroid eye disease, idiopathic orbital inflammatory disease, systemic vasculitis (e.g., Wegener's granulomatosis)
	• Tumors: capillary hemangioma, lymphangioma, optic nerve glioma, myeloid leukemia, histiocytosis, dermoid cyst
	• Vascular anomalies: orbital varices, carotid–cavernous fistula
	• Pseudoproptosis: ipsilateral large globe or lid retraction; contralateral enophthalmos or ptosis; facial asymmetry
Enophthalmos	• Small globe: microphthalmos, nanophthalmos, phthisis bulbi, orbital implant
	• Soft tissue atrophy: post-irradiation, scleroderma, cicatrizing tumors
	• Bony defects: orbital fractures, congenital orbital wall defects

Lymph nodes

Table 19.2 Ophthalmic signs—lymph nodes

Sign	Causes
Enlarged preauricular lymph node	• Infection: viral conjunctivitis, chlamydial conjunctivitis, gonococcal conjunctivitis, Parinaud oculoglandular syndrome
	• Infiltration: lymphoma

Lids

Table 19.3 Ophthalmic signs—lids

Sign	Causes
Madarosis	• Local: cicatrizing conjunctivitis, iatrogenic (cryotherapy, radiotherapy, surgery) • Systemic: alopecia (patchy, totalis, universalis), psoriasis, hypothyroidism, leprosy
Poliosis	• Local: chronic lid margin disease • Systemic: sympathetic ophthalmia, Vogt–Koyanagi–Harada syndrome, Waardenburg syndrome
Lid lump	• Anterior lamella: external hordeolum, cyst of Moll, cyst of Zeis, xanthelasma, papilloma, seborrheic keratosis, keratoacanthoma, nevi, capillary hemangioma, actinic keratosis, basal cell carcinoma, squamous cell carcinoma, malignant melanoma, Kaposi's sarcoma • Posterior lamella: internal hordeolum, chalazion, pyogenic granuloma, sebaceous gland carcinoma
Ectropion	• Involutional, cicatricial, mechanical, paralytic (CN VII palsy), congenital
Entropion	• Involutional, cicatricial, congenital
Ptosis	• True ptosis: Involutional, neurogenic (CN III palsy, Horner's syndrome), myasthenic, myopathic (CPEO group), mechanical, congenital • Pseudoptosis: brow ptosis, dermatochalasis, microphthalmos, phthisis, prosthesis, enophthalmos, hypotropia, contralateral lid retraction
Lid retraction	• Congenital: Down syndrome, Duane syndrome • Acquired: thyroid eye disease, uraemia, CN VII palsy, CN III misdirection, Marcus–Gunn syndrome, Parinaud's syndrome, hydrocephalus, sympathomimetics, cicatrization, lid surgery, large or proptotic globe

Ophthalmic signs: anterior segment (1)

Conjunctiva

Table 19.4 Ophthalmic signs—conjunctiva

Sign	Causes
Hyperemia	• Generalized: conjunctivitis, dry eye, drop or preservative allergy, contact lens wear, scleritis
	• Localized: episcleritis, scleritis, marginal keratitis, superior limbic keratitis, corneal abrasion, FB
	• Circumcorneal: anterior uveitis, keratitis
Discharge	• Purulent: bacterial conjunctivitis
	• Mucopurulent: bacterial or chlamydial conjunctivitis
	• Mucoid: vernal conjunctivitis, dry eye syndrome
	• Watery: viral or allergic conjunctivitis
Papillae	• Bacterial conjunctivitis, allergic conjunctivitis, blepharitis, floppy eyelid syndrome, superior limbic keratoconjunctivitis, contact lens
Giant papillae	• Vernal keratoconjunctivitis, contact lens–related giant papillary conjunctivitis, exposed suture, prosthesis, floppy eyelid syndrome
Follicles	• Viral conjunctivitis, chlamydial conjunctivitis, drop hypersensitivity, Parinaud oculoglandular syndrome
Pseudo-membrane	• Infective conjunctivitis (adenovirus, *Streptococcus pyogenes*, *Corynebacterium diphtheriae*, *Neisseria gonorrhoeae*), Stevens–Johnson syndrome, graft-versus-host disease, vernal conjunctivitis, ligneous conjunctivitis
Membrane	• Infective conjunctivitis (adenovirus, *Streptococcus pneumoniae*, *Staphylococcus aureus*, *Corynebacterium diphtheriae*), Stevens–Johnson syndrome, ligneous conjunctivitis
Cicatrization	• Trachoma, atopic keratoconjunctivitis, topical medication, chemical injury, ocular mucous membrane pemphigoid, erythema muliforme/Stevens–Johnson syndrome/toxic epidermal necrolysis, other bullous disease (e.g., linear IgA disease, epidermolysis bullosa), Sjogren's syndrome, graft-versus-host disease
Hemorrhagic conjunctivitis	• Infective conjunctivitis (adenovirus, enterovirus 70, coxsackie virus A24, *Streptococcus pneumoniae*, *Hemophilus aegyptius*)

Corneal iron lines

These are best seen on slit lamp with cobalt blue light.

Table 19.5 Ophthalmic signs—corneal iron lines

Sign	Causes
Ferry's	Trabeculectomy
Stocker's	Pterygium
Hudson-Stahli	Idiopathic with age (horizontal inferior 1/3 of cornea)
Fleischer	Keratoconus (base of cone)

Cornea (other)

Table 19.6 Ophthalmic signs—cornea (other)

Sign	Causes
Shape	
Thinning	• Central: keratoconus, keratoglobus, posterior keratoconus, microbial keratitis
	• Peripheral: peripheral ulcerative keratitis, marginal keratitis, microbial keratitis, Mooren's ulcer, pellucid marginal degeneration, Terrien's marginal degeneration, chronic exposure keratopathy, neurotrophic keratopathy.
Epithelial	
Punctate epithelial erosions	• Superior: vernal keratoconjunctivitis, superior limbic keratitis, floppy eyelid syndrome, poor contact lens fit
	• Interpalpebral: keratoconjunctivitis sicca, ultraviolet exposure, corneal anesthesia
	• Inferior: blepharitis, exposure keratopathy, ectropion, poor Bell's phenomenon, rosacea, drop toxicity
Punctate epithelial keratitis	• Viral keratitis (adenovirus, HSV, molluscum contagiosum)
	• Thygeson's superficial punctate keratitis
Epithelial edema	• ↑IOP, postoperative, aphakic/pseudophakic bullous keratopathy, Fuchs' endothelial dystrophy, trauma, acute hydrops, herpetic keratitis, contact lens over wear, congenital corneal clouding
Corneal filaments	• Keratoconjunctivitis sicca, recurrent erosion syndrome, corneal anesthesia, exposure keratopathy, HZO
Stromal	
Pannus	• Trachoma, tight contact lens, phlyctenule, herpetic keratitis, rosacea keratitis, chemical keratopathy, marginal keratitis, atopic/vernal keratoconjunctivitis, superior limbal keratoconjunctivitis, chronic keratoconjunctivitis of any cause

Table 19.6 (*Contd.*)

Sign	Causes
Stromal infiltrate	• Sterile: marginal keratitis, contact lens related • Infective: bacteria, fungi, viruses, protozoa
Stromal edema	• Postoperative, keratoconus, Fuchs' endothelial dystrophy, disciform keratitis
Stromal deposits	• Corneal dystrophies: macular, granular, lattice, Avellino • Systemic: mucopolysaccharidoses (some), amyloidosis
Vogt's striae	• Keratoconus
Ghost vessels	• Interstitial keratitis (e.g., congenital syphilis, Cogan syndrome), other stromal keratitis (e.g., viral, parasitic)
Endothelial	
Descemet's folds	• Postoperative, ↓IOP, disciform keratitis, congenital syphilis
Descemet's breaks	• Birth trauma, keratoconus/keratoglobus (hydrops), infantile glaucoma (Haab's striae)
Guttata	• Peripheral: Hassell–Henle bodies (physiological in the elderly) • Central: Fuch's endothelial dystrophy
Pigment on endothelium	• Pigment dispersion syndrome (Krukenberg spindle), postoperative, trauma
Keratic precipitates	• Anterior uveitis: e.g., idiopathic, HLA-B27, Fuchs' heterochromic cyclitis, sarcoidosis, associated with keratitis (e.g., herpetic disciform, microbial, marginal)

Ophthalmic signs: anterior segment (2)

Episclera and sclera

Table 19.7 Ophthalmic signs—episclera and sclera

Sign	Causes
Injection	• Superficial: episcleritis • Deep: scleritis
Pigmentation	• True: nevus, melanocytoma, bilirubin (chronic liver disease), alkaptonuria, pigment spots (at scleral perforations, e.g., nerve loop of Axenfeld) • Pseudo: blue sclera
Blue sclera	• Osteogenesis imperfecta, keratoconus or keratoglobus, acquired scleral thinning (e.g., after necrotizing scleritis), connective tissue disorder (Marfan syndrome, Ehlers–Danlos syndrome, pseudoxanthoma elasticum), other systemic syndromes (Turner's, Russell–Silver, incontinentia pigmenti)

Anterior chamber

Table 19.8 Ophthalmic signs—anterior chamber

Sign	Causes
↑IOP	• Chronic with open angle: primary open angle, normal tension, pseudoexfoliation, pigment dispersion, steroid-induced, angle-recession, intraocular tumor • Chronic with closed angle: chronic primary angle closure, neovascular, inflammatory, ICE syndrome, epithelial downgrowth, phacomorphic, aqueous misdirection • Acute with open angle: inflammatory, steroid-induced, Posner–Schlossman, pigment dispersion, red cell, ghost cell, phacolytic, lens particle, intraocular tumor • Acute with closed angle: primary angle closure, neovascular, inflammatory, ICE syndrome, epithelial down-growth, phacomorphic, lens dislocation, aqueous misdirection
AC leukocytes	• Corneal: keratitis, FB, trauma, abrasion, chemical injury • Intraocular: anterior uveitis, endophthalmitis, tumor necrosis
Hypopyon	• Corneal: severe microbial keratitis • Intraocular: severe anterior uveitis, endophthalmitis, tumor necrosis
Hyphema	• Trauma: blunt or penetrating • Surgery: trabeculectomy, iris manipulation procedures • Spontaneous: iris/angle neovascularization, hematological disease, tumor (e.g., juvenile xanthogranuloma), IOL erosion of iris, herpetic anterior uveitis
Pigment in AC and angle	• Idiopathic (↑ with age), pigment dispersion syndrome, pseudoexfoliation syndrome (Sampaolesi pigment line), intraocular surgery
Blood in Schlemm's canal	• Sturge–Weber syndrome, carotid–cavernous fistula, SVC obstruction, hypotony

Iris/ciliary body

Table 19.9 Ophthalmic signs—iris and ciliary body

Sign	Causes
Iris mass	• Pigmented: iris melanoma, nevus, ICE syndrome, adenoma, ciliary body tumors • Nonpigmented: amelanotic iris melanoma, iris cyst, iris granulomata, IOFB, juvenile xanthogranuloma, leiomyoma, ciliary body tumors, iris metastasis
Rubeosis	• Retinal vein occlusion (usually ischemic CRVO), proliferative diabetic retinopathy, ocular ischemic syndrome, CRAO, posterior segment tumors, long-standing retinal detachment, sickle-cell or other ischemic retinopathy
Heterochromia	• Hypochromic: congenital Horner's syndrome, Fuchs' heterochromic cyclitis (the affected eye is bluer), uveitis, trauma or surgery, Waardenberg syndrome • Hyperchromic: drugs (e.g., latanoprost), siderosis (e.g., IOFB), oculodermal melanocytosis, diffuse iris nevus or melanoma, other intraocular tumors
Transillumination defects	• Diffuse: albinism, post–angle closure, Fuchs' heterochromic cyclitis • Peripupillary: pseudoexfoliation syndrome • Mid-peripheral spoke-like: pigment dispersion syndrome • Sectoral: trauma, post-surgery/laser, herpes simplex or zoster, ICE syndrome, iridoschisis
Leukocoria	• Cataract, retinoblastoma, persistent fetal vasculature syndrome, inflammatory cyclitic membrane, Coats' disease, ROP, *Toxocara*, incontinentia pigmenti, familial exudative vitreoretinopathy, retinal dysplasia (e.g., Norries disease, Patau syndrome, Edward syndrome)
Corectopia	• Iris melanoma, iris nevus, ciliary body tumor, ICE syndrome, posterior polymorphous dystrophy, surgery (e.g., complicated cataract surgery, trabeculectomy), anterior segment dysgenesis, coloboma
Ciliary body mass	• Pigmented: melanoma, metastasis, adenoma • Nonpigmented: cyst, uveal effusion syndrome, medulloepithelioma, leiomyoma, metastasis

Ophthalmic signs: anterior segment (3)

Pupil function

Table 19.10 Ophthalmic signs—pupil function

Sign	Causes
RAPD	• Asymmetric optic nerve disease (e.g., AION, optic neuritis, asymmetric glaucoma, compressive optic neuropathy) or severe asymmetric retinal disease (e.g., CRAO, CRVO, extensive retinal detachment)
Anisocoria	• Abnormal mydriasis: Adie's pupil, iris trauma, iris inflammation, CN III palsy, pharmacological, ischemia • Abnormal miosis: physiological, Horner's, pharmacological, iris inflammation
Light-near dissociation	• Unilateral: afferent defect (optic nerve pathology), efferent defect (aberrant regeneration of CN III) • Bilateral: Parinaud syndrome, Argyll–Robertson pupils, diabetes, amyloidosis, alcohol, myotonic dystrophy, encephalitis

Lens

Table 19.11 Ophthalmic signs—lens

Sign	Causes
Cataract	• Sutural: congenital, traumatic, metabolic (Fabry's disease, mannosidosis), depositional (copper, gold, silver, iron, chlorpromazine) • Nuclear: congenital, age-related • Lamellar: congenital/infantile (inherited, rubella, diabetes, galactosemia, hypocalcemia) • Coronary: sporadic, inherited • Cortical: age-related • Subcapsular: age-related, diabetes, corticosteroids, uveitis, radiation • Polar: congenital • Diffuse: congenital, age-related
Abnormal size	• Microphakia: Lowe syndrome • Microspherophakia: familial microspherophakia, Peters anomaly, Marfan syndrome, Weill–Marchesani syndrome, hyperlysinemia, Alport syndrome, congenital rubella
Abnormal shape	• Coloboma, anterior lenticonus (Alport syndrome), posterior lenticonus (sporadic, familial, Lowe syndrome), lentiglobus
Ectopia lentis	• Congenital: familial ectopia lentis, Marfan syndrome, Weill–Marchesani syndrome, homocystinuria, familial microspherophakia, hyperlysinemia, sulfite oxidase deficiency, Stickler syndrome, Sturge–Weber syndrome, Crouzon syndrome, Ehlers–Danlos syndrome, aniridia • Acquired: pseudoexfoliation, trauma, high myopia, hypermature cataract, buphthalmos, ciliary body tumor
Superficial opacities	• Pseudoexfoliation, Vossius ring (trauma), glaucomflecken (subcapsular opacities from acute-angle closure glaucoma)

Ophthalmic signs: posterior segment (1)

Fundus (chorioretinal)

Table 19.12 Ophthalmic signs—fundus (chorioretinal)

Sign	Causes
Choroid	
Choroidal mass	• Pigmented: e.g., nevus, CHRPE, melanocytoma, metastasis, BDUMP syndrome
	• Nonpigmented: choroidal granuloma, choroidal detachment, choroidal neovascular membrane, hematoma (subretinal, sub-RPE, suprachoroidal), choroidal osteoma, choroidal hemangioma, posterior scleritis, metastasis
Choroidal folds	• Idiopathic, hypermetropia, retrobulbar mass, posterior scleritis, uveitis, idiopathic orbital inflammatory disease, thyroid eye disease, choroidal mass, hypotony, papilledema
Choroidal detachment	• Effusion: hypotony, extensive PRP, extensive cryotherapy, posterior uveitis, uveal effusion syndrome
	• Hemorrhage: intraoperative, trauma, spontaneous
Retina	
Tractional retinal detachment	• ROP, sickle-cell retinopathy, proliferative diabetic retinopathy, proliferative vitreoretinopathy (e.g., trauma or IOFB, intraocular surgery, retinal breaks), vitreomacular traction syndrome, incontinentia pigmenti, retinal dysplasia
Exudative retinal detachment	• Congenital: nanophthalmos, uveal effusion syndrome, familial exudative vitreoretinopathy, disc coloboma or pit
	• Vascular: CNV, Coats' disease, central serous retinopathy, vasculitis, accelerated hypertension, pre-eclampsia
	• Choroidal tumors
	• Inflammatory: posterior uveitis (e.g., VKH), posterior scleritis, orbital cellulitis, postoperative inflammation, idiopathic orbital inflammatory disease
General	
White dots	• Idiopathic white dot syndromes: PIC, POHS, MEWDS, APMPPE, serpiginous choroidopathy, bird-shot retinochoroidopathy, multifocal choroiditis with panuveitis
	• Infective (chorio)retinitis: syphilis, toxoplasma, tuberculosis, candida, HSV
	• Inflammatory (chorio)retinitis: sarcoidosis, sympathetic ophthalmia, VKH

Fundus (vascular)

Table 19.13 Ophthalmic signs—fundus (vascular)

Sign	Causes
Hard exudates	• Diabetic retinopathy, choroidal neovascular membrane, macroaneurysm, accelerated hypertension, neuroretinitis, retinal telangiectasias
Cotton-wool spots	• Diabetic retinopathy, BRVO or CRVO, ocular ischemic syndrome, hypertension, HIV retinopathy, vasculitis
Retinal telangiectasias	• Coats' disease, Leber's miliary aneurysms, idiopathic juxtafoveal telangiectasia, ROP, retinitis pigmentosa, diabetic retinopathy, sickle retinopathy, radiation retinopathy, hypogammaglobulinemia, Eales disease, CRVO or BRVO
Arterial emboli	• Carotid artery disease, atrial thrombus, atrial myxoma, infective endocarditis, fat embolus (long-bone fracture), talc embolus (IV drug abuser), amniotic fluid embolus
Roth's spots	• Septic emboli, leukemia, myeloma, HIV retinopathy
Vasculitis	• Idiopathic retinal vasculitis, intermediate or posterior uveitis (idiopathic), sarcoidosis, MS, Behcet's disease, SLE, toxoplasmosis, tuberculosis, HSV, VZV, CMV, ARN, Wegener's granulomatosis, polyarteritis nodosa, Takayasu's arteritis, Whipple's disease, Lyme disease
Arteritis	• ARN (HSV, VZV); less commonly in other vasculitides

Ophthalmic signs: posterior segment (2)

Macula

Table 19.14 Ophthalmic signs—macula

Sign	Causes
Cystoid macular edema	• Postoperative: cataract, corneal, or vitreoretinal surgery • Post-procedure: cryotherapy, peripheral iridotomy, panretinal photocoagulation • Inflammatory: uveitis (posterior > intermediate > anterior), scleritis • Vascular: retinal vein obstruction, diabetic maculopathy, ocular ischemia, choroidal neovascular membrane, retinal telangiectasia, hypertensive retinopathy, radiation retinopathy • Medication: epinephrine, latanoprost • Other: vitreomacular traction syndrome, retinitis pigmentosa, autosomal dominant CME, tumors of choroid/retina
Macular hole	Idiopathic, trauma, CME, epiretinal membrane, vitreomacular traction syndrome, retinal detachment (rhegmatogenous), laser injury, myopia, hypertension, proliferative diabetic retinopathy
Epiretinal membrane	• Idiopathic, retinal detachment surgery, cryotherapy, photocoagulation, trauma (blunt or penetrating), posterior uveitis, persistent vitreous hemorrhage, retinal vascular disease (e.g., BRVO)
Choroidal neovascular membrane	• Degenerative: ARMD, pathological myopia, angioid streaks • Trauma: choroidal rupture, laser • Inflammation: sarcoidosis, toxoplasmosis, POHS, PIC, multifocal choroiditis, serpiginous choroidopathy, bird-shot retinochoroidopathy, VKH • Dystrophies: Best's disease • Other: idiopathic, chorioretinal scar (any cause), tumor
Central serous detachment	• Central serous retinopathy, optic disc pit, CNV, posterior uveitis (e.g., VKH), malignant hypertension; see also exudative retinal detachment
Bull's eye maculopathy	• Drug: chloroquine group, clofazamine • Macular dystrophies: cone dystrophy, cone-rod dystrophy, Stargardt's • Neurological: Batten's disease
Cherry-red spot	• Systemic: Tay–Sachs disease, Sandhoff disease, GM1 gangliosidoses, Niemann–Pick disease, sialidosis, metachromatic leucodystrophy • Ocular: CRAO
Foveal schisis	• X-linked juvenile retinoschisis

Optic disc

Table 19.15 Ophthalmic signs—optic disc

Sign	Causes
Pallor	• Congenital: Kjer's, Behr's, or Wolfram's optic atrophy • Acquired: compression (optic nerve or chiasm), glaucoma, ischemia, toxins, poor nutrition, inflammation, infection, LHON, trauma, severe retinal disease, post-papilledema
Apparent swelling	• Pseudo: drusen, tilted, hypermetropic, myelinated • True: ↑ICP (usually bilateral) or local causes (may be unilateral), e.g., inflammation, ischemia, LHON, infiltration, tumor
Pit	• Congenital • Acquired: glaucoma

Ophthalmic signs: visual fields

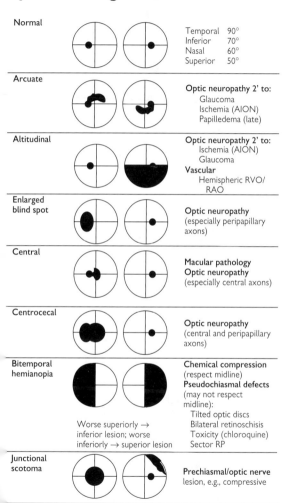

Normal		Temporal 90° Inferior 70° Nasal 60° Superior 50°
Arcuate		**Optic neuropathy 2' to:** Glaucoma Ischemia (AION) Papilledema (late)
Altitudinal		**Optic neuropathy 2' to:** Ischemia (AION) Glaucoma **Vascular** Hemispheric RVO/ RAO
Enlarged blind spot		**Optic neuropathy** (especially peripapillary axons)
Central		**Macular pathology** **Optic neuropathy** (especially central axons)
Centrocecal		**Optic neuropathy** (central and peripapillary axons)
Bitemporal hemianopia		**Chemical compression** (respect midline) **Pseudochiasmal defects** (may not respect midline): Tilted optic discs Bilateral retinoschisis Toxicity (chloroquine) Sector RP
	Worse superiorly → inferior lesion; worse inferiorly → superior lesion	
Junctional scotoma		**Prechiasmal/optic nerve** lesion, e.g., compressive

Figure 19.1 Visual field defects.

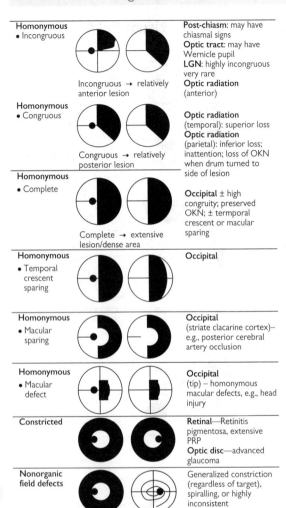

Homonymous • Incongruous	**Post-chiasm**: may have chiasmal signs **Optic tract**: may have Wernicle pupil **LGN**: highly incongruous very rare **Optic radiation** (anterior)
Incongruous → relatively anterior lesion	
Homonymous • Congruous	**Optic radiation** (temporal): superior loss **Optic radiation** (parietal): inferior loss; inattention; loss of OKN when drum turned to side of lesion
Congruous → relatively posterior lesion	
Homonymous • Complete	**Occipital** ± high congruity; preserved OKN; ± termporal crescent or macular sparing
Complete → extensive lesion/dense area	
Homonymous • Temporal crescent sparing	**Occipital**
Homonymous • Macular sparing	**Occipital** (striate clacarine cortex)– e.g., posterior cerebral artery occlusion
Homonymous • Macular defect	**Occipital** (tip) – homonymous macular defects, e.g., head injury
Constricted	**Retinal**—Retinitis pigmentosa, extensive PRP **Optic disc**—advanced glaucoma
Nonorganic field defects	Generalized constriction (regardless of target), spiralling, or highly inconsistent

Figure 19.1 Visual field defects. (*Contd.*)

Vision in context

Low vision: assessment, aids, and support

In the United States, around 15–20% of elderly people over the age of 65 suffer from some visual disability. This represents 7.3 million individuals and will rapidly increase with the aging of the baby-boomer generation.

There is concern that there is a wide-scale lack of access to support and services for patients with visual disorders. It is probable that many of these people may never seek help. However, even those who get to an ophthalmologist may only be rewarded with a delayed diagnosis of an incurable eye disease for which "nothing can be done."

In these circumstances, those involved in eye care must be aware of what *can* be done to optimize the patient's remaining vision and how best to advise and assist the patient. This is often best coordinated in a low-vision aid (LVA) clinic, ideally with access to specialists, optometrists, rehabilitation workers, counselors, and social services.

Assessment

General—what are their concerns?

People are extremely variable in their needs. For some, the priority will be to continue to be able to read or solve the crossword puzzle, whereas others will be afraid of social isolation and lack of independence. Sometimes assessment will also reveal misunderstandings about their condition.

Specific—consider the following:

Reading

Is reading an issue for them? If so, what do they want to read—what size print and in what context (i.e., at home or out-and-about)? The answers to these questions will affect the type of optical devices used.

Television

If this is an issue for patients, consider size of the television, viewing distance, and whether it is standard color or HDTV (higher contrast).

Activities of daily living and recreation

Are patients managing to look after themselves (± dependents)? What about shopping, cooking, and hygiene? Can they still do their hobbies?

Mobility

Do they manage to get around? Do they have access to public transport or rides from family or friends?

Work and financial support

Do patients have the help they need to continue working if they wish to? What resources are available to them for equipment or personal assistance? Do they know how to access any benefits they are entitled to?

Psychosocial

Are they coping emotionally with their visual impairment? Do they have access to local support groups? Would they benefit from talking to a counselor?

Management

General
Optimize lighting conditions (e.g., brighter bulbs, more lights around the house, good reading light). Improve contrast whenever possible.

Registration
If patients are eligible but not yet registered, ensure that the purpose of registration is explained and that it is offered to them.

Support
Ensure that they have access to support from social services and local support groups and that they know how to get help when they need it.

Equipment
Refraction (near and distance) should be optimized. In addition, consider the following issues.

Optical devices (near)
- Reading glasses should be optimized, although they are often not sufficient on their own. Up to +4.00D is usually well tolerated but beyond this, the reading distance is uncomfortably short. Higher reading additions may require a prism to assist convergence.
- Hand magnifiers are usually practical and inexpensive but are limited by a small field of view (especially for the higher powers).
- Stand magnifiers have the advantage of keeping both hands free and keeping the working distance constant but are less transportable.
- Illuminated magnifiers improve contrast (provided that the batteries are charged), but are generally bulkier.
- Reading telescopes may be useful for specific near work because they have a greater working distance than that of reading glasses of an equivalent magnification. However, they are expensive and are unattractive.
- Closed-circuit television: excellent magnification with high contrast can be achieved with a television camera directed down onto reading material(s) and viewed on the adjacent screen. However, it is expensive, not portable, and generally superceded by computer- or scanner-based technology.

Optical devices (distance)
- Distance telescopes can be useful for specific tasks, although generally they are limited by the small field of view. They may be spectacle mounted (useful for static tasks, e.g., watching television, theater, music, sports) or hand-held (used as required, e.g., bus number, direction signs).

Computers and other nonoptical devices
Personal computers (with enlarged text or speech facility) have made a spectacular difference in the lives of many visually impaired people. They provide an easy method of writing, reading (with scanner and optical character recognition) and instant letter communication by e-mail. Web-based facilities also increase access to shopping, entertainment, and support.

Other devices include talking watches and clocks, writing guides, liquid-level indicators (to prevent overfilling cups), tactile controls on domestic appliances, talking scales, and modified games (e.g., large playing cards).

Visual impairment registration

Registration of visual impairment has traditionally had three roles: to formally recognize an individual's vision loss; to identify those patients eligible for assistance due to their disability; and to help eye services, social services, and governmental organizations know the extent and distribution of visual impairment in the community.

However, a recent review showed that for many people the registration process actually excluded or delayed access to services. More than half of those eligible choose not to be registered, and many are unhappy about being registered blind when they have (and are expected to continue to have) residual vision.

Driving standards

Evidence that visual impairment alone causes automobile accidents is surprisingly scarce. The strictness of driving standards varies internationally; this is in part affected by the density of traffic and driving conditions. In some parts of the United States, partially sighted people may drive during daylight hours within a specified radius of their home.

Visual acuity

For Class C vehicle drivers

- 20/40 when both eyes are tested together.
- 20/40 in one eye.
- 20/70, at least in the other eye.
- Uninterrupted visual field of at least 100 degrees in the horizontal meridian.

Commercial vehicle drivers

- At least 20/30 in the better eye AND
- At least 20/40 in the worse eye AND
- Uncorrected acuity in each eye must be at least 20/400

Some drivers who fail these requirements may be permitted to drive under "grandfather rights," which take into account the initial date of the driver's license. The license holder needs to contact the Department of Motor Vehicles (DMV), which will require a certificate of recent driving experience and confirmation of no eyesight-related road accidents in the previous 10 years.

Visual fields

The preferred method of testing is the Humphrey visual field. For those patients who cannot use an automated perimeter, Goldmann testing is acceptable in exceptional circumstances. A maximum of 20% false positives and of three attempts for each test is allowed.

Class C license drivers

- At least 120 feet on the horizontal (Goldmann III4e setting or equivalent) AND
- No significant defect in the binocular field encroaching within 20 feet of fixation above or below the horizontal meridian. "Insignificant" central defects (equivalent to the normal blind spot in a monocular field) comprise
  - Scattered single missed points.
  - A single cluster of 2 or 3 missed points.

When a patient has fully adapted to a static, longstanding defect, the DMV may consider them an "exceptional case" and perform a practical driving assessment.

Commercial drivers

- Full binocular field of vision.
- No missed points in the central 20 feet.

Other

These patients should inform the DMV of their condition.

Monocularity

Patients may drive (Class C vehicles only) when clinically advised that they have adapted to the disability and they satisfy the usual visual acuity requirements and have a normal monocular visual field.

Diplopia

Patients with uncorrected diplopia must not drive. Driving may be resumed if it is controlled; patching is acceptable subject to the above constraints on monocularity. Very rarely, the DMV may permit someone to drive despite uncorrected diplopia if it is stable (>6 months).

Blepharospasm

Patients with severe blepharospasm must not drive. Patients with mild, successfully treated blepharospasm may drive subject to physician approval.

All drivers

If patients fail to reach these standards, they must not drive, and they have a legal requirement to notify the DMV. Failure to comply is a criminal offense and can result in a fine or loss of license.

Professional standards

Pilots (civil aviation authority)

Class 1 pilots (commercial: airplane and helicopter)

Visual acuity
- Distance: at least 20/30 in each eye and 20/20 with both eyes together (best corrected).
- Near: at least N5 at 30–50 cm and N14 at 100 cm (best corrected).

Refractive error and correction
- Refractive error less than +5.0D or −5.0D and anisometropia <2.0D.
- Contact lenses may be used if they can be reliably used for >8 hours/day.
- Refractive surgery: stability of refraction must be demonstrated; usually pilots are unable to fly for 3 months post-LASIK and 1 year after other procedures. Preoperative refractive error may still be a bar to qualification (see above).

Color
- Satisfactory Ishihara testing is required; if patients fail this then they must pass the Lantern test.

Other
- Normal visual fields.
- No diplopia.
- Heterophoria <8Δ exo, 10Δ eso, or 2Δ vertical at 6 meters (20 feet) and <12Δ exo, 6Δ eso, or 1Δ vertical at 33 cm (13 inches): excess of this will require further assessment by an ophthalmologist.
- No ophthalmic or adnexal disease.

Class 2 pilots (private: airplane and helicopter)

Visual acuity
- Distance: at least 20/40 in each eye and 20/20 with both eyes together (best corrected); amblyopes with 20/60 in one eye may be permitted to fly, provided the other eye is at least 20/20 uncorrected.
- Near: at least N5 at 30–50 cm and N14 at 100 cm (best corrected).

Refractive error and correction
- Refractive error less than +5.0D or −8.0D (in the most ametropic meridian) and anisometropia <3.0D.
- Contact lenses may be used if they can be reliably used for >8 hours/day.
- Refractive surgery: stability of refraction must be demonstrated; usually the pilot is unable to fly for 3 months post-LASIK and 1 year after other procedures; preoperative refractive error may still be a bar to qualification (see above).

Color
- Satisfactory Ishihara testing is required. If patients fail this, then they must pass the Lantern test or be restricted to daytime flying.

Other
- Normal visual fields.
- No diplopia.
- Heterophoria will require further assessment by an ophthalmologist.
- No ophthalmic or adnexal disease.

Perioperative care

Preoperative assessment (1)

The following are practical recommendations for patients undergoing cataract extraction and intraocular lens implantation.

General

- Check whether the procedure is appropriate for day surgery (adequate support) or inpatient care and if transportation is needed to the medical facility and to return home.
- Ensure that medical records and any relevant investigations (including biometry, scans, blood tests) are available.
- Check for hazards (e.g., allergies, MRSA, blood-borne diseases, e.g., hepatitis, HIV) and ensure that these are communicated appropriately to the rest of the team.
- Check for special requirements (e.g., interpreter).

Systemic

History

Age

- Past medical history: ask specifically about diabetes, hypertension, ischemic heart disease, asthma/COPD, and any current illnesses.
- Past surgical history: ask about previous surgery and anesthesia (and adverse reactions).
- Systemic review: CVS (e.g., chest pain), respiratory system (e.g., breathlessness on exertion, orthopnea), CNS (e.g., fits), psychological issues (e.g., alcohol, anxiety), ability to lie flat.
- Family history (including problems with anesthesia).
- Medications (mainly anticoagulants) and allergies.

Examination

- CVS: pulse (rate + rhythm), blood pressure.
- Respiratory system: any dyspnea, pulse oximetry saturation, respiratory rate, auscultation.
- Musculoskeletal: neck or back problems (may affect intubation and surgical position).
- CNS: comprehension, cooperation, hearing, tremor, or other abnormal movements.

Ophthalmic

The ophthalmic history and examination should identify any new developments (since the preoperative clinical assessment) that may postpone surgery or might modify the planned operation in any way.

Contraindications

Any identified risk factors should be treated preoperatively (see Box 21.1). This may require postponement of surgery and either coordination with the patient's PCP or referral to an appropriate specialist.

Preoperative workup

- *Operations under local anesthesia:* minimal workup is required unless history and systemic examination suggest significant systemic disease that would be worthy of investigation in its own right.
- *Operations under general anesthesia:* general investigations usually include CBC, UA, glucose, and ECG; specific investigations (CXR, echocardiography) are directed according to patient history and examination. It is common practice to limit routine preoperative testing in healthy younger patients in whom a general history and examination is satisfactory.

Box 21.1 Specific systemic contraindications to ophthalmic surgery

- Uncontrolled BP (e.g., >180/100 mmHg)
- Myocardial ischemia (unstable ischemic heart disease or myocardial infarction (MI) in the last 3 months)
- Uncontrolled hyperglycemia
- Uncontrolled arrhythmias
- Excessive INR
- Acute systemic illness

Preoperative assessment (2)

Preoperative management

- *Patients for intraocular surgery*: appropriate preoperative drops (Table 21.1).
- *Patients for general anesthesia*: nothing by mouth (e.g., from 8 hours before).
- *Patients with diabetes*: normal (or near-normal) regime can be continued in most patients having local anesthesia; a sliding scale may be required in poorly controlled patients or some insulin-requiring patients having general anesthesia (coordinate care with anesthesiologist).
- *Patients with hypertension*: continue antihypertensives (including day of surgery); for example, consider postponing surgery if BP >180/100 mmHg.
- *Patients with ischemic heart disease*: continue usual antianginal medication and ensure their usual prn medication (e.g., sublingual nitroglycerin) is available in the operating room; postpone surgery if within 3 months of myocardial infarct.
- *Patients with valvular heart disease*: antibiotic prophylaxis is not required for intraocular procedures.
- *Patients on aspirin*: continue for intraocular and strabismus surgery; for orbital and oculoplastic surgery, it would ideally be discontinued for 2 weeks prior to surgery. However, this must be discussed with their PCP.
- *Patients on anticoagulants*: ideally the INR should be <3 for intraocular and strabismus surgery but <2 for orbital and oculoplastic surgery (see Table 21.2). This should be checked within 48 hours of surgery. If this is not compatible with their therapeutic target, coordinate care with their hematologist or PCP. They may consider changing to heparin in the perioperative period.

Table 21.1 Common preoperative drop regimes

Cataract surgery	Cyclopentolate 1% + phenylephrine 2.5/10% + diclofenac 0.1%.
Vitreoretinal surgery	Cyclopentolate 1% + phenylephrine 2.5/10% + diclofenac 0.1%.
Penetrating keratoplasty	Pilocarpine 2%

Table 21.2 Target INR levels

Prophylaxis of deep venous thrombosis (DVT)	INR 2.0–2.5
DVT or pulmonary embolism (PE) treatment Atrial fibrillation (AF) Cardioversion Dilated cardiomyopathy Mural thrombus post-MI Rheumatic mitral valve disease	INR 2.5
Recurrent DVT or PE Mechanical heart valve	INR 3.5

Ocular anesthesia (1)

Cataract surgery has become the most commonly performed surgery in the United States. In the 1990s, there was a dramatic shift from general to local anesthesia for the majority of ophthalmic surgeries.

Topical anesthesia

Indications

- Cooperative patient + experienced surgeon + routine suitable operation (usually cataract surgery).

Method

- Repeated preoperative ± intraoperative anesthetic drop.
- Consider also intracameral lidocaine (1% isotonic preservative-free) and an anesthetic-soaked sponge in the inferior fornix.

Complications

- Pain, eye movement, epithelial toxicity; in an uncooperative patient, surgery may be hazardous with increased risk of operative complications.

Subtenon's block

Indications

- Relatively complete anesthesia of the globe and akinesia desired; patient sufficiently cooperative to keep head still during surgery.

Method

Apply topical anesthetic to conjunctiva, ask the patient to look in the opposite direction to the intended injection site (e.g., superotemporally). Open conjunctiva around 8 mm from the limbus (e.g., inferonasally), dissect down to bare sclera with blunt curved scissors, insert subtenon's cannula (blunt curved), and slide cannula posteriorly along the globe. Inject 2.5–3.0 mL lidocaine 2% (or lidocaine 2%/bupivicaine 0.5% mix).

Complications

- Failure (backflow if wide track, leaks out if conjunctiva perforated twice), conjunctival chemosis, conjunctival hemorrhage.

Peribulbar block

Indications

Relatively complete anesthesia of the globe and akinesia is desired. The patient needs to be sufficiently cooperative to keep the head still during surgery. An anesthesiologist trained in the technique is also needed.

Method

The surgeon asks the patient to fix his/her gaze on a target directly ahead and uses a sharp, short needle (27 or 25 gauge, 25–31 mm) to inject a total of 4–8 mL lidocaine 2% (or lidocaine 2%/bupivicaine 0.5% mix) around the globe. This may require a single injection (either inferotemporal extraconal or medial extraconal) or a combined approach if akinesia is insufficient. Ocular compression (e.g., Honan balloon) is administered for 20–30 min.

Complications
- Excessive positive pressure (surgery may become hazardous), ptosis, diplopia, ocular perforation (<0.1% but 0.7% if axial length >26 mm), brainstem anesthesia, oculocardiac reflex (0.03%), orbital hemorrhage.

Ocular anesthesia (2)

General anesthesia

Indications
Complete akinesia and deep anesthesia are required. The patient is unlikely to keep still (mental impairment, children, young adult, very anxious, uncontrolled tremor) or had a previous adverse reaction to local anesthetic. Globe trauma is contraindicative of local anesthesia.

Method
The patient must have adequately fasted (e.g., 8 hours) and all appropriate investigations must have been performed (e.g., CBC, UA, ECG when indicated). General anesthesia requires preoperative assessment (identify and, if possible, minimize anesthetic risk factors), premedication (sedation, amnesia, antiemesis), induction, intubation, maintenance, recovery, and postoperative analgesia.

Effect on IOP

Table 21.3 General anesthesia and IOP

Cause	Effect on IOP
Inhalational anesthetic	↑
Ketamine	None
Opiates, barbiturates, benzodiazepines, neuroleptics	↓
Hyperventilation	↓
Hypoventilation	↑

Complications
These include respiratory depression (→ hypoxia), cardiac depression (→ myocardial ischemia), aspiration of gastric contents, anaphylaxis, malignant hyperthermia, oculocardiac reflex, and difficult recovery (respiratory weaning, psychological problems).

Treatment of anaphylaxis

Anaphylaxis is most commonly encountered by the ophthalmologist when a patient undergoes FA. It is an extreme form of type I hypersensitivity reaction. Severe anaphylaxis occurs in 1 out of every 1900 FAs. Fatal anaphylaxis occurs in 1 out of every 220,000 FAs. Appropriate initial treatment should be instituted by the ophthalmic team while calling for emergency medical support.

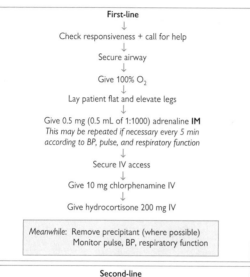

First-line
↓
Check responsiveness + call for help
↓
Secure airway
↓
Give 100% O_2
↓
Lay patient flat and elevate legs
↓
Give 0.5 mg (0.5 mL of 1:1000) adrenaline **IM**
This may be repeated if necessary every 5 min
according to BP, pulse, and respiratory function
↓
Secure IV access
↓
Give 10 mg chlorphenamine IV
↓
Give hydrocortisone 200 mg IV

Meanwhile: Remove precipitant (where possible)
Monitor pulse, BP, respiratory function

Second-line
If hypotensive
↓
Give fluids IV
e.g. 500 mL normal saline over 15 min stat
then titrate according to BP

If respiratory compromise
↓
Give nebulized bronchodilators
e.g., 2.5 mg salbutamol; titrate according to respiratory function

In severe cases the emergency medical/anesthetic team may add in IV aminophylline, perform emergency tracheotomy, or even intubate/ventilate

Figure 21.1 Management of anaphylaxis.

Therapeutics

Ocular medication: general

All doses and frequencies of administration are based on a healthy adult. All medications should be checked in the *Physician Drug Reference Guide* for accuracy, side effects, contraindications, interactions, and appropriate age-adjusted dosing.

When considering patients' medication, it is important to check what they are actually taking rather than what you or anybody else think they are taking. Consider the issue of adherence and compliance, particularly when about to treat a suboptimal response with additional medications or more frequent regimens. For more invasive procedures (e.g., injections), formal consent should be taken.

Topical

Only around 1–10% of most topical agents are absorbed into the eye. Absorption is dependent on ocular contact time, drug concentration, and tissue permeability. Small lipophilic drugs pass through the cornea, whereas larger hydrophilic drugs are generally absorbed through conjunctiva and sclera.

Topical agents may be in aqueous solution (comfortable, no blurring but very short ocular contact time), in suspension (longer ocular contact time, but bottle must be shaken and may cause FB sensation), or in ointment (liquefy at body temperature, longest ocular contact time, but blurs vision).

Technique

- Ensure that patients know how to instill any topical medication and that they can physically manage it.
- If reliable self-administration is not possible, ensure that there is somebody (even a visiting nurse) who can assist them.
- Consider ways of making it easier, e.g., lying flat, mirror positioning, or eyedrop dispensers. Smaller bottles and single-use vials tend to be particularly difficult for the frail and elderly patient.
- Leave at least 5 min between instilling topical medications.
- Keep the eye closed and put pressure over the lacrimal sac for 1–2 min to try to increase ocular and reduce systemic absorption.

Medications

This includes most ophthalmic medications listed on the following page (Tables 22.4–22.17).

Subconjunctival injection

Technique

- Ensure adequate anesthesia (e.g., a couple of drops of proparacaine).
- Under direct vision (or slit lamp or operating microscope), lift an area of conjunctiva to form a small bleb and slowly inject (sharp needle).

Medications

This route is most commonly used for postoperative injections of corticosteroids and antibiotics, but it may be used in acute anterior segment inflammation to deliver mydriatics and corticosteroids.

Subtenon and peribulbar injections

Technique
● See ocular anesthesia, p. 690.

Medications
Although primarily used for ocular anesthesia (e.g., lidocaine, bupivicaine), these routes may be used for delivering corticosteroids (e.g., triamcinolone, methylprednisolone) in posterior segment inflammation, exudation, or macular edema.

Table 22.1 Subtenon and peribulbar corticosteroids

Drug	Dose
Triamcinolone acetonide	40 mg
Methylprednisolone	40 mg

These are nonlicensed uses of the commercial IM preparations of these corticosteroids.

Intravitreal injection

Technique
This should be performed with appropriate anesthesia under sterile conditions. It is either performed immediately after a core vitrectomy to administer intravitreal antibiotics (for endophthalmitis) or may be used for delivering corticosteroids (triamcinolone) or anti-VEGF therapy to treat posterior segment exudation or macular edema.
● Insert a 27 or 30 gauge half-inch needle entering 3.5–4 mm post-limbus (if phakic) or 3.0–3.5 mm (if aphakic/pseudophakic) and directed into the vitreous. At the time of injection, the needle tip should be clearly visualized through the pupil.

Medications

Table 22.2 Intravitreal antimicrobials

Drug	Dose	Reconstituted to
Vancomycin	1 mg	0.1 mL
Amikacin	0.4 mg	0.1 mL
Ceftazidime	2 mg	0.1 mL
Amphotericin	5–10 µg	0.1 mL
Ganciclovir	400 µg	0.1 mL

Table 22.3 Intravitreal corticosteroid

Drug	Dose	Reconstituted to
Triamcinolone acetonide	2–4 mg	0.05–0.1 mL

These are nonlicensed uses of the commercial IV/IM preparations of these corticosteroids.

Topical antibiotics

Table 22.4 Antibacterial agents

Generic	Forms	Pres-free	Frequency	Brand name
Ciprofloxacin	Topical	No	≤4×/hour initially	Ciloxan
Gatifloxacin	Topical	No	4×/day	Zymar
Moxifloxacin	Topical	No	3×/day	Vigamox
Gentamicin	Topical	Available	See below	Garamycin Genticin
Neomycin	Topical ointment	No	See below	Neosporin (neomycin/ gramicidin/ polymyxin B sulfate)
Ofloxacin	Topical	No	See below	Ocuflox
Polymixin B sulfate (PBS)	Combinations only (topical/ ointment)	No	See below	Polyfax (PBS/ bacitracin) Polytrim (PBS/ trimethoprim)
Propamidine isethionate	Topical/ ointment	No	Topical: 4×/day Oinment: 1–2×/ day	Brolene

Frequency: recommendation for antibacterial eyedrops is that they are administered at least every 2 hours, then reduce frequency as infection is controlled and continue for 48 hours after healing. For ointments it is recommended that they be used at night (with drops used during the day) or 3–4×/day if used alone.

Table 22.5 Topical antifungal agents

Generic	Frequency
Amphotericin	≤q1h initially for fungal keratitis, reducing as infection is controlled
Clotrimazole	
Econazole	
Flucytosine	
Itraconazole	
Miconazole	
Natamycin	

Table 22.6 Antiviral agents

Generic	Forms	Pres-free	Frequency	Brand name
Aciclovir	Topical	No	5×/day until healed, then 5×/day for 3 days	Zovirax
Ganciclovir	Gel/topical	No	5×/day until healed, then 3×/day for 1 week	Virgan
Trifluridine	1%	No	9×/day	Viroptic

Frequency: recommend continuing at 5×/day for at least 3 days after healing for aciclovir, and 3×/day for a week after healing for gancyclovir. The aciclovir and gancyclovir ophthalmological formulations are only available in Europe.

Topical anti-inflammatory agents

Corticosteroids

Table 22.7 Corticosteroids

Generic	Conc.	Pres-free	Frequency	Brand name
Betamethasone	0.1% ointment 0.1%	No	≤ hourly	Betnesol Vista-methasone
Dexamethasone	0.1%	Available	≤ half-hourly	Maxidex
Fluorometholone	0.1%	No	≤ hourly	FML
Hydrocortisone acetate	1% ointment 0.5%	No		
Prednisolone	0.5% 1.0%	Available	≤ hourly	Econopred Pred forte/ Omnipred
Rimexolone	1%	No	≤ hourly	Vexol
Difluprednate	0.05%	No	4×/day	Durezol

Frequency: potency and frequency of corticosteroids should be titrated against degree of inflammation to achieve control while minimizing side effects.

Table 22.8 Corticosteroid/antibiotic combinations

Corticosteroid	Antibiotic	Frequency	Brand name
Betamethasone 0.1%	Neomycin 0.5%	≤ 6×/day	Betnesol N Vista-methasone N
Dexamethasone 0.1%	Neomycin 0.35% Polymyxin B sulfate 6000u/mL	≤ 6×/day	Maxitrol
	Tobramycin 0.3%	≤ 6×/day	Tobradex
Predsol 0.5%	Neomycin 0.5%	≤ 6×/day	Predsol-N

Antihistamines and other anti-inflammatory agents

Table 22.9 Topical antihistamines and other antiallergy agents

Generic	Pres-free	Frequency	Brand name
Anti-histamine			
Antazoline sulfate	No	2–3×/day	Otrivine-Antistin
Azelastine hydrochloride	No	2–4×/day	Optivar
Ketotifen	No	2×/day	Zaditor
Levocarbistine	No	2–4×/day	Livostin
Olopatidine	No	2×/day (1×/day)	Patanol/Pataday
Bepotastine	No	2×/day	Bepreve
Other			
Emedastine	No	2×/day	Emadine
Lodoxamide	No	4×/day	Alomide
Nedocromil sodium	No	2–4×/day	Alocril
Sodium cromoglycate	No	4×/day	Opticrom and others

Table 22.10 Other topical anti-inflammatory agents (NSAID type)

Generic	Pres-free	Frequency	Brand name
Diclofenac sodium	Available	4×/day	Voltaren
Flurbiprofen sodium	No	Preoperative Rx	Ocufen
Nepafenac	No	3×/day	Nevanac
Ketorolac	No	3×/day	Acular

Topical glaucoma medications

β-blockers

Table 22.11 β-blockers

Generic	Conc.	Pres-free	Frequency	Brand name
Betaxolol	0.25% or 0.5%	No	2×/day	Betoptic
Carteolol hydrochloride	1%	No	2×/day	Ocupress
Levobunolol	0.5%	No	1–2×/day	Betagan
Metipranolol	0.1%	No	2×/day	Optipranolol
Timolol maleate	0.25% or 0.5% Gel 0.25% or 0.5%	Available No	2×/day 1×/day	Timoptic Timoptic-XE

Prostaglandin analogues

Table 22.12 Prostaglandin analogues

Generic	Conc.	Pres-free	Frequency	Brand name
Bimatoprost	0.03%	No	1×/day	Lumigan
Latanoprost	0.005%	No	1×/day	Xalatan
Travoprost	0.004%	No	1×/day	Travatan/ Travatan Z

Sympathomimetics

Table 22.13 Sympathomimetics

Generic	Conc.	Pres-free	Frequency	Brand name
Apraclonidine	0.5% or 1%	No	Single—3×/day for <1 month	Iopidine
Brimonidine tartrate	0.2% 0.15% 0.1%	No	2×/day	Alphagan/ Alphagan P
Dipivefrin hydrochloride	0.1%	No	2×/day	Propine

Carbonic anhydrase inhibitors

Table 22.14 Carbonic anhydrase inhibitors

Generic	Conc.	Pres-free	Frequency	Brand name
Brinzolamide	1%	No	3×/day	Azopt
Dorzolamide	2%	No	3×/day	Trusopt

Miotics

Table 22.15 Miotics

Generic	Conc.	Pres-free	Frequency	Brand name
Carbachol	3%	No	≤4×/day	Isopto carbachol
Pilocarpine	0.5, 1, 2, 3, or 4% Minims 2 or 4%	Available	≤4×/day	
	Gel 4%		1×/day	Pilogel

Combination drops

Table 22.16 Combinations with timolol

Generic	Conc.	Pres-free	Frequency	Brand name
Timolol + brimonidine	Timolol 0.5% brimonidine 0.2%	No	2×/day	Combigan
Timolol + dorzolamide	Timolol 0.5% dorzolamide 2%	No	2×/day	Cosopt

Topical mydriatics

Mydriatics

Table 22.17 Mydriatics and cycloplegics

Generic	Conc.	Pres-free	Frequency	Brand name
Antimuscarinic				
Atropine sulfate	0.5% or 1% Ointment 1%	Available	Single–1×/day	Isopto atropine
Cyclopentolate	0.5% or 1%	Available	Single–3×/day	Cyclogyl Ak-Pentolate
Homatropine	2% or 5%	No	Single–4×/day	Isopto Homatropine
Tropicamide	0.5% or 1%	Available	Single	Mydriacyl
Sympathomimetic				
Phenylephrine	2.5% or 10%	Available	Single–3×/day	Neo-synephrine Ak-Dilate Mydfrin

Systemic medication: glaucoma

Systemic medication may be required to lower intraocular pressure in the acute setting (e.g., acute angle closure glaucoma) or if topical treatment alone has failed. It is also commonly used prophylactically post-procedure (e.g., acetazolamide after cataract surgery). Acetazolamide may also be used in the treatment of raised intracranial pressure secondary to idiopathic intracranial hypertension.

Table 22.18 Systemic glaucoma medications

Drug	Dose	Route	Contraindications	Side effects
Acetazolamide	250–1000 mg per day in divided doses (2–4×)	IV/PO	Sulfonamide allergy, electrolyte imbalance, renal impairment, hepatic impairment	Nausea Vomiting Diarrhea Paraesthesia Rashes Polyuria Hypokalemia Electrolyte imbalance Mood changes Blood disorders
Methazolamide	50 mg 2×/day	PO	(same as acetazolamide)	
Mannitol 20%	1–2 g/kg over 45 min single dose	IV	Cardiac failure	Fluid overload Fever
Glycerol	1 g/kg in 50% lemon juice single dose	PO	Diabetes mellitus	Hyperglycemia

Systemic corticosteroids: general

Indications and mechanism
In severe ophthalmic inflammation, systemic corticosteroids may be required. Corticosteroids are anti-inflammatory but at higher doses are immunosuppressive. The immunosuppressive role of corticosteroids is via inhibition of NF-kB transcription factor signaling, thus blocking the production of IL-2 and other proinflammatory cytokines.

Routes of administration (systemic)
Oral
The preferred corticosteroid is usually prednisone. This may be started at 1 mg/kg and then titrated down as inflammation is controlled and/or steroid sparing agents are added.

Two forms are available: enteric and nonenteric coated. The enteric-coated form is associated with fewer upper gastrointestinal side effects but its absorption may be less predictable. It is best given in the morning (coincides with physiological morning cortisol peak).

Intravenous
The preferred corticosteroid is usually methylprednisolone. This may be given as a single 500–1000 mg dose or pulsed, e.g., three doses of 500–1000 mg on consecutive or alternate days given in a 100 mL of normal saline over a minimum of 1 hour.

Efficacy

> **Box 22.1 Corticosteroids: equivalent anti-inflammatory doses**
>
> Prednisone 5 mg is equivalent to:
>
> | | |
> |---|---|
> | Dexamethasone | 750 µg |
> | Betamethasone | 750 µg |
> | Methylprednisolone | 4 mg |
> | Triamcinolone | 4 mg |
> | Hydrocortisone | 20 mg |

Contraindications
• Systemic infection (unless covered with appropriate antibiotic(s)).

Monitoring
Pretreatment
Given the profound effects of corticosteroids, a short pretreatment review is advised. This includes selected medical history (varicella status, TB status, pre-existing diabetes or impaired glucose tolerance, hypertension) and examination (weight, BP, glucose). If there is any possibility of tuberculosis, a CXR should be performed.

During treatment
- BP, weight, glucose every 3 months.
- Lipids every year.
- Bone density (DXA or DEXAscan) if steroid course >3 months; repeated scans may be needed for monitoring bone density in at-risk individuals.

Side effects

Table 22.19 Corticosteroid side effects (selected)

Endocrine	Adrenal suppression (risk of Addisonian crisis with withdrawal), Cushing's syndrome, weight gain, moon face
Gastrointestinal	Nausea, indigestion, peptic ulcer, pancreatitis
Musculoskeletal	Myopathy, osteopenia, osteoporosis, avascular necrosis
Skin	Atrophy, bruising, striae, acne, hirsutism
Hematological	Leukocytosis, immunosuppression
Biochemical	Fluid and electrolyte disturbance
Psychiatric	Mood disturbance (high or low), insomnia, psychosis
Neurological	ICP, papilledema, worsening of epilepsy
Cardiovascular	Myocardial rupture after recent MI
Ophthalmic	IOP, posterior subcapsular cataracts, worsening of infection (e.g., viral or fungal keratitis)

Systemic corticosteroids: prophylaxis

Avoiding side effects

Prophylaxis of corticosteroid-induced osteoporosis

Consider prophylaxis (e.g., a bisphosphonate such as alendronic acid) if treating with the equivalent of ≥7.5 mg prednisone per day for ≥3 months in 1) patients >65 years of age, or 2) <65 years of age with previous fragility fracture and/or low DXA scan.

Prophylaxis of gastrointestinal side effects

Consider prophylaxis (e.g., an H2 antagonist such as ranitidine 150 mg 2×/day) if at risk, i.e., higher doses of corticosteroid, history of gastrointestinal disease, coadministration of NSAIDs (avoid if possible).

Withdrawal of corticosteroids

For most patients with short courses (<10 days) of doses ≤40 mg/day prednisone (or equivalent), no tapering is necessary. However, when there is a risk of adrenal suppression (Box 22.2), tapering is required in which the dose is reduced fairly rapidly to physiological levels (equivalent to 7.5 mg prednisone/day) and thereafter reduced more gradually. One suggested tapering approach is given in Box 22.3.

Box 22.2 Increased risk of adrenal suppression from corticosteroid administration

- The daily dose has been >40 mg/day prednisone (or equivalent)
- The duration has been >3 weeks
- The frequency has been >1×/day
- There have been other courses recently or long-term steroid administration within the last year.

Box 22.3 Tapering schedule recommended by Consensus Panel on Immunosuppression for Ocular Disease

- Over 40 mg/day: reduce by 10 mg/day every 1–2 weeks
- 40–20 mg/day: reduce by 5 mg/day every 1–2 weeks
- 20–10 mg/day: reduce by 2.5 mg/day every 1–2 weeks
- 10–0 mg/day: reduce by 1–2.5 mg/day every 1–4 weeks

Reprinted with permission from Jabs DA, et al. (2000). *Am J Ophthalmol* 130:492–513.

Other systemic immunosuppressants

Indications and mechanism

Although corticosteroids are usually the drug of choice in severe systemic or ocular inflammation, other immunosuppressants have an important role as second-line agents in unresponsive cases or in facilitating reduction and withdrawal of corticosteroids to minimize their side effects.

Table 22.20 Immunosuppressants and their mechanisms

Drug	Dose	Route	Mechanism
Antimetabolites			
Azathioprine	50–150 mg/day (2 mg/kg)	PO	Antimetabolite: inhibits purine metabolism
Methotrexate	7.5 mg/week	PO/IM	Antimetabolite: inhibits dihydrofolate reductase
Mycophenolate	1–2 g/day	PO	Antimetabolite: inhibits purine metabolism
Transcription factor inhibitors			
Cyclosporine	2–5 mg/kg/day	PO	NF-AT transcription factor inhibitor: inhibits IL-2 + other cytokines
Tacrolimus	0.1–0.3 mg/day	PO	NF-AT transcription factor inhibitor: inhibits IL-2 + other cytokines
Cytotoxics			
Cyclophosphamide	2–3 mg/kg/day	PO/IV	Alkylating agent: DNA cross-linking blocks cell replication
Biologics			
Infliximab	3–5 mg/kg every 4–8 weeks	IV	Anti-TNF: chimeric antibody against TNF-α
Etanercept	25 mg twice per week	SC	Anti-TNF: Fc fusion protein that binds extracellular TNF-α
Interferon-α	Depends on preparation	SC/IV	Antiviral and anti-tumor: decreases NK cell activity

Cautions

These immunosuppressive agents should only be administered by someone with appropriate experience in their use (normally a PCP, rheumatologist, or immunologist) and with adequate monitoring.

Patient education is essential. This will include the potential side effects, necessary precautions (e.g., contraception during and for a period after taking most of these agents), and warning symptoms that would require urgent medical review (e.g., features suggestive of infection, especially sore throat).

Table 22.21 Immunosuppressants and their side effects

Drug	Side effects (selected)	Suggested monitoring
Antimetabolites		
Azathioprine	Bone marrow suppression GI upset Secondary malignancies Alopecia	Pretreatment: check TPMT levels (low levels increase risk of bone marrow suppression) CBC stat, weekly for 4–8 weeks then at least every 3 months
Methotrexate	Hepatotoxicity Bone marrow suppression GI upset	CBC, UA, LFT stat, weekly until dose stable, then every 2–3 months Commonly folate (1 mg/day or 5 mg/week) is given concurrently
Mycophenolate	Bone marrow suppression GI upset Secondary malignancies	CBC stat, weekly for 4 weeks, then every 2 weeks for 8 weeks, then monthly for first year
Transcription factor inhibitors		
Cyclosporine	Nephrotoxicity Hypertension Hepatotoxicity Gingival hyperplasia Hypertrichosis	UA, LFT, BP stat, then every 2 weeks for 4 weeks, then every 4–6 weeks
Tacrolimus	Nephrotoxicity Hypertension Neurotoxicity Hepatotoxicity	UA, LFT, BP stat, then every 2 weeks for 4 weeks, then every 4–6 weeks
Cytotoxics		
Cyclophos-phamide	Bone marrow suppression Hemorrhagic cystitis GI upset	Intensive specialist supervision required; includes CBC (+differential), LFT weekly for 4 weeks then every 2–4 weeks
Biologics		
Infliximab	Human antichimeric antibodies serum sickness Tuberculosis reactivation	Pretreatment: rule out TB infection (may be latent) CBC (+differential), UA, LFT stat, then every 2 weeks for 4 weeks, then every 4–6 weeks
Etanercept	Tuberculosis reactivation Hypersensitivity reactions	Pretreatment: rule out TB infection (may be latent) CBC (+differential), UA, LFT stat, then every 2 weeks for 4 weeks, then every 4–6 weeks
Interferon-α	Leukopenia Depression Tuberculosis reactivation Flu-like symptoms Nephrotoxicity Hepatotoxicity	CBC (+differential), UA, LFT stat, then every 2 weeks for 4 weeks, then every 4–6 weeks Regular review of mental state

Miscellaneous

Eponymous syndromes

Aarskog's syndrome X-linked; megalocornea, hypertelorism, antimongoloid palpebral fissures; short stature, syndactyly.

Aicardi's syndrome probably X-linked lethal to males; corpus callosal agenesis and other CNS abnormalities, infantile spasms, mental retardation, vertebral, and rib malformations; chorioretinal lacunar defects, colobomata.

Alagille's syndrome Autosomal dominant (Ch20); posterior embryotoxon, optic disc drusen, pale fundi, hypertelorism; intrahepatic bile duct hypoplasia, butterfly vertebrae, congenital heart disease.

Albright syndrome Disorder of G-proteins resulting in polyostotic fibrous dysplasia (of bone), endocrine abnormalities (including precocious puberty), and café-au-lait spots; orbital involvement may cause proptosis, sinus mucoceles, and compressive optic neuropathy.

Alport syndrome Disorder of type IV collagen; X-linked dominant but autosomal inheritance described; anterior lenticonus, anterior polar and cortical cataracts, fleck retina; sensorineural deafness, nephritis.

Alstrom-Olsen syndrome Autosomal recessive; cone-rod dystrophy with features of retinitis pigmentosa, posterior subcapsular cataracts; diabetes mellitus, sensorineural deafness, nephropathy, obesity, acanthosis nigricans.

Anderson–Fabry disease See Fabry's disease.

Apert syndrome. Autosomal dominant (Ch10); craniosynostosis, syndactyly, broad distal phalanx of great thumb/toe, mental handicap; hypertelorism, proptosis, strabismus, keratoconus, ectopia lentis, congenital glaucoma, optic atrophy.

Arnold–Chiari malformation Congenital herniation of the cerebellum/ brainstem through the foramen magnum may cause hydrocephalus, cerebellar signs (e.g., nystagmus, ataxia) and may be associated with syringomyelia.

Bardet–Biedl and Laurence–Moon syndromes Autosomal recessive overlapping conditions; retinitis pigmentosa with early macular involvement; polydactyly, hypogonadism, obesity, microcephaly, nephropathy, ↓IQ.

Bassen–Kornzweig (abetalipoproteinaemia) Autosomal recessive deficiency of triglyceride transfer protein; retinitis pigmentosa, cataract; spinocerebellar degeneration, steatorrhoea, acanthosis (of erythrocytes).

Batten's disease (neuronal ceroid lipofuscinosis). Autosomal recessive metabolic disorder resulting in neurodegeneration. Juvenile form: bull's eye maculopathy, pigmentary retinopathy, optic atrophy, epilepsy, life expectancy <25 years.

Bloch–Sulzberger syndrome (incontinentia pigmenti) X-linked dominant, lethal to males; abnormal peripheral retinal vasculature, gliosis, tractional retinal detachment; abnormal teeth, cutaneous pigment whorls, and CNS anomalies.

Bourneville disease (tuberous sclerosis) Autosomal dominant (Ch9q TSC1, and Ch16p TSC2) phakomatosis with neurocutaneous features and retinal astrocytomas, p. 644.

Brown syndrome Mechanical restriction syndrome attributed to the superior oblique tendon sheath, p. 590.

Caffrey's disease Hyperplasia of subperiosteal bone and proptosis.

Cogan's syndrome Idiopathic, probably autoimmune; interstitial keratitis, sensorineural deafness, tinnitus, vertigo, systemic vasculitis (including life-threatening aortitis).

Crouzon's syndrome Autosomal dominant (Ch10); craniosynostosis, maxillary hypoplasia, prognathism, hooked nose; proptosis, strabismus, micro/megalocornea, iris coloboma, cataract, ectopia lentis, glaucoma.

De Morsier's syndrome Optic nerve hypoplasia; midline brain abnormalities including absent septum pellucidum and corpus callosal hypo/ aplasia.

Down syndrome Trisomy 21; 1 in 650 live births; blepharitis, keratoconus, cataracts; musculoskeletal abnormalities, congenital heart disease, ↓IQ, p. 638.

Duane syndrome Aberrant co-innervation of LR and MR resulting in horizontal-gaze anomalies, p. 590.

Edwards' syndrome Trisomy 18; 1 in 8000 live births; microphthalmos, glaucoma, cataracts; failure to thrive, congenital heart disease; life expectancy <1 year, p. 638.

Fabry disease X-linked; α-galactosidase A deficiency results in glycosphingolipid accumulation; vortex keratopathy, cataracts (posterior cortical and granular), conjunctival and retinal telangiectasia; peripheral neuropathy with painful Fabry crises, renal failure, angiokeratoma corporis diffusum, lymphedema.

Foster Kennedy syndrome Ipsilateral optic atrophy due to compressive optic neuropathy with contralateral disc swelling from ↑ICP.

Friedreich's ataxia Autosomal recessive; triplet repeat expansion (GAA) of noncoding region of the frataxin gene (Ch9); degeneration of spinocerebellar tracts (ataxia, dysarthria, nystagmus), corticospinal tracts (weakness, extensor plantars), posterior columns (proprioception) and peripheral neuropathy (with absent tendon reflexes), pes cavus.

Gardner's syndrome Variant of familial adenomatous polyposis (autosomal dominant) with bone cysts, hamartomas, and soft tissue tumors; atypical CHRPE, p. 510.

Gaucher disease Autosomal recessive; β-glucosidase deficiency; visceromegaly (type I) or neurodegeneration (type II or III); supranuclear palsy (type IIIb).

Gerstmann's syndrome Dominant parietal lobe lesion resulting in finger agnosia, right/left confusion, dysgraphia, acalculia; may be associated with failure of ipsilateral pursuit movements.

Gillespie syndrome Variant of aniridia (PAX-6 mutation) with mental retardation and cerebellar ataxia.

Goldenhar syndrome Accessory auricle, limbal dermoid, hypoplasia of face, vertebral anomaly corneal hyposthesia. Duane's syndrome iris and upper eyelid coloboma.

Goldmann–Favre disease Autosomal recessive; optically empty vitreous, macular retinoschisis, macular changes, peripheral pigmentary retinopathy.

Gorlin's syndrome Autosomal dominant (tumor suppressor gene PATCHED; Ch9q); multiple basal cell carcinomas, jaw cysts, skeletal abnormalities, ectopic calcification (e.g., falx cerebri); hypertelorism, prominent supraorbital ridges.

Gradenigo's syndrome VI nerve palsy and pain in V nerve distribution due to lesion at the apex of the petrous temporal bone; this may be related to chronic middle ear infection.

Gronblad–Strandberg syndrome angioid streaks with pseudoxanthoma elasticum.

Hallermann–Streiff–Francois syndrome micropthalmos, cataract, hypotrichosis, blue sclera; dyscephaly, short stature.

Heerfordt's syndrome: (uveoparotid fever) presentation of sarcoidosis with fever, parotid enlargement, uveitis.

Hermansky–Pudlak syndrome type II oculocutaneous albinism with platelet dysfunction, pulmonary fibrosis, granulomatous colitis.

Kasabach–Merritt syndrome giant hemangioma with localized intravascular coagulation causing low platelets and fibrinogen.

Kearns–Sayre syndrome Mitochondrial inheritance; CPEO, pigmentary retinopathy (granular pigmentation, peripapillary atrophy), and heart block; usually presents before 20 years.

Laurence–Moon syndrome Grouped with Bardet–Biedl syndrome but no obesity or polydactyly.

Leber's congenital amaurosis Autosomal recessive; blind from birth, eye-poking (oculodigital sign), hypermetropia, sluggish or paradoxical pupillary reflexes, macular dysplasia but fairly normal fundus appearance.

Leber's hereditary optic neuropathy Mitochondrial inheritance; rapid sequential visual loss in 20s to 30s due to optic neuropathy, p. 528.

Löfgren syndrome: presentation of sarcoidosis with fever, erythema nodosum, bihilar lymphadenopathy.

Louis–Bar syndrome (ataxia telangectasia) Autosomal recessive (Ch11q, *ATM* gene); conjunctival telangiectasia, progressive oculomotor apraxia; cerebellar ataxia, ↓IQ, immunodeficiency.

Lowe syndrome (oculocerebrorenal syndrome). X-linked disorder of amino acid metabolism; congenital cataract, microspherophakia, blue sclera, anterior segment dysgenesis, glaucoma; ↓IQ, hypotonia, vitamin D–resistant rickets.

Maffucci's syndrome Multiple hemangiomas and enchondromas (which may cause limb deformities), with risk of malignant transformation.

Marfan syndrome Autosomal dominant (Ch15, fibrillin); ectopia lentis, retinal detachment, glaucoma, axial myopia; arachnodactyly, long-limbed, aortic dissection, p. 258.

Meckel–Gruber syndrome Autosomal recessive; coloboma; microcephaly, occipital encephalocele, cleft lip/palate, polydactyly, polycystic kidney disease.

Menke's disease X-linked recessive deficiency of copper transport protein; optic atrophy, retinal dystrophy; wiry hair, ataxia, neurodegeneration.

Mikulicz's syndrome infiltrative swelling of salivary and lacrimal glands.

Millard–Gubler syndrome lesion of the facial colliculus (dorsal pons) resulting in ipsilateral CN VI and VII palsies, ± contralateral hemiparesis.

Miller–Fisher syndrome Variant of Guillan–Barre syndrome characterized by acute external ophthalmoplegia, ataxia, and areflexia.

Niemann–Pick disease Autosomal recessive; deficiency of sphingomyelinase; type A is infantile onset with visceromegaly, neurodegeneration, and cherry-red spot; type B juvenile onset with visceromegaly, rarely cherry-red spot; type C has variable onset, vertical supranuclear gaze palsy, ataxia, and neurodegeneration.

Norrie disease X-linked; retinal dysplasia, retinal detachment, leukocoria, vitreous hemorrhage, cataract, phthisis; ↓IQ, deafness.

Oguchi disease Autosomal recessive; nonprogressive nyctalopia (CSNB), pseudotapetal reflex which normalizes with dark adaptation (Mizuo phenomenon), p. 458.

Parinaud syndrome Lesion of dorsal midbrain resulting in light-near dissociation, supranuclear upgaze palsy, convergence retraction nystagmus, and failure of convergence and accommodation.

Patau syndrome Trisomy 13; 1 in 14,000 live births; cyclopia, colobomata, retinal dysplasia; microcephaly; life expectancy <3 months, p. 638.

Raymond syndrome Lesion of the corticospinal tract in the ventral pons resulting in VI nerve palsy and contralateral hemiparesis.

Refsum's disease Autosomal recessive; deficiency of phytanic acid α-hydrolase results in accumulation of phytanic acid; pigmentary retinopathy, optic atrophy; ichthyosis, deafness, cardiomyopathy, ataxia.

Riley–Day syndrome (familial dysautonomia) autosomal recessive; more common in Ashkenazi Jews; tear deficiency   keratoconjunctivitis sicca, commonly with ulceration, reduced corneal sensation; sensory neuropathy, autonomic dysfunction/crises.

Rubinstein–Taybi syndrome (otopalatodigital syndrome) Developmental abnormality; hypertelorism, colobomas; broad thumbs/big toes, maxillary/mandibular hypoplasia, hypertrichosis, ↓IQ.

Sandhoff's disease Autosomal recessive (Ch 5q, HEXB); GM2 gangliosidosis with deficiency of hexosominadase A and B; cherry-red spot, optic atrophy; splenomegaly, neurodegeneration.

Stargardt's disease (and fundus flavimaculatus) Autosomal recessive (usually Ch1p, ABCA4); most common of the macular dystrophies, with two clinical presentations: Stargardt's ("beaten-bronze" atrophy, yellowish flecks of the posterior pole, significant ↓VA) and fundus flavimaculatus (widespread pisciform flecks with relative preservation of vision), p. 459.

Steele–Richardson–Olszewski (progressive supranuclear palsy) Neurodegenerative disease of the elderly; supranuclear vertical gaze; postural instability, Parkinsonism, pseudobulbar palsy, and dementia.

Stickler's syndrome (hereditary arthro-ophthalmopathy) Autosomal dominant (Ch12q, COL2A1); abnormality of type II collagen; high myopia, optically empty vitreous, retinal detachments, cataract, ectopia lentis, glaucoma; arthropathy, Pierre Robin sequence (micrognathia, high arched/cleft palate), sensorineural deafness, mitral valve prolapse, p. 389.

Sturge–Weber syndrome Phakomatosis with port-wine stain of the face with ocular and CNS hemangiomas, p. 645.

Tay–Sachs disease Autosomal recessive (Ch15q, HEXA); GM2 gangliosidosis with deficiency of hexosominadase A; cherry-red spot, optic atrophy; neurodegeneration.

Treacher–Collins syndrome (mandibulofacial dysostosis) Autosomal dominant (Ch5q); clefting syndrome; antimongoloid palpebral fissures, lower lid colobomas, dermoids; mandibular hypoplasia, zygoma hypoplasia, choanal atresia.

Turcot syndrome Variant of familial adenomatous polyposis (autosomal dominant) with CNS neuroepithelial tumors, especially medulloblastoma and glioma; atypical CHRPE, p. 510.

Turner syndrome XO; 1 in 2000 live female births; antimongoloid palpebral fissures, cataracts, convergence insufficiency; short stature, wide carrying angle, low hair line, webbed neck, primary gonadal failure, congenital heart defects, p. 638.

Vogt-Koyanagi–Harada syndrome Multisystem inflammatory disease; bilateral granulomatous panuveitis; vitiligo, alopecia, deafness, tinnitus, sterile meningoencephalitis and cranial neuropathies, p. 342.

Von-Hippel Lindau Autosomal dominant (Ch3p, *VHL* gene); phakomatosis with retinal capillary hemangiomas, CNS hemangioblastomas, renal cell carcinomas, and other tumors, p. 645.

Waardenburg syndrome Autosomal dominant (PAX3); heterochromia, hypertelorism; white forelock, deafness.

Walker–Warburg syndrome Autosomal recessive; retinal dysplasia; muscular dystrophy, Dandy–Walker malformation.

Wallenberg syndrome (lateral medullary syndrome) Lesion of the lateral medulla (typically posterior inferior cerebellar artery occlusion) resulting in ipsilateral Horner's syndrome, ipsilateral cerebellar signs, ipsilateral palatal paralysis, ipsilateral decreased facial sensation (pain and temperature), contralateral decreased somatic sensation (pain and temperature).

Weill–Marchesani syndrome Autosomal recessive; ectopia lentis, microspherophakia, retinal detachment, anomalous angles; short stature, brachydactyly, ↓IQ, p. 258.

Wildervanck syndrome Klippel–Feil malformation (short neck due to cervical vertebrae anomalies) with deafness and Duane's syndrome.

Wyburn–Mason syndrome Phakomatosis with arteriovenous malformations of retina, orbit, and CNS, p. 645.

Zellweger syndrome (cerebrohepatorenal syndrome) Autosomal recessive; severe end of a spectrum of peroxisomal disorders that includes neonatal adrenoleukodystrophy and infantile Refsum's disease; cataract, optic nerve hypoplasia, pigmentary retinopathy, corneal clouding; high forehead, flat brows; life expectancy <1 year.

Web resources for ophthalmologists (1)

Box 23.1 Ophthalmic and related associations

American Academy of Ophthalmology www.aao.org
Association for Research in Vision and Ophthalmology www.arvo.org
American Society of Cataract and Refractive Surgery www.ascrs.org
American Society of Retina Specialists www.asrs.org
International Council of Ophthalmology (ICO) www.icoph.org
International Society for Clinical Electrophysiology of Vision
www.iscev.org
International Society for Refractive Surgery www.isrs.org

Box 23.2 American Medical Colleges (US)

American Society of Anesthesiologists www.asahq.org
American Academy of Family Physicians www.aafp.org
American College of Obstetricians and Gynecologists www.acog.org
American Academy of Ophthalmology www.aao.org
American College of Pediatricians www.acpeds.org
College of American Pathologists www.cap.org
American College of Physicians www.acponline.org
American College of Surgeons www.facs.org
American College of Radiology www.acr.org
American College of Psychiatrists www.acpsych.org

Box 23.3 Other professional bodies

American Medical Association www.ama-assn.org
United States Department of Health and Human Services www.hhs.gov
National Institute of Health www.nih.gov

Web resources for ophthalmologists (2)

Box 23.4 Ophthalmic and medical resources

PubMED and MEDLINE www.pubmed.com
Cochrane Eye and Vision Site www.cochraneeyes.org
Clinical Evidence www.clinicalevidence.com
Emedicine www.emedicine.com
Internet Ophthalmology www.ophthal.org
Centers for Disease Control and Prevention www.cdc.gov
World Health Organization www.who.int

Box 23.5 Journals

Ophthalmic
American Journal of Ophthalmology www.ajo.com
Archives of Ophthalmology www.archopht.ama-assn.org
British Journal of Ophthalmology www.bjo.bmjjournals.com
Cornea www.cornealjrnl.com
Current Opinion in Ophthalmology www.co-ophthalmology.com
Digital Journal of Ophthalmology www.djo.harvard.edu
Eye www.nature.com/eye
International Ophthalmology Clinics www.internat-ophthalmology.com
Investigative Ophthalmology & Visual Science www.iovs.org
Journal of Cataract and Refractive Surgery www.ascrs.org/publicats/jcrs
Journal of Glaucoma www.glaucomajournal.com
Ophthalmology www.ophsource.org/periodicals/ophtha

General
British Medical Journal www.bmj.bmjournals.com
New England Journal of Medicine www.nejm.org
The Lancet www.thelancet.com

Reference intervals

Hematology

CBC

Hb	13.0–18.0 g/dL
	11.5–16.5 g/dL
Hct	0.40–0.52
	0.36–0.47
RCC	4.5–6.5 × 10^{12}/L
	3.8–5.8 × 10^{12}/L
MCV	77–95 fL
MCH	27.0–32.0 pg
Reticulocytes	50–100 × 10^9/L (0.5–2.5%)
WCC	4.0–11.0 × 10^9/L
Neutrophils	2.0–7.5 × 10^9/L
Lymphocytes	1.5–4.5 × 10^9/L
Eosinophils	0.04–0.4 × 10^9/L
Basophils	0.0–0.2 × 10^9/L
Monocytes	0.2–0.8 × 10^9/L
Platelets	150–400 × 10^9/L
ESR	age/2 (Male)
	(age +10)/2 (Female)

Hematinics

Serum B12	150–700 ng/L
Serum folate	2.0–11.0 µg/L
Red cell folate	160–640 µg/L
Serum ferritin	15–300 µg/L

Clotting

INR	0.8–1.2
PT	12–14 s
APTT ratio	0.8–1.2
APTT	26.0–33.5 s
Protein C	80–135 u/dL
Protein S	80–135 u/dL
Antithrombin III	80–120 u/dL
APCR	2.12–4.0

Biochemistry

Urinalysis and glucose

Sodium (Na)	135–145 mmol/L
Potassium (K)	3.5–5.0 mmol/L
Urea	3.0–6.5 mmol/L
Creatinine	60–125 µmol/L
Glucose (fasting)	3.5–5.5 mmol/L
Glucose (random)	3.5–11.0 mmol/L (normal/IGT)

LFTs and protein

Total protein	63–80 g/L
Albumin	32–50 g/L
Bilirubin	<17 µmol/L
Alkaline phosphatase	100–300 iu/L
ALT	5–60 iu/L
AST	5–42 iu/L
γGT	10–46 iu/L

Bone

Calcium (total)	2.15–2.55 mmol/L
Phosphate	0.7–1.5 mmol/L
Lipids	
Cholesterol	3.9–6.0 mmol/L
Triglycerides	0.55–1.90 mmol/L
ACE	12–71 (age ≥20); 5–87 (age <20)

Iron studies

Iron	14–33 µmol/L
	11–28 µmol/L
TIBC	45–75 µmol/L

Hormones

TSH	0.35–5.5 mU/L
Free T4	9–24 pmol/L
Cortisol (morning)	450–700 nmol/L
FSH	2–8 u/L (luteal); >25 u/L (menopausal)
LH	3–16 u/L (luteal)
Prolactin	<450 u/L
	<650 u/L

Arterial blood gases

PH	7.35–7.45
PaO_2	>10.6 kPa
$PaCO_2$	4.7–6.0 kPa
BE	± 2.0 mmol/L

Immunology

IgG	5.3–16.5 g/L
IgA	0.8–4.0 g/L
IgM	0.5–2.0 g/L
C3	0.9–2.1 g/L
C4	0.12–0.53 g/L
C1 esterase	0.11–0.36 g/L
CH50	80–120%

CSF analysis

Lymphocytes	<4/mL
Neutrophils	0/mL
Glucose	≥2/3 plasma level
Protein	<0.4 g/L
Opening pressure	<20 cmH$_2$O, or <25 cmH$_2$O in the obese

Index